American Academy of Orthopaedic Surgeons

American Academy of Pediatrics

# Essentials
*of*
# Musculoskeletal
# Care
# 3

rd
Edition

**Letha Yurko Griffin, MD, PhD**
**Editor**

Published 2005
by the American Academy of Orthopaedic Surgeons
6300 North River Road
Rosemont, IL 60018

Third Edition
Copyright ©2005
by the American Academy of Orthopaedic Surgeons

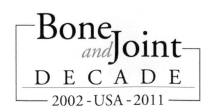

# CONTRIBUTORS

**John F. Dalton IV, MD**
Department of Orthopaedic Surgery
Emory University
Atlanta, Georgia

**Mark Davies, MD**
Department of Orthopaedic Surgery
Kaiser Santa Teresa
San Jose, California

**Craig J. Della Valle, MD**
Assistant Professor
Department of Orthopaedic Surgery
Rush University Medical Center
Chicago, Illinois

**Julie A. Dodds, MD**
Associate Professor
Department of Surgery
Department of Sports Medicine
Michigan State University
East Lansing, Michigan

**Xavier A. Duralde, MD**
Assistant Clinical Professor of Orthopaedic Surgery
Emory University
Peachtree Orthopaedic Clinic
Atlanta, Georgia

**Marcel Gilli, MD**
Staff Anesthesiologist
Piedmont Hospital
Atlanta, Georgia

**Eric Mark Hammerberg, MD**
Assistant Professor
Department of Orthopaedic Surgery
Emory University
Atlanta, Georgia

**Robert H. Haralson III, MD, MBA**
Executive Director of Medical Affairs
American Academy of Orthopaedic Surgeons
Rosemont, Illinois

**Dawn D. Hassinger, MD, PhD**
Atlanta, Georgia

**Thomas R. Johnson, MD**
Orthopedic Surgeons and Sports Medicine
Billings, Montana

**Gregg R. Klein, MD**
Assistant Professor
Department of Orthopaedic Surgery
NYU Hospital for Joint Diseases
New York, New York

**L. Andrew Koman, MD**
Professor and Vice Chair
Associate Director of Surgical Science
Department of Orthopaedic Surgery
Wake Forest University School of Medicine
Winston-Salem, North Carolina

**Joseph M. Lane, MD**
Professor of Orthopaedic Surgery
Assistant Dean, Medical Students
Weill Medical College of Cornell University
New York, New York

**Gary M. Lourie, MD**
Hand Consultant, Atlanta Braves
The Hand Treatment Center
Atlanta, Georgia

**Alexandra Louthan, OTR/L, CHT**
Physiotherapy Associates
Atlanta, Georgia

**Craig S. Mauro, MD**
Department of Orthopaedic Surgery
University of Pittsburgh
Pittsburgh, Pennsylvania

**Tanya Maxwell, MS, L/ATC**
Peachtree Orthopaedic Clinic
Atlanta, Georgia

**Thomas J. Moore, MD**
Assistant Professor
Department of Orthopaedic Surgery
Emory School of Medicine
Atlanta, Georgia

**Scott Olvey, MD**
Department of Hand Surgery/Upper Extremity
Center for Orthopedic Surgery and Sports Medicine
Indianapolis, Indiana

**Douglas G. Smith, MD**
Associate Professor
Director, Prosthetics Research Study
Department of Orthopaedic Surgery
University of Washington
Seattle, Washington

**Margie Scalley Vaught, CPC, CPC-H, CCS-P, ACS-OR**
Healthcare Consultant
Ellensburg, Washington

**James A. Whiteside, MD**
Professor of Sports Medicine
College of Health and Human Services
Troy University
Troy, Alabama

**W. Hayes Wilson, MD**
Chief of Rheumatology
Department of Rheumatology
Piedmont Hospital
Atlanta, Georgia

*To the late Bob Snider, the first editor and inspiration behind* Essentials of Musculoskeletal Care—*may this volume honor your creativity, as have the earlier editions.*

*To Tanya Maxwell—a salute for being the best right-hand woman anyone could have. Your help in this and other projects has always been exemplary.*

*To my family, Jim, Jordyn, and Yurko—my deepest gratitude for doing your own laundry, cooking your own meals, and generally looking after yourselves and the furry inhabitants of our home to provide me the time to participate in this and similar projects.*

*To my mother and father—whose advice regarding life was always, "Never give up; always do your best; and along the way plant a tree to enrich nature, raise a child to foster mankind, and write a book to help repay your debt to society." I miss you.*

# PREFACE

*Essentials of Musculoskeletal Care* is a guide for decision making in the evaluation and treatment of more than 300 common musculoskeletal conditions. The book is organized into a general orthopaedics section; anatomic sections covering the shoulder, elbow and forearm, hand and wrist, hip and thigh, knee and lower leg, foot and ankle, and spine; and a pediatric orthopaedics section. Clinical symptoms, physical examination pearls, diagnostic tests, differential diagnoses, treatment suggestions, adverse outcomes, and referral decisions are listed so that the practitioner will feel comfortable recognizing, evaluating, and treating these conditions.

The third edition of *Essentials of Musculoskeletal Care* has been enhanced with additional charts, tables, and illustrations for improved clarity and ease of reading. The anatomy of each area of the body is now clearly illustrated in classic Netter drawings, and an expanded glossary of orthopaedic terms has been developed for the practitioner to use as a handy reference. Every chapter has been reviewed and updated, and several new chapters have been added, including Anesthesia for Orthopaedic Surgery, Fracture Healing, and Dance Injuries to the Foot and Ankle. In addition, home exercise programs for more than 25 conditions and a general musculoskeletal conditioning program are available in the text and as patient handouts that can be printed from the accompanying DVD. Treatment videos are now available in full-screen DVD format, appropriate for patient viewing in your office. We are excited about the enhancements to the DVD and hope that the practitioner will find it an extremely useful, educational, and time-saving tool in treating patients.

I am indebted to the Board of Directors of the American Academy of Orthopaedic Surgeons (AAOS) for their commitment to excellence in education. My deepest thanks to the Editorial Board for this edition—Jim Andrews, Jody Buckwalter, Joe Chandler, Bob Donatelli, Carol Frey, Chris Harner, Peter Pizzutillo, John Seiler, Dan Spengler, and Joe Zuckerman—for their devotion to this project. It was difficult to improve on the excellence of the second edition, but the Editorial Board accepted and met the challenge through multiple creative additions to the text.

A special thank you to Mina Ferguson and Julie Sawyer, whose expert photography has enhanced the physical examination sections. Thanks also to Laurie Braun and Lynne Shindoll at AAOS, who worked diligently to oversee and guide this venture to ensure a timely and flawless production schedule, and to Marilyn Fox, PhD, Director of the Publications Department, whose wisdom is always inspiring. Additional thanks go to Mary Steermann, Sophie Tosta, Mike Bujewski, and everyone in the Publications Department who contributed to the design and production of this book.

Once again, we are appreciative of the support of the American Academy of Pediatrics, which has been a valuable partner in the *Essentials* project. The comments from this organization as well as from internists, physiatrists, family practitioners, orthopaedic residents, and medical students helped us identify the enhancements included in this third edition. As always, we welcome ongoing dialog with all of you, for it is your suggestions that guide our planning for future editions. Please complete the enclosed comment card, or write to us at *Essentials of Musculoskeletal Care*, AAOS Publications Department, 6300 N. River Road, Rosemont, IL 60018. You may also send e-mail comments to shindoll@aaos.org or lethagriff@aol.com.

Letha Yurko Griffin, MD, PhD
Editor

# How to Use
## *Essentials of Musculoskeletal Care*, 3rd Edition

*Essentials of Musculoskeletal Care* is designed to provide concise content in an easy-to-use format.

**Pain diagram** opens each section. Shows areas of pain and identifies conditions typically associated with each pain location. Names chapter where condition is discussed.

**Table of contents** for section, listing conditions in alphabetic order.

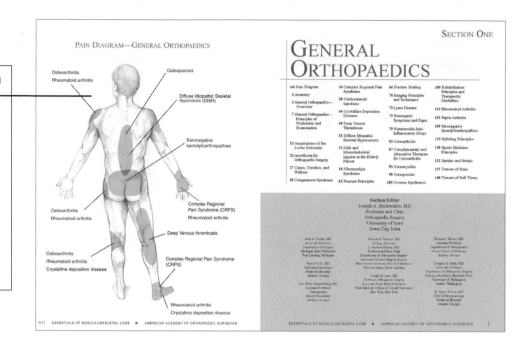

**Netter anatomic art** at beginning of section for handy reference.

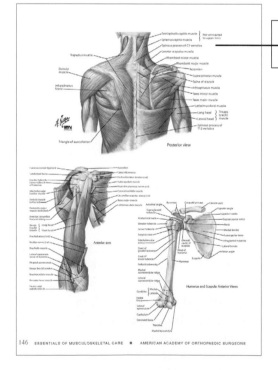

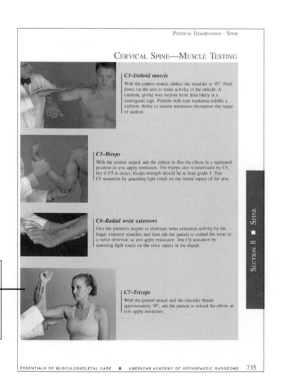

**Physical Examination** presents photographs and step-by-step descriptions of physical examination maneuvers: inspection and palpation, range of motion, muscle testing, and special tests.

# HOW TO USE
## *ESSENTIALS OF MUSCULOSKELETAL CARE*, 3RD EDITION

**Conditions chapters** include:

- ICD-9 codes
- Synonyms
- Clinical symptoms
- Physical examination
- Diagnostic tests
- Differential diagnosis
- Adverse outcomes of the disease
- Treatment
- Physical therapy prescription
- Adverse outcomes of treatment
- Referral decisions/red flags

---

### DIFFUSE IDIOPATHIC SKELETAL HYPEROSTOSIS

**SYNONYMS**
Ankylosing hyperostosis
Vertebral osteophytosis

**ICD-9 Code**
**721.6**
Ankylosing vertebral hyperostosis

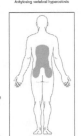

**DEFINITION**
Diffuse idiopathic skeletal hyperostosis (DISH) is an idiopathic disease characterized by striking osteophyte formation in the spine. Patients with DISH have confluent ossification spanning three or more intervertebral disks, most commonly in the thoracic and thoracolumbar spine. The bridging osteophytes follow the course of the anterior longitudinal ligaments and the peripheral disk margins. The disease primarily affects white men (male-to-female ratio is 2:1) who are age 60 years or older.

**CLINICAL SYMPTOMS**
The principal symptom is stiffness in the spine, especially in the morning and evening. Patients often report that symptoms have been present for several months or even years. Nonradicular back pain, especially in the lumbar and thoracolumbar junction area, is relatively mild (Figure 1). Those with cervical spine involvement may notice dysphagia related to a large anterior cervical osteophyte located behind the esophagus. Other weight-bearing joints can be painful, but spinal pain is the most severe.

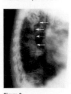
**Figure 1**
Distribution of pain in DISH.

**TESTS**

*Physical Examination*
Examination reveals stiffness in the spine on forward flexion and on extension. Reduced hip motion or associated knee arthritis also is possible.

*Diagnostic Tests*
Radiographs of the thoracic and lumbar spine, especially the lateral view, show confluent ossification spanning the intervertebral disks of at least four contiguous vertebral bodies (three disks) (Figure 2). The intervertebral disk height is preserved in the fused segments. The posterior apophyseal joints and sacroiliac joints are normal as opposed to the findings characteristic of ankylosing spondylitis.

In the cervical spine, ossification of the posterior longitudinal ligament occurs and is the second most common cause of cervical myelopathy (after cervical spondylosis).

**Figure 2**
Lateral radiograph of the thoracic spine showing confluent ossification anteriorly spanning multiple disk levels (arrows).

The pelvis often shows "whiskering" or shaggy hyperostotic bone at the pelvic rim. There may be hyperostotic change in the ribs, as well.
There is no human leukocyte antigen (HLA) association.

**DIFFERENTIAL DIAGNOSIS**
Acromegaly (facial and phalangeal changes)
Ankylosing spondylitis (sacroiliac and apophyseal joint involvement, positive HLA B27)
Degenerative disk disease (reduced disk height)
Paget disease (32% of patients also have DISH)
Polymyalgia rheumatica (muscle and joint pain and stiffness associated with systemic symptoms)

**ADVERSE OUTCOMES OF THE DISEASE**
Spinal stiffness is common. With widespread involvement, a single mobile segment can remain, but it may become unstable and painful.

**TREATMENT**
Walking and exercise programs are the most common initial treatment. Intermittent NSAIDs can help, but pain usually is mild and tolerable.

**ADVERSE OUTCOMES OF TREATMENT**
Heterotopic ossification occurs five times more often following hip replacement surgery in patients with DISH. NSAIDs can cause gastric, renal, or hepatic complications.

**REFERRAL DECISIONS/RED FLAGS**
Symptoms of neurogenic claudication, myelopathy, or dysphagia indicate the need for further evaluation.

---

### HOME EXERCISE PROGRAM FOR FROZEN SHOULDER

Perform the exercises in the order listed. Apply moist or dry heat to the shoulder for 5 or 10 minutes before the exercises and during the external rotation passive stretch. If you experience pain during or after the exercises, call your doctor.

| Exercise Type | Muscle Group | Number of Repetitions/Sets | Number of Days per Week | Number of Weeks |
|---|---|---|---|---|
| External rotation passive stretch | Anterior capsule | 4 repetitions/3 sets | Daily | 3 to 4 |
| Bent over rowing | Posterior deltoid, Middle trapezius | 8 to 10 repetitions/2 sets, progressing to 15 repetitions/3 sets | 3 | 3 to 4 |

Start   Finish

*External Rotation Passive Stretch*
Stand in a doorway, facing the doorjamb. With the affected arm held next to your side and the elbow bent 90°, grasp the edge of the doorjamb. Keeping the hand in place, rotate your upper body as shown in the illustration. Hold the stretch for 30 seconds; then return to the starting position for 30 seconds. Perform 3 sets of 4 repetitions daily, continuing for 3 to 4 weeks.

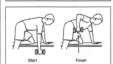

Start   Finish

*Bent Over Rowing*
Stand next to a bench or chair with your knee and hand resting on the bench and your free hand grasping a weight. Lift the weight while you count to 3 slowly by bending the elbow, squeezing the shoulder blade across the back. Lower the weight slowly to a count of 3. Begin with a weight that allows 2 sets of 8 to 10 repetitions without pain. Progress to 3 sets of 15 repetitions. Add weight in increments up to 5 pounds, returning to 8 to 10 repetitions and 2 sets each time weight is added. Perform the exercise 3 days a week, continuing for 3 to 4 weeks.

**Home exercise program** includes:

- Symbol indicating a customizable pdf of the exercise program is available on the DVD
- Handy chart of exercises
- Step-by-step instructions and illustrations

---

### PROCEDURE
#### TENNIS ELBOW INJECTION

The classic tender spot in lateral epicondylitis of the elbow (tennis elbow) is just distal to the lateral epicondyle of the humerus with the elbow in 90° of flexion.
**Note:** Opinions differ regarding single- versus two-needle injection techniques. A two-needle technique is shown on the DVD.

*STEP 1*
Wear protective gloves at all times during this procedure and use sterile technique.

*STEP 2*
Place the patient's arm against the chest or abdomen, with the elbow flexed at least 90° and the forearm fully pronated.

*STEP 3*
Prep the skin with a bactericidal solution.

*STEP 4*
Palpate just distal to the lateral epicondyle and locate the point of maximal tenderness. At this point, insert the 25-gauge needle, make a subcutaneous skin wheal with the local anesthetic, and advance through the tendon of the extensor carpi radialis brevis muscle to inject the remaining 2 to 3 mL of local anesthetic (Figure 1).

**CPT Code**
**20550**
Injection(s); single tendon sheath, or ligament, aponeurosis (eg, plantar "fascia")
**20551**
Injection(s); single tendon origin/insertion
Current Procedural Terminology © 2004 American Medical Association. All Rights Reserved.

*MATERIALS*
Sterile gloves
Bactericidal skin preparation solution
5-mL syringe with a 25-gauge, 1¼" needle
3 to 4 mL of a 1% lidocaine solution without epinephrine
2-mL syringe
1 mL of a corticosteroid preparation
Adhesive bandage

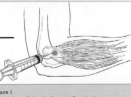

**Figure 1**
Location for needle insertion for tennis elbow injection.

**Procedures** include:

- CPT code(s)
- Symbol indicating video is available on the DVD
- List of materials
- Step-by-step instructions

# PAIN DIAGRAM—GENERAL ORTHOPAEDICS

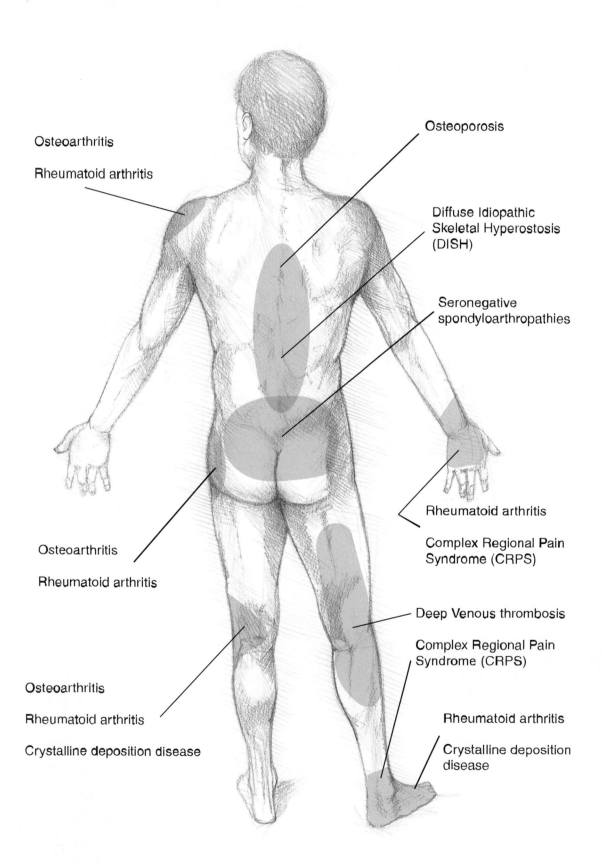

Osteoarthritis

Rheumatoid arthritis

Osteoporosis

Diffuse Idiopathic
Skeletal Hyperostosis
(DISH)

Seronegative
spondyloarthropathies

Rheumatoid arthritis

Complex Regional Pain
Syndrome (CRPS)

Osteoarthritis

Rheumatoid arthritis

Deep Venous thrombosis

Complex Regional Pain
Syndrome (CRPS)

Osteoarthritis

Rheumatoid arthritis

Crystalline deposition disease

Rheumatoid arthritis

Crystalline deposition
disease

# GENERAL ORTHOPAEDICS

**Section Editor**
Joseph A. Buckwalter, MD
Professor and Chair
Department of Orthopaedic Surgery
University of Iowa
Iowa City, Iowa

Julie A. Dodds, MD
Associate Professor
Department of Surgery
Michigan State University
East Lansing, Michigan

Marcel Gilli, MD
Staff Anesthesiologist
Piedmont Hospital
Atlanta, Georgia

Eric Mark Hammerberg, MD
Assistant Professor
Department of Orthopaedic Surgery
Emory University
Atlanta, Georgia

Thomas R. Johnson, MD
Orthopedic Surgeons and Sports Medicine
Billings, Montana

L. Andrew Koman, MD
Professor and Vice Chair
Associate Director Surgical Science
Department of Orthopaedic Surgery
Wake Forest University School of Medicine
Winston-Salem, North Carolina

Joseph M. Lane, MD
Professor, Orthopaedic Surgery
Assistant Dean, Medical Students
Weill Medical College of Cornell University
New York, New York

Thomas J. Moore, MD
Assistant Professor
Department of Orthopaedic Surgery
Emory School of Medicine
Atlanta, Georgia

Douglas G. Smith, MD
Associate Professor
Director, Prosthetics Research Study
Department of Orthopaedic Surgery
University of Washington
Seattle, Washington

W. Hayes Wilson, MD
Chief of Rheumatology
Department of Rheumatology
Piedmont Hospital
Atlanta, Georgia

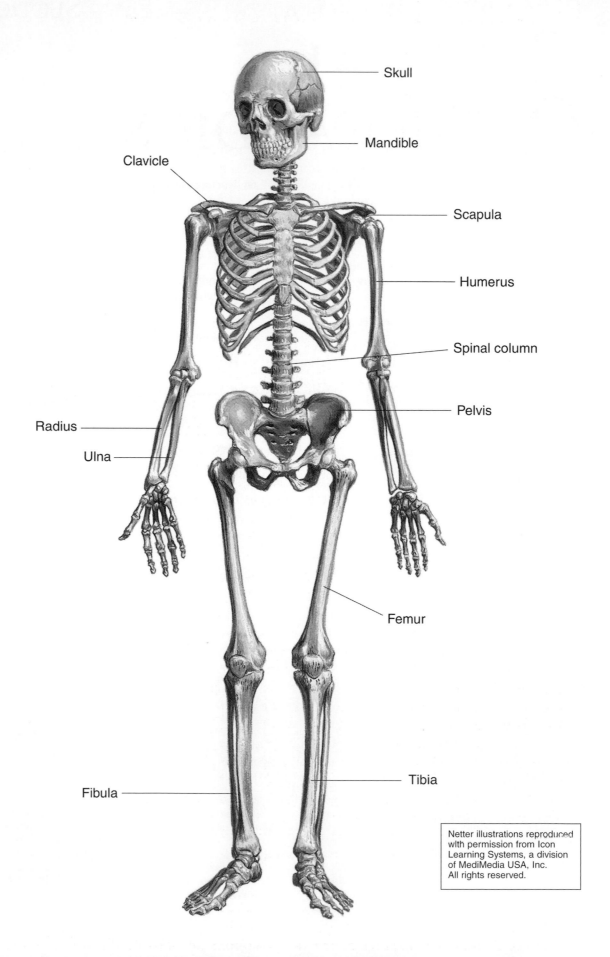

Skull

Mandible

Clavicle

Scapula

Humerus

Spinal column

Pelvis

Radius

Ulna

Femur

Tibia

Fibula

Netter illustrations reproduced
with permission from Icon
Learning Systems, a division
of MediMedia USA, Inc.
All rights reserved.

# GENERAL ORTHOPAEDICS—OVERVIEW

Bone, cartilage, muscle, tendon, ligament, and their supporting nerve and vascular supplies are the specialized structures that make up the musculoskeletal system. In combination, these structures provide remarkable strength, movement, durability, and efficiency. Disease or injury to any of these tissues may adversely affect function and the ability to perform daily activities. This section of *Essentials of Musculoskeletal Care* describes conditions that affect multiple joints, bones, or regions; conditions that have systemic effects; and therapeutic modalities commonly used in the nonsurgical treatment of musculoskeletal conditions. The purpose of this overview is to highlight special conditions and to provide practical advice on diagnosis and treatment. For relevant anatomy, refer to the anatomic drawings that appear at the beginning of each of the sections of this book devoted to particular anatomic areas. A glossary of commonly used orthopaedic terms is provided on pp 996-1013.

## ARTHRITIS

The etiologies of arthritis range from degenerative processes associated with aging (osteoarthritis) to an acute infectious process (septic arthritis). Likewise, disability from arthritis ranges from inconsequential stiffness to severe pain and crippling dysfunction.

The most common type of arthritis, osteoarthritis (also called degenerative joint disease), is a noninflammatory disorder characterized by deterioration of articular cartilage and formation of new bone (sclerosis at the joint surfaces) and osteophytes (outgrowths of new bone at the joint margins). By middle age, virtually everyone experiences some type of degenerative change in the fingers or weight-bearing joints, even though most individuals at this time are asymptomatic. Primary osteoarthritis develops without apparent cause, whereas secondary osteoarthritis can develop as a result of trauma (fracture or repetitive trauma), neuromuscular disorders that cause weakness or loss of proprioception, hemophilia, skeletal dysplasias, hemochromatosis, and other disorders that either injure or overload the articular cartilage. Stiffness and pain with activity are characteristic of osteoarthritis.

Types of inflammatory arthritides include rheumatoid arthritis, the seronegative spondyloarthropathies, crystalline deposition diseases, and septic arthritis. Of these conditions, septic arthritis is the most urgent, as it demands immediate diagnosis and an efficacious treatment plan including appropriate antibiotics and in most cases, surgical drainage and lavage. The crystalline arthropathies present with an abrupt onset of intense pain and swelling. The seronegative spondyloarthropathies are a group of disorders characterized by the following: oligoarticular peripheral joint arthritis, enthesitis, inflammatory changes in axial skeletal joints (sacroiliitis and spondylitis), extra-articular sites of inflammation, association with HLA-B27 antigen, and negative rheumatoid factor. Rheumatoid arthritis is an autoimmune disorder of unknown etiology that is characterized by a destructive synovitis, morning stiffness, and symmetric involvement that primarily affects the joints of the hands, wrists, feet, and ankles.

## BURSITIS AND TENOSYNOVITIS

Sterile inflammation of bursae and tendon sheaths occurs frequently in adults, particularly following an injury or repetitive motion. Characteristic symptoms include localized pain that is exacerbated by specific movements. Patients who have stiffness associated with tendinitis and bursitis may feel better once the tendon or joint is moved because the movement mechanically squeezes out the edema and allows free motion of the parts. With extended activity, however, inflammation develops and the patient notices increasing pain and the return of stiffness.

## OSTEOPOROSIS

Although bone strength and risk of fracture can be affected by diseases such as hyperparathyroidism, osteomalacia, renal osteodystrophy, and other endocrine disorders, primary osteoporosis is the most common and costly bone disease. With the population of people over 65 years increasing, fractures and deformity related to osteoporosis have become epidemic. Preventing excessive bone loss with aging and its disabling consequences and minimizing the risk of fractures should be concerns for all physicians.

## TRAUMA

Trauma is a principal cause of musculoskeletal disorders and is more likely to affect young adults. Appropriate treatment can minimize time lost from work and, more critically, permanent impairment and predisposition to arthritis. Traumatic compartment syndrome is catastrophic if unrecognized and untreated. Appropriate splinting is necessary for all fractures, partly to reduce the likelihood of compartment syndromes, and partly to decrease soft-tissue injury and pain while the patient awaits definitive treatment. The principles used in the initial evaluation and splinting of fractures also can be helpful in the evaluation and initial management of ligament and tendon injuries.

## OTHER PAIN DISORDERS

Three conditions, considered the so-called "fuzzy areas" of arthralgias and periarticular pain, are discussed in this section on General Orthopaedics: fibromyalgia, complex regional pain syndrome, and cumulative trauma disorders also known as overuse syndromes. These processes are as difficult to treat as they are to understand, especially when issues of causation and compensation mix with issues of comfort. Nonorganic symptoms and signs are also discussed. Like the above conditions, these are often misinterpreted as a sign of nondisease, or even malingering; however, nonorganic findings are more likely to be a predictor of the patient's satisfaction with treatment outcomes than an indicator of psychosomatic behavior.

## PATIENT AGE

Trauma and conditions associated with overuse most commonly affect young adults. As adults reach their 40s, degenerative conditions that affect tendons, intervertebral disks, and joints are the source of most presenting symptoms. Common presenting problems in the elderly include fractures, metastatic tumors, and arthritis.

## ABUSE

Abuse involving children, spouses, or the elderly is a complex social and medical problem. Failing to diagnose abuse (false negative) may lead to catastrophic consequences; therefore, it is essential that the appropriate social service agencies be notified if a patient's injuries are potentially from abuse. In the section on Pediatric Orthopaedics, child abuse is discussed in a separate chapter. Spouse or elder abuse may be more difficult to identify. A patient whose history is given wholly by a caregiver may feel unable to talk in the caregiver's presence. In these circumstances, interview the patient and caregiver separately. A caregiver frustrated by an elderly patient's memory problems,

SECTION 1 ■ GENERAL ORTHOPAEDICS

behavior problems, alcoholism, or difficult personality may be abusing the patient regularly. Further, a financially stressed caregiver may be usurping the elderly patient's finances for his or her own benefit.

The complexity of these problems and the seriousness of the consequences demand familiarity with community resources and knowledge of the competence, compassion, and professionalism of those who will investigate the potential abuse.

# General Orthopaedics—Principles of Evaluation and Examination

Patients presenting with musculoskeletal problems usually report pain, deformity, or weakness. In evaluating pain, question the patient about the following:

## History

### Questions about the character of the pain

- Is the pain aching (joint or muscle problem), or is it sharp and associated with numbness or tingling (nerve compression)?
- Is the pain becoming worse, better, or is it relatively stable?
- Is the pain worse on movement in the morning (an inflammatory condition), or is it worse with activity (an injury or degenerative condition)?
- Does the pain wake the patient at night or prevent sleep (neoplasm, infection, or severe arthritis)?
- Does the pain radiate? If so, what course does it take?

### Questions about any type of deformity

- When did the patient first notice the deformity? Was it associated with any injury or disease?
- Is the deformity getting worse?
- Does the deformity affect function, including the ability to work, pursue hobbies, and/or perform activities of daily living?

### Questions about any type of weakness

- What is the extent of the muscle weakness? Does the patient have difficulty placing objects on shelves or climbing steps (proximal muscle weakness and a primary myopathy)?
- Does the patient have any associated sensory abnormalities (a neurologic problem), or does the patient report only weakness (a muscle disorder)?
- Has the patient had any loss of bowel or bladder function, loss of fine motor control (handwriting), or balance function (upper motor neuron involvement)?

Additional questions about the medical history, family history, and a review of systems may reveal clues that suggest the correct diagnosis. For example, weight loss may be a hint that the patient's low back pain is secondary to metastatic disease.

# PHYSICAL EXAMINATION

The principles of examining musculoskeletal problems are similar to evaluating any medical disorder. The specific techniques are detailed in subsequent sections, but the general principles used for inspection, palpation, range of motion, muscle testing, motor and sensory evaluation, and special tests are outlined below. When examining the extremities, comparison with the opposite, asymptomatic extremity is often helpful in defining the specific abnormalities in the symptomatic extremity.

## Inspection/Palpation

The examination starts with inspection. Ask the patient to place one finger on the one spot that hurts the most (**Figure 1**). This simple request will localize the problem and narrow the differential diagnosis. Look for swelling, ecchymosis, and muscular atrophy. Note the patient's body habitus and standing posture. Compare the affected extremity with the opposite extremity. This comparison is important to define subtle abnormalities and to rate the severity of the problem.

Watch the patient walk. Analyze the stance and swing phases of gait. Look for an antalgic gait, which is characterized by limited stance phase on the affected extremity. Weakness of the swing-phase muscles, eg, weakness of the ankle dorsiflexors (peroneal nerve dysfunction), is manifested by a drop foot gait.

The affected area should be palpated for tenderness, abnormal masses, or temperature changes (increased heat from inflammation secondary to injury, infection, or other inflammatory process).

## Range of Motion

Measuring joint motion is important for several reasons. In acute illnesses, the degree of joint mobility is a clue to the diagnosis. For example, hip motion is restricted in children with septic arthritis of the hip or transient synovitis of the hip, but this loss of motion is much greater in patients with septic arthritis. In chronic conditions such as osteoarthritis, the degree of joint motion provides an index to the severity and progression of the disorder, as well as providing important information concerning the results of treatment.

### Basic principles

Joint motion is an objective measurement that can be simply done. Therefore, the parameters for rating musculoskeletal disability, whether for governmental or other agencies, are based largely on the degree that joint motion is impaired.

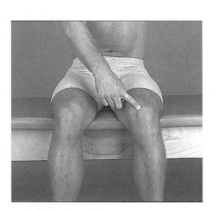

**Figure 1**

Patients can best localize a problem by identifying the one spot that hurts the most.

Joint motion can be estimated visually; however, a goniometer enhances accuracy and is preferred at the elbow, wrist, finger, knee, ankle, and great toe. In measuring hip and shoulder motion, the overlying soft tissue does not allow the same degree of precision with a goniometer.

### Zero Starting Position

Knowing the accepted Zero Starting Position for each joint is necessary to provide consistent communication between observers. The Zero Starting Position for each joint is described in the examination chapter of each section and on the inside covers of this book. For most joints, the Zero Starting Position is the extended anatomic position of the extremity.

To measure joint motion, start by placing the joint in the Zero Starting Position. Place the central axis of the goniometer at the center of the joint. Align one arm of the goniometer with the proximal segment and the other end of the goniometer with the bony axis of the distal segment (**Figure 2**). The upper end of the goniometer is held in place while the joint is moved through its arc of motion. The lower arm of the goniometer is then realigned with the axis of the extremity, and the degree of joint motion is read off the goniometer.

### Definitions of limited motion

The terminology for describing limited motion is illustrated in **Figure 3**. The knee joint depicted in this photograph can be neither fully extended nor fully flexed. The restricted motion is recorded as follows: (1) the knee flexes from 30° to 90° (30° → 90°), or (2) the knee has a 30° flexion contracture with further flexion to 90° (30° FC → 90° or 30° FC W/FF 90°).

Range of motion is slightly greater in children, particularly those younger than age 10 years. Decreased motion occurs as adults age, but the loss of motion is relatively small in most

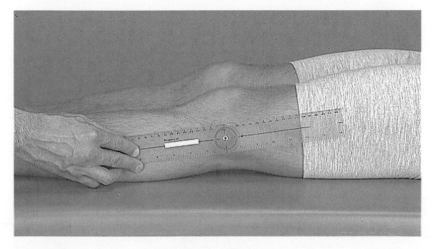

**Figure 2**
The correct position of the goniometer in the Zero Starting Position.

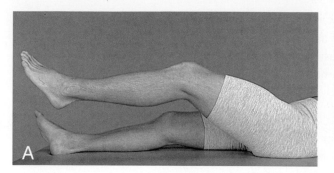 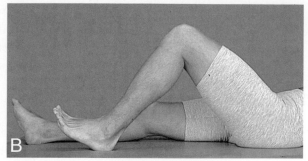

**Figure 3**
**A,** The knee flexes from 30° to 90°. **B,** The knee has a 30° flexion contracture with further flexion to 90°.

joints. Except for motion at the distal finger joints, it is safe to say that any substantial loss of mobility should be viewed as abnormal and not attributable to aging.

Finally, motion of an injured or diseased joint is often painful. In such a situation, it is better to observe active motion first. The examiner will then know how much support to provide the limb as the passive arc of motion is analyzed.

## Muscle Testing

The examination techniques used in muscle testing start with placing the muscle in a shortened position and then proceed with the examiner resisting the movement. For example, when testing the biceps muscle, the patient should position the elbow in flexion and supination, and then the examiner should test resistance of the biceps by attempting to push the elbow into extension.

| Table 1 | Grading of Manual Muscle Testing | |
|---|---|---|
| Numeric Grade | Descriptive Grade | Description |
| 5 | Normal | Complete range of motion against gravity with full or normal resistance |
| 4 | Good | Complete range of motion against gravity with some resistance |
| 3 | Fair | Complete range of motion against gravity |
| 2 | Poor | Complete range of motion with gravity eliminated |
| 1 | Trace | Muscle contraction but no or very limited joint motion |
| 0 | Zero | No evidence of muscle function |

Manual muscle testing provides a semi-quantitative measurement of muscle strength (**Table 1**). The key differentiation is grade 3. For example, a patient's passive knee range of motion is normally 0 to 135°. However, if the patient can actively extend or lift the knee to only 20° of flexion, then, by definition, the quadriceps strength is less than grade 3.

## Motor and sensory evaluation

Nerve root function should be tested if the patient's presenting symptoms suggest a neck or back problem. Peripheral nerve function should be tested if the disorder is localized to the extremities. In either case, the examination should be thorough and efficient. This is most readily accomplished by evaluating one muscle and one area of sensation for either a nerve root or peripheral nerve. The guidelines for assessing nerve root function are presented under Physical Examination in the Spine section, p 722.

Evaluation of peripheral nerves is outlined in **Table 2**. Basically, each peripheral nerve that crosses an acute injury or chronic disorder of the extremity should be evaluated. This examination can be done quickly and completely by evaluating one distal muscle group and one distal area of sensation.

## Special Tests

One basic principle to keep in mind when examining patients with joint and/or muscle pain is that stretch exacerbates pain or

**SECTION 1 ■ GENERAL ORTHOPAEDICS**

### Table 2  Evaluation of Peripheral Nerves

| Nerve | Muscle and Function | Sensory Area |
|---|---|---|
| **Upper extremity** | | |
| Axillary | Deltoid–shoulder abduction | Lateral aspect arm |
| Musculocutaneous | Biceps–elbow flexion | Lateral proximal forearm |
| Median | Flexor pollicis longus–thumb flexion | Tip of thumb, volar aspect |
| Ulnar | First dorsal interosseous–abduction | Tip of little finger, volar aspect |
| Radial | Extensor pollicis longus–thumb extension | Dorsum thumb web space |
| **Lower extremity** | | |
| Obturator | Adductors–hip adduction | Medial aspect, midthigh |
| Femoral | Quadriceps–knee extension | Proximal to medial malleolus |
| Peroneal | | |
|    Deep branch | Extensor hallucis longus–great toe extension | Dorsum first web space |
|    Superficial branch | Peroneus brevis–foot eversion | Dorsum lateral foot |
| Tibial | Flexor hallucis longus–great toe flexion | Plantar aspect foot |

contracture of an injured or deformed structure. Furthermore, if a muscle/tendon crosses two joints, then both joints must be positioned to stretch the injured part. For example, if the hamstrings are injured, their involvement is elucidated by placing these structures on stretch (eg, flexing the hip to 90° and then extending the knee). Pain and/or limited knee extension typically occurs with this maneuver when a patient has an injury or contracture of the hamstring muscles.

Tests specific to individual anatomic injuries are described in the appropriate section.

Of note, as the physician becomes familiar with the musculoskeletal examination, combining different elements of inspection, palpation, range of motion, etc will make the evaluation more efficient.

# AMPUTATIONS OF THE LOWER EXTREMITY

## DEFINITION

Limb amputation is the removal of all or part of an extremity by cutting through the bone. Disarticulation is the removal of all or part of an extremity by cutting through the joint.

## INDICATIONS

Disease states, particularly diabetes mellitus, severe infections, and peripheral vascular disease, are the cause of approximately 70% of all lower extremity amputations. In fact, these conditions account for more than 100,000 lower extremity amputations performed yearly in the United States. Each year, trauma accounts for approximately 20% of lower extremity amputations and tumors for another 5%, with another approximately 5% of amputations related to congenital limb deficiency. Prevalence data, obtained through surveys of all individuals living with limb loss, show that approximately 55% of lower limb amputees and 85% of upper limb amputees experienced limb loss as a result of trauma. The differences between the incidence and prevalence data can be explained by understanding that traumatic amputations more often occur in younger individuals, who typically live with the amputation for many more years than do individuals who undergo amputation because of chronic disease.

Amputations frequently are performed after the patient has undergone extensive medical or surgical intervention to salvage the limb. In these situations, the patient and even the medical team may have a negative attitude concerning the amputation and subsequent rehabilitation, regarding it as a sign of failure. This attitude is inappropriate, however, because most lower extremity amputees regain functional ambulation. Almost 90% of transtibial (below-knee) amputees achieve a functional ambulatory capacity that approaches their preamputation level. Therefore, the physician should maintain a positive attitude and should aggressively pursue early rehabilitation, including prosthesis fitting, to allow patients to resume their normal daily activities.

The energy requirements of walking generally increase with more proximal levels of amputation. Therefore, amputations should usually be performed at the most distal level possible. Sometimes, however, good prosthetic management requires amputation at a more proximal level. For example, an amputation performed at the hindfoot often compromises prosthetic function. In this case, an amputation at the next higher level (ankle disarticulation) may provide better function.

**ICD-9 Code**

**997.60**
Amputation stump complication, unspecified

SECTION 1 ■ GENERAL ORTHOPAEDICS

# LEVELS OF AMPUTATION AND PROSTHETIC CONSIDERATIONS

## Toe Amputation

Dysvascular amputees note no significant loss of function after toe amputation because of their low baseline activity level. Young, active adults with traumatic toe amputations lose some propulsive function but have little significant walking difficulty. Isolated amputation of the second toe should retain the base of the proximal phalanx whenever possible to prevent hallux valgus. In elderly patients, toe amputations often indicate a foot at high risk of ulceration or pressure problems from standard shoes because of poor vascular perfusion and difficulty healing minor injuries and wounds. Therefore, shoes for these individuals should include extra depth and extra width and, often, custom-molded insoles to accommodate and protect a high-risk foot. Following trauma, patients are typically most comfortable in shoes with a more rigid sole and wide toe box to minimize pressure on the amputation site.

## Ray Resection

A ray resection includes a toe and all or part of the corresponding metatarsal. A single-ray resection of ray 2, 3, 4, or 5 functions well in either standard shoes or diabetic footwear, depending on the shape and size of the remaining foot. Ray amputations of the first ray or resection of more than one ray leads to a residual foot that is more difficult to manage. A custom-molded, multi-durometer orthosis is required to load the remaining metatarsal shafts and to unload the amputation site and the remaining metatarsal heads, and can help improve comfort and lessen the chance of re-ulceration. This type of orthosis almost always requires the use of footwear with extra depth and extra width.

## Midfoot Amputation

Amputation of the midfoot is performed at either the transmetatarsal or tarsometatarsal level. Muscle rebalancing at the time of surgery and postoperative physical therapy can help prevent the two most common postoperative contractures of the foot, equinus and varus. Prosthetic requirements vary tremendously at this level. A widened foot at the amputation site is almost universal, and tenderness at the end of the amputation is very common. Because of the increased width of the foot, accommodative footwear and prosthetic/orthotic management are usually needed. A low-profile prosthetic device that cups the heel and provides a long footplate will prevent the shoe from folding and putting pressure on the amputation site. If the foot is hypersensitive, or if balance and weakness are major symptoms, a prosthetic device that encloses the calf may improve function.

## Hindfoot Amputation

Poor function and difficult prosthetic management are common after amputations in the hindfoot. The retained talus and calcaneus frequently are pulled into equinus, and attempts at weight bearing put excessive pressure directly on the amputation site. Surgical muscle rebalancing consists of reattachment of the anterior tendons and a complete release of the Achilles tendon. Advances in prostheses have improved function, especially for elderly individuals, and household ambulation and transfer skills can be very successful. Even with state-of-the-art prostheses, however, aggressive walking and impact activities are still very compromised with a hindfoot amputation.

## Ankle Disarticulation

Removing the entire foot at the ankle and using the heel pad to cover the amputation site is known as a Syme ankle disarticulation. Cutting the bony malleoli flush with the articular cartilage creates a very smooth weight-bearing surface. When combined with durable heel pad coverage, the resulting residual limb ("stump") can often tolerate direct pressure and end weight bearing. A prosthesis is required for routine walking, but the amputation site can usually tolerate transfer pressure and the pressure required for a limited number of steps for bathroom activities without a prosthesis, a benefit to many amputees. The prosthesis socket extends up to the proximal tibia region, very similar to a transtibial prosthesis. The foot component must be very low profile because the amputated limb is almost as long as the nonamputated limb. The gait pattern is stable and requires minimal training. The major disadvantage of a Syme procedure is that the prosthesis is quite wide at the ankle area and looks much less cosmetic than a transtibial prosthesis.

## Transtibial Amputation

This type of amputation is also referred to as a below-knee, or BK, amputation. Various surgical methods are used, but a long posterior flap usually results in more durable padding over the distal end of the tibia and a cylindrical shape, which tolerates prosthetic fitting better than a dramatically tapered residual limb. This durable padding can be very important for minimizing residual limb ulcerations, particularly in patients with diabetes mellitus or peripheral vascular disease. The optimal length recommended was traditionally 12 to 15 cm below the knee joint, but many amputation teams now recommend longer transtibial amputations when the vascular status and skin condition are adequate. Amputation in the lower third of the tibia is not recommended because the padding is simply not adequate below the level of the calf muscle.

Even if walking is expected to be minimal, providing a simple prosthesis and a wheelchair can enhance a transtibial amputee's functional independence if safe transfer skills can be achieved. New developments in flexible sockets are providing a more comfortable fit and better proprioception through improved suspension. The spring-like design of dynamic-response feet both absorbs the shock and rotation of impact and actually returns energy at the end of each stride.

## Knee Disarticulation

This amputation extends through the knee joint itself. Like the Syme disarticulation at the ankle joint, the goal is to create a smooth surface that can directly tolerate end weight bearing, improving function. Early prostheses had major drawbacks: they were bulky around the knee area, and the prosthetic knee joint attached below the socket at a level lower than that of the opposite, normal knee. Newer prosthetic knee joints minimize these disadvantages and have greatly improved the walking function of patients with knee disarticulations. For individuals who are nonambulatory because of paraplegia, neurologic conditions, or other chronic diseases, knee disarticulation is preferable to a more proximal amputation because it maintains a full-length thigh to maximize sitting support and can improve function. It also minimizes the risk of skin problems associated with more distal amputations.

## Transfemoral Amputation

An amputation through the thigh is commonly referred to as an above-knee, or AK, amputation. Contractures are common following this surgery because the muscle attachments at the hip pull the residual thigh into flexion and abduction. Rebalancing the muscles surgically by attaching the adductor muscle and hamstrings can minimize postoperative problems associated with severe hip joint contractures. Aggressive physical therapy is also helpful. The energy requirements of walking are significantly higher with this level of amputation than with more distal amputations, and many dysvascular transfemoral amputees do not have adequate cardiac function for functional ambulation using a prosthesis. Also, the transfemoral amputation loses the power of the knee joint, which the prosthesis cannot replace. Therefore, the decision whether to prescribe a prosthetic limb is more difficult in these patients.

The weight of a transfemoral prosthesis acts as an anchor and makes transfer more difficult. Therefore, to be a candidate for a prosthetic limb, a high-level amputee should have three skills: (1) being able to independently transfer from bed to chair; (2) being able to independently rise from sitting to standing; and (3) being able to ambulate with a one-legged gait up and down the parallel bars. Many transfemoral amputees master these skills within days or weeks of surgery, but others simply cannot. Being able to go a short distance without a prosthesis in the parallel bars or with a walker is an excellent indication that the transfemoral amputee will have the energy to use a prosthesis safely.

## Hip Disarticulation

Amputations and disarticulations at the hip and pelvic level lead to significant loss of function. For many individuals, sitting balance and sitting support to prevent decubitus ulcers are the first priority, followed by learning independent transfer and safe toilet skills. Even young adults with this level of amputation find use of a prosthesis very challenging because of the high energy requirements and the need to control three joints (hip, knee, and ankle). Many individuals with amputations at this level therefore prefer walking with crutches rather than using a prosthesis. Educating patients about the importance of mastering the three vital independence skills listed above under transfemoral amputation before proceeding with a prosthesis can help set task-oriented goals. The success of the patient in meeting these goals can guide the difficult decision of whether to proceed with prosthetic fitting.

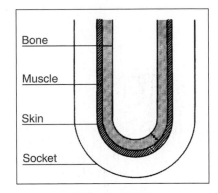

**Figure 1**

The soft-tissue envelope acts as an interface between the bone of the residual limb and the prosthetic socket. Ideally, it should be composed of a mobile, nonadherent muscle mass and full-thickness skin that will tolerate the direct pressures and pistoning within the prosthetic socket.

# PRINCIPLES OF PROSTHETIC FITTING

The soft-tissue envelope over the end of the amputation site is the interface, or cushion, between the bone of the patient's residual limb and the prosthetic socket (**Figure 1**). Disarticulations at the ankle and knee levels can allow weight bearing directly through the end of the residual limb because the bone surface is broad and smooth. The soft-tissue envelope acts as a cushion, and the function of the prosthetic socket is simply to prevent the prosthesis from falling off (**Figure 2**).

In amputations at the transtibial and transfemoral levels, the bone is transected through the diaphysis and cannot accept much direct force at the end. With these amputations, the socket distributes the load over the entire surface of the residual limb. With transtibial amputations, much more load is directly proximal to the amputation site over the sides of the amputated limb and the contours of the knee; with transfemoral amputation, the load is placed on the hip area (**Figure 3**). Intimate fit of the prosthetic socket is crucial. If the patient loses weight or the residual limb atrophies, the limb will "bottom out," or drop down in the socket, resulting in the

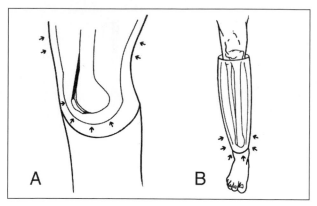

**Figure 2**

Load transfer in knee disarticulation and Syme ankle disarticulations. Weight bearing is accomplished directly through the end of the residual limb in knee disarticulations (**A**) and Syme ankle disarticulations (**B**).

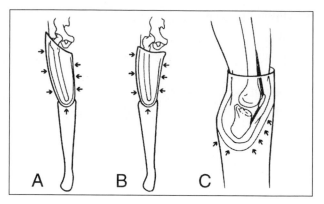

**Figure 3**

Load transfer in transfemoral and transtibial amputations. Indirect load transfer is required in transfemoral amputations. This is accomplished with either a standard quadrilateral socket (**A**) or an adducted narrow medial-lateral socket (**B**). The transtibial amputation socket (**C**) transfers weight indirectly with the knee flexed approximately 10°.

development of a pressure ulcer due to increased end-bearing pressure. In many cases, a prosthetist can add pads inside a socket that is too big to improve the fit. Conversely, if the patient gains weight, the residual limb will not fit down into the socket and the end of the limb will swell into the void and create tender, weeping skin lesions from lack of any distal contact. Unfortunately, a socket that is too small cannot be modified easily and needs to be replaced.

Perfect, intimate prosthetic fit is impossible; therefore, all amputees experience pistoning within the prosthetic socket. Pistoning produces shear forces. Good surgical technique produces a residual limb composed of mobile muscle and durable skin; however, if the soft-tissue envelope is thin (eg, composed of split-thickness skin graft or adherent to bone), blisters and shearing ulcers will develop. In this situation, the prosthetist attempts to compensate by using pressure- and shear-dissipating materials and by maximizing the suspension of the prosthesis to the residual limb.

A prosthetic socket can be expected to last 18 months to 3 years, but it should be modified or replaced if the fit is poor. Socket liners should be replaced when torn or worn out, and they do not last as long as the socket itself. Liners made of foam may last 6 to 24 months, but the new elastomeric and silicon liners often tear within 3 to 4 months of normal use. Prosthetic components such as feet, ankle units, and knee units should be replaced when they are broken or show signs of fatigue failure. Typically, the components should last 3 to 5 years, and many have warranties for this time span.

# ADVERSE OUTCOMES

If pain or pressure problems develop, referral to an amputee clinic, a certified prosthetist, or a rehabilitation physician should be considered. The initial approach for most pain- and pressure-related problems is to adjust the residual limb/prosthesis interface by modifying the socket. If problems persist, heterotopic bone, bone spurs, increased pressure or bruising of the residual nerve ending, or the formation of symptomatic neuromas may be the cause.

## Residual Limb Ulcers or Infection

Most blisters, ulcers, and infections are caused by an inadequate residual limb soft-tissue envelope or poor prosthetic fit. If these problems develop, the patient should stop wearing the prosthesis until it can be adjusted. Often, simply modifying the socket will relieve pressure points, and this modification, combined with simple, nonbulky dressings, will allow the wounds to heal. Antibiotics are necessary only if the patient has signs of local or systemic infection. Surgical revision of the amputation is indicated when superficial wounds fail to heal within 4 to 8 weeks following prosthetic modification, when infection fails to resolve with appropriate antibiotics, or when wounds become deep, exposing muscle, tendon, or bone.

## Skin Conditions

The environment within the prosthetic socket is closed, so excessive sweating or poor hygiene will lead to dermatologic eruption on the residual limb. To prevent this, the prosthetic socket and residual limb should be kept clean and dry. Absorbent powders (other than talcum powder) or creams should be used for this purpose.

Folliculitis, which typically develops in the groin of a transfemoral amputee or in the popliteal area of a transtibial amputee, may be just a nuisance or it may be painful, and it can compromise prosthetic fit. Good hygiene, including keeping the prosthesis clean, can help minimize folliculitis. Treatment with warm soaks and topical agents resolves many mild cases. If cellulitis is present, oral antibiotics may be required. When folliculitis becomes chronic or cystic lesions develop, surgical excision of the involved skin may be required.

Extreme swelling of the residual limb, similar in appearance to severe venous insufficiency disease, may develop if the socket fit is not intimate. The hyperemic, weeping skin may become very painful and develop superficial infection. Treatment includes topical agents and antibiotics as well as improving the fit of the socket.

## Amputation-Related Sensation

Various types of pain are experienced by individuals with limb loss, including nonpainful phantom limb sensations, phantom limb pain, residual limb pain, and back and neck pain. Nonpainful phantom limb sensations may include sensations such as a feeling that a missing foot is wrapped in cotton or that a missing limb is actually present. These sensations can take a variety of forms such as touch, pressure, temperature, itch, posture, or location in space. They can also involve feelings of movement in the phantom limb. "Telescoping," the sensation that the distal part of the phantom limb is moving progressively closer to the residual limb, sometimes occurs. Phantom limb sensations may initially be frightening or annoying, but most individuals adjust to these sensations, and they rarely require treatment.

Phantom limb pain refers to painful sensations in the phantom, or missing, portion of the amputated limb. Although early reports in the literature suggested that the incidence of chronic phantom limb pain was low, it is now thought that as many as 55% to 85% of limb amputees will continue to experience phantom limb pain from time to time. Fortunately, however, severe, persistent phantom limb pain is unusual. Phantom limb pain tends to be more episodic and more intense than nonpainful phantom limb sensations. Persistent symptoms are best controlled with antiseizure membrane-stabilizing drugs, such as gabapentin. Modalities such as transcutaneous electrical nerve stimulation have been reported as helpful for some individuals, especially for short-term flare-ups, but surgery has not been successful. As in many chronic pain syndromes, treatment often requires multiple modalities. Unrelenting phantom limb pain is best managed as a major causalgia with guidance from a specialist in pain management.

Residual limb pain is pain in the portion of the amputated limb that is still physically present. Existing studies disagree regarding the prevalence of chronic residual limb pain after wound healing. Localized residual limb pain may be caused by poor prosthetic socket fit or alignment, and evaluation and adjustment by a prosthetist often resolves the problem. When persistent residual limb pain is caused by bone spurs, which can be visualized on plain radiographs, surgical excision is indicated. Painful nodules or masses that cause an electrical sensation when palpated or taped may indicate symptomatic nerve endings or neuromas. Prosthetic modification to relieve local pressure should be tried initially, but if it is not successful, surgical excision with repositioning of the end of the nerve can help.

Back and neck pain are common following amputation of an extremity. Likely contributing factors are asymmetric pelvic motion, weight shifts, and shoulder motion during gait; asymmetric standing posture; and overuse of the remaining extremities. Such back and neck pain is often more functionally limiting than is phantom limb pain or residual limb pain. A careful examination for spine-related causes of pain is necessary. Treatment typically consists of physical therapy, stretching, and other physical modalities.

## REFERRAL DECISIONS/RED FLAGS

Referral for amputation may be required for vascular disease, trauma, diabetes-related ulceration or infection, or for amputation site complications. Orthopaedic surgeons, vascular surgeons, general surgeons and plastic surgeons all have training in amputation-related care. Orthopaedic surgeons and rehabilitation medicine specialists typically have the most experience with prosthetic rehabilitation and complications. Typically the choice is made based on finding an individual with a particular interest in the care and management of limb loss.

SECTION 1 ■ GENERAL ORTHOPAEDICS

# ANESTHESIA FOR ORTHOPAEDIC SURGERY

## ANESTHETIC TECHNIQUES

### General Anesthesia

General anesthesia has become quite safe thanks to the introduction of modern anesthetic agents (propofol, desflurane, sevoflurane) and the laryngeal mask airway, which allow for fast induction and speedy recovery. In addition, infiltration of local anesthetic agents into the wound or the use of peripheral nerve blocks may reduce the need for potent opioids, decreasing the occurrence of postoperative nausea and vomiting, sleepiness, or respiratory depression.

### Epidural and Spinal Anesthesia

Epidural and spinal anesthetic techniques are very popular for procedures involving the lower extremities because they reduce postoperative cognitive dysfunction in the elderly and allow for perioperative pain relief. Despite certain advantages of these types of regional anesthesia, no prospective studies have shown better outcomes compared with general anesthesia. Also, according to current practice, neuraxial regional anesthesia is contraindicated in patients taking low-molecular-weight heparin and/or potent antiplatelet medication.

### Peripheral Nerve Blocks

Peripheral nerve blocks of the upper and lower extremity are highly effective and may be used alone or in combination with general anesthesia or monitored anesthesia care (MAC). The correct use of a modern peripheral nerve stimulator minimizes patient discomfort and is highly successful for nerve blocks. Peripheral nerve blocks are performed with the patient awake or lightly sedated in order to avoid intraneural injection and traumatic nerve injury. Nerve blocks of the brachial plexus at the level of the interscalene groove, the infraclavicular location, or in the axilla are the most commonly performed procedures for surgery of the upper extremity. Pain from lower extremity surgery can be managed easily with femoral and/or sciatic nerve blocks in the groin, the popliteal fossa, or at the ankle.

### Intravenous Regional Anesthesia

Intravenous regional anesthesia is safe, easy to perform, and highly effective for short procedures on the forearm, wrist, and hand.

# PREOPERATIVE EVALUATION

Many large medical centers and outpatient facilities have developed their own preoperative testing and screening guidelines based on risks and benefits in their particular patient populations. The American Society of Anesthesiologists (ASA) Physical Status Classification System (**Table 1**) is widely used. In general, healthy patients (ASA class 1 or 2) undergoing routine inpatient or outpatient surgery are unlikely to benefit from extensive testing, but patients in ASA class 3, 4, or 5 might benefit from tests that confirm or better define severe underlying medical conditions. The integration of medical information and risk factors will guide the anesthesiologist to a care plan that should include consideration of the following factors:

- Patient education and preferences
- Anesthetic techniques: regional versus general anesthesia, peripheral nerve block
- Strategies for postoperative pain management
- Perioperative pharmacologic interventions: anxiolysis, antacids, beta blockers, inhalers

The anesthesiologist and surgeon should discuss anticoagulation during the perioperative period because the use of newer anticoagulants and antiplatelet drugs for the prevention of thromboembolic events has raised important questions about the use of regional anesthesia in those patients.

# SURGICAL PROCEDURES

Orthopaedic surgical procedures differ in terms of the typical physical status of the patient and the anesthetic requirements of the patient and of the procedure. These factors are summarized in **Table 2**.

| Table 1 | ASA Physical Status Classification System |
| --- | --- |
| Class 1 | A normal healthy patient |
| Class 2 | A patient with mild systemic disease |
| Class 3 | A patient with severe systemic disease |
| Class 4 | A patient with severe systemic disease that is a constant threat to life |
| Class 5 | A moribund patient who is not expected to survive without the operation |
| Class 6 | A declared brain-dead patient whose organs are being removed for donor purposes |

(Reprinted from the ASA website, www.asahq.org/clinical/physicalstatus.htm)

**Table 2  Anesthetic Considerations for Selected Orthopaedic Surgical Procedures**

| Procedure | Typical Patient/Procedure Characteristics | Common Anesthesia Technique |
|---|---|---|
| Repair of hip fracture | Older patient<br>Abnormal mental and/or nutritional status<br>Analgesia required for positioning<br>At risk for thromboembolism, hypothermia, cognitive dysfunction | General |
| Hip or knee replacement | Predominantly older patients, but some < 40 years<br>Congenital, rheumatic, or traumatic joint changes and reduced mobility<br>Disabling pain, history of chronic pain therapy<br>Overweight<br>At risk for thromboembolism, intraoperative reaction to acrylic bone cement<br>Significant postoperative pain | Regional anesthesia usually requested by patient |
| Knee arthroscopy/ ACL reconstruction | Younger patient<br>Outpatient setting<br>Short procedure<br>Minimal blood loss<br>Significant postoperative pain | General plus local anesthetic and/or nerve block |
| Shoulder procedures | Younger and older patients<br>Arthroscopic or open procedures<br>Beach chair or lateral position<br>Painful postoperative period | General plus brachial plexus block |
| Procedures involving the extremities | Any age<br>Varying health status | Depends on patient and procedure |
| Spine surgery | Chronic pain<br>Potential for difficult airway control<br>Potential for blood loss<br>Need for specialized monitoring | General |

## Hip Fracture

The typical patient who undergoes surgery for a hip fracture is an elderly individual who sustained the fracture as a result of a minor fall. Induction of general anesthesia must take into consideration the mental and nutritional status of the patient and may be done before the patient is moved onto the fracture table. The choice of airway, anesthetic drugs, and extent of intraoperative monitoring is most often determined by the preoperative patient profile.

## Hip or Knee Replacement Surgery

Most patients who undergo hip or knee replacement surgery request a regional anesthesia technique. Spinal/epidural anesthesia may reduce intraoperative blood loss as well as postoperative thromboembolic events and probably contributes less to abnormal mental function in the elderly than does general anesthesia. Appropriate use of postoperative spinal or epidural opioids is safe, but effective monitoring by a dedicated pain management team as well as properly trained nursing staff is mandatory. Besides patient preferences, certain medical conditions such as an abnormal coagulation profile, morbid obesity, and heavy preoperative use of pain medication favor the use of general anesthesia. Intravenous patient-controlled analgesia (PCA) provides adequate and satisfactory postoperative pain management.

## Knee Arthroscopy/ACL Reconstruction

General anesthesia is ideal for the typically young, healthy patient undergoing a knee arthroscopy or ACL reconstruction. This type of anesthesia allows for fast recovery and discharge from the outpatient center. Intra-articular injection of local anesthetics by the surgeon or the administration of a suitable nerve block often provides excellent analgesia for many hours. Preoperative administration of the popular "three-in-one" block (femoral, lateral femoral cutaneous, obturator nerves) significantly reduces the amount of general anesthetic needed and provides excellent analgesia during and after ACL reconstruction. The reduced need for postoperative narcotics may contribute to less nausea and vomiting.

## Shoulder Procedures

General anesthesia is the technique of choice for most procedures involving the shoulder joint. The addition of a brachial plexus block at the interscalene groove provides excellent long-lasting perioperative pain relief. The beach chair/ lateral decubitus position requires careful positioning of the head and neck as well as meticulous protection of the face and the eyes. Intraoperative surges in heart rate or blood pressure may be the result of epinephrine-containing irrigation fluid being absorbed in the bloodstream.

Shoulder joint replacement surgery is a complex surgical procedure usually performed in elderly patients. Because of the length of the surgery and the potential for significant blood loss, close monitoring and adequate intravenous access are required. Postoperative pain control is best achieved with a brachial plexus block or PCA.

## Surgical Procedures Involving the Extremities

Surgical procedures involving the extremities are quite variable. Patients cannot be characterized by a consistent set of features, as their age and health status varies widely. Therefore, depending on the particular surgical procedure and the particular patient, any of a wide variety of anesthetic techniques and agents may be appropriate.

SECTION 1 ■ GENERAL ORTHOPAEDICS

Most patients presenting for surgery of the upper extremity or of the foot or ankle will do well with the modern agents used for general anesthesia. Short and minimally invasive procedures can be accomplished by using a peripheral/field block and MAC. Intravenous regional anesthesia (Bier block) lends itself perfectly for short procedures on the hand, wrist, or forearm, and brachial plexus blocks (interscalene, infraclavicular, axillary) provide excellent and long-lasting anesthesia of the upper extremity. An ankle block alone or in combination with general anesthesia or MAC creates excellent surgical conditions for most interventions on the foot, at the same time reducing postoperative pain, nausea, and vomiting.

## Spine Surgery

The most common procedures on the spine are related to instability and herniation of intervertebral disks. Patients often have a long-standing history of back or neck pain that requires chronic administration of narcotic analgesics, which is most likely to be continued in the immediate postoperative period. After induction of general anesthesia, control of the airway may require fiberoptic intubation because of cervical instability or malformation. In addition, the conflicting needs for surgical exposure and for control and maintenance of ventilation and circulation can make positioning of the patient very challenging. Somatosensory evoked potentials (SSEPs) are useful in assessing spinal cord function during major corrective surgeries of the spine. Potential problems for the anesthesiologist include major blood loss, air embolism, pneumothorax, ventilation perfusion mismatch, and injury to the face and eyes when the patient is in the prone position. Postoperative bleeding with formation of hematoma in the neck requires immediate decompression, as would any bleeding in or around the spinal canal that compromises cord function. Postoperative pain can be very significant and is probably best treated with PCA, often requiring help from a pain consultant.

# CANES, CRUTCHES, AND WALKERS

Canes, crutches, and walkers (in that order) reduce weight-bearing stresses on the lower extremities and also augment balance and stability during walking. As such, these devices are helpful in the treatment of arthritic conditions and lower extremity injuries. They also improve balance and stability in elderly patients and in patients who have had a stroke, reducing the risk of a fall or fracture.

## CANES

Canes are lightweight and are easily stored. For long-term use, a spade handle is easier on the hand than the standard crook handle. A "quad" or four-footed cane has four prongs at its base; it is more cumbersome than a single-tipped cane but provides a wider base of support and can be quite useful to patients after a stroke when they have only one functional upper extremity.

A cane should be used on the contralateral side to maximize reduction in stress on an arthritic hip.

A cane that is too long causes excessive flexion of the elbow and increases the demand on the triceps muscle, which is a major stabilizer of the upper extremity when using a cane. A cane that is too short provides inadequate support and compromises walking. The optimal length of a cane will position the elbow in 20° to 30° of flexion when the tip of the cane is placed approximately 6″ in front of and 6″ lateral to the little toe.

## CRUTCHES

Crutches offer more support than a cane but less than a walker. For short-term use, wooden axillary crutches are satisfactory and economical. Aluminum crutches are more durable but cost more and are therefore prescribed for chronic conditions. Forearm crutches extend only to the forearm and, therefore, are less bulky but require better balance and upper extremity strength. These crutches typically are used for patients with chronic conditions. Platform crutches allow forces to be transmitted through the forearm and are useful when patients have arthritic or traumatic conditions of the hand or wrist.

Crutches must be properly fitted, and the patient should receive education in their proper use (**Figure 1**). Crutches that are too long or that are used improperly can cause axillary artery or venous thrombosis or a brachial plexus compression neuropathy (primarily the radial nerve). The hand piece should

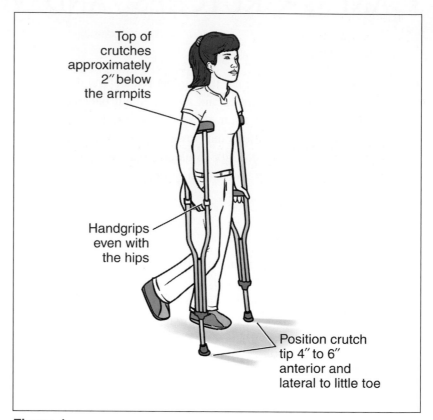

**Figure 1**

Properly fitted crutches. The tops of the crutches are approximately 2″ below the patient's armpits when the patient stands erect, and the hand pieces are even with the patient's hips and allow 25° to 30° of flexion at the elbow.

be positioned to provide optimal function of the triceps and latissimus dorsi muscles. Depending on the height of the patient, position the crutch tip 4″ to 6″ anterior and lateral to the little toe. In that position, adjust the length of the crutch to allow approximately 2″ of clearance between the anterior axillary fold and the top of the crutch. Adjust the hand piece to position the elbow in 25° to 30° of flexion. As a general guideline, the length of the crutch should be 77% of the patient's height. Caution the patient against wrapping towels around the axillary pad.

## WALKERS

Walkers have four points of contact and provide the greatest support and balance. Patients with balance problems more or less carry the walker, while those with arthritic conditions reduce the stress on their lower extremities by transmitting more load onto the walker. The bulkiness of a walker is its major disadvantage. Some walkers fold, making storage in cars easier, but these models are more fragile. Rolling walkers require less energy to use. If balance reactions are adequate, a rolling walker may be advantageous for a patient with significant cardiopulmonary restrictions.

The same principles used for fitting crutches apply for adjusting the height of a walker (ie, the hand grip should be positioned to allow 30° flexion at the elbow when the patient is in a neutral standing position).

Gait techniques for crutches are described in **Table 1**. Following injury to the lower extremity, the technique most commonly prescribed is a non–weight-bearing, swing-through gait. Walking on level ground using this method is easy to teach because it involves simply advancing both crutches, followed by a forward step with the uninjured leg. Ascending or descending steps is more difficult, but the key is to advance the crutches first when going down stairs and to advance the sound leg first when going up. A training session with a physical therapist often is helpful.

**Table 1  Gait Patterns Used with Crutches**

| Type | Instructions |
| --- | --- |
| Swing-to | Advance both crutches. |
| | Lift the body to advance both feet on line with the crutches. |
| Swing-through | Advance both crutches. |
| | Lift the body to advance both feet beyond the crutches. |
| Non–weight-bearing, swing-through | Advance both crutches. |
| | Shift weight and advance the sound leg. |
| Four-point | Move one crutch forward, then advance the opposite foot, followed by the ipsilateral crutch, then the contralateral foot. (Three points of contact are always maintained.) |
| Alternating two-point | Advance one crutch and the contralateral foot at the same time. |
| | Shift weight and advance the other foot and crutch. |
| | (A progression of the four-point gait.) |

SECTION 1  ■  GENERAL ORTHOPAEDICS

# COMPARTMENT SYNDROME

**ICD-9 Codes**

**355.8**
Mononeuritis of lower limb, unspecified (Chronic compartment syndrome)

**958.8**
Other early complications of trauma (Acute compartment syndrome)

## DEFINITION

A muscle compartment is defined as a group of one or more muscles and their associated nerves and vessels surrounded by fascia that is relatively unyielding (**Figure 1**). Compartment syndrome occurs when vascular perfusion of the muscle and other tissues within a compartment decreases to a level that is inadequate to sustain the viability of these tissues.

Compartment syndrome usually is acute in onset and follows trauma, especially fractures of the tibia or other long bones. Patients with severe crush injuries and/or systemic hypotension are particularly susceptible. Patients with peripheral vascular disease also are at risk, as their poor tissue perfusion leads to mild ischemia and transudation of fluid, which increases the local compartment pressure. Acute compartment syndrome also may develop after direct blows that cause only muscular injury and hemorrhage. Exertional compartment syndrome results

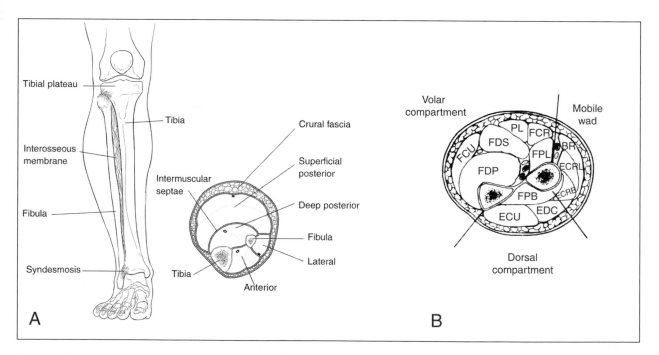

**Figure 1**

**A,** The muscle compartments of the leg are enveloped by strong septae. Swelling within a compartment increases the pressure on the nerves and compromises the perfusion of the muscles. **B,** Cross section of the midportion of the forearm shows the location of the various compartments. BR = brachioradialis; ECRB = extensor carpi radialis brevis; ECRL = extensor carpi radialis longus; ECU = extensor carpi ulnaris; EDC = extensor digitorum communis; EPB = extensor pollicis brevis; FCR = flexor carpi ulnaris; FDP = flexor digitorum profundus; FDS = flexor digitorum superficialis; FPL = flexor pollicis longus; PL = palmaris longus.

(A, Reproduced from Bernstein J (ed): *Musculoskeletal Medicine.* Rosemont, IL, American Academy of Orthopaedic Surgeons, 2003, pp 175-187. B, Reproduced from Whitesides TE, Heckman MM: Acute compartment syndrome: Update on diagnosis and treatment. *J Am Acad Orthop Surg* 1996;4:209-218.)

when muscles that are metabolically active during exercise swell pathologically, compressing neurovascular structures within the same compartment.

Chronic compartment syndrome may develop in long-distance runners, new military recruits, or others involved in a major change in activity level. In these patients, the symptoms are less acute and tend to improve with rest following exercise.

As a compartment syndrome develops, the intracompartmental tissue pressure becomes elevated, producing a secondary elevation in venous pressure that obstructs venous outflow. This causes an escalating cycle of continued increases in intracompartmental tissue pressure and a resultant decrease in arterial flow. The end result is necrosis of muscle and nerve tissues that can occur in as few as 4 to 8 hours.

Failure to recognize an acute compartment syndrome can lead to a tragic outcome with necrotic muscle that is replaced by fibrotic scar tissue, muscular contracture, and permanent dysfunction of all nerves traveling through the compartment. Prevention of this outcome requires early recognition and, in most cases, early surgical intervention.

## CLINICAL SYMPTOMS

The anterior compartment of the leg and the volar aspect of the forearm are the most commonly affected muscular compartments. Pain that is disproportionate to the injury and sensory hypoesthesia distal to the involved compartment (ie, deep peroneal nerve distribution in the foot and median nerve distribution in the hand) are characteristic early symptoms. Other findings may include paresthesias, weakness, and pallor.

## TESTS

### Physical Examination

The most important physical sign is extreme pain on stretching of the long muscles that pass through a compartment. For example, extension of the fingers will stretch the volar forearm muscles, and plantar flexion of the ankle and toes will place the anterior leg muscles on stretch. The inability to actively contract these muscles, as when making a fist or dorsiflexing the toes, is an indication of paralysis.

While passive or active stretching of muscles around fractured bones is always painful, it is usually tolerable; if it is not, the patient may have a compartment syndrome. A patient who has an extraordinary amount of pain in the leg or forearm should be examined carefully.

Examination of a patient who is wearing a cast or dressing begins by removing the cast and any padding to carefully evaluate the muscle compartments. Palpation of increased compartment pressure is subjective, but normally compartments are soft, not tight or rigid. Assess motor and sensory function of the peripheral nerves passing through the compartments, as well as passive stretch of the involved muscles.

Pulselessness indicates arterial trauma—not compartment syndrome—although a compartment syndrome may exist in combination with vascular ischemia. Pulses are typically completely normal in early compartment syndrome because, at that time, the intracompartmental pressure rarely exceeds systolic pressure levels.

## Diagnostic Tests

When necessary, compartment pressures can be measured directly (**Figure 2**). A compartment syndrome usually is present when the diastolic pressure minus the intracompartmental pressure is less than or equal to 30 mm Hg.

# DIFFERENTIAL DIAGNOSIS

Arterial injury (pulse deficit)
Muscle contusion (local soft-tissue bleeding)
Shin-splints (exercise-induced weakness and pain)

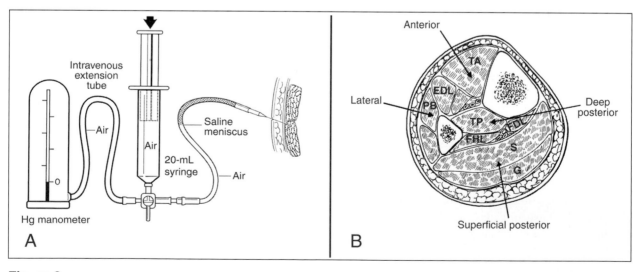

**Figure 2**

Testing compartment pressure. **A,** The Whitesides infusion technique. **B,** Cross section of the proximal half of the leg shows the direction of needle insertion for testing each compartment. EDL = extensor digitorum longus; FDL = flexor digitorum longus; FHL = flexor hallucis longus; G = gastrocnemius; PB = peroneus brevis; S = soleus; TA = tibialis anterior; TP = tibialis posterior.

(Reproduced from Whitesides TE, Heckman MM: Acute compartment syndrome: Update on diagnosis and treatment. *J Am Acad Orthop Surg* 1996;4:209-218.)

## ADVERSE OUTCOMES OF THE DISEASE

Without immediate treatment, compartment syndrome can result in permanent loss of function. The muscles die, scar, and shorten; fingers and toes are often clawed and have little motion. The wrist is held in flexion, and sensation is impaired. Late reconstructive surgery has little chance of restoring original, normal function.

## TREATMENT

Because muscle necrosis can develop within as few as 4 to 8 hours, there is little time to delay treatment. Even a suspicion of compartment syndrome probably requires treatment, especially if intracompartmental pressure measurements support the diagnosis. Surgical fasciotomy of the compartment is essential. The wound is left open, with delayed closure or skin grafting performed after swelling subsides.

Strict instructions must be given to patients to call at any hour, day or night, if the pain is unbearable or if they are unable to actively extend the long extensors of the fingers or toes. Patients must be able to actively extend their fingers or toes before leaving the emergency department or office so that either they or their parents/guardians know what is acceptable motion and usage.

Elevating the lower extremity on pillows placed under the calf will help reduce edema. Elevating the upper extremity with a pillow also is appropriate. Excessive elevation should be avoided because this increases hydrostatic pressure and can lower arterial pressure enough to decrease compartment perfusion.

## ADVERSE OUTCOMES OF TREATMENT

There is very little negative risk in treating an acute compartment syndrome with fasciotomy, except that the scar may be unsightly. However, failure to perform a fasciotomy could be disastrous for the patient.

## REFERRAL DECISIONS/RED FLAGS

Even a tentative diagnosis of compartment syndrome requires urgent evaluation so that surgical decompression by emergency fasciotomy can be considered.

SECTION 1 ■ GENERAL ORTHOPAEDICS

# Complex Regional Pain Syndrome

**ICD-9 Codes**

**337.21**
Reflex sympathetic dystrophy of the upper limb

**337.22**
Reflex sympathetic dystrophy of the lower limb

## SYNONYMS

Causalgia
Pain dysfunction syndrome
RSD
Shoulder-hand syndrome
Sudeck's atrophy
Sympathetically maintained pain (SMP)

## DEFINITION

Complex regional pain syndrome (CRPS), also known as reflex sympathetic dystrophy, algodystrophy, and causalgia, is a clinical diagnosis comprising pain, autonomic dysfunction, trophic changes, and functional impairment. CRPS is classified as type 1 (reflex sympathetic dystrophy, algodystrophy) if there is no identifiable nerve injury or type 2 (causalgia) if there is an identifiable nerve lesion. Part of the spectrum of pain dysfunction syndromes, CRPS is characterized by pain that is generally out of proportion to what would be expected after the original injury and that persists despite the absence of ongoing cellular damage or death. CRPS is the abnormal prolongation of normal postinjury physiologic responses and involves, in part, receptor dysfunction. It is a dynamic process that is initiated and manifested in the extremity but is affected by spinal cord and cortical events. The precise etiology of CRPS has not been defined, and no pathognomonic marker has been identified.

The worldwide incidence of CRPS is unknown; however, one report from Minnesota showed an incidence of 5.5 and a prevalence of 20.7 per 100,000 population. Women are affected at a rate three to four times that of men, and smokers are at increased risk. Individuals between the ages of 30 and 50 years are most likely to be affected, although CRPS does sometimes occur in children. No identifiable psychological profile or psychiatric disorder is linked causally to CRPS.

Although CRPS is classically associated with the upper extremity, the lower extremity is affected almost as often. Injuries that commonly precipitate CRPS include fracture of the distal radius and injuries of the infrapatellar branch of the saphenous nerve; the latter occurs after contusion or arthroscopy. Up to 30% of patients have no apparent injury, indicating the innocuous nature of the events that may precipitate CRPS in some individuals, and a persistent and associated nociceptive focus—either neural or mechanical—is identifiable in less than 50% of patients. Early, appropriate treatment is important for the best prognosis. With the exception of CRPS after fracture of the distal radius (in which poor finger function 3 months following the fracture correlates significantly with the presence of components of algodystrophy after 10 years), 80% of patients who are diagnosed and treated within 1 year of the injury improve significantly, whereas 50% of patients in whom treatment is initiated after 1 year have significant long-term morbidity. Some patients, however, deteriorate and manifest long-term disability in spite of early diagnosis and appropriate intervention.

## CLINICAL SYMPTOMS

The clinical presentation of CRPS varies from classic dystrophy to indolent forms. Classic CRPS becomes obvious at 3 to 10 days after the initiating event, with the affected area progressing from painful/hot/swollen to painful/cold/stiff to stiff/atrophic. Variant forms are common, and classic staging with time intervals is often unreliable. Symptoms include pain, swelling, cold sensitivity, hypersensitivity, allodynia, and difficulty sleeping. The hallmark pain of CRPS is described as "burning," "tearing," "searing," and "throbbing"; is associated with allodynia (pain caused by a normally nonpainful stimulus), hyperpathia (perception of pain that is delayed and extends beyond the normal nerve distribution), and hypesthesia; and is not managed adequately with narcotics. Extremities often appear hot and swollen or cold and stiff with varying manifestations.

## TESTS

The use of functional and health-related quality-of-life instruments such as the DASH (disabilities of the arm, shoulder, and hand) questionnaire, the SF-36 (Short Form-36 Health Survey), and the McGill Pain Questionnaire may be helpful.

### Physical Examination

Signs include swelling, hypersensitivity, abnormal sweating, stiffness, contracture, temperature change, and/or atrophy of hair, skin, and soft tissue. Evaluation for underlying nociceptive foci—coexistent carpal tunnel syndrome, etc—is important and should be done both before and after sympatholytic intervention.

### Diagnostic Tests

Plain radiographs may show spotty areas of osteopenia or demineralization in the bones of the affected extremity. Three-phase bone scans may show increased uptake in the extremity, especially in the third phase of the scan. Autonomic function may be evaluated with temperature and laser Doppler fluxmetry after cold stress testing and QSART (quantitative sudomotor axon reflex testing). Functional impairment may be quantified with endurance testing. Nutritional flow may be analyzed with vital capillaroscopy. Response to sympatholytic oral or injectable drugs should be evaluated to assess whether the patient has sympathetically maintained pain (SMP) or sympathetically independent pain (SIP). Pain relief after sympatholysis from intravenous phentolamine defines SMP, which has a more favorable prognosis than SIP. Similarly, response to stellate block, other autonomic blocks, and/or oral agents supports the diagnosis and suggests SMP. It should be remembered, however, that CRPS is a dynamic process, and the pain of CRPS can change from SMP to SIP.

## Differential Diagnosis

Other neuropathic pain disorders (localized to the site of nerve damage)

Factitious syndromes (SHAFT—sad, hostile, anxious, factitious, tenacious—syndrome, Munchausen syndrome, etc), malingering (skin breakdown, unexplainable and massive edema, recurrent and mixed flora infections, abnormal posturing, spread to other areas)

## Adverse Outcomes of the Disease

Chronic, possibly debilitating, pain; joint contractures and stiffness; and skin and muscle atrophy may develop. Loss of function in the affected extremity, osteopenia, and delayed healing also may occur.

## Treatment

Early recognition and prompt treatment are important. Treatment includes physical therapy, oral medications, biofeedback, therapeutic modalities, parenteral medications, and surgery. Generally, several modalities are used simultaneously, starting with less invasive treatment and progressing to more invasive if the response to treatment is unsatisfactory.

Initial management frequently includes oral medications and physical therapy. Although analgesics (nonnarcotic and narcotic) and NSAIDs treat pain from underlying nociceptive insults and trauma, pharmacologic management of CRPS is designed to block sympatholytic events and/or improve nutritional blood flow. This is accomplished by multiple drug classes, none of which is FDA-labeled for chronic pain. Commonly used drug classes include antidepressants (tricyclic and serotonin-reuptake inhibitors), anticonvulsants, membrane stabilizers, and calcium channel blockers. Effective oral medications include prednisone, amitriptyline, gabapentin, phenytoin, amlodipine besylate, clonidine, and calcitonin. The use of two or more oral agents is common. Therapy includes passive range of motion but emphasizes active range of motion, including stress loading. Frequently, adaptive modalities such as contrast baths, transcutaneous electrical nerve stimulation (TENS), or iontophoresis are used.

Psychological counseling may be helpful and often incorporates coping techniques and biofeedback to control the autonomic functions of the body that regulate sweating, skin temperature, and blood flow. Acupuncture and injections of corticosteroid and local anesthetic into trigger points also can provide transient relief.

Parenteral medications such as bupivacaine may be used for stellate blocks or continuous brachial plexus autonomic blocks for diagnosis and/or management. Continuous intrathecal drugs such as clonidine are used as salvage treatment for refractory symptoms, as are dorsal column stimulators, brain stem stimulators, and other implanted central nervous system devices. Phenol or partial radiofrequency stellate ganglion interruption can be palliative, but nerve transection should be avoided because of receptor up-regulation and potential late exacerbation of symptoms.

In acute CRPS, identification and surgical management of associated nerve injury or compression or mechanical injury is desirable. Perioperative continuous or intermittent autonomic block may be used to prevent dystrophic exacerbation if less invasive modalities are ineffective. It is appropriate to operate on patients with CRPS during all stages of the process. The sequelae of CRPS, including joint contractures and deformity, can be managed surgically, using appropriate monitoring and pharmacologic management as needed.

## Adverse Outcomes of Treatment

Side effects of treatment are minimal when used judiciously. Undertreatment is common. Significant side effects of stellate ganglion blocks, which include hoarseness, weakness, numbness in the arm, pneumothorax, and possible seizure from vertebral artery injection, are infrequent. Use of narcotics may lead to addiction, and excessive use of NSAIDs may result in gastric, hepatic, and renal symptoms. Fractures also may occur from too-vigorous manipulations.

Section 1 ■ General Orthopaedics

# REFERRAL DECISIONS/RED FLAGS

If symptoms fail to respond to initial pharmacologic and therapeutic treatments, consider consultation with a pain specialist. Additional evaluations at a center where a multidisciplinary team is available to treat this difficult problem should be used as needed.

# CORTICOSTEROID INJECTIONS

## GENERAL GUIDELINES

Corticosteroid injections have an accepted role in the treatment of acute and chronic inflammatory diseases. In general, these injections can decrease inflammation and improve function, but they also may occasionally cause significant adverse effects. In addition, the indications for their use in some musculoskeletal conditions are not well defined.

Many long-acting corticosteroid ester preparations enhance anti-inflammatory actions and reduce undesirable hormonal side effects. The most widely used compounds are listed in **Table 1**.

The choice of agent depends somewhat on the desired effect. For an acute condition that requires immediate effect (eg, carpal tunnel syndrome), a fast-acting agent would be appropriate. For chronic inflammatory conditions, a long-acting agent is preferred. Triamcinolone compounds often are used for intra-articular injections, particularly of intermediate or large joints, but because these agents are more likely to cause local tissue necrosis, other preparations often are chosen for small joint and tendon injections.

## HOW CORTICOSTEROIDS WORK

Corticosteroids suppress inflammation. They decrease collagenase and prostaglandin formation and formation of granulation tissue. They are catabolic promoters that block glucose uptake in the tissues, enhance protein breakdown, and decrease new protein synthesis in muscle, skin, bone, connective tissue, and lymphoid tissue (predominantly T cells).

**Table 1   Common Injectable Corticosteroids**

| Medication | Relative Potency | Onset | Duration |
|---|---|---|---|
| Hydrocortisone (Cortisol) | 1 | Fast | Short |
| Prednisolone terbutate (Hydeltra) | 4 | Fast | Intermediate |
| Methylprednisolone acetate (Depo-Medrol) | 4 | Slow | Intermediate |
| Triamcinolone acetonide (Kenalog) | 5 | Moderate | Intermediate |
| Triamcinolone hexacetonide (Aristospan) | 5 | Moderate | Intermediate |
| Betamethasone (Celestone) | 25 | Fast | Long |

# USE OF INTRA-ARTICULAR INJECTIONS

An optimal intra-articular dose of corticosteroid is the maximum amount that can be held locally. However, it should be noted that some of the locally injected steroid is absorbed systemically and may produce transient systemic effects. Usual doses of methylprednisolone or equivalent are listed in **Table 2**.

## Rheumatoid Arthritis

Use of an intra-articular injection for active synovitis associated with rheumatoid arthritis and other inflammatory arthritides improves symptoms in the injected joint about 50% of the time and lasts from several days to several weeks. Repeated injections to suppress rheumatoid synovitis are generally effective in the knees, elbows, and interphalangeal joints. Long-term studies are limited but do not show accelerated destructive changes in the injected joints when compared with control joints.

## Osteoarthritis

Intra-articular corticosteroid injection is less effective, and its effects are of shorter duration, in patients with osteoarthritis than in those with rheumatoid arthritis. The joints most often helped are the knee and the interphalangeal or metacarpophalangeal joints of the hand.

## Crystal-Induced Arthritis

Use of an intra-articular corticosteroid injection in patients with gout or pseudogout can be especially helpful for those whose comorbid conditions or allergies prohibit use of systemic medications.

| Table 2 | Usual Doses of Methylprednisolone or Equivalent by Site |
|---|---|
| **Dose (mg)** | **Anatomic Site** |
| 5 to 10 | Phalangeal joints |
| 20 to 30 | Wrist |
| 20 to 30 | Elbow and ankle |
| 40 to 80 | Shoulder, hip, or knee |

## Tenosynovitis and Bursitis

Both flexor tenosynovitis in the hand (trigger finger) and de Quervain tenosynovitis at the wrist respond well to injections of corticosteroids into the tenosynovial sheath (not the tendon). Bursitis associated with shoulder impingement often responds well to a single injection. Trochanteric bursitis usually responds well to injection (usually no more than three), and few adverse effects have been reported with multiple injections. Lateral epicondylitis and plantar fasciitis may respond well to corticosteroid injection.

Injections into ligaments or tendons carry the risk of spontaneous rupture of the tendon or ligament and usually are quite painful. The Achilles and patellar tendons should not be injected in the substance of the tendon. Pain in these structures usually indicates interstitial tears, which have already reduced their tensile strength.

## Entrapment Neuropathies

Carpal tunnel syndrome is often treated with injections into the carpal canal, but there is a substantial relapse rate and a chance of intraneural injection.

## Ganglia

Injection of corticosteroids into ganglia is not necessary. Use a large-bore needle and make multiple punctures to decompress the ganglion. Recurrence of the ganglion is common.

# IMPROPER USES OF INJECTIONS

Acute trauma

Injection into a tendon, ligament, or nerve

Injection into an infected joint, tendon, or bursa

Multiple injections (except as noted) in conditions other than rheumatoid arthritis

# ADVERSE OUTCOMES

Adverse systemic effects include transient serum cortisol suppression and transient hyperglycemia (a particular problem in patients with diabetes). Significant effects are uncommon with doses of 25 to 50 mg of methylprednisolone. Postinjection infectious arthritis is uncommon (perhaps 1 in 13,000 injections or fewer) but potentially catastrophic.

Local side effects after injection include lipodystrophy, loss of skin pigmentation, tendon rupture, and possible accelerated joint degeneration, although recent evidence suggests this is unlikely. Up to 10% of treated patients can experience a transient flare or increased pain for 24 to 48 hours following an injection.

Nerve injection injuries can be catastrophic. Extrafascicular injection usually results in no permanent damage, but intrafascicular injection can temporarily or even permanently interfere with nerve function and cause severe pain. Injection of dexamethasone results in minimal damage; triamcinolone acetonide and methylprednisolone result in moderate damage. The damage has been blamed on the carrier agent, but the effect of these agents has not been distinguished from the corticosteroid.

Patients should be advised that the site of injection might be uncomfortable for a few hours after injection. Application of ice helps relieve the discomfort. Patients also should be advised that the potential beneficial effects of the steroid will not be apparent for several hours or days, although the patient typically will experience immediate but transient relief from the local anesthetic.

It is not possible to establish a safe dose of corticosteroid because of individual variability regarding sensitivity to the drug.

Olecranon and prepatellar intrabursal injections carry an increased risk for infection. These structures should be injected only when the patient's problem has not resolved with time and there is clearly no evidence of underlying infection.

Patients with diabetes mellitus are at risk for serious infection and for systemic effects of absorbed corticosteroids.

# INJECTION PRINCIPLES

Prior to injecting a corticosteroid, review the following guidelines:

1. Scrub the intended injection site with a bactericidal solution. Wear sterile gloves and handle the syringes and needles with strict aseptic technique. Observe universal precautions.

2. Cleanse the top of the solution vial with an antiseptic solution.

3. Use an 18- or 20-gauge needle for easy withdrawal of solution. Discard this needle.

4. Consider anesthetizing the injection site with ethyl chloride or a small amount of local anesthetic given with a 25- or 27-gauge needle.

5. Do not use local anesthetics that contain epinephrine when injecting the hand or foot; these can cause arterial constriction and infarction of a digit.

6. Corticosteroid and local anesthetic solutions can be mixed in the same syringe, usually in a 1:2 ratio. Injection of the site with 2 to 3 mL of a rapid-acting local anesthetic solution, advancing the same needle into the joint or tendon shcath, and injecting additional local anesthetic followed by the steroid through the same needle is less traumatic to the patient. Large joints (knee and shoulder) may need an additional 4 mL of local anesthetic.

7. Short- and long-acting local anesthetics also may be mixed in the same syringe.

8. Inject anesthetic or corticosteroid preparation with a sterile 22- to 25-gauge needle.

9. Do not inject anesthetic or corticosteroid into a nerve, a tendon, a ligament, or subcutaneous fat.

10. Use multiple injections only if clear improvement has occurred. Limit the number to three injections.

11. Following the injection, have the patient rest the extremity for 24 hours and avoid the precipitating cause of the problem.

SECTION 1 ■ GENERAL ORTHOPAEDICS

# CRYSTALLINE DEPOSITION DISEASES

**ICD-9 Codes**

**274.0**
Gouty arthropathy

**712.2**
Chondrocalcinosis due to pyrophosphate crystals

**712.3**
Chondrocalcinosis, unspecified

## SYNONYMS

Calcium pyrophosphate deposition disease (CPDD)
Gout
Podagra
Pseudogout

## DEFINITION

Crystalline deposition diseases are secondary to deposition of crystals in the synovium and other tissues and the subsequent inflammatory response. The arthritis is characterized by abrupt episodes of severe joint pain involving a single joint. In time, more than one joint may be involved, and joint destruction may occur.

Gout is secondary to monosodium urate crystal deposition. The disease is relatively common and increases with age and with increasing serum uric acid concentrations. The most frequent manifestation of gout is arthritis, but the uric acid crystals also may be deposited in other tissues such as bursae, tendon sheaths, skin, heart valves, and kidneys with resultant tophi, renal stones, and gouty nephropathy. Acute arthritis is the most common presentation of gout, but in some patients, nephrolithiasis is the first manifestation of the disorder.

Calcium pyrophosphate dihydrate crystals reside in cartilage and are shed into the joint, causing calcium pyrophosphate deposition disease (CPPD). How these crystals affect the joint varies widely, and CPPD can be confused with gout, osteoarthritis, rheumatoid arthritis (RA), and neuropathic (Charcot) arthropathy. Chondrocalcinosis, pseudogout, and chronic arthropathy are common manifestations of CPPD.

## CLINICAL SYMPTOMS

Acute gouty arthritis typically begins in a single joint, with symptoms first appearing at night. The pain and swelling are intense. Patients often note that the joint is so painful that even the weight of a sheet is intolerable. The overlying erythema may be confused with cellulitis or a septic joint. The metatarsophalangeal joint of the great toe (podagra) is most commonly affected, accounting for approximately 50% of the initial episodes of gouty arthritis. Other frequent sites of involvement include the ankle, tarsal joints, and the knee. Patients often also have fever and chills. As the inflammation subsides, desquamation of the skin overlying the affected joint may be noted.

Pseudogout tends to manifest itself in larger joints and is typically less explosive and dramatic in presentation, although, like gout, it can present as a suddenly acute, painfully swollen joint. Approximately 50% of the episodes of pseudogout affect the knees. Other commonly involved joints include the elbows, wrists, ankles, hips, and shoulders. In the elderly, pseudogout is the most common cause of acute arthritis involving a single joint.

Tophi are soft-tissue masses resulting from urate crystal deposition that are noted several years following the onset of gout. They can develop in many locations, including the olecranon bursa, extensor surface of the forearm, Achilles tendon, or tendon sheaths in the hand. Tophi may be confused with rheumatoid nodules.

Chondrocalcinosis is calcification of articular cartilage or meniscus, usually at the periphery of the joint. The calcifications do appear on radiographs, but most patients are asymptomatic or have only mild arthritic symptoms. This disorder is more common in women and increases with age, affecting approximately half of the population over the age of 80 years.

Chronic pyrophosphate arthropathy is more common in older women. The knees, wrists, shoulders, elbows, hips, and hands are frequently affected. Symptoms include stiffness on arising and multiple joint involvement. CPPD arthropathy may be confused with RA, but patients do not have bony erosions or other features of RA, such as tenosynovitis. The symptoms also mimic osteoarthritis, but the inflammatory aspects and history of acute exacerbations help to distinguish it from osteoarthritis.

# TESTS

## Physical Examination
Document the degree of swelling, surrounding erythema, and limited motion.

## Diagnostic Tests
For acute arthritis, joint aspiration and analysis of synovial fluid are most critical. Examination of joint fluid under polarized microscopy reveals the characteristic negatively birefringent urate crystals or weakly positive, birefringent rhomboid-shaped calcium pyrophosphate crystals (**Figure 1**). Cell counts can be quite variable in acute gouty arthritis. Because septic arthritis is a consideration, obtain a Gram stain and culture of the synovial fluid.

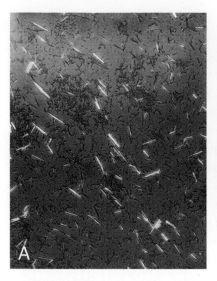 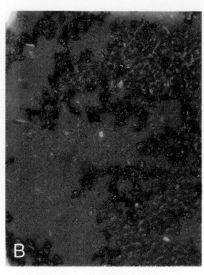

**Figure 1**

**A,** Monosodium urate crystals as seen under polarized light. These crystals are characteristic of gout and are found in the fluid of the inflamed joint and in other affected tissues. **B,** Birefringent rhomboid-shaped calcium pyrophosphate crystals, characteristic of pseudogout. **(Courtesy of Ann Faber, photographer.)**

Radiographs are normal except for soft-tissue swelling at the onset of acute gouty arthritis, but punctate or linear calcification of articular cartilage and internal joint structures, such as menisci in the knee or the triangular fibrocartilage in the wrist, are characteristic of pseudogout (**Figure 2**). Radiographs of established gout are characterized by subchondral bony erosions and peripheral articular spurs (**Figure 3**).

Serum uric acid levels should be checked with suspicion of gout; however, these levels may be normal during an acute episode. Plasma urate levels are variable in acute episodes, but a state of asymptomatic hyperuricemia exists prior to development of these episodes and in the intervals between them.

Some metabolic disorders, such as hyperparathyroidism, hemochromatosis, hypophosphatasia, and hypothyroidism, are associated with CPPD and should be ruled out.

# DIFFERENTIAL DIAGNOSIS

Cellulitis (joint not involved and motion only mildly affected by overlying skin infection)

Lyme arthritis (chronic fatigue, memory loss, history of rash, IgM or IgG antibody titer)

Neuropathic arthropathy (underlying neurologic disorder such as diabetes, insignificant pain)

Osteoarthritis (less acute, pain proportionate to activity)

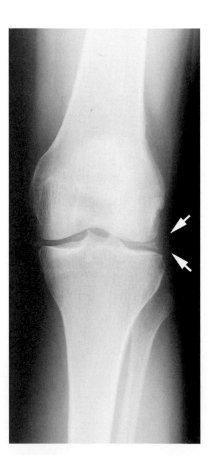

**Figure 2**

AP view of the knee of a 48-year-old patient with pseudogout. Note the characteristic crystals in the meniscal cartilage (arrows).

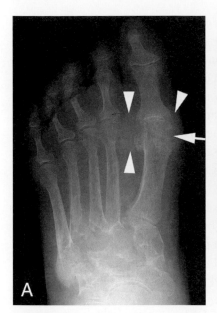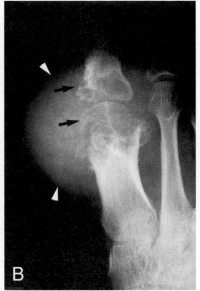

**Figure 3**

**A,** AP view of the foot of a patient with gout. Note the erosions with sharp margins, the overhanging edge in the metatarsophalangeal joint of the great toe (arrow), and a soft-tissue mass around the first metatarsal consistent with a deposit of sodium urate (arrowheads). **B,** AP view of the great toe of a patient with advanced gout. The black arrows indicate large, well-marginated erosions on both sides of the metatarsophalangeal joint, and the white arrowheads indicate a large soft-tissue mass, findings consistent with advanced gout.

Reproduced from Johnson TR, Steinbach LS (eds): *Essentials of Musculoskeletal Imaging.* Rosemont, IL, American Academy of Orthopaedic Surgeons, 2004, p 627.

Rheumatoid arthritis (younger age, multiple joint involvement, associated tenosynovitis)

Septic arthritis (severe pain, systemic signs, positive Gram stain and culture)

Trauma (history, hemarthrosis, or fracture)

## ADVERSE OUTCOMES OF THE DISEASE

Before effective control of hyperuricemia was common, development of tophi and chronic gouty arthritis was the expected course. Chronic hyperuricemia also leads to nephropathy and renal stones. End-stage arthritis may occur with CPPD, but this is infrequent.

## TREATMENT

Treatment of acute episodes first focuses on relieving the inflammation and then minimizing the risk of recurrence and other complications. Colchicine can be quite effective in treating acute gouty arthritis whether given orally or intravenously, but the side effects are significant. Indomethacin also can be quite effective, with an initial dose of 75 to

SECTION 1 ■ GENERAL ORTHOPAEDICS

100 mg, followed by 50 mg every 6 hours until symptoms subside. Other NSAIDs can be used, as well. The joint also can be aspirated and injected with a corticosteroid.

Long-term treatment of gout is aimed at limiting hyperuricemia with drugs such as allopurinol and preventing recurrent acute episodes with small daily doses of colchicine or early use of indomethacin at the first sign of joint inflammation. Attention to any underlying disease in cases of secondary gout is important. Dietary discretion may help reduce the frequency of episodes.

Joint aspiration alone may relieve acute episodes of pseudogout. NSAIDs also can be effective with acute episodes of pseudogout. These medications, combined with a program of exercise, weight reduction, and canes, may be helpful in the long-term management of CPPD. Injection of intra-articular steroid may be required for a severe acute episode.

## ADVERSE OUTCOMES OF TREATMENT

NSAIDs can interfere with drugs used concomitantly for control of hypertension and often produce gastrointestinal side effects. Complications of corticosteroid use are well known.

## REFERRAL DECISIONS/RED FLAGS

Joint deformity or destruction, large tophaceous masses, or drainage of tophaceous material may require surgical attention.

# DEEP VENOUS THROMBOSIS

## DEFINITION

Deep venous thrombosis (DVT) is characterized by hypercoagulation, obstruction of venous outflow, and/or endothelial trauma that precipitates venous clot formation. Proximal propagation of clots can lead to pulmonary embolism and even death. Major musculoskeletal procedures (eg, total hip arthroplasty, total knee arthroplasty, hip fracture surgery), multiple trauma, and spinal cord injuries increase the likelihood of DVT and subsequent pulmonary embolism. Other risk factors include previous thrombosis; immobilization; stroke; congestive heart failure; malignancy; deficiencies in antithrombin III, protein C, or protein S; myeloproliferative diseases; estrogen use; inflammatory bowel disease; diabetes; obesity; and age older than 40 to 50 years.

## CLINICAL SYMPTOMS

Many patients with DVT are asymptomatic, but some report pain or swelling in the calf or thigh. Patients with pulmonary embolism often report dyspnea, pleuritic or substernal chest pain, and hemoptysis.

## TESTS

### Physical Examination

Clinical signs of venous thrombosis often are nonspecific. Swelling, whether painful or not, is common. However, clots may be asymptomatic, and pulmonary embolism can occur without any prior warning. Patients with superficial saphenous vein thrombophlebitis have a tender, warm, ropy vein, which may be serious if it extends into the common femoral vein. A positive Homans' sign is calf pain with forced ankle dorsiflexion.

The clinical signs of pulmonary embolism include dyspnea, hemoptysis, tachycardia, pleural rub, tachypnea, and sometimes circulatory collapse.

### Diagnostic Tests

If patients report swelling and pain, duplex ultrasound is highly accurate in diagnosing proximal clot formation. However, the role of a duplex scan in screening for asymptomatic thrombi remains controversial. Venography remains the gold standard to confirm DVT but is an invasive procedure that may cause pain, allergic reactions to contrast medium, or, rarely, DVT.

**ICD-9 Code**

**451.1**
Phlebitis and thrombophlebitis, of deep vessels of lower extremities

SECTION 1 ■ GENERAL ORTHOPAEDICS

## Differential Diagnosis

Baker cyst (ruptured popliteal cyst) (no history of prior trauma or surgery)

Cellulitis (erythema, superficial tenderness)

Contusion of calf muscles (direct blow, subsequent ecchymosis and tenderness)

Lymphedema (nontender, diffuse swelling)

Strain of the calf or thigh muscles (history of injury, pain with stretch of the involved muscle)

## Adverse Outcomes of the Disease

Both distal and proximal clots can lead to pulmonary embolism and/or death. Symptomatic proximal leg vein thromboses may have silent pulmonary emboli in as many as 50% of patients. Other possible problems include postthrombotic syndrome with venous stasis ulceration, chronic edema, venous claudication, and recurrent thromboses.

## Treatment

### Prophylaxis

Most patients who die of a pulmonary embolism do so within 30 minutes of the acute event, which is too soon for therapeutic anticoagulation to be effective. Consequently, prophylaxis is needed to reduce the incidence of thromboembolism or prevent proximal propagation of the clots. There is no universally accepted regimen (agent or duration) for prophylaxis in orthopaedic surgical conditions. The effect of early hospital discharge on the duration of prophylaxis and the impact on the prevalence of symptomatic thromboembolism following discharge are unclear. Effective prophylaxis can be obtained with both pharmacologic and mechanical methods. There is general agreement that patients undergoing total hip or knee arthroplasty and multiple-trauma patients require DVT prophylaxis. There is, however, disagreement concerning the preferred approach.

The ultimate goal of prophylaxis is to prevent a symptomatic pulmonary embolism or chronic venous insufficiency. Warfarin may be given the night following surgery, although some physicians prefer to give a low dose before surgery. The dose of warfarin is adjusted to keep the international normalized ratio (INR) between 1.8 and 2.5. Warfarin prophylaxis usually continues for 2 to 3 weeks. The prophylaxis regimen used with the low-molecular-weight heparins depends on the particular drug being prescribed. In general, these drugs have a very short half-life and therefore should not be administered immediately after

Section 1 ■ General Orthopaedics

surgery. Depending on the drug used, the first dose is started 6 to 24 hours postoperatively. Monitoring of INR or partial thromboplastin time (PTT) is not necessary with the low-molecular-weight heparins. Low-molecular-weight heparin has been found to be more effective than warfarin in reducing the overall rates of asymptomatic DVT, but no difference has been noted in reducing the prevalence of death from pulmonary emboli.

The duration of prophylaxis remains controversial. After total hip arthroplasty, hip fracture, and total knee arthroplasty, 7 to 10 days of prophylaxis has been recommended, although some physicians recommend a longer course of prophylaxis (28 to 30 days) after total hip arthroplasty and hip fracture.

Pneumatic compression boots or plantar arch compression devices reduce the overall risk of DVT and should be applied during and after surgery. The advantage to using these devices is that they do not require laboratory monitoring, and there is no risk of bleeding. However, patient compliance can be a problem, and the efficacy of these devices in limiting proximal clot formation in patients undergoing total hip arthroplasty requires further study. These devices can serve as an adjunct to pharmacologic prophylaxis.

Effective prophylaxis after total hip arthroplasty includes warfarin and low-molecular-weight heparin. Effective prophylaxis after total knee arthroplasty includes low-molecular-weight heparin, warfarin, pneumatic compression boots, and plantar compression devices. Low-molecular-weight heparin also provides effective prophylaxis for most multiple-trauma patients.

## Treatment of Distal Clots

The risk of pulmonary embolism and of death from pulmonary embolism is significantly less for a distal clot than for a proximal clot, and therefore many physicians do not treat distal clots. Instead, they follow them with serial duplex ultrasound imaging and, if the clot migrates proximally (as occurs in 20% of patients), they treat the proximal clot. No consensus exists as to how long to follow patients, though one accepted regime recommends following patients every 7 to 10 days for 3 weeks, discontinuing follow-up if the clot does not progress.

## Treatment of Proximal Clots

Anticoagulation is recommended in patients diagnosed with a proximal venous thrombosis. This can be done by hospitalization for intravenous heparin, or as an outpatient for low-molecular-weight heparin, until oral Coumadin doses can be adjusted within the therapeutic range (INR of 2 to 3). Popliteal clots are considered as proximal clots. Continue warfarin therapy for at least 3 months.

SECTION 1 ■ GENERAL ORTHOPAEDICS

Contraindications of long-term warfarin therapy include pregnancy, liver insufficiency, severe liver disease, noncompliance, severe alcoholism, uncontrolled hypertension, active major hemorrhage, and inability to return for monitoring.

## Treatment of Acute Pulmonary Embolism

Admission to the hospital for intravenous heparin, supplemental oxygen, and close monitoring is advised. Coumadin therapy is initiated, and when INR levels reach the therapeutic range, the intravenous heparin may be discontinued.

# Adverse Outcomes of Treatment

Bleeding has been associated with all anticoagulants. Thrombocytopenia occurs with standard heparin but occurs infrequently with low-molecular-weight heparin. However, bleeding risks are low, and it is important that high-risk patients receive prophylaxis despite these potential problems. Skin necrosis can develop with warfarin but is uncommon.

# Referral Decisions/Red Flags

None

# Diffuse Idiopathic Skeletal Hyperostosis

## Synonyms

Ankylosing hyperostosis
Vertebral osteophytosis

## Definition

Diffuse idiopathic skeletal hyperostosis (DISH) is an idiopathic disease characterized by striking osteophyte formation in the spine. Patients with DISH have confluent ossification spanning three or more intervertebral disks, most commonly in the thoracic and thoracolumbar spine. The bridging osteophytes follow the course of the anterior longitudinal ligaments and the peripheral disk margins. The disease primarily affects white men (male-to-female ratio is 2:1) who are age 60 years or older.

## Clinical Symptoms

The principal symptom is stiffness in the spine, especially in the morning and evening. Patients often report that symptoms have been present for several months or even years. Nonradicular back pain, especially in the lumbar and thoracolumbar junction area, is relatively mild (**Figure 1**). Those with cervical spine involvement may notice dysphagia related to a large anterior cervical osteophyte located behind the esophagus. Other weight-bearing joints can be painful, but spinal pain is the most severe.

## Tests

### Physical Examination
Examination reveals stiffness in the spine on forward flexion and on extension. Reduced hip motion or associated knee arthritis also is possible.

### Diagnostic Tests
Radiographs of the thoracic and lumbar spine, especially the lateral view, show confluent ossification spanning the intervertebral disks of at least four contiguous vertebral bodies (three disks) (**Figure 2**). The intervertebral disk height is preserved in the fused segments. The posterior apophyseal joints and sacroiliac joints are normal as opposed to the findings characteristic of ankylosing spondylitis.

In the cervical spine, ossification of the posterior longitudinal ligament occurs and is the second most common cause of cervical myelopathy (after cervical spondylosis).

**ICD-9 Code**
**721.6**
Ankylosing vertebral hyperostosis

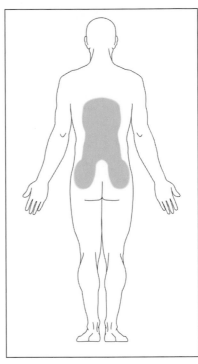

**Figure 1**
Distribution of pain in DISH.

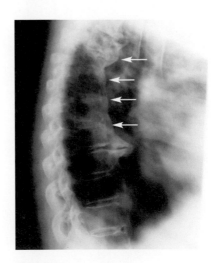

**Figure 2**
Lateral radiograph of the thoracic spine showing confluent ossification anteriorly spanning multiple disk levels (arrows).

Section 1 ■ General Orthopaedics

The pelvis often shows "whiskering" or shaggy hyperostotic bone at the pelvic rim. There may be hyperostotic change in the ribs, as well.

There is no human leukocyte antigen (HLA) association.

## DIFFERENTIAL DIAGNOSIS

Acromegaly (facial and phalangeal changes)

Ankylosing spondylitis (sacroiliac and apophyseal joint involvement, positive HLA-B27)

Degenerative disk disease (reduced disk height)

Paget disease (32% of patients also have DISH)

Polymyalgia rheumatica (muscle and joint pain and stiffness associated with systemic symptoms)

## ADVERSE OUTCOMES OF THE DISEASE

Spinal stiffness is common. With widespread involvement, a single mobile segment can remain, but it may become unstable and painful.

## TREATMENT

Walking and exercise programs are the most common initial treatment. Intermittent NSAIDs can help, but pain usually is mild and tolerable.

## ADVERSE OUTCOMES OF TREATMENT

Heterotopic ossification occurs five times more often following hip replacement surgery in patients with DISH. NSAIDs can cause gastric, renal, or hepatic complications.

## REFERRAL DECISIONS/RED FLAGS

Symptoms of neurogenic claudication, myelopathy, or dysphagia indicate the need for further evaluation.

# FALLS AND MUSCULOSKELETAL INJURIES IN THE ELDERLY PATIENT

## DEFINITION

The elderly are the fastest growing segment of the population. Fall prevention is a critical wellness issue in this age group because nearly one third of all elderly people fall each year. Of these, 50% fall repeatedly. One percent of falls result in a hip fracture. Falls also are responsible for 40% of nursing home admissions.

Intrinsic factors causing falls are those associated with the aging body, as follows:

- visual changes (often due to diseases such as glaucoma, macular degeneration, diabetic retinopathy, and improper use of corrective lenses)
- hearing problems and/or vestibular dysfunction
- neurologic conditions (such as Parkinson disease, weakness from stroke, transient ischemic attacks)
- cardiovascular problems (arrhythmia, hypertension, hypotension, peripheral vascular disease)
- dementia
- musculoskeletal conditions (arthritis, stiffness, osteoporosis)
- systemic illness (leading to metabolic defects or malignancy causing pathologic fractures).

Extrinsic factors causing falls are related to the environment and include obstacles or design flaws in the home, poor supervision, weather conditions, and improper footwear. The elderly often do not have adequate assistance with their daily routine; as a result, they may be forced to engage in risky behavior, such as climbing to reach objects in the kitchen or closet. Bathing also poses numerous hazards, most notably a slippery, wet floor. Obstacles such as furniture or rugs can contribute to falls, particularly at night. Cracks in sidewalks and ice contribute to outdoor falls. Assistance in and out of the home can decrease these risks. Attention to layout in the home, including clearing obstructed pathways and installing handrails and traction pads in the bathroom, can decrease the risk of falls.

Many elderly patients present in poor nutritional condition and/or are weakened and confused as a result of multiple drug use (polypharmacy). The use of sedatives specifically in the elderly is associated with an increased risk of falls and injury. Communicating with elderly patients can be difficult because of poor hearing, poor eyesight, or confusion. Despite the frustrations in communication, it is important to treat elderly patients with dignity and respect.

## CLINICAL SYMPTOMS

The most common fractures involve the hip, wrist, shoulder, and spine. Specific information about these different fractures is detailed in individual chapters.

Recent data suggest that more than 350,000 individuals sustain hip fractures in the United States each year. Hip fracture is a common injury in the elderly, with significant morbidity and mortality, and should be suspected when a fall results in the inability to walk. Surgical treatment is optimal for nearly all hip fractures. Mortality has been shown to increase significantly with a surgical delay of more than 3 calendar days following injury. Following surgery, early mobilization is ideal.

Wrist fractures most often follow a fall on an outstretched hand. Presenting symptoms include pain, swelling, and obvious deformity. Many wrist fractures can be treated by closed reduction and splinting or casting for approximately 6 weeks.

Proximal humerus fractures typically occur following low-energy trauma such as a simple fall. Patients report shoulder pain that becomes worse with motion. Treatment typically is immobilization in a sling or shoulder immobilizer; early motion is encouraged. Occasionally, surgical treatment with open reduction and internal fixation or prosthetic replacement is necessary. While the patients are usually pain-free following fracture union, they are often left with functional limitations.

Vertebral compression fractures in the elderly are nearly synonymous with osteoporosis. These fractures typically occur in the low thoracic and/or upper lumbar region, often after minimal trauma. Though pain and deformity occasionally occur, neurologic injury is rare. Vertebral compression fractures are usually treated by a short period of rest and pain medication, followed by early mobilization and short-term bracing.

## TESTS

Clinical and diagnostic tests depend on the specific conditions.

## ADVERSE OUTCOMES OF THE DISEASE

Elderly patients are susceptible to many medical complications following fracture. Ability to manage without assistance and/or to ambulate may deteriorate despite optimal fracture care and may result in loss of independence.

## TREATMENT

All the intrinsic causes of these injuries are a natural part of aging, but many can be prevented or mitigated by appropriate medical intervention. Pharmacologic treatment of osteoporosis has been shown to prevent or delay decrease in bone density. Medical management of chronic conditions such as diabetes can improve vision. Proper nutrition and exercise throughout life can decrease the incidence of cardiovascular disease. Medications, particularly antihypertensives and sedatives, must be closely monitored to prevent orthostatic hypotension, syncope, and oversedation.

The goal of fracture treatment is to restore the preinjury level of function. Therefore, treatment must be tailored to the patient and the specific injury. The patient's ability to actively participate and comply with a rehabilitation program factors into the treatment decision. Evaluate polypharmacy, vision, balance, and associated medical conditions. Ask a friend or family member of the patient to remove throw rugs or other objects that may cause the patient to trip. Also advise the removal of obstacles from hallways or frequently traveled pathways. Recommend that the patient obtain a prescription for single-vision glasses (without bifocals) for ambulation to the bathroom at night. Emphasize the importance of handrails for the toilet and bathtub and nonslip mats in the bathtub.

The medical condition of elderly patients also impacts on fracture management. Because cardiovascular and pulmonary disease are so common in this population, the risks associated with surgery and general anesthesia are significant. These risks must be considered when deciding on treatment options.

## ADVERSE OUTCOMES OF TREATMENT

Medications must be continuously monitored in elderly patients to avoid polypharmacy, oversedation, and adverse drug interactions. Postoperative complications are common; therefore, frequent, careful monitoring of cerebrovascular, cardiovascular, neurologic, and hematologic function is mandatory.

## REFERRAL DECISIONS/RED FLAGS

Pain with walking may signal a hip problem that requires evaluation. If initial radiographs are inconclusive, then a second series or adjunctive studies such as a bone scan or MRI may be indicated. Osteoporosis affects fracture management. Surgical fixation is more difficult in a patient with osteoporosis because of the difficulties in obtaining stable fixation in weak bone.

SECTION 1 ■ GENERAL ORTHOPAEDICS

# FIBROMYALGIA SYNDROME

**ICD-9 Code**

**729.1**
Myalgia and myositis, unspecified

## DEFINITION

Fibromyalgia syndrome (FMS) is a chronic condition characterized by generalized pain, fatigue, and tender areas in the soft tissues. The joints, however, are spared. Women between the ages of 20 and 60 years are at greatest risk. The cause is unknown, and a cure is not available.

## CLINICAL SYMPTOMS

In 1990, the American College of Rheumatology established the following criteria for the diagnosis of fibromyalgia:

- Widespread pain that has been present for 3 months.
- Pain is considered widespread when all of the following are present: pain in the left side of the body, pain in the right side of the body, pain above the waist, and pain below the waist. In addition, axial skeletal pain must be present (neck, anterior chest, or thoracic or low back). By definition, shoulder and buttock pain is considered as pain for each involved side. Low back pain is considered pain below the waist.
- Pain and tenderness at 11 or more of 18 trigger point sites on digital palpation with an approximate force of 4 kg. For a tender point to be considered positive, the patient must state that the palpation was "painful" in contrast to "tender" (**Figure 1**).

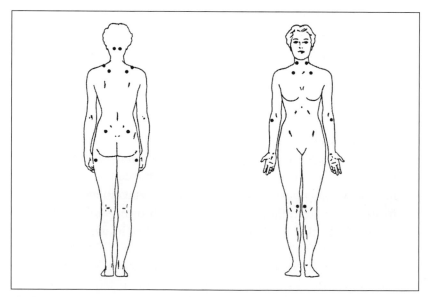

**Figure 1**

Posterior and anterior trigger points.

(Reproduced with permission from the Arthritis Foundation, Atlanta, GA.)

## Posterior Trigger Point Sites

Occiput: Bilateral, at the occipital muscle insertions

Supraspinatus: Bilateral, at origins, above the scapular spine near the medial border

Trapezius: Bilateral, at the midpoint of the upper border

Gluteal: Bilateral, in upper outer quadrants of buttocks in anterior fold of muscle

Greater trochanter: Bilateral, posterior to the trochanteric prominence

## Anterior Trigger Point Sites

Low cervical: Bilateral, at the anterior aspects of the intertransverse spaces at C5-7

Second rib: Bilateral, at the second costochondral junctions, just lateral to the junctions on upper surfaces

Lateral epicondyle: Bilateral, 2 cm distal to the epicondyles

Knee: Bilateral, at the medial fat pad proximal to the joint line

A wide variety of symptoms can accompany FMS. Sleep disturbances and stiffness often are present. Short-term memory loss may be reported. Fatigue, which is worse in the morning and late in the day, is a common complaint. Mood changes include depression and anxiety and often develop concurrently with multiple somatic complaints, such as migraine and tension headaches, substernal chest pain, bursitis and tendinitis, cystitis, irritable bowel syndrome, urinary frequency, and paresthesias in the hands and feet.

# TESTS

## Physical Examination

Examination reveals tenderness to palpation over several of the 18 tender point sites. Sufficient pressure should be applied so that the patient's skin blanches under the examiner's fingers. These tender points are limited to the soft tissues (muscle, tendon, ligament, or bursa); examination of the joints is normal.

## Diagnostic Tests

No radiographs or laboratory tests are diagnostic of FMS.

# DIFFERENTIAL DIAGNOSIS

AIDS (blood test)

Bursitis or tendinitis (usually single joint or extremity)

Complex regional pain syndrome (usually a single extremity)

Hypothyroidism (abnormal thyroid function tests)

Lyme disease (serology test)

Multiple sclerosis (abnormal MRI of the brain)

SECTION 1 ■ GENERAL ORTHOPAEDICS

Polymyalgia rheumatica (elevated erythrocyte sedimentation rate)

Polymyositis (skin rash)

Rheumatoid arthritis (positive rheumatoid factor)

Systemic lupus erythematosus (antinuclear antibodies, elevated erythrocyte sedimentation rate)

Tenosynovitis (single focus, associated with tendon motion)

## ADVERSE OUTCOMES OF THE DISEASE

The chronic pain associated with FMS can result in depression, anxiety, and inactivity. The multiple tests ordered and the multiple clinicians consulted to make the correct diagnosis can be expensive.

## TREATMENT

Patients should be advised that FMS is not a life-threatening or progressive disease. No cure is available, but symptom relief is possible. The optimal treatment program is multifaceted. Tricyclic antidepressants and NSAIDs can be helpful in controlling the pain. Amitriptyline in doses of 10 to 50 mg or cyclobenzaprine in doses of 10 to 40 mg, taken at bedtime, can be useful. Fluoxetine, taken in the morning, is useful to reduce a severe depression. Short-term or intermittent NSAIDs may help diminish pain, but corticosteroids and narcotic analgesics are contraindicated. The nonnarcotic analgesic tramadol taken in divided doses of 50 to 400 mg per day has been shown to help the pain in FMS. Topical agents such as capsaicin cream applied to the tender point areas may be beneficial.

Patients should be instructed in a stretching program to increase flexibility. Exercise programs for FMS should begin slowly and increase gradually to build endurance while minimizing pain. In addition, initiation of an aerobic exercise program to increase cardiac fitness is recommended. Referral to a dietitian for weight loss supervision often is indicated. Many patients will benefit from participation in FMS support groups, which are a useful source of information and encouragement. Many larger medical centers have established FMS clinics, which use a multidisciplinary approach in the treatment of these patients.

## ADVERSE OUTCOMES OF TREATMENT

Patients can become dependent on narcotics and tranquilizers. Medications also have side effects, including drowsiness, dry mouth, change in appetite, and constipation. Tachyphylaxis (decreased response) can develop with long-term use of amitriptyline and/or cyclobenzaprine.

## REFERRAL DECISIONS/RED FLAGS

Severe symptoms that interfere with the patient's ability to work or the presence of serious psychiatric problems indicates the need for evaluation at an FMS treatment center.

# FRACTURE PRINCIPLES

## DEFINITION

A fracture is a disruption in the continuity of bone that occurs as a result of a direct blow to the bone or an indirect force applied to the limb. Most fractures result in gross interruption of the bone matrix. Fractures, however, may occur at a microscopic level, as seen in stress fractures.

## CLINICAL SYMPTOMS

The classic symptoms of acute fractures are swelling, pain that is aggravated by movement, deformity, and decreased function. Nondisplaced fractures may not exhibit any obvious deformity. Stress fractures often present with the indolent onset of mild swelling and tenderness and pain with weight bearing. **Table 1** lists the defining characteristics of specific types of fractures.

## TESTS

### Physical Examination

Examination reveals localized tenderness, swelling, and often deformity. A complete examination should include an evaluation of the surrounding skin integrity, stability of the adjacent joints, and function of the nerves and vessels distal to the site of injury. *Any laceration or abrasion of the skin should be considered an open fracture.* All suspected open fractures require further evaluation for exploration and débridement.

### Diagnostic Tests

Radiographs usually identify an acute fracture. With stress fractures and some nondisplaced fractures, the injury may not be visible on radiographs until bone resorbs from the fracture ends (1 to 4 weeks). Carpal navicular fractures often are missed for this reason. Tomography, CT, and MRI usually are not indicated in the initial assessment of fractures unless the diagnosis cannot be confirmed with routine radiographs or unless further definition of a complex fracture is required before surgical stabilization.

## DIFFERENTIAL DIAGNOSIS

Dislocation (marked deformity, disruption of normal joint alignment on radiographs)

Infection (no history of trauma, fever, elevated erythrocyte sedimentation rate)

Sprain (normal radiographs)

Tumor (gradual onset, bone destruction evident on radiographs)

## Table 1   Fracture Classification

| Location in the bone | Description |
|---|---|
| Epiphyseal | The end of the bone, forming part of the adjacent joint |
| Metaphyseal | The flared portion of the bone at the ends of the shaft |
| Diaphyseal | The shaft of a long bone |

| Orientation/Extent of the fracture line(s) | Description |
|---|---|
| Transverse | A fracture that is perpendicular to the shaft of the bone |
| Oblique | An angulated fracture line |
| Spiral | A multiplanar and complex fracture line |
| Comminuted | More than two fracture fragments |
| Segmental | A completely separate segment of bone bordered by fracture lines |
| Intra-articular | The fracture line crosses the articular cartilage and enters the joint |
| Torus | A buckle fracture of one cortex, often seen in children |
| Compression | Impaction of bone, such as in the vertebrae or proximal tibia |
| Greenstick | An incomplete fracture with angular deformity, seen in children |
| Pathologic | A fracture through bone weakened by disease or tumor |

| Amount of displacement of the fracture fragments | Description |
|---|---|
| Nondisplaced | A fracture in which the fragments are in anatomic alignment |
| Displaced | A fracture in which the fragments are no longer in their usual alignment |
| Angulated | A fracture in which the fragments arc malaligned |
| Bayonetted | A fracture in which the distal fragment longitudinally overlaps the proximal fragment |
| Distracted | A fracture in which the distal fragment is separated from the proximal fragment by a gap |

| Integrity of the skin and soft-tissue envelope around the fracture | Description |
|---|---|
| Closed | The skin over and near the fracture is intact |
| Open | The skin over and near the fracture is lacerated or abraded by the injury. |

## ADVERSE OUTCOMES OF THE DISEASE

Any fracture can exhibit delayed union (slower healing than normal), nonunion (failure to heal by bone), or malunion (healing with unacceptable deformity). Limb function can be adversely affected by nearby joint contractures, stiffness, limb shortening, or malalignment to such a degree that the patient cannot easily compensate using the nearby joints. Osteomyelitis may develop if the fracture is open. In severe fractures, nerve and/or vascular damage may jeopardize the viability or usefulness of the extremity. A compartment syndrome can develop if there is excessive swelling. This complication requires early recognition and emergency treatment. Complex regional pain syndrome can develop but is rare.

## TREATMENT

Treatment is guided by the four Rs: Recognition, Reduction, Retention of reduction while achieving union, and Rehabilitation. The key to recognition is awareness of the subtle injuries that may occur at different anatomic locations. Reduction is not necessary with nondisplaced or minimally displaced injuries. For fractures with significant displacement, however, reduction will be required. Some fractures can be

---

### Table 2 ■ Factors That Influence Fracture Healing

**Factors that increase fracture stability, facilitate treatment, and offer a good prognosis**

Skeletal immaturity—thick periosteum, faster rate of healing, potential for remodeling

Single bone fractures in forearm (radius or ulna) or lower leg (tibia or fibula)

Nondisplaced pelvic fractures

Transverse fractures—tend to be stable when reduced

Presence of adjacent bone for support (eg, finger buddy taped to adjacent finger)

Thoracic spine fractures

**Factors that decrease fracture stability and render fracture more difficult to treat**

Skeletal maturity—thin periosteum and poor potential for remodeling

Both-bone fractures of forearm or lower leg

Comminuted, displaced pelvic fractures

Oblique fractures

Marked displacement (indicates severe soft-tissue stripping)

Unstable cervical and lumbar spine fractures

Comminuted and segmental fractures

Fractures involving a joint

manipulated to an acceptable position by closed techniques, whereas others require open reduction and internal fixation. Retention of reduction may involve a splint, circular cast, or internal fixation device. Rehabilitation is extremely important. Even nondisplaced fractures treated by splinting result in muscle atrophy and adjacent joint stiffness. Many patients can be treated by a gradual increase in activities and simple instructions in range-of-motion and strengthening exercises. **Table 2** lists factors that influence fracture healing

## ADVERSE OUTCOMES OF TREATMENT

Malunion, nonunion, stiffness, arthritis, or vascular or nerve injury is possible. One of the most devastating problems is unrecognized compartment syndrome from the injury or from a cast that is too tight.

## REFERRAL DECISIONS/RED FLAGS

Patients with open, unstable, or irreducible fractures, suspected compartment syndrome, or nerve, vascular, or muscle damage need further evaluation. Most patients who have displaced fractures require further evaluation, as even fractures that appear innocuous may be associated with poor outcomes.

SECTION 1 ■ GENERAL ORTHOPAEDICS

# FRACTURE HEALING

## DEFINITION

Unlike most tissues, which heal with scar formation, bone is capable of complete functional regeneration after injury. Fracture healing involves a complex biologic cascade that is mediated by a variety of bioactive cells and proteins. Although most fractures heal without difficulty, certain fractures have a propensity for either delayed healing or nonunion. Enhancement of fracture healing has evolved significantly over the last decade.

## PRINCIPLES OF FRACTURE HEALING

### Primary Fracture Healing

Primary, or intramembranous, fracture healing can occur only with rigid fixation of a fracture that produces absolute stability at the fracture site, which usually is achievable only with a surgical approach that includes internal fixation by compression plating. With primary fracture healing, no intermediate cartilaginous callus forms. Rather, bone heals directly across the fracture site, and no bridging callus is visible radiographically (**Figure 1**). The presence of significant callus indicates that the construct was unstable, allowing motion at the fracture site.

### Secondary Fracture Healing

Secondary, or enchondral, fracture healing involves the indirect formation of bone from uncommitted mesenchymal cells through the formation and remodeling of an intermediate cartilaginous callus. This type of fracture healing is enhanced by controlled motion at the fracture site, such as occurs in a cast or a functional brace and with some types of surgical fracture fixation. Uncontrolled motion at a fracture site can result in a fibrous nonunion.

Secondary fracture healing comprises three overlapping phases (**Figure 2**). The first (inflammatory) phase is rapid, lasting for approximately 48 hours. During this phase, bioactive proteins and cells migrate into the fracture site. In the second (reparative) stage, bridging callus is formed. The third phase is remodeling, which occurs over a variable time period and is more important in children than in adults.

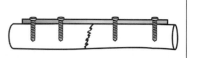

**Figure 1**
Primary fracture healing.
**A,** Diagram of primary fracture healing. **B,** Radiograph showing intramembranous fracture healing following rigid fixation. Note lack of callus.

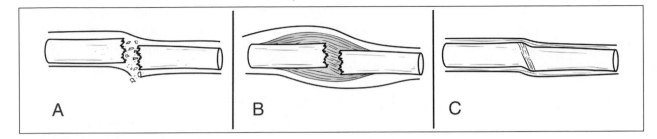

**Figure 2**
Stages of secondary fracture healing. **A,** Inflammatory phase: migration of bioactive cells. **B,** Reparative phase: formation of bridging callus. **C,** Remodeling phase: fracture remodels, often with a faint fracture line visible.

## ADVANTAGES AND DISADVANTAGES OF TYPES OF FRACTURE TREATMENT

Preservation of the biologic environment in treatment of fractures has been found to enhance fracture healing. With surgical treatment using compression plates, the required dissection may threaten the blood supply to the fractured bone. Treating a fracture by closed means, such as casting of a tibia fracture, causes a minimum of disruption to the biologic environment. Indirect reduction by traction or manipulation and percutaneous fixation provides a compromise, conferring stability to the fracture site while preserving the blood supply.

## IMPAIRED FRACTURE HEALING

### Nonunion

The definitions of delayed fracture healing and nonunion are controversial. Traditionally, delayed union has been defined as a fracture that has not healed after 16 to 20 weeks and nonunion as a fracture that has not healed after 9 months. A better criterion for nonunion, however, is absence of radiographic evidence of progression of callus formation over a 3- to 5-month period.

Risk factors for nonunion include smoking, indolent infection, and inadequate immobilization. Smoking results in vasoconstriction and diminished blood supply to the fracture site. In addition, nicotine has been shown to have a direct inhibitory effect on osteoblasts in vitro. Malnutrition also may play a role in nonunion, as may the use of NSAIDs, by interfering with the inflammatory phase of fracture healing. Several fractures intrinsically have a high incidence of nonunion because the regions of bone involved have a threatened or tenuous blood supply. These include femoral neck fractures, fractures of the scaphoid in the wrist, fractures of the talus, and fractures of the odontoid in the cervical spine. **Table 1** lists these possible risk factors for nonunion.

| Table 1   Possible Risk Factors for Nonunion |
| --- |
| Smoking |
| Indolent infection |
| Inadequate immobilization |
| Malnutrition |
| NSAID use |
| Fracture in bone with tenuous blood supply |

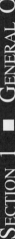

SECTION 1 ■ GENERAL ORTHOPAEDICS

Both surgical and nonsurgical methods are used to enhance bone healing in the presence of the risk of nonunion or after nonunion has occurred. Several of these methods are summarized in **Table 2**.

# SURGICAL TREATMENT

Various substances have been used in the surgical treatment of bone defects and to enhance fracture healing. These modalities have different properties. An osteogenic (bone-forming) substance contains cells that have osteogenic properties. Only autogenous bone graft (bone taken from the patient) can be said to be truly osteogenic. An osteoinductive substance enhances osteogenesis by inducing the differentiation of mesenchymal cells into bone-forming cells. An osteoconductive substance provides structural stability to the defect and provides a microscopic scaffold on which bone-forming cells can build.

Autogenous bone graft is the most common substance used surgically to stimulate bone formation. It is osteogenic, osteoinductive, and osteoconductive. Autogenous bone graft is limited in quantity, however, and harvesting autogenous bone graft creates significant morbidity. Iliac crest autograft using cancellous bone (the spongy portion of the bone) has been considered the gold standard when evaluating the efficacy of other substances intended to enhance fracture healing. Bone marrow injected into fracture sites is a type of autogenous bone graft and is osteogenic and osteoinductive.

## Table 2   Enhancers of Bone Healing

| Methods | Indications | Advantages | Disadvantages |
|---|---|---|---|
| **Surgical** | | | |
| Autogenous bone | Smaller bone defects | Most effective, biologically compatible | Limited availability, harvesting causes morbidity |
| Allographic bone | Large bone defects, tumor reconstruction | Allows reconstruction of large defects | High infection rate |
| Synthetic bone substitutes | Large bone defects | Unlimited supply | Fracture must be stabilized |
| Bioactive cells and proteins | Refractory nonunions | Accelerate bone and wound healing, decrease infection | Expensive |
| **Nonsurgical** | | | |
| Electrical stimulation | Nonunions | Noninvasive | Expensive |
| Ultrasound | Nonunions, acceleration of healing of acute fractures | Noninvasive | Expensive |

Allographic bone substitutes (cadaver bone) have become safer and are being used more commonly as improved processing techniques have minimized the risk of viral and bacterial transmission during transplantation. Demineralized bone matrix is a type of allograft in which cadaver bone is processed and bone morphogenic proteins are extracted. Bulk allografts are used primarily in tumor reconstruction. They have a significant infection rate because they involve large, relatively avascular implants and because many of the patients who receive these grafts are immunosuppressed.

Synthetic bone substitutes have been used increasingly for significant bony defects. The most commonly used bone substitutes are ceramics, such as calcium phosphate; purified sea coral; and various hydroxyapatites, which comprise the matrix of bone. These synthetic bone substitutes have varying osteoinductive potential and can be used only in fractures that have been stabilized, usually surgically.

Other substances have been used to enhance bone formation. Platelet growth factor, obtained from centrifuged blood, has been used to accelerate fracture healing. Recently, certain recombinant bone morphogenic proteins have been shown to not only accelerate bone healing but also to improve wound healing and decrease infection in open fractures.

# NONSURGICAL TREATMENT

It has long been known that an electrical potential exists in bone, especially at a fracture site. Electrical stimulation, either by external application or implanted electrodes, has been shown by well-devised prospective studies to aid in the healing of nonunions. Low-intensity ultrasound external stimulation has also been successful in treating nonunions, as has been high-intensity ultrasound stimulation administered in a single setting, usually with anesthesia. Because of its potential to accelerate healing, low-intensity ultrasound also has been approved for acute fracture care.

SECTION 1 ■ GENERAL ORTHOPAEDICS

# IMAGING PRINCIPLES AND TECHNIQUES

Imaging studies are expensive and time consuming and may be painful for the patient. The simplest studies should be ordered and interpreted before more specialized studies are considered. MRI, CT, and other specialized studies are rarely needed in the initial evaluation. *Essentials of Musculoskeletal Imaging*, another volume in this series, describes appropriate imaging studies for more than 300 musculoskeletal conditions.

## RADIOGRAPHY

Plain radiographs are the mainstay of bone and joint imaging (**Table 1**). Radiographic examination of a long bone for fracture should meet the following criteria:

- Any radiograph of a long bone should include the joints above and below to avoid missing a dislocation associated with a fracture.
- Images should be obtained in at least two planes perpendicular to each other (eg, AP and lateral). Standard positioning should be used because radiographs of a joint may be confusing if the extremity is in a nonstandard position. In children, the presence of open physes (growth plates) may make it difficult to determine if a fracture is present. In these instances, obtaining views of the asymptomatic limb may help.

### Indications

Deformity of a bone or joint, inability to use the extremity or a joint, or unexplained pain and localized tenderness in a bone or joint indicates the need for radiographic examination. Children and women of child-bearing age should be protected with lead shields whenever possible.

## MAGNETIC RESONANCE IMAGING

MRI offers the advantage of seeing soft-tissue detail (muscle, ligaments, tendons, menisci, disks, etc) and often identifies the extent of tumors. MRI is an excellent technique for imaging the spine, joints, and soft tissues.

### Indications

MRI often is very valuable in preoperative planning, especially in certain soft-tissue conditions, tumors, or chronic osteomyelitis; however, the underlying diagnosis usually can be made by less expensive means. MRI also is valuable in situations of diagnostic dilemma. Patients whose conditions are associated with issues of liability, such as personal injury or workers' compensation claims, can require MRI to determine

## Table 1   Standard Radiographic Views

| Region | Views | Special Considerations |
|---|---|---|
| Hand | PA, lateral, and oblique | |
| Wrist | PA and lateral | |
| Elbow/forearm | AP and lateral | Comparison views may be helpful (opposite elbow) |
| Shoulder | AP of shoulder, AP of glenohumeral joint, axillary | Transscapular lateral view if unable to obtain axillary view |
| Cervical spine | AP and lateral | Include from C1 through C7 in the lateral view; swimmer's view may help visualize C7 |
| Thoracic | AP and lateral | Swimmer's view may help visualize C7-T5 |
| Lumbar spine | AP and lateral | Spot lateral of L5 if not seen well on standard lateral; try to see from T12-sacrum |
| Pelvis | AP | |
| Hip | AP and groin lateral or true lateral | |
| Knee | Weight-bearing AP in full extension and 30° flexion in patients older than 40 years; otherwise, standard AP, lateral, and bilateral axial (Merchant) views | |
| Ankle | AP, lateral, and mortise | |
| Foot | Weight-bearing AP and lateral, supine oblique (45°) | |

the anatomic extent of injury or disease for purposes of claim settlement. Claustrophobic patients can generally be accommodated by the use of open MRI units.

## COMPUTED TOMOGRAPHY

CT offers axial visualization of bone, muscle, and fat tissues. Bone visualization is usually excellent and soft-tissue structures less so.

### Indications

CT is helpful in preoperative planning for bony procedures to help localize lesions and appreciate the scope of bony changes. Complex or extensive fracture patterns, especially those with joint involvement, also are best visualized with CT. This imaging technique often is used with myelography in patients who have degenerative spine disease.

# ARTHROGRAPHY

Arthrography is an invasive but less expensive technique than CT or MRI in which a contrast medium is injected into the joint to evaluate the joint capsule and articular surface integrity. At times, arthrography is combined with CT or MRI. Arthrography is associated with a risk of infection and allergic reaction to the contrast material.

## *Indications*

Rotator cuff tears, interosseous ligament tears at the wrist, and meniscal tears are conditions well evaluated by arthrography; however, MRI often provides superior imaging of these conditions.

# BONE SCAN

Bone scan, or scintigraphy, is a radioisotope technique that shows blood flow and metabolic activity in the bone, thereby indicating bone formation or destruction.

## *Indications*

A bone scan is useful for identifying infection, tumor, and fractures.

# LYME DISEASE

## DEFINITION

Lyme disease is a multisystem illness with acute and chronic manifestations caused by the spirochete *Borrelia burgdorferi* that is borne by the deer tick *Ixodes dammini*. Lyme disease is named after a town in Connecticut where, in 1975, several children developed a mysterious arthritis of unknown cause that was subsequently found to be caused by this spirochete. Lyme disease is the most prevalent vector-borne illness in the United States, with nearly 50,000 cases reported since 1982. The incidence is highest in the Northeast (Maryland to northern Massachusetts), the upper Midwest (Wisconsin and Minnesota), and the far West (northern California and Oregon). Lyme disease has been reported in 48 states, as well as in Asia and Europe.

## CLINICAL SYMPTOMS

Patients with Lyme disease initially have variable constitutional and flulike symptoms. In adults, these symptoms are commonly accompanied by a distinctive skin lesion (erythema migrans) originating and expanding from the site of the tick bite (**Figure 1**). A subacute or intermediate stage of Lyme disease can follow the acute episode and is characterized by arthralgia and arthritis in up to 80% of untreated patients. The knee is most commonly affected. Multiple joint involvement is rare. Cardiovascular involvement occurs in 4% to 8% of patients at this stage, and neurologic symptoms develop in 15% of patients. Half of these neurologic complications are either Bell palsy or other types of cranial nerve paralysis. Dermatologic and ocular symptoms also may occur in the intermediate phase. The chronic stage of Lyme disease often does not appear for several months or even years after the initial episode and is characterized by chronic arthritis and recurrent arthralgias. Other symptoms include chronic fatigue, polyradiculopathy, and encephalopathy with loss of memory and inability to concentrate.

## TESTS

### *Physical Examination*
Patients with arthralgia should be examined for synovitis and restricted joint motion.

**ICD-9 Code**
088.81
Lyme disease

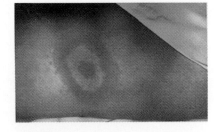

**Figure 1**
Appearance of lesion following bite by tick infected with Lyme disease.

Reproduced from Browner BD, Pollak AN, Gupton CL (eds): *American Academy of Orthopaedic Surgeons Emergency Care and Transportation of the Sick and Injured*, ed 8. Boston, MA, Jones and Bartlett, 2002, p 427.

## *Diagnostic Tests*

Lyme disease is a clinical diagnosis, but serologic testing for *Borrelia* titer is important, particularly in the later stages of the disease.

# DIFFERENTIAL DIAGNOSIS

Acute rheumatic fever

Idiopathic Bell palsy (physical examination)

Meningitis (lumbar puncture)

Multiple sclerosis (abnormal MRI of the brain)

Peripheral neuritis (specific nerve involvement)

Reiter syndrome (iritis, urethritis)

# ADVERSE OUTCOMES OF THE DISEASE

Lyme disease can be complicated by arthritis in major weight-bearing joints, facial paralysis, chronic fatigue, concentration defects, cardiac conduction block, and peripheral neuritis.

# TREATMENT

When diagnosed early, Lyme disease is effectively treated with antibiotics. Doxycycline 100 mg twice a day for 10 to 30 days or amoxicillin 500 mg three times a day for 10 to 30 days has been shown to be effective. For children younger than age 8 years, amoxicillin 20 mg/kg in divided doses is indicated.

People in high-risk areas should avoid or minimize walking in the woods. Those living in heavily wooded areas should wear long-sleeved shirts tucked into trousers with the trouser legs tucked into socks. Most importantly, the skin and clothing should be checked for ticks. If the tick is removed within 24 to 36 hours, the risk of Lyme disease is minimal. Tick removal is best done by carefully teasing with fine tweezers. Heat and chemicals should not be used on the tick as these can cause the tick to burst or regurgitate and expel fluid onto the skin.

# ADVERSE OUTCOMES OF TREATMENT

Allergic reactions or adverse drug interactions to antibiotics can occur.

# REFERRAL DECISIONS/RED FLAGS

Patients with suspected Lyme disease may require evaluation by an infectious disease specialist.

# NONORGANIC SYMPTOMS AND SIGNS

## SYNONYMS
Psychosomatic illness
Functional overlay

**ICD-9 Code**

**ICD-9**
lists psychophysiologic disorders
according to body system.

## DEFINITION
Patient responses or symptoms that do not fit known patterns of illnesses or injury are considered nonorganic. These findings are not considered malingering; rather, they often are the way that some patients communicate their perception of the seriousness of their problem or their perception that they are not receiving the care they think they need. True malingering is rare and typically is a manifestation of bizarre social behavior.

Nonorganic findings should not be construed as indicating lack of concomitant disease because significant underlying pathology can be present. Nonorganic findings occur three to four times more often in situations where workers' compensation and litigation are issues than in situations where they are not.

## CLINICAL SYMPTOMS
Pain or symptoms that appear to "travel" from one side or area of the body to another in a nonanatomic fashion and global pain are characteristic. Nonsegmental numbness (ie, numbness that does not fit a nerve root or peripheral nerve pattern) also occurs.

## TESTS

### Physical Examination
Exaggerated responses: Light touch causes a jerk or withdrawal. Other findings include grimacing, groaning, and grabbing the affected extremity during examination when there is no obvious trauma or medical problem.

Axial loading (low back pain): With the patient standing, place both hands on the head and push down, asking if it causes pain. Low back pain elicited in this position is a nonorganic finding; however, neck pain may be a legitimate finding.

Axial rotation (spine): With the patient's hands on the iliac crests, grasp and rotate the pelvis, asking the patient if this causes back pain. This maneuver should not elicit back pain, since the motion occurs at the hips, not in the back. Because

SECTION 1 ■ GENERAL ORTHOPAEDICS

this test may be positive in 20% of patients, it is not as sensitive in identifying nonorganic behavior as are exaggerated responses and axial loading.

Flip sign: This sign is elicited with the patient seated and leaning slightly forward, with his or her hands on the edge of the examination table. While asking if the patient has knee problems, lift the foot and extend the knee. This maneuver increases tension on the sciatic nerve, and patients with lower lumbar herniated disks or other similar conditions will involuntarily "flip" back against the wall, reporting back and leg pain. A negative flip sign in the presence of a supine straight-leg raising test that produces leg and back pain at less than 45° of leg elevation is a significant nonorganic finding, as these maneuvers are the same test.

Distraction: A provocative test (such as palpation) may be negative when the patient is distracted with conversation, but positive when attention is drawn to the test or body part.

Giving way: During muscle testing, a nonorganic finding is a lack of sustained effort. Typically, the patient "gives way" or "lets go" in a ratchety, uneven pattern. Another variant is the patient who gives a poor effort on muscle testing and then, with coaxing, may intermittently contract the muscle, then let go.

Stocking or nonanatomic numbness: Some patients report hypoesthesia that affects the extremity in a circumferential (stocking-glove) distribution or covers nonanatomic patterns. Patients with diabetes mellitus or multiple sclerosis may develop sensory abnormalities in a stocking-glove or nonsegmental pattern.

Pain diagram: On a diagram of the body, ask the patient to draw representations of symptoms, using dashes, slashes, Xs, etc. Bizarre drawings do not indicate malingering or mental disease. Many people have perceptual disorders that blunt the scientific validity of these drawings, but they often yield insight into how pain is perceived by patients, and what areas of the body they believe are related in their current problem (**Figure 1**).

The kneeling bench test of Burns: This is another test of exaggerated response. Ask a patient who reports back pain to kneel on a stool. Hold the patient's ankles to ensure confidence and ask the patient to bend forward and touch the floor. Patients who are exaggerating symptoms will bend forward a few degrees and then grab their back, saying they cannot bend. Note that these patients are already bending forward significantly.

A thorough neurologic examination is required to give the above tests perspective and to rule out concomitant disease.

## Diagnostic Tests
None

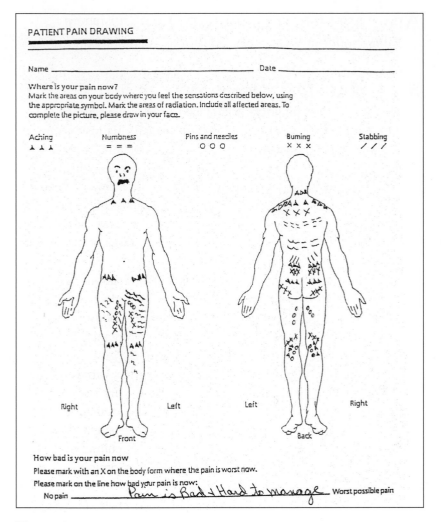

**Figure 1**
Pain diagram for patient with nonorganic physical findings.

# DIFFERENTIAL DIAGNOSIS

Acute injury (withdrawal from a painful examination maneuver may be an appropriate response)

Diabetes mellitus (stocking-type peripheral neuropathy)

Multiple sclerosis (bizarre sensory patterns that are not segmental)

Stroke or other central lesions with altered sensory appreciation

# TREATMENT

Rule out serious disorders that may be masked by these symptoms and discuss the absence of specific disorders with the patient. Because patients with this condition often are indirectly indicating that they are not getting the support or help they need, discuss psychological and social support interventions and inquire about contributing factors such as occupational stress and marital difficulties.

## Adverse Outcomes of Treatment

Failure to identify an associated serious condition is possible.

## Referral Decisions/Red Flags

True diminished pinprick, diminished light touch with or without areflexia, clonus, or spasticity usually indicates neurologic involvement.

Section 1 ■ General Orthopaedics

# Nonsteroidal Anti-Inflammatory Drugs

## Definition

Nonsteroidal anti-inflammatory drugs (NSAIDs) are a group of drugs used to treat inflammatory conditions such as arthritis, bursitis, and tendinitis. Aspirin is a nonsteroidal anti-inflammatory drug, but the term NSAID usually is reserved for the newer aspirin-like agents that were developed to decrease the severity of gastritis associated with long-term use of aspirin.

Inflammation is an essential, normal protective mechanism associated with injury to the musculoskeletal system, but in addition to trauma, inflammation may also be triggered by infection, allergy, or an autoimmune response, as in rheumatoid arthritis. The inflammatory response is mediated by chemicals, such as prostaglandins, which are released from mast cells, granulocytes, and basophils. NSAIDs block prostaglandin by interfering with the action of the enzyme cyclooxygenase (COX). Corticosteroids also block the formation of prostaglandins but do so at a different step in the production chain.

In addition to their anti-inflammatory properties, all NSAIDs exhibit analgesic and antipyretic activity. These drugs also decrease platelet adhesiveness and may inhibit the production of prothrombin.

NSAIDs vary in chemical structure, cost, frequency of side effects, and duration of action (**Table 1**). Effective use of these drugs often requires some experimentation because patients may respond to certain NSAIDs but not to others, and an initial good response may wane with time. Switching to another class of NSAIDs as opposed to switching within the class is likely to be more effective, and for this reason, Table 1 is organized by class.

Two forms of COX have been identified. COX-1 is expressed in many tissues, but COX-2 is an enzyme that primarily mediates the inflammatory response. Most NSAIDs inhibit COX-1 and COX-2 production, thereby affecting gastric mucosa, renal blood flow, and platelet aggregation as well as inflammation. Recently developed COX-2 inhibitors selectively affect COX-2 enzymes and, therefore, are less likely to cause gastric ulcers and bleeding. Renal and hepatic complications have been reported in patients taking COX-2 inhibitors. COX-2 inhibitors also have been associated with an increased risk of stroke and myocardial infarction and should be used with great caution in a susceptible patient population.

## Table 1   Types of NSAIDs

| Drug | Strength (mg) | Trade Name | Typical Dosage |
|------|---------------|------------|----------------|
| *Salicylates* | | | |
| Aspirin | 300, 325, 600, 650 | Several | 325 mg qid |
| Choline magnesium trisalicylate | 500, 750, 1000 | Trilisate | 1,500 mg bid |
| Salsalate | 500, 750 | Disalcid | 1,000 mg tid, 1,500 mg bid |
| Diflunisal | 500 | Dolobid | 250 mg bid or tid, 500 mg bid |
| *Propionic acids* | | | |
| Naproxen sodium | 220 | Aleve | 220 mg bid |
| | 375, 500 | Naprelan 375, 500 | 750-1,000 mg/day |
| | 275, DS 550 | Anaprox | 275 mg bid or tid |
| | | | 550 mg bid |
| Naproxen | 250, 375, 500 | Naprosyn | 250, 375, or 500 mg bid |
| Naproxen EC | 375, 500 | EC Naprosyn | 375 or 500 mg/day |
| Flurbiprofen | 50, 100 | Ansaid | 100 mg bid |
| Oxaprozin | 600 | Daypro | 600-1,200 mg/day |
| Ibuprofen | 400, 600, 800 | Motrin | 400-800 mg bid or tid |
| Ibuprofen (OTC) | 200 | Motrin IB, Advil, Rufin, Nuprin | 200-400 mg bid or tid |
| Ketoprofen | 25, 50, 75 | Orudis | 50 mg qid, 75 mg tid |
| Ketoprofen extended release | 100, 150, 200 | Oruvail | 200 mg/day |
| Ketorolac tromethamine | 10 | Toradol Oral | 10 mg qid; 5 days max of oral and IM combined |
| *Indolacetic acids and related compounds* | | | |
| Sulindac | 150, 200 | Clinoril | 150-200 mg bid |
| Indomethacin | 25, 50 | Indocin | 25-50 mg tid |
| Indomethacin sustained release | 75 | Indocin SR | 75 mg/day |
| Etodolac | 200-500 | Lodine | 200-400 mg tid, 500 mg bid |

## Side Effects

NSAIDs cause similar side effects, but in varying degrees. Minor dyspepsia is common, even with COX-2 drugs. Gastric ulcers and bleeding are less common but more serious. In patients older than 65 years, approximately 30% of hospitalizations and deaths from gastrointestinal hemorrhage are secondary to NSAID treatment.

Reversible hepatotoxicity is observed with some NSAIDs in 10% to 15% of patients with long-term usage. Nephrotoxicity is less common but can develop early in treatment and results from loss of the vasodilatory effects of renal prostaglandins. Fluid retention can increase blood pressure in susceptible patients. The inhibition of prostaglandin synthesis also can be responsible for hives and acute episodes of asthma in some patients.

## Choice of Therapeutic Agents

Cost, side effects, the dosage schedule, and physician familiarity are all factors to consider. Once or twice daily dosage schedules are optimal for patients with poor compliance. Although long-term use in patients with rheumatoid arthritis or osteoarthritis is standard practice, short-term use for most other conditions is encouraged. For osteoarthritis that has a minimal inflammatory component, the use of acetaminophen for primary management with intermittent use of NSAIDs for breakthrough pain can help reduce gastric complications.

In general, all NSAIDs should be taken with food to decrease gastric irritation. Oral hypoglycemic agents or warfarin sodium may be unfavorably potentiated by some NSAIDs in some patients. Full-dose aspirin or other NSAIDs should not be taken at the same time as another NSAID; however, low-dose aspirin often is used with other NSAID medications in patients with cardiac disease. NSAIDs should be used with caution in patients with hypertension; indomethacin is particularly hazardous in elderly patients.

Patients who are at risk for gastric complications can choose from the following alternatives, in addition to those described previously:

- A nonacetylated NSAID such as salsalate (Disalcid) appears to cause less mucosal injury.
- NSAIDs that are nonacidic (such as nabumetone)
- Prodrugs (drugs that must undergo biotransformation to an active metabolite) are reported to decrease gastric injury.
- NSAIDs of the pyranocarboxylic acid class, such as etodolac (Lodine), are appropriate in high-risk patients.

- COX-2 inhibitors should cause the lowest incidence of gastritis but are more expensive than generic NSAIDs that inhibit both COX-1 and COX-2. In light of recent findings of increased risk of cardiovascular events and stroke associated with COX-2 inhibitors, caution must be exercised when prescribing these anti-inflammatories.

# OSTEOARTHRITIS

## SYNONYMS

Degenerative joint disease
Osteoarthrosis
Wear and tear arthritis

## DEFINITION

Osteoarthritis (OA), or perhaps more appropriately osteoarthrosis, is a progressive, currently irreversible condition involving loss of articular cartilage that leads to pain and sometimes deformity, principally in the weight-bearing joints of the lower extremities and the spine. It is the most common type of arthritis and is most often associated with age, obesity, and previous trauma or other disorders that change the mechanics of the joint.

## CLINICAL SYMPTOMS

The common symptoms are stiffness, pain, and deformity. Even when there is a joint effusion, patients more commonly report stiffness rather than swelling. Until the later stages of the disease, the pain of OA usually is relieved by rest. Osteophytes (spurs) may physically block joint motion in advanced disease.

## TESTS

### Physical Examination

Osteophytes are often palpable at the joint margins in the knee, ankle, elbow, hand, foot, and digits (**Figure 1**). An effusion

SECTION 1 ■ GENERAL ORTHOPAEDICS

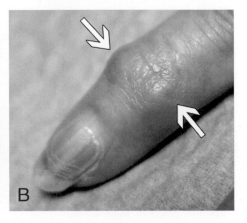

**Figure 1**
**A,** Photograph of hands of patient with OA. Note the prominences at the distal interphalangeal joint of the fingers, caused by osteophytes. These are called Heberden's nodes and are characteristic of OA of the hands.
**B,** Close-up of little finger with Heberden's nodes (arrows).

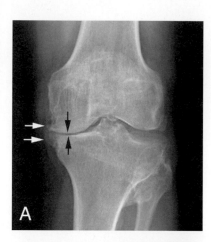
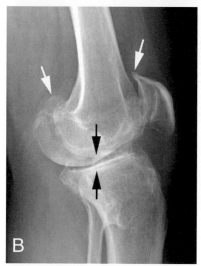

**Figure 2**

**A,** AP view of the knee shows joint space narrowing in the medial compartment (black arrows) and osteophyte formation (white arrows), characteristic of OA. **B,** Lateral view of a knee with OA shows joint space narrowing (black arrows) and osteophyte formation in the posterior femur and off the superior aspect of the patella (white arrows).

Reproduced from Johnson TR, Steinbach LS (eds): *Essentials of Musculoskeletal Imaging.* Rosemont, IL, American Academy of Orthopaedic Surgeons, 2004, p 531.

sometimes is present but is typically mild. Range of motion is decreased. The loss of motion usually is mild unless the disease is severe. Genu varum (bowleg) or genu valgum (knock-knee) are common findings. With OA of the hip, the patient often walks "toes out" with the limb externally rotated and tilts or lurches to the affected side with each step.

### Diagnostic Tests

Radiographs of the affected joint usually demonstrate loss of joint space, sclerosis, subchondral cysts, and/or osteophytosis or spurs at the joint margin (**Figures 2** and **3**).

## DIFFERENTIAL DIAGNOSIS

Charcot joint (primarily foot and ankle, diabetic neuropathy)

Chondrocalcinosis (crystals in joint aspirate)

Degenerative changes secondary to inflammatory arthritis (positive rheumatoid factor)

Epiphyseal dysplasia (short stature)

Hemochromatosis (abnormal liver function studies)

Hemophilia (bleeding tendency)

## ADVERSE OUTCOMES OF THE DISEASE

Pain, deformity, loss of joint motion, loss of limb function, and joint instability are possible.

## TREATMENT

Continued reassurance, patient education, and avoiding activities that cause intense torsional and impact loading of joints are critical. Simply telephoning patients periodically can often help them cope with this irreversible disorder. Gentle, regular joint exercises help maintain function and manage pain. Water exercise, bicycling, and non–weight-bearing exercises can help to reduce symptoms and preserve muscle support in the affected joints. Isometric exercises help improve strength if patients are unable to tolerate exercises involving joint motion.

Weight loss is important, especially for the joints of the lower extremity, not only to reduce symptoms but also to improve the survival of joint implants, placed when symptoms are intolerable. Shock-absorbing heel inserts can help decrease weight-bearing stress to the joints of the lower extremities. Braces may also be helpful occasionally.

Acetaminophen, propoxyphene, or salicylates and nonsteroidal anti-inflammatory drugs (NSAIDs) can be used for pain management, as may locally applied analgesic creams or ice. Glucosamine and chondroitin sulfate are other popular options for pain management. (See Complementary and

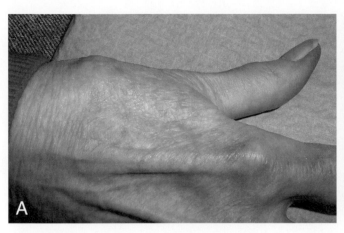
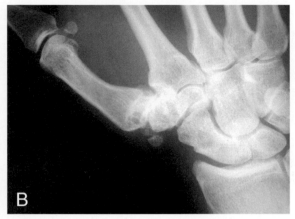

**Figure 3**

OA of the CMC joint at the base of the thumb. **A,** Clinical photograph. Note the bony prominence at the location of the osteophyte. **B,** Radiograph demonstrates sclerosis (dense bone), joint space narrowing, osteophytic spur, and cystic changes.

Alternative Therapies for Osteoarthritis, pp 87-92, for further discussion of these options.) Many elderly patients are better able to cope with symptoms if they can manage their pain. Simple medications may allow them to postpone or avoid surgery and its associated risks.

Intra-articular corticosteroids often relieve symptoms, but the duration of relief may be short (1 to 2 weeks) in the lower extremities, the shoulder, or the elbow. In the hand, intra-articular steroids may relieve symptoms for months. No more than two injections should be given in any weight-bearing joint. Viscosupplement injections are useful for OA at the knee (see Complementary and Alternative Therapies for Osteoarthritis, pp 87-92).

Surgery, typically joint replacement or arthrodesis, is appropriate when patients have pain at rest, pain at night, or unacceptable loss of joint function. Hip, knee, ankle, and shoulder replacement surgery is especially effective in reducing pain and increasing function.

## ADVERSE OUTCOMES OF TREATMENT

Salicylates and NSAIDs often help but can cause renal, hepatic, or gastric problems. In addition, NSAIDs may inhibit joint repair by interfering with prostaglandin synthesis. This is currently only a theoretic consideration.

Removal of prosthetic implants due to infection or loosening is possible. Patients who have an earlier, preemptive procedure, such as an arthroscopic joint débridement or osteotomy, may ultimately require a second operation (ie, joint replacement).

# REFERRAL DECISIONS/RED FLAGS

Patients who have pain at rest, pain at night, a rapid onset of disabling pain, or unacceptable loss of joint function need further evaluation.

# COMPLEMENTARY AND ALTERNATIVE THERAPIES FOR OSTEOARTHRITIS

Osteoarthritis (OA) is the most common form of arthritis and is a leading cause of disability in adults. NSAIDs are commonly used to alleviate the symptoms of OA, but these medications can have significant side effects. For this and other reasons, the field of complementary and alternative medicine (CAM) has grown exponentially, especially as it relates to OA. A telephone survey in 1997 found that more than 40% of Americans used some form of CAM, accounting for 629 million visits to CAM providers and far exceeding the 386 million visits to primary care physicians that same year. This chapter reviews just a few of the complementary and alternative practices sought out by patients for the treatment of OA.

## CAM PROVIDERS

Certification and/or licensing is available in specific CAM specialties (**Table 1**). The amount of training required for licensing or certification varies from hundreds of hours to several years.

## CHIROPRACTIC CARE

Chiropractic care is the most widely used CAM modality in the United States, used by more than 50 million Americans per

### Table 1   Complementary and Alternative Medicine Providers

| | |
|---|---|
| Acupuncturist | The acupuncturist inserts fine needles at points along the body's meridians to correct the flow of life energy, or "chi," to restore health and relieve pain. |
| Ayurvedic practitioner | Ayurveda focuses on wellness and healthy living through diet, exercise, moderation, and meditation; practitioners advise patients on practices to restore mental, physical, and spiritual well-being. |
| Chiropractor | Chiropractic is based on the theory that misalignment of vertebrae is the cause of most neuromuscular and related functional diseases and disorders. Chiropractors use spinal manipulation to restore proper vertebral alignment. |
| Chinese herbalist | Herbalists prepare various formulations of herbs in an attempt to restore balance to the body. |
| Homeopath | Homeopathy is based on the theory that "like cures like." Homeopaths administer minuscule amounts of natural substances such as herbs, minerals, and animal products in serially diluted preparations in an attempt to induce the patient's body to heal itself. |
| Massage therapist | Massage uses manual touch to improve health and well-being. |
| Naturopath | Naturopathy encourages healthy living habits, especially proper nutrition, and allowing the body to heal itself. Naturopaths often work closely with physicians and other health providers. |

year. The most common use of chiropractic care is for back pain and arthritis, but chiropractors often also treat extremity pain, including pain symptomatic of OA. The main focus of chiropractic treatment is manipulation, or "adjustment," aimed at realigning spinal segments. Chiropractic treatment may be beneficial in shortening the duration of acute back pain, but caution must be exercised in applying manipulative therapy to patients with OA and osteoporosis because of the risk of fracture.

## ACUPUNCTURE

Acupuncture is an ancient Chinese practice consisting of the placement of needles in specific acupuncture points on the body to promote the flow of "chi," or body energy, in pathways throughout the body called meridians. Acupuncture has been used for a variety of purposes, including weight loss and the cessation of smoking, as well as decreasing pain and swelling such as associated with OA. Several studies have shown that acupuncture can ease the pain of arthritis, back pain, and fibromyalgia.

## QI XIONG AND TAI CHI

Qi xiong and tai chi have recently gained popularity for increasing the activity level and enhancing the feeling of well-being of elderly patients. These ancient Chinese practices are based on meditation and gentle movements based on the movements of animals in nature. These practices have been credited with decreasing the rate of falls and hip fractures, increasing circulation, and improving mobility in the elderly.

## MAGNET THERAPY

Relatively inexpensive and easy to use, magnets have become a $1.5 billion a year business. They have been used to minimize pain and swelling associated with OA. It is said that Cleopatra slept with a magnet to prevent aging. Magnets often come with wraps or bandages to hold them in place. Little scientific evidence supports the claims that magnets alleviate arthritis symptoms, although anecdotal evidence abounds.

## NUTRITIONAL SUPPLEMENTS

In the United States, more than one third of the population use nutritional supplements for health purposes, spending more than $3.5 billion annually. Unfortunately, the content of these supplements is poorly regulated, and potential interactions of these supplements with prescribed medications are not well publicized. Also, many supplements are contraindicated in the presence of certain medical conditions. Some studies have shown nutritional supplements to be beneficial, but the physician should exercise caution when recommending any supplement. **Table 2** lists commonly used herbal supplements and the potential hazards they pose.

## Glucosamine and Chondroitin

Articular cartilage is composed of chondrocytes, water, collagen, and proteoglycans. OA is associated with a breakdown of the proteoglycans, resulting in increased water permeability and deterioration of cartilage. Glycosaminoglycans are an important component of proteoglycans.

Glucosamine is hexosamine sugar and a building block for glycosaminoglycans. The nutritional supplement is extracted from cow tracheas and is sold in either a sulfate or hydrochoride form. Chondroitin sulfate is a glycosaminoglycan that is found in proteoglycans. The nutritional supplement is usually derived from shellfish. Glucosamine and chondroitin are often sold in combination as over-the-counter supplements, with recommended dosages of 1,500 mg/day and 1,200 mg/day, respectively. Only mild side effects such as dyspepsia have been reported in humans, but glucosamine has been shown to increase blood glucose levels in laboratory animals, and there is some concern that chondroitin may increase clotting times in patients taking anticoagulants. Both substances, either alone or in combination, are proposed to have an articular cartilage protective function. At the time of the publication of this book, the National Institutes of Health had initiated a double-blinded, randomized controlled trial of glucosamine and chondroitin sulfate in patients with OA of the knee. Until the results of that study are known, patients should be advised that these compounds appear to be safe and may be effective in treating OA, but that there is little scientific proof of their benefits.

## S-Adenosyl-L-Methionine (SAMe)

SAMe is available as an over-the-counter dietary supplement used to treat OA and depression. The usual dosage is 200 to 400 mg three times a day. SAMe is synthesized in the body from the essential amino acid methionine. SAMe is theorized to augment cartilage formation by forming sulfur compounds. Some clinical studies have shown SAMe to be as effective as NSAIDs in relieving pain and to have fewer side effects, but more evidence is needed to prove whether it promotes cartilage repair.

**Table 2  CAM Herb/Drug Interactions***

| Herbal Supplement | Common Uses | Potential Problems | Potential Interactions With |
|---|---|---|---|
| Dong Quai (*Angelica*) | To treat menopausal symptoms, PMS, dysmenorrhea | Enhances bleeding | Anticoagulants |
| Echinacea | To treat colds, flu, and mild infections, especially upper respiratory infections | Hepatotoxicity; Intestinal upset | Other hepatotoxic drugs; Anabolic steroids; Methotrexate |
| Ephedra (*Ma Huang, Ephedrine, Pseudo-ephedrine*) | To treat asthma, cough, and to induce weight loss | Seizures; Adverse cardiovascular events, hypertension | Cardiac glycosides; General anesthesia; MAO inhibitors; Decongestants, stimulants |
| Garlic | To decrease cholesterol and blood clot formation | Enhances bleeding | Anticoagulants |
| Ginger | To relieve nausea | Enhances bleeding; CNS depression; Hypotension; Cardiac Arrhythmia; Hypoglycemia | Anticoagulants; Enhances the effects of barbiturates; Antihypertensives; Cardiac drugs; Hypoglycemic drugs |
| Ginkgo Biloba | To improve circulation, especially to brain; For memory loss, dizziness, and headache | Enhances bleeding; Cramps, muscle spasms | Anticoagulants |
| Ginseng | To increase energy and reduce stress | Enhances bleeding; Tachycardia and hypertension; Mania | Anticoagulants; Stimulants; Antihypertensives; Antidepressants/Phenelzine; Digoxin; Potentiates the effects of corticosteroids and estrogens |
| Goldenseal | Used as a mild antibiotic to treat sore throats and upper respiratory infections | Increases fluid retention; Hypertension; Nausea; Nervousness | Diuretics; Antihypertensives |
| Kava Kava | To treat anxiety, nervousness, and insomnia | Upset stomach; Allergic skin reaction, yellow discoloration of skin; Central nervous system depression, liver toxicity | Potentiates the effects of antidepressants, barbiturates, and benzodiazepines; Skeletal muscle relaxants; Anesthetics |
| Licorice | To treat hepatitis and peptic ulcers | Hypertension; Hypokalemia; Edema | Antihypertensives; Potentiates the effects of corticosteroids |
| SAM-e (*S-adenosyl-L-methionine*) | To treat depression or osteoarthritis | Mimics serotonin; Nausea, upset stomach | Drugs that can increase or mimic serotonin, such as antidepressants |

**Table 2   CAM Herb/Drug Interactions\* (Continued)**

| Herbal Supplement | Common Uses | Potential Problems | Potential Interactions With |
|---|---|---|---|
| St. John's Wort | To treat mild depression, anxiety, seasonal affective disorder | Enhances bleeding; hastens metabolic breakdown of drugs; contraindicated for organ transplant recipients | Anticoagulants; Antidepressants; Decreases the effectiveness of cyclosporine, antiviral drugs; Digoxin; Dextrometorphan; Prolongs the effects of general anesthetics; MAO inhibitors |
| Valerian | To treat insomnia, anxiety | Sedation; Digestion problems | Potentiates the effects of barbiturates |

\*This table was compiled by the AAOS Committee on Complementary and Alternative Medicine. The information contained here is based on literature searches conducted in July and August of 2001 and was updated in 2003, and it may not be exhaustive. User physicians should rely on their own judgment concerning the care of specific patients and should use this table for general guidance only. Common medical practice is that patients cease using most of these preparations at least 2 weeks prior to surgical interventions.

*Methyl Sulfonyl Methane (MSM)*

MSM is a sulfur compound formed in the breakdown of dimethyl sulfoxide (DMSO). It is sold as an over-the-counter nutritional supplement and lotion that has been touted as a "cure" for arthritis. DMSO has been widely used in veterinary medicine for musculoskeletal problems, including arthritis. Both DMSO and MSM are proposed to act as potent anti-inflammatories.

## VISCOSUPPLEMENTATION

A relatively recent development in the treatment of OA is viscosupplementation. This involves injecting hyaluronic acid into a joint to improve joint function and decrease pain. Hyaluronic acid (HA) is a large glycosaminoglycan usually produced by chondrocytes and type B synoviocytes. It is essential for synovial viscoelasticity, joint lubrication, and joint motion. Patients with OA have a diminished concentration of hyaluronic acid within the affected joint(s). Because it is poorly absorbed in the gastrointestinal tract, HA must be injected into the joint rather than taken orally. Possible mechanisms by which HA may be therapeutic include (1) providing additional lubrication of the synovial membrane; (2) controlling permeability of the synovial membrane, thus diminishing joint effusions; and (3) directly blocking inflammation by scavenging free radicals. Several clinical trials have shown pain relief, but it is not known whether viscosupplementation will delay the progression or reverse the cartilage wear seen in OA.

Currently, the US Food and Drug Administration (FDA) approves viscosupplementation for OA of the knee only. These are produced either from rooster combs or from bacterial cultures. Intra-articular injections are administered weekly, for 3 or 5 weeks. Local reactions of increased joint pain, swelling, erythema, and itching have been reported. Viscosupplementation has been most effective in less severe OA (ie, OA without bone-on-bone changes). **Table 3** lists several of these preparations.

**Table 3   Comparative Prescribing Information for Selected Viscosupplements**

| | Hyalgan*<br>Sodium<br>Hyaluronate | Orthovisc*<br>High-Molecular-<br>Weight<br>Hyaluronan | Supartz*<br>Sodium<br>Hyaluronate | Synvisc*<br>Hylan G-F 20 |
|---|---|---|---|---|
| FDA-Approved Course of Therapy | 5 injections | 3 or 4 injections | 5 injections | 3 injections |
| Dose per injection | 20 mg | 30 mg | 25 mg | 16 mg |
| Description | High-molecular-weight fraction of purified natural sodium hyaluronate in buffered physiologic sodium chloride | High-molecular-weight, ultra-pure natural hyaluronan extracted from rooster combs, dissolved in physiologic saline | A sterile, nonphylogenic solution of purified, high-molecular-weight sodium hyaluronate | Hylan polymers produced from chicken combs by cross-linking of hyaluronan molecules (hylan A + B) |
| Molecular Weight (x $10^6$ D) | 0.5 to 0.73 | 1.0 to 2.9 | 0.62 to 1.17 | 6 (hylan A only) |
| Hyaluronic Acid Concentration (mg/mL) | 10 | 15 | 10 | 8 |
| Needle Gauge | 20 | 18 to 21 | 22 to 29 | 18 to 22 |
| Syringe Cap | Latex rubber | Nonlatex rubber | Latex rubber | Latex rubber |
| Syringe Content | Sodium hyaluronate 20 mg, sodium chloride 17 mg, monobasic sodium phosphate 0.1 mg, dibasic sodium phosphate 1.2 mg, water for injection up to 2 mL | Hyaluronan 30 mg, sodium chloride 18 mg, water for injection up to 2 mL | Sodium hyaluronate 25 mg, sodium chloride 21.25 mg, dibasic sodium phosphate dodecahydrate 1.343 mg, sodium dihydrogen phosphate dihydrate 0.04 mg, water for injection up to 2.5 mL | Hylan polymers (hylan A + hylan B) 16 mg, sodium chloride 17 mg, disodium hydrogen phosphate 0.32 mg, sodium hydrogen phosphate monohydrate 0.08 mg, water for injection up to 2.5 mL |

Refer to Hyalgan, Orthovisc, Supartz, and Synvisc prescribing information. The information given here is not intended to imply a comparison of efficacy or safety.

# OSTEOMYELITIS

## SYNONYM
Bone infection

### ICD-9 Code
**730**
Osteomyelitis, periostitis and other infections involving bone

## DEFINITION
Bone, like any other tissue, is susceptible to invasion by microorganisms. Osteomyelitis usually is caused by pyogenic organisms, but other sources such as tuberculosis, syphilis, and viral or fungal elements also are causative of osteomyelitis. The infecting agent creates an inflammatory response that progresses to an abscess that then destroys bone. The organism usually reaches the bone by hematogenous spread but can also infect the bone by direct spread of a soft-tissue infection or by a penetrating wound, eg, an open fracture. *Staphylococcus aureus* is the most common causative organism, with hemolytic streptococci next.

## CLINICAL SYMPTOMS
Unrelenting pain is the first symptom. The patient may report a history of an injury, which can delay the diagnosis. Fever develops early, followed by other symptoms, including localized tenderness, particularly over the metaphyseal area of the bone, generalized aches and pains, and a flushed appearance. In a neonate or infant, diagnosis is more difficult, and the bone infection may accompany other infectious causes such as meningitis, septicemia, or pneumonia.

## TESTS

### Physical Examination
Patients, including neonates, will not use the limb and often hold it in a protective manner. Motion is possible but painful. Gentle attempts at motion can be used to help differentiate osteomyelitis from a septic joint, as motion is extremely painful in an infected joint. Focal bone tenderness leads to the diagnosis and also to the site for possible aspiration. More established lesions will demonstrate swelling, erythema, and increased localized warmth. These findings typically are less dramatic with chronic osteomyelitis or osteomyelitis caused by nonpyogenic organisms. However, the latter may be associated with soft-tissue ulceration or draining sinuses.

SECTION 1 ■ GENERAL ORTHOPAEDICS

## Diagnostic Tests

Obtain a white blood cell count, erythrocyte sedimentation rate, C-reactive protein, AP and lateral radiographs of the affected area, blood culture, and aspiration of the suspected site for culture. Early radiographs will be negative or will show only soft-tissue swelling but should be obtained to rule out other conditions. A bone scan usually is not necessary in the acute situation but indicates osteomyelitis very early. MRI also is usually not necessary but can provide early diagnosis in complicated cases.

The most important diagnostic step is aspiration of the suspected site, which provides material for culture and identification of the organism. Even a tiny drop of pus may be adequate for culture and Gram stain.

# DIFFERENTIAL DIAGNOSIS

Septic arthritis (extremely painful joint motion)

Trauma (deformity, open wound)

Tumor (Ewing sarcoma, eosinophilic granuloma) (persistent localized pain, pain at rest)

# ADVERSE OUTCOMES OF THE DISEASE

In the preantibiotic era, osteomyelitis often resulted in death—quickly in the case of hematogenous disease and more slowly in chronic disease. Delay in treatment can still lead to death or serious compromise of growth and function of the extremity. Pathologic fracture or progression of the acute illness to the chronic stages with persistent drainage, repeated episodes of pain and fever, and soft-tissue destruction are avoided by early, aggressive treatment.

# TREATMENT

After diagnostic aspiration has been attempted, parenteral antibiotic treatment with bactericidal drugs should be initiated. Do not wait for culture results but consider that *S aureus* or *Streptococcus* are the likely causative organisms and use appropriate intravenous antibiotics against these organisms while awaiting culture and sensitivity reports. Negative results on aspiration do not exclude the diagnosis.

If a dramatic decrease in temperature and diminished pain and tenderness do not occur within 24 to 36 hours, surgical decompression is indicated. Different antibiotic regimens and surgical treatments are indicated for nonpyogenic cases or for chronic conditions.

## ADVERSE OUTCOMES OF TREATMENT

Damage to the physis or adjacent joint by needle aspiration, bone biopsy, or open surgery is possible. Serious allergic reaction to penicillin or other antibiotics also is possible.

## REFERRAL DECISIONS/RED FLAGS

Most patients with acute osteomyelitis should be hospitalized. Aspiration or surgical decompression usually requires specialty consultation. Infectious disease consultation may be helpful when dealing with unusual organisms.

# OSTEOPOROSIS

## DEFINITION

Osteoporosis is a disease characterized by low bone mass leading to microarchitectural deterioration. As a result, there is increased fragility of the bone and an increased risk of fracture. Other adverse outcomes include deformity, pain, loss of independence, and premature death, particularly following hip fracture. Approximately 10 million Americans over the age of 50 years have osteoporosis, and the disease is associated with 1.5 million fractures and health care costs of $18 billion per year. Although osteoporosis has long been considered an inevitable consequence of aging, the natural history can be altered by diet and treatment strategies.

Osteoporosis is defined as primary (type I or II) or secondary. Type I osteoporosis, frequently called postmenopausal osteoporosis, is six times more common in women than in men. Estrogen deficiency in women and testosterone deficiency in men lead to trabecular bone loss. These patients commonly present with vertebral compression fractures or fractures of the distal radius. Type II osteoporosis, previously called senile osteoporosis, is twice as frequent in women as in men, and it occurs more commonly in individuals over the age of 70 years. Altered calcium metabolism and intrinsic problems in bone formation lead to a decrease in formation of new bone. Hip and pelvic fractures are common in this group. In secondary osteoporosis, an identifiable agent or disease process causes loss of bone.

## CLINICAL SYMPTOMS

Osteoporosis frequently is not recognized until a patient seeks medical attention for back pain, fracture, loss of height, or spinal deformity (**Figure 1**). Over the past decade, however, with the greater availability of dual-energy x-ray absorptiometry (DXA or DEXA) and quantitative ultrasound, screening examinations for osteoporosis, especially in women with risk factors, is becoming more common. **Table 1** summarizes risk factors for osteoporotic fractures.

Secondary osteoporosis is seen commonly in patients taking long-term steroid therapy. It is also seen in a wide range of disorders such as hormone abnormalities (hyperthyroidism, hyperparathyroidism), neoplastic disorders (multiple myeloma), metabolic abnormalities (osteomalacia), and connective tissue diseases (osteogenesis imperfecta). Among men with osteoporosis, most have secondary osteoporosis. It is a serious problem for patients who require prolonged immobilization.

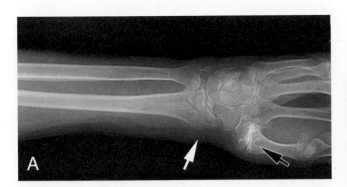
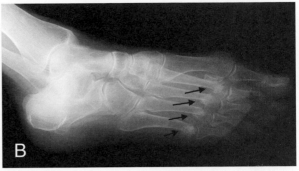

**Figure 1**

**A,** Radiograph of the forearm and wrist of a 74-year-old woman who fell on her outstretched hand, sustaining a fracture of the distal radius and ulna (white arrow). Carpometacarpal arthritis of the thumb (black arrow) is an incidental finding. **B,** Radiograph of the right foot and ankle of an 82-year-old woman who sustained fractures of the necks of metatarsals 2 through 5 (arrows). In both patients, the generalized lack of BMD is suggestive of osteopenia or frank osteoporosis, and further studies to evaluate BMD are indicated.

---

**Table 1    Risk Factors for Osteoporotic Fracture**

**Nonmodifiable**

*Personal history of fracture as an adult\**

*History of fracture in a first-degree relative\**

Caucasian or Asian race (recent data suggest that African- and Hispanic Americans are at a significant risk, as well)

Advanced age

Female gender

Dementia

Poor health/fragility\*\*

**Potentially modifiable**

*Current cigarette smoking\**

*Low body weight (< 127 lb)\**

Estrogen deficiency

Early menopause (< age 45) or bilateral ovariectomy

Prolonged premenopausal amenorrhea (> 1 year)

Low calcium intake (lifelong)

Use of certain medications such as corticosteroids and anticonvulsants

Alcoholism

Impaired eyesight despite adequate correction

Recurrent falls

Inadequate physical activity

Poor health/fragility\*\*

\*These items in italics are major factors in determining the risk of hip fracture, independent of bone density.

\*\*Note that poor health and fragility may or may not be modifiable and thus occur under both headings.

Adapted from National Osteoporosis Foundation: *Physician's Guide to the Prevention and Treatment of Osteoporosis.* Washington, DC, National Osteoporosis Foundation, 1998.

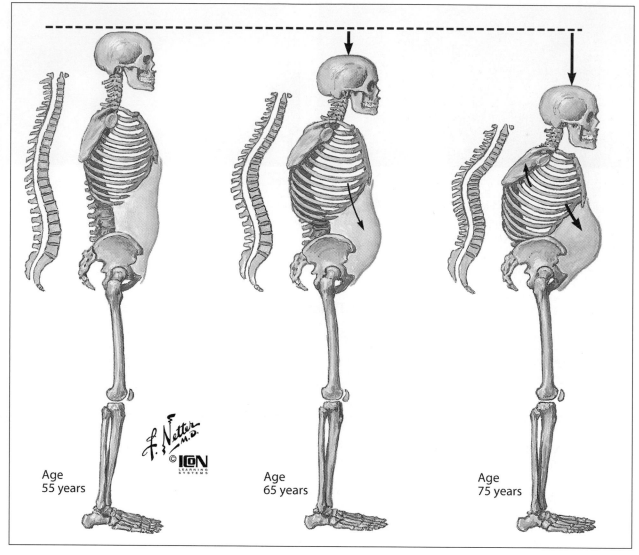

Age
55 years

Age
65 years

Age
75 years

**Figure 2**

Progressive spinal deformity in osteoporosis. Compression fractures of thoracic vertebrae lead to loss of height and progressive thoracic kyphosis (dowager's hump). The lower ribs eventually rest on the iliac crests, and downward pressure on the viscera causes abdominal distention.

(Reproduced with permission from Icon Learning Systems, Inc.)

# TESTS

## *Physical Examination*

The physical examination is normal in the early stages. In advanced disease, findings may include tenderness to palpation over an area of fracture, spinal deformity, loss of height (often more than 2 inches), lax abdominal musculature with a protuberant abdomen, hypermobility, and exaggerated thoracic kyphosis (dowager's hump) (**Figure 2**).

Female athletes, particularly those participating in endurance activities, gymnastics, skating, and dance, may develop low bone density and subsequent stress or overt fractures because of

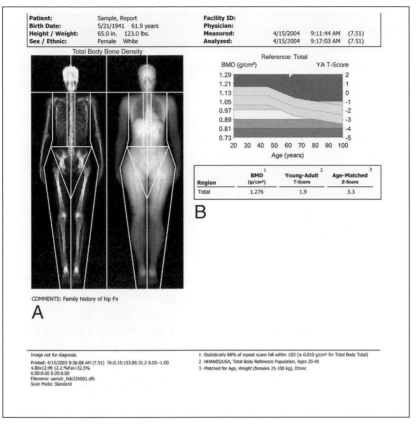

**Figure 3**

DXA scan (**A**) and report (**B**) for a 61-year-old white woman. The report provides a reference database of BMD as a function of age. The middle line is the mean BMD, and the lines above and below the line represent 1 SD above and below the mean, respectively. Findings are compared with young adults (T scores) and with age-matched adults (Z scores). The World Health Organization (WHO) bases management guidelines on T scores. According to WHO, a T score at or above −1.0 SD is normal; a T score between −1.0 and −2.5 indicates osteopenia; and a T score at or below −2.5 SD indicates osteoporosis.

overtraining, inadequate diet, and menstrual cessation. It is imperative to thoroughly question female athletes about their menstrual history and to question all athletes about their diet and exercise habits.

## Diagnostic Tests

Diagnostic tests are performed to identify the presence and severity of the disease, measure response to therapeutic interventions, and rule out secondary causes of osteoporosis.

Because there is no specific measurement for bone strength, bone mineral density (BMD) is used as a surrogate. DXA is currently the gold standard for BMD measurement (**Figure 3**). This quick, painless test helps estimate bone strength and predict future fracture risk. It is fast, reproducible, and involves very low radiation exposure. Bone mass is reported as areal density and compared with both peers (Z score) and young normal individuals (T score). Z and T scores represent standard deviations (SDs) below the comparison group. Bone density is characterized by the lowest value at either the spine, femoral neck, trochanter, or total femur. Values of 0 to −1 are normal; −1 to −2.5 indicate osteopenia; less than −2.5 indicates osteoporosis. DXA currently is the best test for monitoring the results of osteoporosis treatment. For reasons of cost, speed, and availability, however, quantitative ultrasound may be used as a screening tool in younger patients.

Because osteoporosis typically is a "silent" disease, the decision to test should be based on a patient's risk profile. The National Osteoporosis Foundation recommends BMD testing for the following individuals:

- All women age 65 years or older, regardless of risk factors;
- Postmenopausal women under age 65 years who have one or more of the following risk factors: family history of osteoporosis, personal history of low-trauma fracture after age 45 years, current cigarette smoker, or low body weight (less than 127 lb);
- Men with a history of a low-trauma fracture or of treatment with a GnRH agonist for prostate cancer;
- Individuals with primary hyperparathyroidism, on long-term glucocorticoid treatment, with diseases or conditions known to cause bone loss, or using medications known to cause bone loss.

Osteoporosis may be either high-turnover osteoporosis (increased rate of absorption) or low-turnover osteoporosis (decreased rate of bone formation). The NTx test measures bone collagen breakdown products, with a high NTx level indicating high turnover and a low NTx level indicating low turnover. Tests to rule out secondary causes of osteoporosis include a complete blood cell count, erythrocyte sedimentation rate, C-reactive protein, serum protein level, and immunoelectrophoresis (serum/urine) to rule out a bone marrow disorder. Thyroid function tests and parathyroid hormone (PTH) level tests are performed to rule out hyperthyroidism or hyperparathyroidism. Cushing disease and diabetes are ruled out by history. Tests for serum levels of calcium, phosphorus, alkaline phosphatase, and 25-hydroxyvitamin D (along with PTH levels) rule out osteomalacia. Other studies include renal and liver function tests and a 24-hour urine calcium test.

# DIFFERENTIAL DIAGNOSIS

Disuse osteopenia (history of prolonged immobilization or bed rest)

Multiple myeloma (anemia, elevated sedimentation rate, bone pain, immunoelectrophoresis results)

Osteomalacia (deformity, renal osteodystrophy) (bone pain, low hydroxyvitamin D level, high intact PTH level, elevated alkaline phosphatase, low calcium, low urinary calcium)

Poor imaging technique on radiographs (overpenetration) (overpenetration may be suspected when soft tissues are not visible on radiograph; all radiographic diagnoses optimally confirmed by DXA)

Primary osteoporosis (type I or type II) (by exclusion, all low-energy fracture patients, loss of more than 2 inches in height)

Secondary osteoporosis (history, occurs in men)

## ADVERSE OUTCOMES OF THE DISEASE

Adverse outcomes of osteoporosis include fracture, deformity, chronic pain, social withdrawal, loss of independence, and death, particularly following hip fracture.

## TREATMENT

### Prevention

Because peak bone mass is reached before the age of 25 to 28 years, women should be encouraged to maximize bone formation during youth through proper diet and exercise and minimize bone loss during adulthood. Recommendations for the general population include an adequate intake of calcium and vitamin D, regular weight-bearing exercise, and avoidance of tobacco use and alcohol abuse.

Older patients should be educated about the importance of maintaining their body weight and reducing their risk factors for falls by walking for exercise, avoiding long-acting benzodiazepams, minimizing caffeine intake, and treating impaired visual function (Table 1).

Standards for the optimal type and duration of exercise have not been established. The ideal exercise program includes impact-loading exercise (such as walking), strength training, and balance training (such as tai chi).

Recommendations for calcium intake are listed in **Table 2**. Most Americans consume far less calcium than is recommended, particularly in their elder years. Calcium supplements are frequently required. The two main forms of calcium are carbonate and citrate. Carbonate requires an acid environment to dissolve; H2 blockers and indigestion impair its availability. Citrate forms dissolve at all pH levels and decrease the risk of kidney stones. As a consequence, citrate is preferred to carbonate unless chewed.

SECTION 1 ■ GENERAL ORTHOPAEDICS

**Table 2  Dietary Reference Intake Values for Calcium by Life-Stage Group**

| Life-stage group* | Adequate intake (mg/day) |
|---|---|
| 0 to 6 months | 210 |
| 6 to 12 months | 270 |
| 1 through 3 years | 500 |
| 4 through 8 years | 800 |
| 9 through 13 years | 1,300 |
| 14 through 18 years | 1,300 |
| 19 through 30 years | 1,000 |
| 31 through 50 years | 1,000 |
| 51 through 70 years | 1,200 |
| > 70 years | 1,200 |
| **Pregnancy** | |
| ≤ 18 years | 1,300 |
| 19 through 50 years | 1,000 |
| **Lactation** | |
| ≤ 18 years | 1,300 |
| 19 through 50 years | 1,000 |

*All groups except Pregnancy and Lactation are both males and females

Adapted from National Osteoporosis Foundation: *Physician's Guide to the Prevention and Treatment of Osteoporosis.* Washington, DC, National Osteoporosis Foundation, 1998.

Vitamin D is essential for intestinal absorption of calcium, and requirements increase with age because skin production of this vitamin decreases even with adequate sun exposure. Current recommendations for vitamin D intake are 400 IU/day in young adults and 800 to 1,200 IU/day in the elderly. Fractures resulting from falls can be decreased by 20% with 800 units of vitamin D per day. Combination vitamin D and calcium can decrease the risk of hip fracture in the elderly by approximately 25%.

## Intervention

In the best circumstances, treatment of osteoporosis is initiated before a fracture occurs. Physicians should encourage all patients to follow the prevention strategies listed above. The National Osteoporosis Foundation (NOF) recommends pharmacologic intervention for osteoporosis in white women whose BMD scores are 2 standard deviations below those of a "young normal" adult in the absence of risk factors and in women whose BMD scores are 1.5 standard deviations below those of a "young normal" adult if other risk factors are present. The NOF also notes that white women over age 70 with multiple risk factors (especially those with previous nonhip, nonspine fractures) are at high enough risk of fracture to initiate treatment without BMD testing.

All interventions include appropriate calcium and vitamin D intake. Treatment classes include antiresorptive agents (bisphosphonates [alendronate, risedronate], SERMS [selective estrogen receptor modulators], calcitonin), prescribed for patients with high NTx levels; and anabolic agents (intermittent PTH), prescribed for patients with low NTx levels (**Table 3**). Both alendronate and risedronate are taken once a week and decrease the fracture risk in all bones at least 50%. Although estrogen prevents fractures, it is no longer recommended by the FDA for the treatment of osteoporosis because of its increased risk for myocardial infarct, stroke, breast cancer, and possibly

## Table 3    Drugs Used in Treatment of Osteoporosis

| Drug | Dosage/ Administration | Side Effects | Contraindications |
|---|---|---|---|
| **Antiresorptive agents (indication: high NTx)** | | | |
| Bisphosphonates (alendronate, risedronate) | Taken once weekly, orally, on empty stomach (alendronate 70 mg; risedronate 35 mg) | Upper GI disturbances | Premenopausal or pregnant women; patients with esophagitis or esophageal dysfunction |
| SERMs (raloxifene) | 60 mg daily | Phlebitis, pulmonary embolism | Premenopausal women; history of phlebitis or pulmonary embolism; does not prevent hip fractures |
| Calcitonin | 1 spray (200 units)/day | Nosebleed | Does not prevent hip fractures |
| Pamidronate | 30 mg intravenously 4 times/year | | |
| Zoledronic acid | 4 mg intravenously 4 times/year | | |
| **Anabolic agents (indication: low NTx)** | | | |
| PTH | 20 µg daily, subcutaneously | Cramps, orthostatic hypotension in very elderly | Children; patients with prior radiation therapy; patients with Paget disease |

dementia. Raloxifene is a SERM that enhances spinal bone mass and decreases vertebral fractures. It does not prevent hip fractures. Calcitonin gives minor spinal fracture protection and possibly some pain relief, but it affords no nonvertebral fracture protection. For individuals who cannot tolerate oral bisphosphonates, intravenous forms developed for cancer (pamidronate and zoledronic acid) are efficaceous in protecting bone mass.

Anabolic agents are recommended for low-turnover states, failures of bisphosphonates, premenopausal women, and in the setting of fresh diaphyseal fractures. Intermittent PTH (1-34 amino acids) is given only intravenously and results in marked enhancement of bone mass, fracture protection comparable to bisphosphonates, and enhancement of fracture healing. It is contraindicated in children, patients with prior radiation, and patients with Paget disease.

## ADVERSE OUTCOMES OF TREATMENT

Estrogen hormone replacement therapy is associated with an increased risk of breast cancer, heart disease, and deep venous thrombosis. Side effects can include vaginal bleeding, breast tenderness, mood disturbances, and gallbladder disease. Consequently, estrogen is not recommended for osteoporosis. Bisphosphonate must be taken on an empty stomach, and some patients report upper gastrointestinal disturbance. Also, some animal studies suggest a delay of maturation during fracture healing. Calcitonin has fewer side effects but is minimally effective and only for the spine. Raloxifene has been shown to increase the risk of deep venous thrombosis at the same rate as estrogen, and it provides no hip fracture protection. It also causes hot flashes and does not treat menopausal symptoms. PTH may cause cramps and orthostatic hypotension in the very elderly.

## REFERRAL DECISIONS/RED FLAGS

Osteoporosis and fragility fractures are not inevitable in any age group. All appropriate patients should be referred for BMD testing and offered treatment.

Many physicians may feel uncomfortable evaluating BMD studies, ruling out secondary causes of osteoporosis, or initiating pharmacologic treatment. Referral to an osteoporosis specialist may be appropriate.

# OVERUSE SYNDROMES

## SYNONYMS
Cumulative trauma disorder
Occupational arm pain
Occupational stress syndrome
Repetitive strain injury
Work-related pain disorder
Writer's cramp

**ICD-9 Code**
**729.5**
Pain in limb

## DEFINITION
Overuse injuries are caused or aggravated by repetitive motion or sustained exertion of a particular body part, resulting in microtrauma to a musculotendinous unit. Overuse syndrome is an umbrella term that encompasses specific conditions such as carpal tunnel syndrome, tennis elbow, wrist flexor and extensor tendinitis (de Quervain disease), Achilles and posterior tibial tendinitis, patellar tendinitis, stress fractures of the lower extremity, shin-splints, exertional compartment syndromes, epicondylitis, and flexor tendinitis, as well as generalized myofascial pain. While more attention has been focused on overuse syndromes in the upper extremity, some conditions, such as stress fractures and exertional compartment syndromes, are actually more common in the lower extremity.

Overuse syndromes reflect an interplay of physical, psychosocial, and sociopolitical factors. While the exact cause of overuse syndromes remains controversial, contributing factors may include repetitive tasks, forceful exertions, exposure to vibration or cold temperatures, awkward postures in the workplace, the ergonomic environment, lack of job satisfaction, psychological makeup, boredom, the state's workers' compensation laws, and the social environment.

## CLINICAL SYMPTOMS
Unfortunately, a precise definition of overuse syndromes is lacking, and there is no agreement concerning the diagnostic criteria. Likewise, whether certain jobs or occupations cause overuse syndromes remains controversial. The many synonyms listed above illustrate the confusion that surrounds these conditions. Overuse syndromes develop over time—from a few weeks to years. Frequently, the onset is insidious, and patients may not report their problems early on in anticipation that the condition will improve.

Typical symptoms include pain, fatigue, numbness, or any combination of the above. Although patients often have difficulty localizing their pain, they may report specific symptoms related to carpal tunnel syndrome, lateral elbow epicondylitis, or flexor tenosynovitis in the palm, associated with vague and nonanatomic discomfort elsewhere in the arm. Patients with overuse syndromes may report numbness in a nonanatomic or nondermatomal distribution. Patients also may report a sensation of swelling in the extremity, although it is not generally apparent on examination.

Certain individuals are at risk for overuse syndromes, principally those with exposure to physical stresses (eg, repetition, force, awkward postures, temperature extremes, and vibration) and those with psychosocial stresses (eg, fast work pace, inflexibility in the workplace, monotonous demanding tasks, and depression). At least 25% of adult athletes also experience overuse injuries. Certain jobs and occupations appear to predispose workers to overuse syndromes. Professional dancers, musicians, grocery store checkers, computer keyboard operators, and dental hygienists are particularly susceptible. Women with serious psychosocial problems, such as a history of physical and sexual abuse, are at increased risk for unexplained musculoskeletal pain. Individuals who are poorly educated or who work in mundane, low-paying jobs also are at risk. Note, too, that highly skilled individuals who believe that they are overworked, underpaid, overstressed, and unappreciated also are at higher risk.

# Tests

## Physical Examination

Patients should be asked specific job-related questions, including questions about job satisfaction; working conditions; the relationship with the supervisor and coworkers; exposure to repetitive and forceful exertions, vibration, or cold temperature; and job harassment. Identifying the type of industry and specific job also is important, as the incidence of claims for overuse syndromes is higher for certain industries and jobs, such as meat packers, assembly line workers, grocery store checkers, and clerical workers.

Many of the conditions listed in the differential diagnosis may be present concomitantly.

## Diagnostic Tests

Radiographs are indicated if there is a clear history of trauma, but they are often normal. A bone scan may be necessary to identify a stress fracture. Likewise, nerve conduction velocity studies can be ordered to rule out carpal tunnel syndrome or ulnar nerve entrapment at the elbow, but results of these studies usually are normal. Exertional compartment syndrome can be confirmed by measuring compartment pressure after exercise.

## DIFFERENTIAL DIAGNOSIS

Angina with referred arm pain (abnormal electrocardiogram)

Claudication (decreased peripheral pulses)

Deep vein thrombosis (abnormal venogram)

Fibromyalgia (11 of 18 tender points in four body quadrants)

Herniated cervical or lumbar disk (abnormal spine radiographs, myelogram, and MRI)

## ADVERSE OUTCOMES OF THE DISEASE

With these disorders, patients often lose time from work and experience psychological changes. They may even change occupations or simply never return to work.

## TREATMENT

A satisfactory outcome for the patient depends on the cooperative efforts of the employer, the insurance carrier, and a physician-directed health care team that might include physical and occupational therapists, occupational health nurses, and vocational rehabilitation counselors. A case manager, such as an occupational health nurse, can be invaluable in coordinating the efforts of these groups to return the patient to work.

Initial treatment should include ice and rest of the affected part, along with a progressive exercise program of subsymptomatic stresses to strengthen the extremity. At the workplace, modify tasks and work schedules, and consider job change if the symptoms persist.

NSAIDs and analgesic creams may reduce the musculoskeletal pain associated with these conditions. Narcotics should be avoided because of the possibility of addiction. Antidepressants can be a useful adjunct if depression is a significant part of the clinical picture.

Although surgery may be indicated, it is seldom urgent. The results of surgery are less predictable in these patients. Better results are obtained when the overuse has caused a specific, clearly identifiable syndrome such as carpal tunnel syndrome. Lack of job satisfaction and depression are also important predictors of recovery. Poor prognosis is associated with both long-standing disability (longer than 6 months) and litigation.

## ADVERSE OUTCOMES OF TREATMENT

Drug dependence from narcotics or antidepressants is possible. If the patient has had multiple, ill-advised surgeries, persistently tender scars may be left.

## REFERRAL DECISIONS/RED FLAGS

Once a diagnosis of overuse syndrome is suspected, treatment by a team of health care professionals may be the best way to manage these difficult problems.

# REHABILITATION PRINCIPLES AND THERAPEUTIC MODALITIES

## DEFINITION

The goals of rehabilitation are to return the patient to maximal function as quickly as possible after injury. Through advances in knowledge in the fields of anatomy, joint mechanics, muscle physiology, soft-tissue healing, neurology, and kinesiology, rehabilitation has evolved into an evidence-based, multidisciplinary profession. The American Board of Physical Therapy Specialties certifies therapists in seven specialty areas: Orthopedics, Sports, Pediatrics, Cardiovascular and Pulmonary, Geriatrics, Neurologic, and Clinical Electrophysiologic.

The patient care rendered by the rehabilitation specialist should be recognized as an integral part of treatment. For many patients, the care begins with the physician. It is important for the physician to start the patient on a basic range-of-motion (ROM), stretching, and strengthening exercise program. If the patient does not recover quickly with a home program monitored by the physician or the physician's assistant, the patient should be referred to a rehabilitation specialist or a multidisciplinary health care team.

## TREATMENT

Restoring full function starts with regaining ROM. Stretching exercises, passive low-load stretching devices, and manual therapy are the most successful approaches to restoring full ROM. Isometric exercises may also be initiated, along with active or passive stretching exercises. As the ROM improves, strengthening exercises starting with light resistance and higher repetitions can be added to assist in the reeducation of the muscles surrounding the joint and to increase their endurance. Strength training with heavier weights and lower repetitions may be initiated as long as no pain is present during the exercise. Progressively more advanced strengthening and ROM exercises are needed to return the patient to sports- or work-related activities.

Modalities that decrease swelling and pain are useful adjuncts. These modalities are frequently used to prepare the soft tissue prior to manual therapy or passive and active stretching exercises. They are also used as an adjunct to strengthening exercises to enhance the treatment effectiveness. For example, there is good evidence that high-frequency electrical stimulation used in conjunction with a closed kinetic chain anterior cruciate ligament rehabilitation program enhances the strength of the quadriceps muscle. Research also has demonstrated that use of a superficial hot pack during low-load prolonged stretching lasting 30 to 40 minutes produces more permanent changes in ROM than does stretching alone. **Table 1** lists indications for various therapeutic modalities and exercises.

## ADVERSE OUTCOMES OF TREATMENT

Rarely, overaggressive therapy used at the wrong point in the healing process may damage the healing soft-tissue structures.

## REFERRAL DECISIONS/RED FLAGS

Complex problems, lack of progression, or the need for special rehabilitation equipment indicates referral to a physical therapist. Patients who are not able to do therapy on their own also benefit from referral. When ordering physical therapy, the physician should specify the diagnosis and the limitations of the patient.

## Table 1  Use of Therapeutic Modalities, Exercises, and Equipment

| Symptoms and Physical Findings | Modalities | Exercise | Equipment | Comment |
|---|---|---|---|---|
| Acute swelling | Ice<br>EGS | In noninjured areas only | Compression<br>Braces and splints for immobilization | |
| Chronic inflammation | Ice<br>Phonophoresis<br>Iontophoresis<br>NSAIDs | Stretching<br>Joint mobilization<br>Isometric and short-arc strengthening | Tape<br>Soft braces<br>Neoprene sleeves | |
| Restricted joint motion with inflammation | Ice | Isometric strengthening<br>Active exercises in ROM without pain | Compression wraps<br>Functional braces | Assess for intra-articular pathology |
| Restricted joint motion without inflammation | Heat<br>Ultrasound | Active ROM exercises<br>Passive ROM exercises<br>Active-assist ROM exercises | Progressive splints to maintain motion<br>Night splints | Rule out systemic disease, CRPS |
| Joint instability | None, unless swelling present | Strengthening in ROM without pain<br>Closed-chain kinetic exercises<br>Proprioception exercises | Immobilize acute injury<br>Functional braces later | Distinguish between static and functional instability |
| Muscle atrophy | EGS | PREs | Weights and tubing for home exercise program | Distinguish between disuse and neurologic injuries |
| Muscle imbalances | Objective measurement | Selective strengthening exercises | | Distinguish between disuse and neurologic injuries |
| Loss of flexibility with injury | Ice<br>EGS<br>Ultrasound | Static stretching<br>Massage<br>PREs | Compression with and without immobilization | |
| Loss of flexibility without injury | | Active stretching, with and without assistance<br>Massage<br>Myofascial release | | Address underlying cause of muscle tightness |
| Proprioceptive deficit | | Balance and proprioceptive exercises<br>Functional exercises | Neoprene sleeve for warmth<br>Neoprene sleeve or wrap for tactile input<br>Balance board | Modified Romberg test |

EGS = electrogalvanic stimulation; NSAIDs = nonsteroidal anti-inflammatory drugs; ROM = range of motion; CRPS = complex regional pain syndrome; PREs = progressive resistive exercises

Reproduced from Anderson SJ: Principles of rehabilitation, in Sullivan JA, Anderson SJ (eds): *Care of the Young Athlete*. Rosemont, IL, American Academy of Orthopaedic Surgeons, 2000, pp 267-280.

# RHEUMATOID ARTHRITIS

**ICD-9 Code**

**714.0**
Rheumatoid arthritis

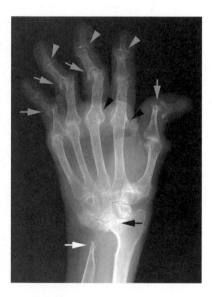

**Figure 1**

PA view of the left hand of a
42-year-old woman with advanced
RA. Note the ulnar translocation
of the carpus (black arrow);
the pencil shape of the ulna (white
arrow); the dislocation of the
metacarpophalangeal joints of the
index and middle fingers (black
arrowheads); the destruction of the
interphalangeal joint of the thumb
and the proximal interphalangeal
joints of the long, ring, and
little fingers (gray arrows); and the
arthritic changes in the distal
interphalangeal joints (gray
arrows).

Reproduced from Johnson TR, Steinbach LS
(eds): *Essentials of Musculoskeletal
Imaging.* Rosemont, IL, American Academy of
Orthopaedic Surgeons, 2004, p 394.

## DEFINITION

Rheumatoid arthritis (RA) is a systemic autoimmune disorder
characterized by an inflammatory synovitis that can erode and
ultimately destroy the articular cartilage. The etiology is
unknown, but most likely an unknown agent activates an
immune response in synovial tissue.

RA affects women more often than men, and the prevalence
increases with age, with peak onset in the late 40s and early 50s.
The arthritis typically is symmetrical and most often involves the
joints of the hands, wrist, feet, and ankles (**Figure 1**).

## CLINICAL SYMPTOMS

By definition, symptoms of RA must be of at least 6 weeks'
duration. Pain, morning stiffness, swelling, and systemic
symptoms are common. The 1987 revised criteria of the
American College of Rheumatology require at least four of the
following seven criteria to be satisfied before a diagnosis can be
established.

- Morning stiffness that is periarticular and lasts at least
  1 hour
- Arthritis (synovitis with periarticular soft-tissue swelling) of
  three or more joints for at least 6 weeks
- Arthritis of hand joints (wrist, metacarpophalangeal, or
  proximal interphalangeal) for at least 6 weeks
- Symmetric arthritis for at least 6 weeks
- Rheumatoid nodules (subcutaneous nodules over extensor
  surfaces or bony prominences)
- Positive serum rheumatoid factor
- Radiographic changes

Extra-articular symptoms include generalized malaise,
fatigue, tenosynovitis (particularly of the hands and feet) that
may be complicated by carpal tunnel syndrome or other
tenosynovitis manifestations, vasculitis manifested by palpable
purpura, dry eyes secondary to keratoconjunctivitis sicca,
pulmonary nodules, and inflammatory pericarditis.

The hypertrophic synovium stretches the ligaments and joint
capsules. As a result, these supporting structures become less
effective. Erosion of the articular cartilage in combination with the
ligamentous changes results in deformity and contractures such as
ulnar drifting and subluxation of the metacarpophalangeal joints in
the hand, and hallux valgus and claw toe deformities in the foot.
With progression of the disease, pain and deformity increase.

Patients with severe RA typically have multiple affected joints in the upper and lower extremities. Joints of the cervical spine may be involved as well. Neck pain and stiffness occur, and with atlantoaxial subluxation, cervical myelopathy may develop.

# TESTS

## Physical Examination

Joint contractures, joint effusions, deformity (genu valgum or knock-knee), and painful motion are common. Swelling of the proximal interphalangeal joints and stiffness in the hands usually occur early. An associated carpal tunnel syndrome, manifested by severe neuritic-type pain and a positive Phalen test, may appear acutely.

Most joints show increased warmth and synovial bogginess. Joint aspirations often produce less fluid than expected because much of the enlargement comes from synovial hypertrophy.

Rheumatoid nodules often appear, especially along the extensor aspect of the arm.

## Diagnostic tests

Rheumatoid factors (mostly IgM antibodies against the Fc portion of IgG) are elevated in 75% to 90% of patients. This test, however, is not specific for RA, because rheumatoid factors also are elevated in chronic inflammatory conditions that cause sustained elevation of IgG. The erythrocyte sedimentation rate and C-reactive protein level usually are elevated.

Radiographs often show periarticular osteopenia and bony erosion at the joint margin (correlates with insertion site of synovium). Lateral flexion and extension views of the neck may demonstrate C1-2 instability secondary to erosion of the ligaments that hold the odontoid in place. These findings are important if the patient is anticipating any surgery that involves intubation or manipulation of the neck, as it could lead to quadriparesis or death.

# DIFFERENTIAL DIAGNOSIS

Hepatitis (abnormal liver function tests)

Lyme disease (serology, rash, anemia)

Seronegative arthropathies (HLA tests, abnormal radiographs, urethritis)

Systemic lupus erythematosus (antinuclear antibodies, peripheral blood smear)

## ADVERSE OUTCOMES OF THE DISEASE

Joint contractures, pain, loss of function, loss of ambulation, and multisystem disorders leading to death are possible. Osteoporosis is common, in part related to the disease, inactivity, and steroid use.

## TREATMENT

Describing complete medical treatment for this condition is beyond the scope of this text. Commonly, salicylates, NSAIDs, splinting, and oral and intra-articular corticosteroids are used to treat the polyarthralgias and pain. Disease-modifying agents, such as hydroxychloroquine, methotrexate, and gold are used at earlier stages of the disease. Corticosteroid injections into selected joints and the carpal tunnel may relieve acute synovitis and carpal tunnel syndrome. Splints can help manage acute episodes of pain associated with synovitis as well as positioning joints to minimize progressive deformity. Custom shoes are helpful with severe foot deformities. Physical therapy in the form of range-of-motion and strengthening exercises and other modalities is important. Selective surgical intervention by synovectomy or tenosynovectomy may prevent tendon rupture and progression of joint deformity. End-stage arthritis requires total joint arthroplasty or arthrodesis.

## ADVERSE OUTCOMES OF TREATMENT

Infection secondary to injection or surgery; gastric, hepatic, or renal complications associated with NSAID use; and osteonecrosis of bone or osteoporosis associated with steroid use are possible. Skin rash and other side effects of various medications also can develop.

## REFERRAL DECISIONS/RED FLAGS

Patients whose symptoms persist for more than 3 months, who have uncontrollable joint pain at rest, or who have deformity need further evaluation. Patients with foot deformities not responsive to custom shoes also need additional evaluation, as do those in whom extra-articular manifestations develop.

# Septic Arthritis

## Definition

Septic arthritis usually occurs as a result of inoculation of bacteria into a joint. The inoculation can occur as a hematogenous event, by direct penetration of a joint, or by spread from an adjacent focus of infection. Septic arthritis has a wide variety of presentations depending on the age and general health of the patient, virulence of the infecting organism, and circumstances of the inoculation, eg, tissue necrosis with a penetrating injury.

Septic arthritis occurs most commonly in children as a result of hematogenous spread of bacteria. When hematogenous septic arthritis occurs in adults, there is often an associated arthritic condition such as rheumatoid arthritis or an underlying medical condition that affects the immune system. Gonococcal infections also may cause septic arthritis.

## Clinical Symptoms

An infant or child with septic arthritis often appears seriously and acutely ill, with a high fever, tachycardia, irritability, and pain with any motion of the limb. Children who previously have been walking may now refuse to walk. Older patients with sepsis secondary to a total joint arthroplasty might have only a vague sense of discomfort in the joint and a variable history of pain on weight bearing or motion. Between these two extremes, symptoms of discomfort, limited joint motion, swelling, or deformity vary widely depending on the type of organism. The onset of symptoms with fungal or mycobacterial infections is quite indolent compared with that of pyogenic bacteria.

## Tests

### Physical Examination

Examination of a patient with suspected septic arthritis should include a general physical examination to identify a source of the infection, such as a furuncle or abscessed tooth, or the site of a penetrating wound near the joint. Note swelling and the position of the joint. With septic arthritis, the patient holds the joint in a position of comfort, such as flexion of the hip or knee. Passive motion of the joint causes severe pain. Palpate the joint for increased warmth and effusion. With a chronic infection, hypertrophy of the synovium will be present.

**ICD-9 Code**
**711.0**
Pyogenic arthritis

*Diagnostic Tests*

A white blood cell count (WBC), erythrocyte sedimentation rate (ESR), C-reactive protein (CRP), screening AP and lateral radiographs, blood culture, and aspiration of joint fluid for analysis, Gram stain, and culture are standard. The WBC may be normal or elevated, and the ESR and CRP are frequently but not always elevated. Radiographs usually are normal or show only soft-tissue swelling but are useful in ruling out other pathologic conditions. Blood cultures are important because this study may identify the causative organism when joint fluid cultures are negative. Analysis of the synovial fluid typically shows a WBC >50,000/mm$^3$, and often the WBC is >100,000/mm$^3$. However, the WBC of the joint fluid typically is less elevated in gonococcal arthritis. Culture of joint fluid mandates special considerations when *Haemophilus influenzae* or *Neisseria gonorrhoeae* is considered.

With chronic infections, cultures should include study for acid-fast and fungal organisms, as well as pyogenic bacteria. A negative culture does not necessarily exclude septic arthritis, particularly in chronic cases that may be caused by organisms of low virulence or that are fastidious in their growth.

# DIFFERENTIAL DIAGNOSIS

Acute rheumatic fever (migratory arthralgia, carditis, increased antistreptolysin titer, group A streptococcal infection)

Juvenile rheumatoid arthritis (morning stiffness, usually mild joint swelling)

Lyme disease (indolent onset, erythema migrans, cardiac and neurologic manifestations)

Osteoarthritis (evident on radiographs)

Rheumatoid arthritis (morning stiffness, symmetric involvement, positive rheumatoid factor, elevated erythrocyte sedimentation rate)

Transient synovitis of the hip (pediatric disorder, limited hip motion, afebrile)

# ADVERSE OUTCOMES OF THE DISEASE

The most serious associated outcomes clearly are generalized sepsis or death. In infants and children, joint destruction or physeal damage is possible. In older patients, loss of joint function is usually less dramatic, but chronic infection may never be eradicated. In these situations, arthrodesis of the joint or even amputation of the extremity may be necessary.

**Table 1    Likely Infecting Organism and Early Antibiotic Treatment of Septic Arthritis**

| Age | Likely Organism | Initial Antibiotic Regimen |
|---|---|---|
| Neonate | *S aureus*, group B *Streptococcus* | Oxacillin plus gentamicin |
| Child < 5 years | *S aureus*, group A *Streptococcus*, *Streptococcus pnemoniae*, *H influenzae* | Second-generation cephalosporin |
| Child 5 years to adolescence | *S aureus* | Oxacillin |
| Adolescence to adults | *N gonorrhoeae*, *S aureus* | Ceftriaxone (third-generation cephalosporin) |
| Older adults | *S aureus* | Oxacillin or cefazolin, aminoglycoside |

# TREATMENT

Antibiotics also must be started immediately, beginning with broad-spectrum coverage based on age-related factors until culture and sensitivity results are known (**Table 1**). Surgical decompression and drainage by arthroscopic or open arthrotomy should be considered at presentation with either a severely involved joint or for all cases of hip joint infection (to prevent osteonecrosis). Surgical drainage also should be considered in patients who do not demonstrate a clinical response to antibiotic therapy in 24 to 48 hours.

# ADVERSE OUTCOMES OF TREATMENT

Allergic reactions or adverse drug interactions related to antibiotics can occur. Strict aseptic technique must be followed in aspiration of joints to avoid additional contamination or joint injury.

# REFERRAL DECISIONS/RED FLAGS

Acute septic arthritis requires emergent antibiotic treatment and consideration of surgical drainage. Patients with chronic septic arthritis may require evaluation by an infectious disease specialist.

# SERONEGATIVE SPONDYLOARTHROPATHIES

## ICD-9 Codes

**696.0**
Psoriatic arthropathy

**711.1**
Arthropathy associated with Reiter disease and nonspecific urethritis

**713.1**
Arthropathy associated with gastrointestinal conditions other than infections

**720.0**
Ankylosing spondylitis

## SYNONYMS

Ankylosing spondylitis
Arthritis of inflammatory bowel disease
Psoriatic arthritis
Reiter disease

## DEFINITION

The seronegative spondyloarthropathies are a group of arthritides that have common clinical and genetic features. The genetic factor is an association with the HLA-B27 antigen. The associated clinical features include involvement of the spine and sacroiliac joints, oligoarticular peripheral joint arthritis, enthesitis (inflammation at sites of tendon and ligament insertion into bone), and unique eye, skin, and intestinal manifestations. The seronegative spondyloarthropathies are not associated with rheumatoid factor or antinuclear antibodies.

### Ankylosing Spondylitis

Ankylosing spondylitis affects 1 in every 2,000 persons. In the past, ankylosing spondylitis was thought to primarily affect men, but studies now indicate a more equivalent gender ratio, but with milder disease in women. Ankylosing spondylitis particularly involves the sacroiliac joints and the spine (**Figure 1**). Involvement of peripheral joints correlates with the severity of the disease but typically is less than that observed in the other seronegative spondyloarthropathies. The association with the HLA-B27 antigen is high, particularly in white patients, who have an HLA-B27–positive rate of approximately 95%. Uveitis, carditis, or enthesitis may occur.

### Reiter Disease

Reiter disease is a seronegative arthritis that develops after urethritis, cervicitis, or dysentery. It is considered to be a reactive arthritis that is typically an asymmetric oligoarthritis of the lower extremities that starts 2 to 8 weeks after an infection. Other musculoskeletal manifestations include enthesitis of the Achilles tendon or plantar fascia, dactylitis ("sausage digit" with swelling of an entire toe or finger), and sacroiliitis. Conjunctivitis commonly develops. Other associated lesions include iritis and cutaneous manifestations such as balanitis circinata and keratoderma blennorrhagica. Chronic, recurrent episodes of arthritis are most common, but some patients have no recurrence of joint problems while others have unremitting arthritis.

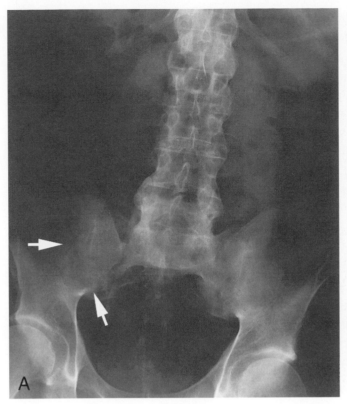 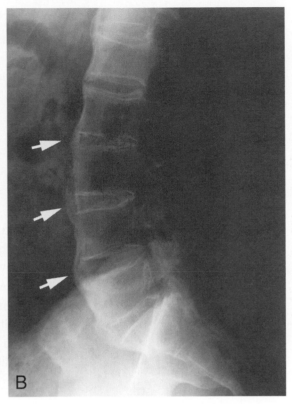

**Figure 1**
**A,** AP radiograph of the pelvis demonstrating advanced sacroiliitis (which is associated with seronegative spondyloarthropathies) with narrowing of the joint, sclerosis, and spurring (arrows). **B,** Lateral radiograph of the lumbar spine demonstrating bridging syndesmophytes (arrows), seen in ankylosing spondylitis.

## Psoriatic Arthritis

Psoriatic arthritis affects approximately 5% to 10% of patients who have psoriasis. The gender ratio is approximately equal. Skin disease usually, but not always, precedes joint symptoms. Patients with joint problems have a high association of nail disorders, including pitting, ridging, and oncolysis (**Figure 2**). Iritis may develop.

## Arthritis Associated With Inflammatory Bowel Disease

Arthritis associated with inflammatory bowel disease occurs in patients with ulcerative colitis or Crohn disease. The incidence is 10% to 20% and is more common in patients with Crohn disease. In those who develop arthritis, the HLA-B27 incidence is 50% to 70%. Sacroiliitis, spondylitis, and arthritis of the knee and ankle are common. The peripheral arthritis usually parallels the course of the bowel disease, but the severity of the spondylitis bears no relation to the activity of the bowel disorder.

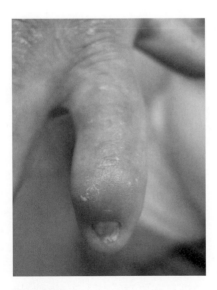

**Figure 2**
Finger of patient with psoriatic arthritis. Note the pitting, ridging, and oncolysis of the nail.

# CLINICAL SYMPTOMS

Back pain may be the presenting complaint, particularly in young men with ankylosing spondylitis. Stiffness may be worse in the morning, with patients needing up to 30 minutes to "warm up" on arising. Enthesitis is common, particularly at the Achilles tendon insertion and origin of the plantar fascia (heel pain). Extraskeletal manifestations such as iritis, conjunctivitis, and urethritis may occur.

# TESTS

## Physical Examination

With spondylitis, limited spinal motion is common. The FABER maneuver (flexion, abduction, and external rotation of the hip) will place stress across the sacroiliac joint, and patients with sacroiliitis will have increased pain. Examine the patient for enthesitis (inflammation of the tendon insertion, evidenced by swelling and restricted motion), particularly of the lower extremity joints, and abnormalities of the digits and nails.

## Diagnostic Tests

Although HLA-B27 antigen is positive in many of these patients, this relatively expensive test usually is not needed to make the diagnosis. A detailed history and examination are more important. In patients with sacroiliitis, radiographs demonstrating narrowing of the sacroiliac joints can be helpful (Figure 1). With spondylitis, early radiographic findings in the spine include squaring of the superior and anterior margins of the vertebral bodies, thought to be caused by enthesitis at the attachment of the anulus fibrosus (ligament surrounding the disk) into the vertebral body. Later findings include ossification of the anterior longitudinal ligament of the spine and autofusion of the facet joints leading to the classic "poker spine," which may be fused along the entire length of the spine.

# DIFFERENTIAL DIAGNOSIS

Degenerative disk disease (no associated symptoms, normal skin distraction on flexion of the spine)

Localized Achilles tendinitis or plantar fasciitis (no associated symptoms)

Rheumatoid arthritis (positive rheumatoid factor, peripheral joint involvement)

## ADVERSE OUTCOMES OF THE DISEASE

Severe spinal deformity may occur in ankylosing spondylitis. End-stage arthritis may affect the peripheral joints. Uveitis with visual impairment may occur. Occasionally, carditis may cause aortic insufficiency in patients with ankylosing spondylitis.

## TREATMENT

NSAIDs, particularly indomethacin, are effective in controlling symptoms in many patients. Tetracycline is appropriate for suspected *Chlamydia* infections associated with Reiter disease. Topical treatment of psoriatic skin lesions is important. Methotrexate has been used with success for both skin and joint lesions in psoriatic arthritis. Methotrexate also may be useful for severe Reiter disease. Regular exercise is important, particularly for patients with ankylosing spondylitis. Surgery (total joint replacement) can provide relief of end-stage arthritic pain. An occasional patient may require a spinal osteotomy for correction of deformity associated with ankylosing spondylitis.

## ADVERSE OUTCOMES OF TREATMENT

Postoperative infection and/or loosening of total joint implants following surgery is possible, while heterotopic ossification can complicate total hip arthroplasty. NSAIDs can cause gastric, renal, or hepatic complications.

## REFERRAL DECISIONS/RED FLAGS

Patients with kyphosis, pain at rest, or pain at night in a weight-bearing joint need further evaluation. Accompanying problems with the eyes, skin, or pulmonary system may require additional attention.

SECTION 1 ■ GENERAL ORTHOPAEDICS

# SPLINTING PRINCIPLES

Splinting of fractures, dislocations, or tendon ruptures often is required as part of initial emergency management. A well-applied splint reduces pain, bleeding, and swelling by immobilizing the injured part. Splinting also helps prevent a number of problems:

- Further damage of muscles, nerves (including the spinal cord), and blood vessels by the sharp ends of fractured bones
- Laceration of the skin by sharp fracture ends
- Constriction of vascular structures by malaligned bone ends
- Further contamination of an open wound

## GENERAL PRINCIPLES OF SPLINTING

1. Remove clothing from the area of any suspected fracture or dislocation to inspect the extremity for open wounds, deformity, swelling, and ecchymosis.
2. Note and record the pulse and capillary refill and neurologic status distal to the site of injury.
3. Cover all wounds with a dry, sterile dressing before applying a splint. If further evaluation is necessary, notify the receiving physician of all open wounds.
4. Ensure that the splint immobilizes the joints above and below the suspected fracture.
5. With injuries in and around the joint, ensure that the splint immobilizes the bones above and below the injured joint.
6. Pad all rigid splints to prevent local pressure.
7. During application of the splint, use your hands to minimize movement of the limb and to support the injury site until the splint has set and the limb is completely immobilized.
8. Align a severely deformed limb with constant gentle manual traction so that it can be incorporated into a splint.
9. If you encounter resistance to limb alignment when you apply traction, splint the limb in the position of deformity.
10. When in doubt, splint.

## MATERIALS

Although prefabricated plastic, fabric, or metal splints are available, they generally are unsatisfactory except for very brief periods of emergency treatment. If a splint is expected to be effective and to remain in place for more than a few hours, custom application of a well-padded plaster or fiberglass splint is preferred. Plaster is cheaper, but fiberglass is lighter, stays cleaner, and is more durable. Caution: Many-layered "homemade" splints or thick commercial plaster splints can generate enough heat to burn the patient during application. See **Table 1** for the materials needed for splinting. Store these materials in a dry cabinet or closet.

**Table 1   Splinting Materials**

| Thumb/Finger | Wrist and Forearm | Arm |
|---|---|---|
| 1 to 2 rolls 4″ cast padding (adults) or 3″ cast padding (children) | 2 rolls 4″ cast padding (adults) or 3″ cast padding (children) | 2 or 3 rolls 4″ cast padding (adults) or 3″ cast padding (children) |
| 4″ x 15″ splints, six thicknesses (adults), or 3″ roll folded into splint of appropriate length (children) | 5″ x 30″ splints, six thicknesses (adults), for "sugar tong"; or 4″ x 15″ splints, six thicknesses (children), for simple dorsal or volar splint | 5″ x 30″ splints, six thicknesses (adults), or 4″ roll folded to necessary length (children) |
| 2″ or 3″ elastic bandage | 2″ or 3″ elastic bandage | 3″ or 4″ elastic bandage |
| Tepid water (≈24°C) | Tepid water (≈24°C) | Tepid water (≈24°C) |
| Nonsterile gloves | Nonsterile gloves | Nonsterile gloves |

| Long leg splint | Short leg splint |
|---|---|
| 3 to 4 rolls 6″ cast padding | 2 rolls 4″ to 5″ cast padding |
| 3 to 4 rolls 5″ or 6″ wide plaster or 5″ x 45″ plaster splints | 12 to 14 thicknesses of 5″ x 30″ or 5″ x 45″ plaster strips |
| One roll each of 4″ and 6″ elastic bandages | One 3″ to 4″ wide roll of plaster |
| One bucket of tepid water (≈24°C) | One roll 4″ elastic bandage |
| Nonsterile gloves | One bucket of tepid water (≈24°C) |
| | Nonsterile gloves |

*Sidebar (vertical):* SECTION 1 ■ GENERAL ORTHOPAEDICS

# SPLINTING THE UPPER EXTREMITY
## *Fractures or Injuries of the Hand or Wrist*

1. Position the patient supine or sitting and have an assistant hold the patient's thumb and/or index fingers.

2. Loosely wrap cast padding from the palm to the elbow, making sure that there are three layers of padding at any bony prominence.

3. Place a 4″ x 15″ preassembled splint in the palm and carry it up the volar aspect of the forearm to just below the elbow (**Figure 1, A**).

4. If the injury involves the thumb, wrap it separately with 2″ or 3″ of cast padding. Place the splint on the volar or radial aspect and fold the plaster around the thumb, extending across the wrist to the proximal forearm. Leave the dorsal or ulnar side open for swelling (**Figure 1, B**).

5. Wrap the cast padding loosely over the plaster, then wrap an elastic bandage loosely over the cast padding as you mold the splint.

6. Trim the palmar portion of the splint back to the distal palmar flexion crease, proximal to the metacarpophalangeal (MP) joint.

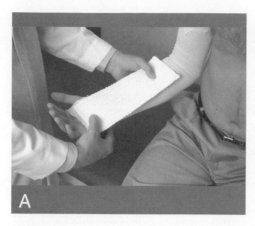
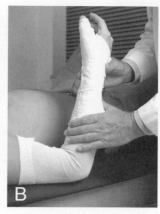

**Figure 1**

Splinting an injury of the hand or wrist. **A,** Begin in the palm and extend up the volar surface of the forearm to below the elbow. **B,** Apply the splint along the volar aspect of the thumb, extending across the wrist to the proximal forearm.

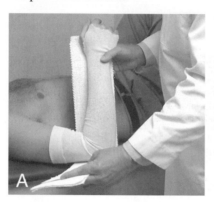
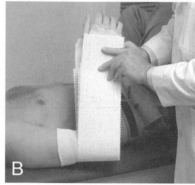

**Figure 2**

Splinting an injury of the elbow and forearm. **A,** Begin in the palm and extend proximally around the posterior elbow. **B,** Complete the splint distally on the extensor aspect of the forearm to the dorsum of the hand.

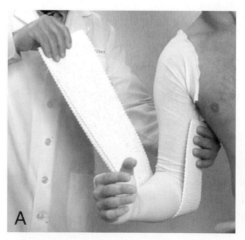
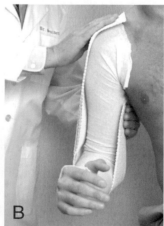

**Figure 3**

Splinting an injury of the humerus. **A,** Begin the splint below the axilla, extending it under the elbow, then up the lateral aspect of the arm. **B,** For unstable humeral fractures, continue the splint over the top of the shoulder.

## Fractures or Injuries of the Forearm and Elbow

1. With the patient sitting or supine, have an assistant support the patient's hand with the elbow flexed to 90°. If sitting, the patient should lean slightly to the affected side so that the elbow falls away from the body.

2. Loosely wrap cast padding from the palm to above the elbow, taking care to avoid creating a constriction in the antecubital fossa. Make sure that there are three layers of padding at any bony prominence, such as the wrist and elbow.

3. Begin the splint in the palm, carry it up the forearm to the elbow, around the posterior elbow, then distally on the extensor aspect of the forearm to the dorsum of the hand (sugar tong) (**Figure 2**). Use multiple 4″ x 15″ preassembled splints, or a 5″ x 30″ preassembled splint if that size is appropriate.

4. Wrap cast padding loosely over the plaster, then wrap an elastic bandage loosely over the cast padding as you mold the splint.

5. Trim the palmar portion of the splint back to the distal palmar flexion crease, proximal to the MP joint.

## Fractures or Injuries of the Humerus

1. With the patient sitting, have an assistant support the patient's hand with the elbow flexed to 90°. The patient should lean slightly to the affected side so that the elbow falls away from the body.

2. Loosely wrap cast padding from the palm to the upper arm. Begin the splint below the axilla, carry it under the elbow, then up the lateral aspect of the arm.

3. For unstable humeral fractures, continue the splint over the top of the shoulder, cover the plaster with a layer of cast padding, and then loosely wrap the entire arm with an elastic bandage (elephant ear splint) (**Figure 3**).

4. For lower humeral fractures or elbow injuries, end the splint below the lateral shoulder, cover the plaster with a layer of cast padding, and then loosely wrap the entire arm with an elastic bandage (coaptation splint). Provide the patient with a strap sling that loops around the wrist, then around the neck, and back to the wrist (**Figure 4**). The sling should be long enough to allow the elbow to be maintained at 90°.

5. Ensure that the sling has padding at the neck and wrist; these straps do not slide at night and can be adjusted for different arm lengths.

# PATIENT INSTRUCTIONS

Patients should be advised to protect the splint for 24 hours, until the plaster cures and hardens (fiberglass splints harden faster than plaster splints). A splinted arm should not be placed on any plastic-covered surfaces (including pillows) until the plaster has cooled. Patients also should be reminded to watch for changes in skin color (circulation), sensation, and motion in the hand.

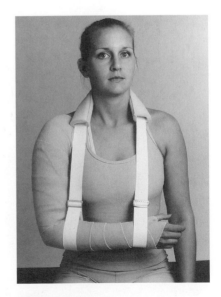

**Figure 4**
Proper positioning of a sling to maintain the elbow at 90°.

# SPLINTING THE LOWER EXTREMITY

## *Long Leg Splint*

1. For unstable fractures of the leg or ankle, a long leg splint with the knee flexed slightly (25° to 30°) and the ankle flexed 90° should be used.

2. The patient should be supine, with the buttock on the affected side at the edge of the table, allowing the entire leg to hang suspended as an assistant holds the patient's forefoot. Ask the patient to allow the heel to sink so that the foot will be maintained at 90° during splinting.

3. Use either a stirrup-type splint or a long posterior splint. For a stirrup splint, have an assistant hold the patient's forefoot as you wrap the leg with three layers of 6″ cast padding. Place extra padding over the kneecap and lateral knee (fibular head).

4. Begin the 5″ x 45″ plaster splint (10 to 12 thicknesses) on the lateral aspect of the thigh, extend it down the lateral aspect of the leg, under the heel, and then back up the medial side (**Figure 5, A**).

5. Start a second splint medially, and extend it beneath the foot and up the lateral side.

6. Apply a layer of cast padding over the plaster, and wrap a 5″ or 6″ elastic bandage over the padding as you mold the splint.

7. Ensure that the knee is positioned in slight flexion (approximately 25° to 30°) and the foot is positioned at 90° to the tibia (**Figure 5, B**).

Avoid folds in the plaster over the area of the peroneal nerve below the lateral knee (fibular head) or around the ankle. Preassembled foam padded splints are convenient, but use them with caution, as they may develop folds or ridges in critical areas.

Use tepid or cool—never hot—water when applying the splint. The heat generated by the reaction of the plaster, if

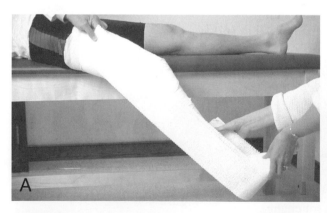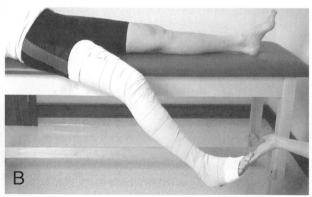

**Figure 5**

Long leg splint. **A**, Applying the splint. This is followed by a second splint and a layer of cast padding and then is wrapped with an elastic bandage. **B**, Maintain the knee in 25° to 30° of bend and the ankle at 90° as the splint hardens.

coupled with the use of hot water, can seriously burn the skin. For the same reason, place the leg on a cloth (not plastic) pillow and leave it uncovered for about 10 minutes following application to allow better convection of the heat.

Hold the splint in place with a loosely applied elastic bandage or bias-cut stockinet, rolled on with almost no tension. As the splint hardens, maintain the ankle at 90°. Mold or support the splint with the flat of the hand—only while it hardens—to avoid causing dents. Dents not only make the splint uncomfortable, but can cause cast sores or peroneal nerve palsy and foot drop.

## Short Leg Splint

1. With the patient sitting, have an assistant hold the forefoot to maintain the ankle at 90°. Wrap the foot, ankle, and leg loosely with three thicknesses of cast padding.

2. Use either 5″ × 45″ cast padding or fashion a splint with 4″ or 5″ rolls folded to length.

3. Begin the splint laterally, three fingerbreadths below the knee flexion crease, and extend it down and wrap it under the heel and then up the medial side of the leg (**Figure 6, A**).

4. Apply the splint like a stirrup, extending material under the foot, covering the heel and arch.

5. Place a single layer of cast padding over the splint, and loosely wrap a 4″ elastic bandage to secure the splint as you mold it to the extremity.

6. Maintain the ankle at 90° as the splint hardens (**Figure 6, B**).

7. An additional splint may be placed posteriorly if needed. Leave the plaster open in front and/or back for swelling, so the patient can unwrap the elastic bandage and spread the splint if needed.

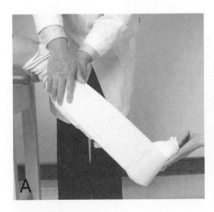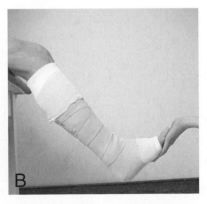

**Figure 6**

Short leg splint. **A**, Begin the splint laterally, three fingerbreadths below the knee flexion crease, and extend it down and wrap it under the heel and then up the medial side of the leg. **B**, Maintain the angle of the ankle at 90° as the splint hardens.

# PATIENT INSTRUCTIONS

Patients should be advised to keep their injured leg elevated to the level of their heart as much as possible. Sitting in a reclining chair with a pillow beneath the leg is useful for this. In addition, ice bags should be kept on the injured leg intermittently for the next 2 to 3 days to reduce pain and minimize swelling.

If the pain becomes a lot worse, the foot begins to feel numb or like it is "going to sleep," or the patient cannot move his or her toes up and down, the splint should be loosened by unwrapping the elastic bandage and tearing the padding down the front of the leg. If the leg does not feel better in 20 to 30 minutes, the patient should be advised to call the doctor because problems with circulation to the leg may be developing, which can have serious consequences.

The splint must be kept dry. To bathe, patients should be advised to place a plastic bag or commercially available cast cover over their leg, prop their leg on the side of the tub, and fill the tub around them, keeping the splinted leg out of the water. They should not shower.

Patients should be advised to contact the physician if they notice any places where the splint feels as though it is chafing or digging into the skin. Patients also should be reminded to watch for changes in skin color (circulation), sensation, and motion in the foot.

# ADVERSE OUTCOMES OF TREATMENT

Compartment syndrome, burns, nerve compression injuries, and pressure sores can occur in splinted upper or lower extremities. Plantar flexion contractures of the ankle can develop if the ankle is splinted for prolonged periods with the ankle plantar flexed beyond the neutral position.

# Sports Medicine Principles

## Definition

The term "sports medicine" means different things to different people. A general definition is the application of professional training to the understanding, prevention, care, and rehabilitation of sports-related problems. This necessarily makes sports medicine a multidisciplinary field that encompasses other disciplines, such as physical therapy, athletic training, and exercise physiology. Thus, all areas of general and specialized primary care and internal medicine, as well as all surgical specialties, have legitimate roles in the management of sports-related problems.

Being a team physician involves coordination of preparticipation physical evaluations; determining readiness for participation; ensuring medical coverage of high-risk practices and competitions; arranging regular visits to the training room to evaluate and monitor problems; arranging appropriate referrals; communicating with parents, coaches, and administrators; and ensuring that adequate records are kept.

The fact that these patients are athletes on teams does not change their status as patients, and physicians providing their care must keep the best interests of the athlete-patient in mind, regardless of the relationship with the team.

## General Issues of Importance in Sports Medicine

- If you are responsible for covering sports practices and games, create an emergency response plan and make it available to the entire athletic and sports medicine staff. Make certain an individual who is qualified to administer CPR and first aid is available at all practices and games. The emergency plan needs to address such issues as who calls 911 in an emergency, who attends the athlete, where the emergency response equipment is kept, what equipment is available, etc.

- Know and appreciate the importance of sports and/or fitness participation to athlete-patients. Communicate your understanding and commitment to helping them return to participation as effectively and safely as possible.

- Competitive athletes and serious fitness participants need a prompt diagnosis and treatment plan; they also need to know the prognosis. If they are part of a team, all concerned must understand these issues and the anticipated lost playing time as soon as possible so appropriate team planning can be initiated. Parents need to know this information for their peace of mind.

- Communication plays a critical role. Prompt, authoritative, and efficient communication among parents, coaches, trainers, and involved colleagues is essential. Telephone calls can be notoriously inefficient. An immediately available sports injury report form with multiple copies can be a big help.

- Personal coverage of competitions is optimal for team physicians but is not always feasible. When not physically present, a team physician needs to be available for timely communication with coaches, trainers, parents, or athletes.

- Provide a team approach to the care of the athlete. Coordinated involvement of all concerned with the athlete and the team (athletes, parents, coaches, trainers, colleagues, and therapists) optimizes outcomes.

- Recognize public interest in the status of injured athletes. Treating physicians frequently are approached by the media for information about prominent athletes who are injured. It is important to protect physician-patient confidentiality. A practical, successful approach is to prepare a brief factual statement that includes no details that should remain confidential. This statement can be released upon request, with the proviso that any additional information has to come from the team or the athlete.

- Many more nonsurgical illnesses and injuries are encountered than surgical. Nonsurgical treatment does not mean no treatment. Aggressive nonsurgical treatment is the mainstay of sports medicine.

- Sports-oriented physical therapy plays a critical role by providing an understanding of the extent of recovery required to return safely and effectively to competitive sports. Many of these needs apply to virtually all sports and fitness activities, but many others are sport-specific, and some are also position-specific. Traditional physical therapy rarely provides adequate or timely rehabilitation for an in-season or preseason competitive athlete.

## CLINICAL SYMPTOMS

Symptoms are exactly the same for athletes as for nonathletes in situations of sprains/strains, tendinitis, or fractures. Certain injuries are somewhat specific to athletics, such as turf toe or myositis ossificans. Shoulder and elbow tendinitis in baseball players and tennis players is another example.

## TESTS

Physical examination and appropriate radiographs are needed, as indicated for the specific situation.

# Treatment

Sports-oriented rehabilitation includes four phases: initial, functional, sport-specific, and graduated return to play. It is essential that the injured structures be protected to the extent necessary and that the injury not be aggravated. The principles of rest, ice, compression, and elevation (RICE) should be followed. Pain control modalities and electrical stimulation also can be helpful. Joint range of motion; muscle flexibility, strengthening, and endurance; and apparatus-based functional and aerobic activities are initiated as tolerated. It is not possible to make injuries heal faster, but the healing process should not be impaired. Athletes and serious fitness participants can maintain their aerobic fitness by doing other activities that do not aggravate or jeopardize the injury.

Functional rehabilitation begins when the healing status is appropriate and when joint motion, muscle flexibility, strength, and endurance are adequate. The program should be disciplined and independent and should emphasize normal form. A gradual running program is initiated for lower extremity problems. It should begin with straight-line running, progressing from jogging to half speed to three-quarter speed to sprinting as tolerated. Agility drills are then added, starting at half speed and progressing to three-quarter speed and to full speed as tolerated. Jumping activities are added last.

For upper extremity and spine injuries, individual programs that apply general and sport-specific principles should be used. Once a general functional program has been successfully completed, sport-specific and position-specific drills can be initiated.

Graduated return to play should include transition to increasing partial practice and then to full practice as tolerated. A helpful guideline is to require at least two full practices without restriction and without problems before returning to full competition. This helps the athlete, coaches, and family to know that the athlete is truly ready to return to competition effectively and safely.

# SPRAINS AND STRAINS

## DEFINITION

Sprains and strains are both injuries, but they differ in the tissue that is affected. A sprain involves the supporting structures of a joint and therefore is a stretching or tearing of a ligament or joint capsule. A strain involves muscle or, more precisely, the muscle-tendon unit. A strain is a stretching or partial tear of a muscle. A complete tear of a muscle or tendon typically is described as a rupture.

Sprains may occur in patients of any age, but they are much more common in older adolescents, young adults, and middle-aged adults. In children, the physis is the weak link, and similar forces or injuries result in a fracture of the growth plate. In older adults, the bone again is the weak link and similar injuries cause a fracture.

Strains likewise may occur in patients of any age but are more common in middle-aged and older adults. With aging, the collagen in a muscle-tendon unit changes. As a result, muscles have decreased elasticity and are more susceptible to injury.

## CLINICAL SYMPTOMS

Sprains usually are a result of sudden trauma, such as a fall causing an inversion stress to the ankle resulting in tearing of the lateral ligaments of the ankle. Patients often report a pop or snap at the time of the acute event, followed by pain, swelling, stiffness, and difficulty bearing weight. Ecchymosis can appear within 24 to 48 hours.

Strains and muscle ruptures commonly result from a sudden stretch on a muscle that is actively contracting. For example, a strain or rupture of the quadriceps muscle commonly occurs when a person falls and lands with the knee flexed and the quadriceps contracting to absorb the energy of the fall. Severe strains also are associated with a snap or tearing sensation; however, pain and swelling with a mild strain may not be noted on the day of injury.

## TESTS

### Physical Examination

Swelling, tenderness, and ecchymosis at the site of the torn ligament or capsule usually are seen early and persist until healing is well underway in joints that are superficial. Swelling, tenderness, and ecchymosis are not as well defined with muscle injuries or with sprains of joints that are deep and covered by muscles.

Palpate the injured area for the site of maximal tenderness. This leads to or narrows the diagnostic possibilities. Gently place the injured structure on stretch. This increases the pain and provides additional information concerning what structure has been injured. For example, for a patient who has tenderness over the medial aspect of the proximal tibia after a fall, gently stress the knee into valgus. If the pain is increased with a valgus stress and the radiographs are negative for a fracture, then the patient has a sprain of the medial collateral ligament of the knee. Likewise, the diagnostic test for a patient who reports acute pain in the posterior thigh while running is to position the limb so that the hamstring muscles are put on stretch (flex the hip to 90° and then extend the knee).

With a sprain, the degree of injury and stability of the joint should be assessed. This assessment is not always precise, particularly if the patient has marked swelling and tenderness. Some ligamentous injuries require unique clinical maneuvers to determine injury and instability. When possible, however, classifying sprains provides useful information concerning the degree of disability and requirements for treatment (**Table 1**). For example, a grade I sprain is a partial tear of the ligament.

With a muscle injury, it is important to distinguish a strain from a complete rupture. The latter sometimes requires surgical repair. If the patient can move the joint, that is suggestive evidence of a strain. For example, a patient with a strain of the quadriceps muscle can hold the knee extended, but with a complete rupture of the quadriceps tendon, the patient is unable to straighten the knee. Pain and resultant inhibition of muscle contraction sometimes make this clinical test imprecise.

## Diagnostic Tests

Radiographs are helpful only in the negative sense. Thus, they should be obtained only if a fracture is suspected. The Ottawa

**Table 1   Classification of Sprains**

| Grade | Degree of Injury | Treatment Principles |
|-------|------------------|----------------------|
| I | Partial tear but no instability, or opening of the joint on stress maneuvers | Symptomatic treatment only |
| II | Partial tear with some instability indicated by partial opening of joint on stress maneuvers | Immobilization to protect injured part, but full healing expected |
| III | Complete tear with complete opening joint on stress | Immobilization or possibly repair |

guidelines are useful in patients with suspected foot or ankle sprain. These guidelines delineate that radiographs of the ankle are necessary only if there is pain near the malleoli or if either of the following findings are present: inability to bear weight (four steps) both immediately and in the emergency department; or bony tenderness at the posterior edge or tip of the malleoli. Similarly, radiographs of the foot are necessary only if there is midfoot pain and either of the following conditions: inability to bear weight (four steps) both immediately and in the emergency department; or bony tenderness at the navicular or the base of the fifth metatarsal.

## DIFFERENTIAL DIAGNOSIS

Fracture (evident on radiographs)
Soft-tissue contusion

## ADVERSE OUTCOMES OF THE DISEASE

The tissue damaged as a result of a sprain might not heal, resulting in a chronic condition, such as chronic ankle instability. Prolonged weakness, tightness, and tenderness can follow a muscle strain or tear. Complex regional pain syndrome (CRPS) can develop after a seemingly minor strain or sprain. Compartment syndrome occasionally occurs.

## TREATMENT

Rest, ice, compression, and elevation (RICE) are the mainstays of treatment. Heat can be helpful later, but ice should be used initially. NSAIDs are useful for the first few days. Grade I sprains need immobilization only for comfort. Grade II and III sprains should be protected. Most grade III sprains can be treated nonsurgically, but certain injuries require surgical repair.

## ADVERSE OUTCOMES OF TREATMENT

Overemphasis on treatment in the suggestible patient can lead to chronic impairment and disability, particularly in workers' compensation situations.

## REFERRAL DECISIONS/RED FLAGS

Patients with grade III sprains, severe grade II sprains, or complete muscle-tendon ruptures require further evaluation. Patients whose symptoms are out of proportion to their injury and findings can be at risk for chronic conditions or CRPS, and a second opinion should be sought early. Equivocal radiographs should be repeated in these cases.

# TUMORS OF BONE

## SYNONYMS
Bone cancer
Bone lesion
Malignancy
Neoplasm

**ICD-9 Code**
**238.0**
Neoplasm of uncertain behavior of other and unspecified sites and tissues, bone and articular cartilage

## DEFINITION
Bone tumors are classified as either benign or malignant. Benign tumors of bone and bone cysts are relatively common, but primary malignant tumors of bone are rare. Bone, however, is a common site for metastasis, and any malignant lesion of bone in a patient older than age 40 years must be considered as a possible skeletal metastasis.

Bone tumors also are classified by their tissue of origin: benign and malignant tumors can develop from cartilage, bone, fibrous tissue, and marrow elements.

Age is an important factor in predicting the type of bone tumor. Gender, history of trauma, and site are of limited or no diagnostic benefit (**Table 1**).

SECTION 1 ■ GENERAL ORTHOPAEDICS

## Table 1 Bone Tumors and Tumor-like Conditions by Age

| 1 to 5 years | 6 to 18 years | 19 to 40 years | 40+ years |
| --- | --- | --- | --- |
| Osteomyelitis | Simple bone cyst | Ewing sarcoma | Metastases |
| Metastatic neuroblastoma | Aneurysmal bone cyst | Giant cell tumor | Multiple myeloma |
| Leukemia | Nonossifying fibroma | Osteosarcoma | Chondrosarcoma |
| Eosinophilic granuloma | Ewing sarcoma | | Fibrosarcoma |
| Simple bone cyst | Osteomyelitis | | Malignant fibrous histiocytoma |
| | Osteosarcoma | | Chordoma |
| | Enchondroma | | |
| | Chondroblastoma | | |
| | Chondromyxoid fibroma | | |
| | Osteoblastoma | | |
| | Fibrous dysplasia | | |
| | Osteofibrous dysplasia | | |

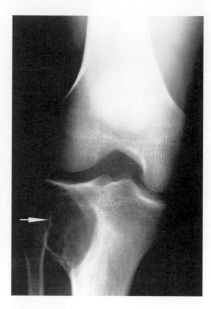

**Figure 1**

Lytic tumor destroying bone of proximal lateral tibia.

Reproduced from Kasser JR (ed): *Orthopaedic Knowledge Update 5. Rosemont, IL, American Academy of Orthopaedic Surgeons, 1996,* pp 133-48.

# CLINICAL SYMPTOMS

Pain is the usual presenting complaint. Malignant tumors are associated with a constant, deep aching pain that does not go away with rest and is present at night. However, certain benign tumors also cause night pain. This is particularly true of osteoid osteoma, but it also occurs with benign tumors that are relatively large and have weakened the bone. A sudden increase in pain following trivial trauma that was preceded by a history of mild, dull, aching pain suggests a pathologic fracture.

The presence of a mass also may be the presenting complaint. If the mass is painless, it is most likely benign. Bony tumors may press on adjacent nerves and cause radicular symptoms. The size and locations of some tumors interfere with joint and muscle function.

Ask about fever, malaise, weakness, weight loss, and other constitutional symptoms that are more common with malignant tumors, particularly Ewing sarcoma, primary tumors of bone that have metastasized, and secondary skeletal metastasis.

# TESTS

## *Physical Examination*

Physical examination should focus on identifying masses, sites of tenderness, reduced range of motion, a limp, and regional adenopathy. In patients older than age 40 years, careful examination of other systems, particularly the lungs, breasts, prostate, kidneys, and thyroid, should be done to rule out a metastatic carcinoma.

## *Diagnostic Tests*

AP, lateral, and oblique radiographs usually identify the location of the lesion. Associated findings can include the following: the characteristics of the borders of the lesion (well circumscribed or not well delineated); periosteal elevation and reactive bone formation adjacent to the lesion; the presence of calcification within the lesion; and whether the lesion is eccentric or central and lytic or blastic. These factors help to distinguish the lesion and, most importantly, whether the mass is benign or malignant (**Figure 1**).

The goal in staging a bone neoplasm is to determine the extent of the disease before performing a biopsy and initiating definitive treatment. CT is excellent for demonstrating bony changes and degree of calcification within the lesion and, therefore, is often better for benign bony lesions (**Figure 2**). MRI is better for malignant tumors because of its superiority in defining extension of the lesion through the medullary canal and into the surrounding muscle compartments. Bone scans are

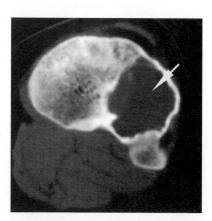

**Figure 2**

CT scan of tumor shown in Figure 1.

Reproduced from Kasser JR (ed): *Orthopaedic Knowledge Update 5. Rosemont, IL, American Academy of Orthopaedic Surgeons, 1996,* pp 133-48.

helpful in identifying the presence or absence of other skeletal lesions. If a malignant tumor is suspected, a chest radiograph, bone scan, and usually CT of the chest also should be obtained.

Routine laboratory tests are of limited value in the diagnosis of many bone tumors, but with certain tumors they can help to narrow the differential diagnosis. With suspected malignant tumors, laboratory studies can provide baseline values for patients who need chemotherapy. The following laboratory studies usually are obtained: CBC with differential, erythrocyte sedimentation rate, C-reactive protein, serum electrolytes, blood urea nitrogen, creatinine, calcium, phosphorus, and alkaline phosphatase. Tests for patients age 40 years and older include the following additional studies: urinalysis, urine and serum protein electrophoresis, and prostate specific antigen (PSA) for men.

A biopsy is performed to determine if the lesion is benign or malignant, to determine the cell type of lesion, and to determine the grade of the lesion. The biopsy should be performed by a surgeon who has the training to perform the definitive surgical procedure.

# DIFFERENTIAL DIAGNOSIS (PARTIAL LIST)

## Benign Cartilaginous

Chondroblastoma (age 8 to skeletal maturity, rare, located in epiphysis)

Chondromyxoid fibroma (adolescents, eccentric, metaphyseal, tibia)

Enchondroma (young adults, phalanges and metacarpals, speckled calcification)

Osteochondroma (children and teenagers, cartilaginous cap on bony stalk)

## Benign Bony

Osteoblastoma (children, young adults, rare, spine)

Osteoid osteoma (children and teenagers, night pain relieved by NSAIDs, small size)

## Benign Marrow Elements

Eosinophilic granuloma (young children, "hole in a bone")

## Benign Fbrous Tissue

Fibrous dysplasia (age 6 years to maturity, diaphyseal, bone deformity, limb shortening)

Nonossifying fibroma (children and teenagers, eccentric metaphyseal location)

### Benign With Tissue of Uncertain Origin

Aneurysmal bone cyst (children and teenagers, metaphyseal, expansile)

Giant cell tumor (young adults, epiphysis and metaphysis, eccentric and lytic)

Simple bone cyst (children and teenagers, metaphyseal, lytic)

### Malignant Cartilaginous, Bony, and Fibrous Tissue Origin

Chondrosarcoma (age over 40 years, central metaphyseal location, calcification)

Fibrosarcoma/malignant fibrous histiocytoma (older adults, metaphyseal, lytic)

Osteosarcoma (second decade, metaphyseal, long bones, mixed blastic and lytic areas)

Secondary osteosarcoma (originates in Paget disease or irradiated bone)

### Malignant Tumors of Marrow Origin

Ewing sarcoma (second decade, may simulate osteomyelitis, lytic)

Leukemia (in young children may present as bone lesion in limbs or spine)

Lymphoma

Multiple myeloma or plasmacytoma (age over 40 years, spine and pelvis, lytic)

## ADVERSE OUTCOMES OF THE DISEASE

Pathologic fracture (minimal trauma, poor healing), disability, and even death are possible.

## TREATMENT

Observation is appropriate for benign bone tumors that are causing minimal symptoms, that are not likely to enlarge, and for which the diagnosis is clear on radiographs. Other benign bony tumors should be excised. Malignant lesions usually require surgery, often in conjunction with chemotherapy and radiation therapy.

## ADVERSE OUTCOMES OF TREATMENT

Disability, disfigurement, pathologic fracture, infection, failure of implant, nerve and vascular deficits, and death are possible and depend on the size and growth potential of the tumor.

# Referral Decisions/Red Flags

Suspicious bone or soft-tissue masses, unusual pain or night pain, constitutional symptoms in association with bone pain or lytic or blastic changes of bone, soft-tissue calcification, or periosteal reaction on radiography all require further evaluation.

Section 1 ■ General Orthopaedics

# TUMORS OF SOFT TISSUE

**ICD-9 Code**

**238.1**
Neoplasm of uncertain behavior of other and unspecified sites and tissues, connective and other soft tissue

## DEFINITION

Soft-tissue tumors of the extremities can be classified as benign or malignant. Benign soft-tissue tumors are much more common than malignant tumors (ratio of more than 100:1). Some benign lesions, such as ganglia, popliteal cysts, and epidermoid cysts, although classified as tumors, are not neoplastic but result from degenerative changes. Compared to bony tumors, malignant soft-tissue tumors cannot be clearly distinguished from benign lesions. For example, lipomas and hemangiomas can occur anywhere on the extremity or even on the trunk and may resemble malignant tumors. However, sarcomas arising in the soft tissue of the extremities are more likely with lesions that are at least 5 cm in diameter, fixed to the surrounding tissues, and deep to the fascia. Pain, however, is not a defining characteristic of malignant soft-tissue somatic tumors. All soft-tissue masses should be considered as neoplasms because failure to do so can have serious consequences. Although most musculoskeletal tumors are benign, the possibility of malignancy always should be considered.

## CLINICAL SYMPTOMS

Most soft-tissue tumors are asymptomatic, except for the presence of an enlarging mass. A much smaller mass will be discovered earlier in the hand or foot than around the pelvis or shoulder. Mild pain and tenderness may be present.

## TESTS

### Physical Examination

Inspect the limb for swelling and adherence of the surrounding structures. Palpate the lesion to determine size, discreetness, and texture. Benign lesions tend to be more discreet with well-defined margins, while malignant lesions can be less well defined. A lipoma has a rubbery consistency, while a fibroma is firm. Auscultation can yield the sound of a bruit or the to-and-fro murmur of an arteriovenous fistula. Cystic lesions may transilluminate, which distinguishes them from solid tumors.

### Diagnostic Tests

Routine laboratory studies are nonspecific. If a malignant lesion is possible, obtain a baseline CBC with differential, erythrocyte sedimentation rate, C-reactive protein, routine blood chemistries, and radiographs of the involved area. MRI is the best imaging study to define the extent and characteristics of a soft-tissue malignancy; however, a biopsy is often necessary to make a definitive diagnosis.

# DIFFERENTIAL DIAGNOSIS (PARTIAL LIST)

## Benign Tumors

Angiomyoma (middle-aged adults, lower limbs, small, subcutaneous)

Ganglia (children, teenagers, and young adults, degenerative lesions arising from joint capsule or tendon sheath, may transilluminate)

Giant cell tumor of tendon sheath (middle-aged adults, hand and foot, close proximity to the tendon sheath)

Hemangioma and vascular malformations (children and adolescents)

Lipoma (adults, most common soft-tissue tumor, lobular nature, rubbery consistency)

## Malignant Tumors

Angiosarcomas

Fibrosarcoma (young and middle-aged adults, subfascial)

Liposarcoma (young, middle-, and older-aged adults, subfascial)

Malignant fibrous histiocytoma (middle- and older-aged adults, often deep but may be superficial to fascia)

Nerve cell sarcomas

Rhabdomyosarcoma (children and teenagers, subfascial)

Synovial cell sarcoma (teenagers and young adults, small focal calcification)

# ADVERSE OUTCOMES OF THE DISEASE

Continued growth, discomfort, and impaired function due to location of the mass or patient concerns about the identification of the mass may necessitate removal. Malignant soft-tissue tumors have a variable prognosis depending on several factors, but loss of limb or even death can be the end result.

# TREATMENT

If the diagnosis is reasonably certain, many benign soft-tissue tumors can be observed for signs of growth, change in character, or interference with function. Patients, however, are often uncomfortable with this approach and prefer biopsy and, if indicated, surgical excision. For malignant lesions, surgical excision, in conjunction with chemotherapy, radiation, or immunotherapy, is indicated, with a variable response depending on the patient's age, tumor type, duration, and location.

## ADVERSE OUTCOMES OF TREATMENT

Aside from injury to adjacent nerves or other structures and a cutaneous scar, few adverse effects are associated with excision of a small, benign tumor. Disfigurement, disability, loss of more vital neurovascular structures, and extensive scarring may be the consequence of the much more extensive surgery required for malignant lesions.

## REFERRAL DECISIONS/RED FLAGS

All but the smallest, clearly benign lesions in nonthreatened locations require further evaluation.

# PAIN DIAGRAM—SHOULDER

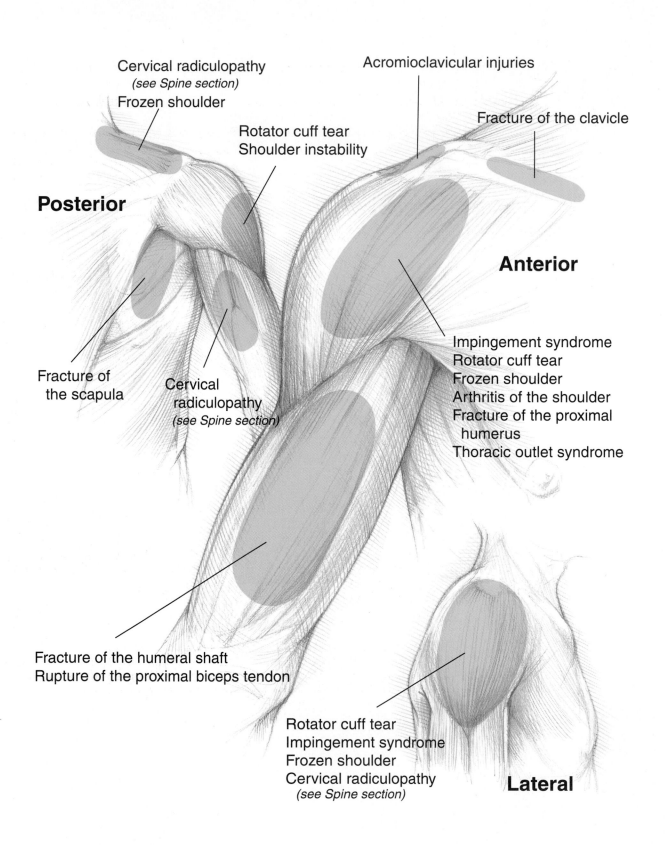

Cervical radiculopathy
*(see Spine section)*
Frozen shoulder

Acromioclavicular injuries

Fracture of the clavicle

Rotator cuff tear
Shoulder instability

**Posterior**

**Anterior**

Fracture of
the scapula

Cervical
radiculopathy
*(see Spine section)*

Impingement syndrome
Rotator cuff tear
Frozen shoulder
Arthritis of the shoulder
Fracture of the proximal
  humerus
Thoracic outlet syndrome

Fracture of the humeral shaft
Rupture of the proximal biceps tendon

Rotator cuff tear
Impingement syndrome
Frozen shoulder
Cervical radiculopathy
*(see Spine section)*

**Lateral**

# SHOULDER

**Section Editor**
James R. Andrews, MD
Medical Director
American Sports Medicine Institute
Birmingham, Alabama

Mark Davies, MD
Department of Orthopaedic Surgery
Kaiser Santa Teresa
San Jose, California

Robert Donatelli, PhD, PT, OCS
National Director of Sports Rehabilitation
Physiotherapy Associates
Las Vegas, Nevada

James A. Whiteside, MD
Professor of Sports Medicine
College of Health and Human Services
Troy University
Troy, Alabama

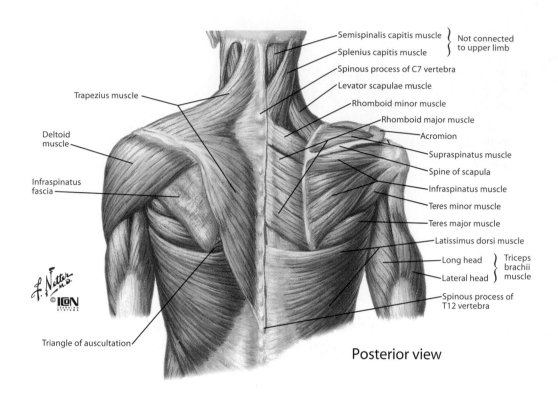

Semispinalis capitis muscle } Not connected to upper limb
Splenius capitis muscle
Spinous process of C7 vertebra
Levator scapulae muscle
Rhomboid minor muscle
Rhomboid major muscle
Acromion
Supraspinatus muscle
Spine of scapula
Infraspinatus muscle
Teres minor muscle
Teres major muscle
Latissimus dorsi muscle
Long head }
Lateral head } Triceps brachii muscle
Spinous process of T12 vertebra

Trapezius muscle
Deltoid muscle
Infraspinatus fascia
Triangle of auscultation

Posterior view

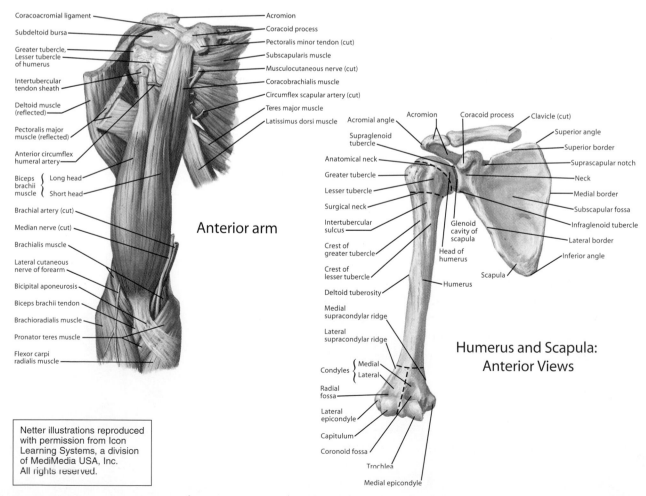

Coracoacromial ligament
Subdeltoid bursa
Greater tubercle, Lesser tubercle of humerus
Intertubercular tendon sheath
Deltoid muscle (reflected)
Pectoralis major muscle (reflected)
Anterior circumflex humeral artery
Biceps brachii muscle { Long head
Short head
Brachial artery (cut)
Median nerve (cut)
Brachialis muscle
Lateral cutaneous nerve of forearm
Bicipital aponeurosis
Biceps brachii tendon
Brachioradialis muscle
Pronator teres muscle
Flexor carpi radialis muscle

Acromion
Coracoid process
Pectoralis minor tendon (cut)
Subscapularis muscle
Musculocutaneous nerve (cut)
Coracobrachialis muscle
Circumflex scapular artery (cut)
Teres major muscle
Latissimus dorsi muscle

Anterior arm

Acromial angle
Acromion
Coracoid process
Clavicle (cut)
Supraglenoid tubercle
Superior angle
Superior border
Anatomical neck
Suprascapular notch
Greater tubercle
Neck
Lesser tubercle
Medial border
Surgical neck
Subscapular fossa
Intertubercular sulcus
Infraglenoid tubercle
Glenoid cavity of scapula
Lateral border
Crest of greater tubercle
Head of humerus
Inferior angle
Crest of lesser tubercle
Scapula
Deltoid tuberosity
Humerus
Medial supracondylar ridge
Lateral supracondylar ridge

Humerus and Scapula: Anterior Views

Condyles { Medial
Lateral
Radial fossa
Lateral epicondyle
Capitulum
Coronoid fossa
Trochlea
Medial epicondyle

# SHOULDER—OVERVIEW

This section of *Essentials of Musculoskeletal Care* focuses on the common conditions affecting the shoulder girdle in adults. These include acute injuries (fractures, dislocations, and acute tendon ruptures), chronic or repetitive injuries (impingement syndrome and most rotator cuff tears and biceps tendon ruptures), and degenerative, inflammatory, or idiopathic conditions (glenohumeral and acromioclavicular [AC] arthritis, frozen shoulder). Most shoulder disorders can be diagnosed from a careful history, a thorough physical examination, and plain radiographs.

A concise differential diagnosis often is achieved by evaluating the chief symptom in the context of its chronicity and the patient's age. The chief symptom is usually related to pain or instability. Decreased motion, power, or function sometimes accompanies pain or instability but only rarely is the chief symptom.

## PAIN

Patients with acute symptoms (less than 2 weeks' duration) usually have sustained an injury, such as a fracture or a dislocation, a rotator cuff tear, or a biceps tendon rupture. Common physical findings include local tenderness, deformity, swelling, and ecchymosis. Determining the mechanism and magnitude of the injury and the anatomic location of the symptoms helps in making the diagnosis. For example, a football player who has severe pain and deformity at the superior aspect of the shoulder after falling directly on that shoulder most likely has an AC joint separation.

Similarly, for patients with chronic shoulder pain, knowledge of the activities related to the onset of symptoms and the location and character of symptoms often leads to the correct diagnosis. Pain localized to the top of the shoulder suggests AC joint arthritis or chronic separation. This pain often is exacerbated by cross-body adduction in the horizontal plane. Pain from subacromial bursitis, frozen shoulder, or rotator cuff pathology is typically referred to the lateral deltoid region and may radiate to the lateral aspect of the upper arm. Overhead activities most commonly exacerbate this pain. In contrast, shoulder pain arising from cervical nerve root irritation usually follows a dermatomal distribution, is associated with numbness and/or tingling, and is often relieved by placing the forearm on top of the head. Degenerative arthritis of the glenohumeral joint may cause pain along the anterior and posterior joint lines.

Both rotator cuff tears and arthritis may cause night pain, which makes sleeping on the affected side difficult.

# INSTABILITY

Instability can be classified by the frequency of symptomatic episodes, as well as the direction and degree of instability. An acute injury may be a first-time dislocation or a recurrent episode. The instability episode may be partial (subluxation) with spontaneous reduction, or it may be complete (dislocation). The instability can be anterior, posterior, inferior, or multidirectional. Most traumatic dislocations are anterior. Multidirectional instability should be considered in patients who present with recurrent episodes of subluxations or dislocations and no history of significant trauma.

# RANGE OF MOTION, MUSCLE STRENGTH, AND FUNCTION

In assessing motion, it is important to determine if there is a discrepancy between active and passive motion. Patients with rotator cuff tears primarily lose active elevation and external rotation, although some loss of passive range of motion can occur secondary to disuse. Equal losses of active and passive range of motion may be secondary to soft-tissue contracture, as in frozen shoulder, or the result of joint incongruity from trauma or arthritis.

Muscle strength should be assessed and compared with the opposite shoulder. Tears of the rotator cuff and neurologic injury may produce weakness. Pain inhibition can affect the accuracy of muscle testing.

Functional status relates to a patient's ability to perform his or her normal activities. The level of functional disability depends on the specific type and intensity of activities the patient normally performs. Motivation and the ability to adapt to impairment also play a significant role.

# PATIENT AGE

## Younger Patients

Patients younger than 30 years most commonly present with traumatic injuries or instability such as glenohumeral dislocations and AC joint separations. Impingement syndrome and rotator cuff tears rarely occur in this age group.

### Middle-aged Patients

Impingement syndrome and rotator cuff tears are common in this group. These must be distinguished from the early onset of adhesive capsulitis, commonly known as frozen shoulder. Often it is difficult to distinguish between impingement syndrome and early adhesive capsulitis, and, adding to the confusion, the two diagnoses often coexist. Glenohumeral dislocations are much less common and must be treated with a high index of suspicion for a concomitant rotator cuff tear (50% of patients over 40 years of age will have an acute tear).

### Older Patients

Patients older than 50 years commonly have symptoms related to rotator cuff dysfunction and present as an impingement syndrome. Rotator cuff tears and degenerative arthritis of the AC joint, the glenohumeral joint, or both are also common in this group. Acute pain following a fall in an elderly, frail patient with osteoporosis most commonly indicates a fracture of the proximal humerus.

# RADIOGRAPHS

The standard trauma series starts with two good-quality radiographs of the shoulder taken orthogonally (at a 90° angle) to one another. A scapular Y view or axillary view is needed to assess the position of the humeral head in the glenoid. A transthoracic lateral is often added. In younger patients, an AP view of the shoulder in internal rotation can usually be obtained without too much patient discomfort.

SECTION 2 ■ SHOULDER

# PHYSICAL EXAMINATION SHOULDER

## INSPECTION/PALPATION

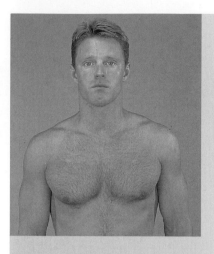

### Anterior view

Look for abnormal contours and bony prominences. An AC separation produces a "step-off" deformity with prominence of the distal clavicle. An anterior shoulder dislocation produces a prominent acromion and anterior fullness of the deltoid, and the arm typically is held in slight abduction and external rotation. By contrast, with a posterior dislocation, the coracoid and anterior acromion are prominent, there is posterior fullness, and the arm is held in adduction and internal rotation.

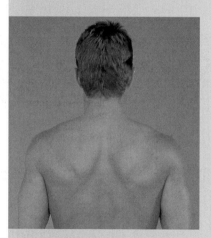

### Posterior view

Note symmetry of shoulder heights and contours (the dominant shoulder often rests slightly lower than the opposite shoulder). Look for muscle atrophy, particularly of the trapezius, deltoid, and supraspinatus/infraspinatus muscles. Diminished posterior contour from neck to shoulder indicates atrophy of the trapezius. With atrophy of the supraspinatus/infraspinatus muscles, loss of lateral shoulder contour occurs at the deltoid, and a prominent suprascapular ridge can be seen.

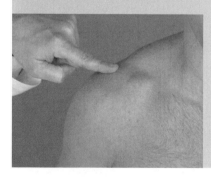

### AC joint

Palpate the end of the clavicle and the acromion for tenderness or spurs. Tenderness usually is most pronounced at the posterior joint interval and is exaggerated when the patient adducts the arm toward the opposite shoulder.

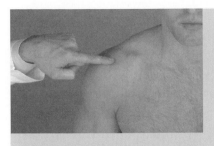

### Subacromial bursa

Palpate the anterolateral portion of the acromion, moving down toward the deltoid until you feel the acromiohumeral sulcus. Tenderness in this area usually is related to subacromial bursitis or a rotator cuff tear (supraspinatus tendon).

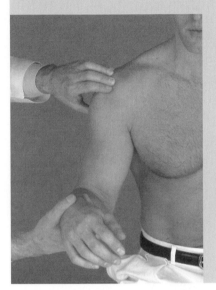

### Long head of the biceps tendon

Palpate over the humeral head in the region of the bicipital groove. With tendinitis, there is tenderness and swelling, and the area of tenderness should move with the humeral head as the shoulder is rotated.

## RANGE OF MOTION

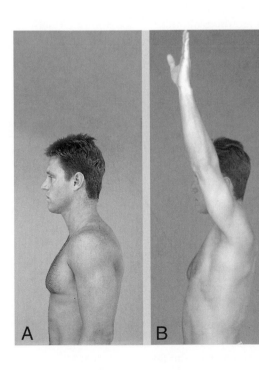

### Flexion: Zero Starting Position

The shoulder has greater mobility than any other joint in the body. Normal shoulder motion is a composite movement that couples glenohumeral motion with rotation of the scapula on the thorax. Shoulder motion also includes minor contributions from motion at the AC and sternoclavicular joints. Shoulder mobility is efficiently assessed by measuring four planes of motion.

The Zero Starting Position (**A**) is with the arm at the side of the body. Flexion, sometimes called elevation, is upward motion of the arm (**B**). Slight external rotation and abduction are required to reach maximal elevation. These accessory motions are permitted because maximal elevation correlates well with functional impairment. Ask the patient to raise the arm in the most comfortable plane, and then measure active and passive motion in reference to the trunk. Normal shoulder flexion is 160° to 180°.

SECTION 2 ■ SHOULDER

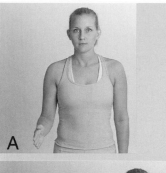

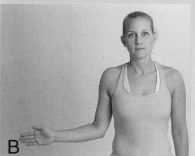

### External rotation, arm at the side

The Zero Starting Position (**A**) is with the arm held comfortably against the thorax, the elbow flexed to 90°, and the forearm parallel to the sagittal plane of the body. Measure external rotation by evaluating the maximum outward rotation of the arm (**B**). Restricted rotation in this position is often observed in patients with degenerative arthritis of the shoulder.

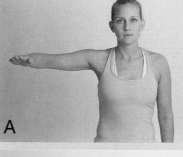

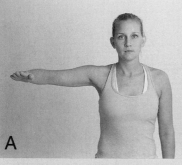

### External rotation, arm abducted 90°

The Zero Starting Position is with the arm abducted 90° and aligned with the plane of the scapula, the elbow flexed 90°, and the forearm parallel to the floor. Measure external rotation in this position by evaluating how many degrees the forearm moves away from the floor. Limited external rotation in this position is seen in some athletes who emphasize strengthening exercises without including an appropriate stretching program and in patients who have had reconstructive surgery of the shoulder.

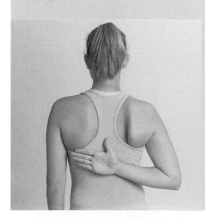

### Internal rotation

Internal rotation is measured by evaluating the patient's posterior reach, noting the highest midline spinous process that can be reached by the hitchhiking thumb. This maneuver is simple and easy to reproduce, but it represents a composite motion that depends on shoulder extension as well as elbow, wrist, and thumb motion. Internal rotation may be severely limited in patients with adhesive capsulitis or degenerative arthritis. In these patients, the thumb may reach only to the sacrum, gluteal region, or greater trochanter. Young adults typically can reach beyond the interior tip of the scapula (approximately T7 level).

# MUSCLE TESTING

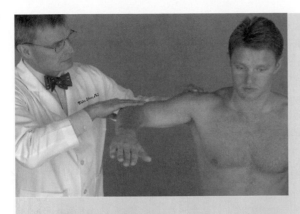

### Deltoid

Place the arm in 90° of abduction with the elbow flexed 90° and the forearm parallel to the floor. Push down on the arm as the patient resists this pressure. This position also activates the supraspinatus and, to some degree, the other rotator cuff muscles. The anterior deltoid is isolated by moving the arm forward. The posterior deltoid is isolated by moving the arm backward and then performing the muscle test.

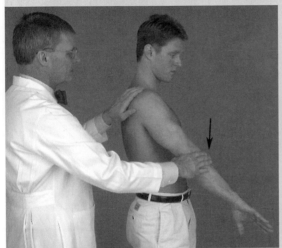

### Supraspinatus

Place the arm in 90° of abduction, 30° of forward flexion, and internal rotation with the elbow extended (the "thumbs down" position). Push down on the arm as the patient resists this pressure.

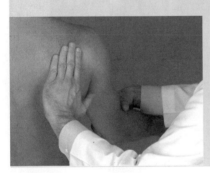

### Infraspinatus and teres minor

With the patient's arm at the side and externally rotated 30° and with the elbow flexed, apply pressure to the forearm and resistance to external rotation to test strength in the infraspinatus and teres minor.

SECTION 2 ■ SHOULDER

SECTION 2 ■ SHOULDER

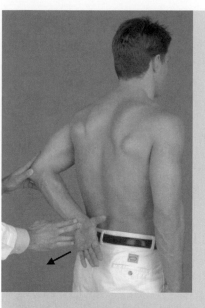

### Subscapularis

Test subscapularis strength and possible tendon rupture by asking the patient to place a hand behind the back, palm facing away from the body, and then lift it away from the back against resistance (lift-off test).

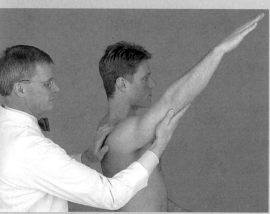

### Serratus anterior

Test serratus anterior strength by asking the patient to elevate the arm as you depress the arm with one hand and palpate the scapula with the other. With normal strength of the serratus anterior, the scapula remains in position on the chest wall. Winging and prominence of the vertebral border occurs with a weak serratus anterior muscle. Stretch or avulsion injuries of the long thoracic nerve with resultant paralysis of the serratus anterior also cause winging of the scapula and fatigue with overhead activities.

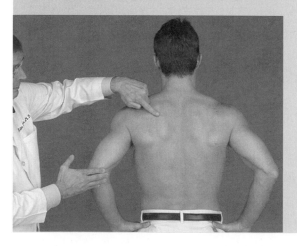

### Rhomboid

Test rhomboid function by asking the patient to place both hands on the side of the iliac crest as you push the patient's arm forward with your hand and palpate the vertebral border of the scapula with the other hand. An intact rhomboid maintains the scapula against the chest wall.

# SPECIAL TESTS

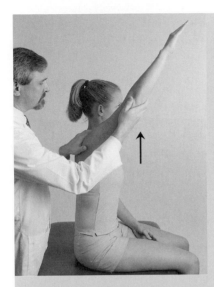

## Neer impingement sign

With the patient seated, depress the scapula with one hand while elevating the arm with the other. This maneuver compresses the greater tuberosity against the anterior acromion and elicits discomfort in patients who have a rotator cuff tear or impingement syndrome.

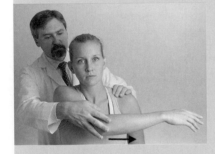

## Hawkins impingement sign

This test reinforces a positive Neer impingement sign. Elevate the patient's shoulder to 90°, flex the elbow to 90°, and place the forearm in neutral rotation. Support the arm and then internally rotate the humerus. Pain elicited with this test is indicative of rotator cuff tear or impingement syndrome.

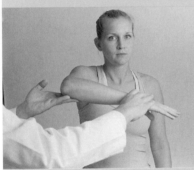

## Cross-body adduction

Elevate the shoulder to 90° and then adduct the arm across the body in the horizontal plane. Pain over the AC joint suggests arthritis of this joint.

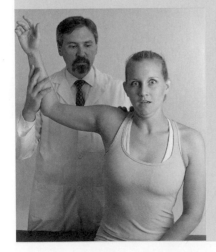

## Apprehension sign for anterior instability

Place the arm in 90° of abduction and then maximal external rotation. Patients with anterior instability may report apprehension and a sense of impending dislocation. A report of pain without apprehension is less specific.

SECTION 2 ■ SHOULDER

SECTION 2 ■ SHOULDER

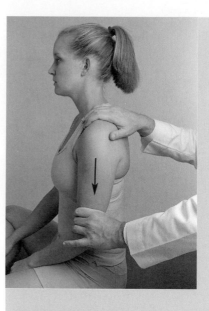

### Sulcus sign

Apply traction in an inferior direction with the arm relaxed at the patient's side. In patients with inferior shoulder laxity, this maneuver causes inferior subluxation of the humeral head and a widening of the sulcus between the humerus and acromion.

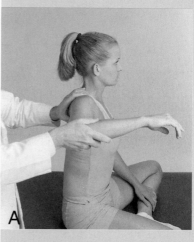

A

### Jerk test for posterior instability

Place the arm in 90° of flexion and maximum internal rotation with the elbow flexed 90° (A). Adduct the arm across the body in the horizontal plane while pushing the humerus in a posterior direction (B). The test is positive if a posterior subluxation or dislocation occurs. If this maneuver causes a dislocation, the humeral head can be felt to clunk back into the joint as the arm is then abducted.

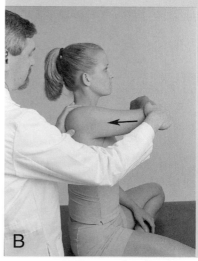

B

# ACROMIOCLAVICULAR INJURIES

## SYNONYMS

Acromioclavicular separation

Shoulder separation

### ICD-9 Code

**831.04**
Closed dislocation acromioclavicular joint

## DEFINITION

Acromioclavicular (AC) injuries commonly result from a fall onto the tip of the shoulder. A common example is a fall off a bicycle. When the acromion is driven into the ground, variable degrees of ligamentous disruption occur.

These injuries can be classified as one of six types based on the severity of injury and the degree of clavicular separation (**Figure 1**). In type I injuries, the AC joint ligaments are partially or completely disrupted, but the strong coracoclavicular (CC) ligaments are intact. As a result, there is no superior separation of the clavicle from the acromion. In type II injuries, the AC ligaments are torn and, in addition, the CC ligaments are partially disrupted. As a result, there is partial separation of the clavicle from the acromion. This superior separation may not be apparent unless the joint is stressed. In type III injuries, the CC ligaments are completely disrupted,

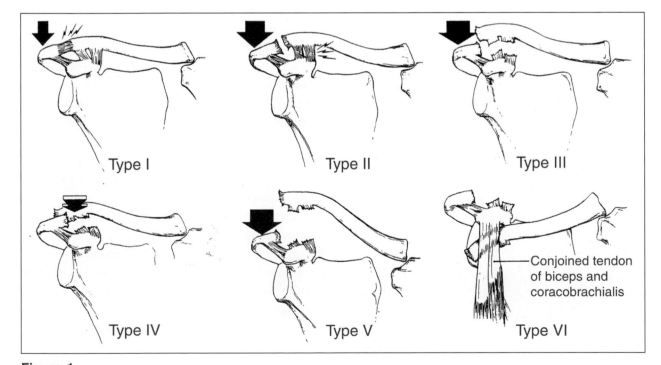

**Figure 1**

Classification of AC separations.

Adapted with permission from Rockwood CA Jr: Subluxation and dislocations about the shoulder, in Rockwood CA Jr, Green DP (eds): *Rockwood and Green's Fractures in Adults*, ed 3. Philadelphia, PA, JB Lippincott, 1988.

SECTION 2 ■ SHOULDER

and there is complete separation of the clavicle from the acromion. Types IV through VI are uncommon. In these injuries, the periosteum of the clavicle and/or the deltoid and trapezius muscle are also torn, causing wide displacement.

# Clinical Symptoms

Patients report pain over the AC joint and pain on lifting the arm. With type III and higher injuries, there is an obvious deformity.

# Tests

## Physical Examination

Patients support the arm in an adducted position, and any motion, especially abduction, causes pain. Tenderness to palpation can be elicited over the AC joint. The distal end of the clavicle may be prominent and slightly superior to the acromion in type II injuries, and there is an obvious deformity in types III and higher. Elevating the arm or depressing the clavicle will temporarily reduce the AC joint, except in types IV and VI injuries, in which there is soft-tissue and bony interposition, respectively.

## Diagnostic Tests

AP radiographs of both shoulders will confirm type II or higher AC separations. A weighted radiographic view in which a 10-lb weight is strapped to each wrist can aid in diagnosis by increasing the separation in the injured shoulder.

Type I injuries are sprains; therefore, patients have pain and tenderness, but radiographs are normal.

Type II injuries display some AC joint widening on radiographs. However, the distance between the clavicle and coracoid remains normal.

Type III injuries show complete displacement of the clavicle above the superior border of the acromion with a 30% to 100% increase in the CC interspace.

Type IV injuries may show superior displacement of the clavicle on AP radiographs, but an axillary lateral view will clearly show the predominant posterior displacement.

Type V injuries show the CC interspace to be increased over 100% of that seen in the opposite shoulder without the application of weights.

Type VI injuries are rare and show the distal end of the clavicle to lie either in the subacromial or subcoracoid space.

# DIFFERENTIAL DIAGNOSIS

Fracture of the acromion (evident on radiographs)

Fracture of the end of the clavicle (evident on radiographs)

Rotator cuff tear (most tenderness over the subacromial space, not the AC joint; no visible deformity or radiographic findings)

# ADVERSE OUTCOMES OF THE DISEASE

Cosmetic deformity, weakness on lifting the arm, chronic shoulder pain, and numbness in the arm are possible. Arthritis of the AC joint may eventually develop.

# TREATMENT

Nonsurgical treatment of type I and II injuries consists of wearing a sling for a few days until the pain subsides. Ice is helpful for the first 48 hours, and analgesics can be used to control severe pain. Patients may resume everyday activities as pain allows, with a full return to normal activities and sports within 4 weeks. Treatment of type III injuries is controversial. Many type III injuries can be treated nonsurgically with good functional results. However, surgical repair may be considered in a young manual laborer who does heavy overhead work. Types IV, V, and VI injuries require evaluation for surgical repair.

# PHYSICAL THERAPY PRESCRIPTION

The functional goal of rehabilitation for a patient with an AC injury is to reduce the pain and protect the joint from further damage. After the shoulder has been immobilized in a sling for an appropriate period of time, a home exercise program (see pp 161-162) that includes basic pain-free exercises to promote rotation of the glenohumeral joint should be started. Exercises for the scapula rotators are also initiated, especially scapula retractions and protractions. The patient should be able to perform the exercise without pain. To restore normal shoulder function, exercises should be performed with strict adherence to the exercise instructions.

Formal physical therapy should be ordered if the patient continues to report pain or limited mobility after performing the home exercise program for 2 to 3 weeks. The prescription should include evaluation of the strength of the glenohumeral and scapula rotators and the mobility of the AC joint. The physical therapist should also supervise the exercise program to ensure that the patient is using proper technique and is not experiencing pain. Mobilization of the AC joint is indicated if joint motion is limited.

## ADVERSE OUTCOMES OF TREATMENT

Following prolonged immobilization in a sling, stiffness may develop; use of a sling or tape also may cause skin breakdown. AC arthritis can be a late sequela of any grade of injury, regardless of treatment.

## REFERRAL DECISIONS/RED FLAGS

Patients with types IV, V, or VI injuries; some athletes (baseball throwers and football quarterbacks on an individual basis); and laborers with type III injuries may be candidates for early surgical repair. Injuries that remain painful warrant further evaluation.

# Home Exercise Program for Acromioclavicular Injuries

Perform the exercises in the order listed. To prevent inflammation, apply ice, such as a bag of crushed ice or frozen peas, to the shoulder for 20 minutes after performing all the exercises. You should not experience any pain with the exercises. If you are unable to perform any of the exercises because of pain or stiffness, call your doctor.

| Exercise Type | Muscle Group | Number of Repetitions/Sets | Number of Days per Week | Number of Weeks |
|---|---|---|---|---|
| External rotation | Infraspinatus Teres minor | 8 to 10 repetitions/2 sets, progressing to 15 repetitions/3 sets | 3 | 2 to 3 |
| Internal rotation | Subscapularis Teres major | 8 to 10 repetitions/2 sets, progressing to 15 repetitions/3 sets | 3 | 2 to 3 |
| Scapular retraction/protraction | Middle trapezius Serratus | 8 to 10 repetitions/2 sets, progressing to 15 repetitions/3 sets | 3 | 2 to 3 |

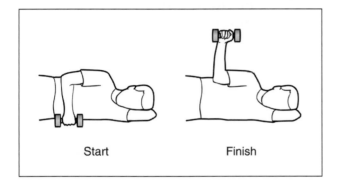

Start          Finish

## *External Rotation*

Lie on your side on a firm, flat surface with the unaffected arm under you, cradling your head. Hold the injured arm against your side as shown, with the elbow bent at a 90° angle. Slowly rotate the arm at the shoulder, keeping the elbow bent and against your side, to raise the weight to a vertical position, and then slowly lower the weight to the starting position to a count of 5. Begin with weights that allow 2 sets of 8 to 10 repetitions, and progress to 3 sets of 15 repetitions. Add weight in 1-pound increments to a maximum of 5 pounds, starting over at 2 sets of 8 to 10 repetitions each time weight is added. Perform the exercise 3 days a week. Continue for a total of 2 to 3 weeks.

SECTION 2 ■ SHOULDER

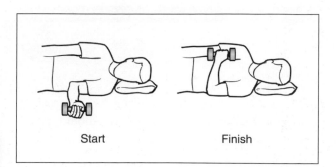

Start          Finish

## Internal Rotation

Lie on your side on a firm, flat surface with the affected arm under you and with a pillow or folded cloth under your head to keep your spine straight. Hold the injured arm against your side as shown, with the elbow bent at a 90° angle. Slowly rotate the arm at the shoulder, keeping the elbow bent and against your torso, to raise the weight to a vertical position, and then slowly lower the weight to the starting position. Begin with weights that allow 2 sets of 8 to 10 repetitions, and progress to 3 sets of 15 repetitions. Add weight in 1-pound increments to a maximum of 5 pounds, starting over at 2 sets of 8 to 10 repetitions each time weight is added. Perform the exercise 3 days a week, continuing for a total of 2 to 3 weeks.

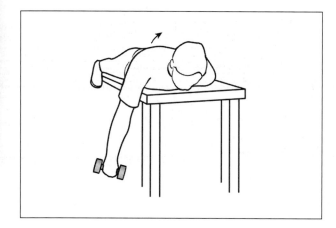

## Scapular Retraction/Protraction

Lie on your stomach on a table or bed with the injured arm hanging over the side. Keeping the elbow straight, lift the weight slowly by moving the scapula toward the opposite side as far as possible. Do not shrug the shoulder. Then slowly return to the starting position. Begin with a weight that allows 2 sets of 8 to 10 repetitions without pain. Progress to 3 sets of 15 repetitions. Then add weight in 1-pound increments to a maximum of 5 pounds, starting over at 2 sets of 8 to 10 repetitions each time weight is added. Perform the exercise 3 days a week, continuing for a total of 2 to 3 weeks.

# ARTHRITIS OF THE SHOULDER

## SYNONYM
Glenohumeral arthritis

## DEFINITION
Arthritis of the shoulder is characterized by destruction of joint cartilage with loss of joint space (**Figure 1**). Like arthritis in other joints, glenohumeral arthritis generally affects patients over age 50 years and occurs as a result of many conditions. Common etiologies include osteoarthritis, rheumatoid arthritis, and posttraumatic arthritis. Less common causes include osteonecrosis, infection, seronegative spondyloarthropathies, and rotator cuff tear arthropathy (a type of arthritis that results from large, long-standing rotator cuff tears) (**Figure 2**).

### ICD-9 Codes
**714.0**
Rheumatoid arthritis

**715.11**
Primary osteoarthritis, shoulder

**715.21**
Secondary osteoarthritis, shoulder (rotator cuff arthropathy)

**716.11**
Traumatic arthropathy, shoulder

**716.91**
Arthropathy, unspecified, shoulder

SECTION 2 ■ SHOULDER

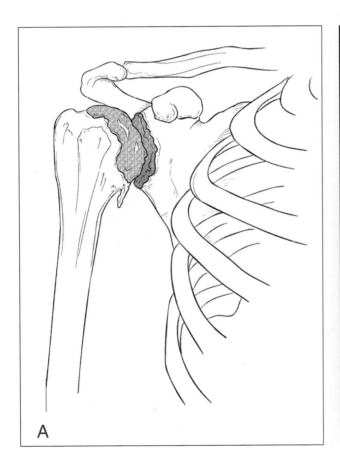

A

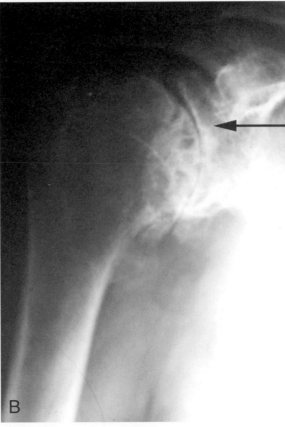

B

**Figure 1**

Diagram (**A**) and AP radiograph (**B**) showing osteoarthritis of the shoulder. Note cystic changes, sclerosis, and decreased joint space (arrow).

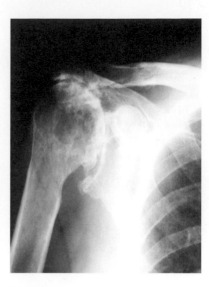

**Figure 2**
Radiograph of shoulder with end-stage rotator cuff arthropathy demonstrates superior migration of the humeral head.

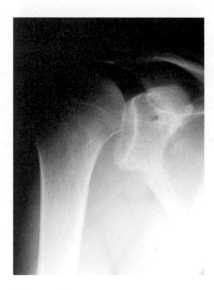

**Figure 3**
Radiograph of shoulder demonstrates superior migration of the humeral head secondary to a chronic rotator cuff tear.

# CLINICAL SYMPTOMS

Patients sometimes report diffuse or deep-seated pain but most often localize the worst pain to the posterior aspect of the shoulder. Initially, the pain is aggravated by any strenuous activity. As the disease progresses, any movement of the shoulder causes pain, and rest and night pain are reported.

Along with pain, range of motion is progressively limited. As a result, activities of daily living, such as dressing, combing the hair, and reaching overhead, are increasingly difficult.

Osteoarthritis typically involves a single joint in an older patient, whereas multiple and symmetric joint involvement and a positive rheumatoid factor suggest rheumatoid arthritis. Generally, there is no apparent relationship between the development of osteoarthritis in the shoulder and the patient's previous level of physical activity. A history of previous fracture or dislocation suggests posttraumatic arthritis or osteonecrosis. Superior migration of the humeral head can develop in association with long-standing rotator cuff tears, which results in eccentric loading of the glenoid and can lead to rotator cuff tear arthropathy (**Figure 3**).

# TESTS

## *Physical Examination*

Examination may reveal generalized atrophy of the muscles about the shoulder. Swelling within the shoulder joint is not common and is difficult to detect. Palpation elicits tenderness over the front and back of the shoulder. Bone-on-bone crepitus is commonly present with rotation or flexion of the shoulder. Range of motion is usually decreased. Patients with concomitant rotator cuff tears often have less active than passive range of motion.

## *Diagnostic Tests*

AP and axillary views of the shoulder are indicated. The axillary view most reliably demonstrates the joint space narrowing that is indicative of cartilage destruction. Other radiographic findings that support a diagnosis of osteoarthritis include flattening of the humeral head, an inferior osteophyte, and posterior erosion of the glenoid. Rheumatoid arthritis is suggested by the presence of periarticular erosions, osteopenia, and central wear of the glenoid. Superior migration of the humeral head suggests a large rotator cuff deficiency.

# DIFFERENTIAL DIAGNOSIS

Adhesive capsulitis (normal radiographs)

Charcot joint (gross destruction of the joint without trauma and relatively little pain)

Fracture of the humerus (history of trauma, evident on radiographs)

Herniated cervical disk (unilateral or bilateral radicular pain, positive Spurling test)

Infection (acute onset, systemic symptoms, elevated WBC)

Rotator cuff tear (normal radiographs, pain mostly with overhead use)

Tumor of the shoulder girdle (variable presentation, radiographic lesion)

# ADVERSE OUTCOMES OF THE DISEASE

Chronic shoulder pain and loss of strength and motion can develop. Severe losses of strength and motion can be difficult to recover, even with joint replacement surgery.

# TREATMENT

Nonsurgical treatment is recommended initially, including use of NSAIDs and application of heat and/or ice to relieve symptoms, and gentle stretching exercises to preserve motion. A trial of glucosamine and/or chondroitin sulfate can be considered, but their efficacy needs further investigation. Activity modifications are beneficial in reducing pain. Corticosteroid injections may provide relief, particularly in some patients with inflammatory (ie, rheumatoid) arthritis. Clinical studies are underway to study the efficacy of injected hyaluronics ("hylans") in osteoarthritis of the shoulder.

For advanced arthritis, total shoulder replacement or hemiarthroplasty (the choice of which procedure to use remains controversial) offers a very satisfactory solution, even in younger patients (30 to 50 years of age) who do not use their shoulders for strenuous activities. Manual laborers may be better served by glenohumeral arthrodesis because the heavy demands placed on their shoulders often lead to early loosening of the prosthetic components.

# ADVERSE OUTCOMES OF TREATMENT

Because addiction to narcotic pain medication is also a possibility, consider other alternatives when treating patients with chronic pain secondary to arthritis. NSAIDs may cause gastric, renal, and hepatic complications. Corticosteroid injection has a small risk of causing an infection in the joint that may preclude or compromise later joint replacement. Patients who undergo shoulder replacement surgery may also experience perioperative complications, including limb thrombophlebitis and possible embolus. Narcotics should be used for short-term postoperative pain relief only.

## REFERRAL DECISIONS/RED FLAGS

Patients with intolerable shoulder pain and/or a progressive loss of motion that does not respond to at least 3 months of nonsurgical treatment need further evaluation. In some cases, surgery may be indicated.

# Burners and Other Brachial Plexus Injuries

## Synonyms
Brachial plexopathy
Stingers

**ICD-9 Codes**

**353.0**
Brachial plexus lesions

**723.4**
Brachial neuritis or radiculitis NOS

## Definition

Brachial plexus injuries include a broad array of neurologic dysfunction ranging from momentary paresthesias to completely flail extremities. The mechanism of injury is equally diverse, from high-energy motor vehicle crashes, falls from a height, and gunshot wounds to lower-energy injuries such as most athletic injuries.

Burners or stingers (transient brachial plexopathy) are transient injuries to the upper trunk of the brachial plexus involving the C5 and C6 nerve roots. The most common mechanism of injury is a traction force when the shoulder is forcefully depressed and the head and neck are tilted toward the opposite side or by compression of the upper plexus between a shoulder pad and the scapula. These injuries are relatively common among college and professional athletes in contact sports, especially football.

Brachial plexus injuries involving axonal disruption can be further categorized as occurring proximal to the dorsal root ganglion in the spinal foramen (preganglionic) or anywhere distal to the ganglion (postganglionic) (**Figure 1**). This distinction is important because surgical repair is impossible and the prognosis for recovery is poor for preganglionic root avulsions.

## Clinical Symptoms

The symptoms of a brachial plexus injury depend on the position of the plexus when it is injured. The mechanism of injury to the upper and middle trunks (C5, C6, and C7, respectively) usually involves a direct blow to the top of the shoulder accompanied by tilt of the head in the opposite direction, causing traction on the plexus with the arm adducted at the side. Lower trunk injuries (C8, T1) occur when these nerves are stretched with the arm abducted, as when grabbing onto a ledge when falling from a height. Injuries involving the entire plexus result from extreme traction from a major trauma.

A typical presentation is a football player injured by a direct blow to the head, neck, or shoulder. The classic symptom is sharp, burning shoulder pain that radiates down the arm.

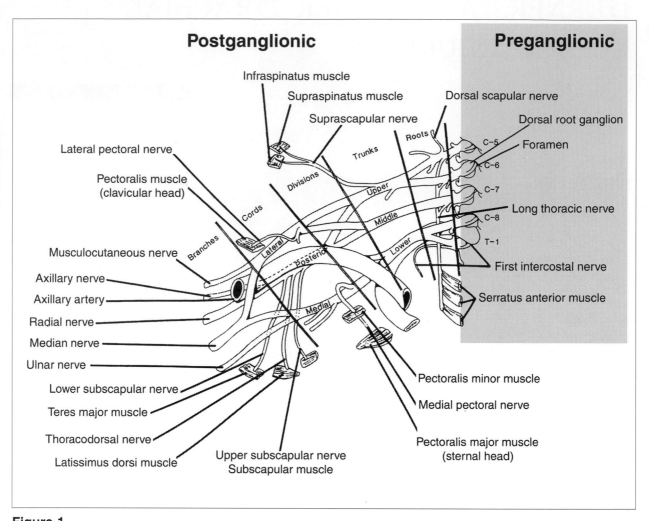

**Postganglionic** | **Preganglionic**

Infraspinatus muscle
Supraspinatus muscle
Suprascapular nerve
Dorsal scapular nerve
Dorsal root ganglion
Roots
Trunks
C-5 Foramen
C-6
C-7
C-8
T-1
Lateral pectoral nerve
Pectoralis muscle (clavicular head)
Divisions
Upper
Middle
Long thoracic nerve
Cords
Lower
First intercostal nerve
Musculocutaneous nerve
Branches
Lateral
Posterior
Serratus anterior muscle
Axillary nerve
Axillary artery
Radial nerve
Median nerve
Medial
Ulnar nerve
Lower subscapular nerve
Pectoralis minor muscle
Teres major muscle
Medial pectoral nerve
Thoracodorsal nerve
Pectoralis major muscle (sternal head)
Latissimus dorsi muscle
Upper subscapular nerve
Subscapular muscle

**Figure 1**

The brachial plexus.

Adapted from *Athletic Training and Sports Medicine*, ed 2. Rosemont, IL, American Academy of Orthopaedic Surgeons, 1991, p 238.

Weakness is also common, and the patient often is seen holding the arm on the affected side, which often is hanging limply at the side. Burners usually last seconds to minutes, although some lasting several weeks have been reported.

# TESTS

## *Physical Examination*

A detailed neurologic examination is the cornerstone of an accurate diagnosis. At a minimum, sensation to light touch, motor power, and deep tendon reflexes should be tested. Deficits should be mapped out by nerve root and peripheral nerve distribution. The neurologic examination also should include evaluation of the lower extremities because spasticity or weakness in the ipsilateral leg suggests a concomitant spinal cord injury.

Injuries to C8 and T1 are more likely to be preganglionic, which is confirmed by the presence of an ipsilateral ptosis, myosis, anhydrosis, and enophthalmos (Horner syndrome). Because the dorsal scapular nerve and the long thoracic nerve arise from the C5 and C5-7 nerve roots, respectively, intact function of the rhomboids and serratus anterior muscles in upper plexus injuries indicates that the injury is distal to these nerves and hence is postganglionic.

Examination of the neck (with cervical spine precautions if indicated) and shoulder, as well as a general examination, is indicated to rule out associated injuries such as cervical spine fractures or disk herniations; clavicle, scapula, or humerus fractures; or scapulothoracic dissociation.

As with other plexus injuries, the sideline evaluation of a burner should include the cervical spine and a neurologic examination of the extremities. Bilateral upper extremity burners or radicular symptoms into the legs should be treated as a spinal cord injury until proven otherwise.

### Diagnostic Tests

Plain radiographs should be obtained if injury to the cervical spine or shoulder girdle is suspected. Although some controversy still exists, many experts suggest that anyone experiencing a burner or stinger needs cervial spine radiographs, including flexion and extension lateral views, to rule out instability, congenital anomaly, or cervical stenosis (assessed by the relative width of the cervical body and the spinal canal). MRI is helpful in patients with abnormal plain radiographs or when symptoms persist.

## DIFFERENTIAL DIAGNOSIS

Cervical spine fracture or instability (evident on radiographs)

Peripheral nerve injury (isolated weakness or sensory deficit confined to a specific nerve distribution)

Transient quadriplegia (neurapraxia of the cervical spinal cord producing bilateral paresthesias and weakness)

## ADVERSE OUTCOMES OF THE DISEASE

Burners, by definition, resolve spontaneously, although recurrent episodes may suggest cervical stenosis and an associated increased risk for catastrophic spinal cord injury. Depending on the location and severity of a brachial plexus injury, persistent pain, sensory loss, paresthesias, and weakness, paralysis, or even amputation is possible.

SECTION 2 ■ SHOULDER

# TREATMENT

Complete resolution of pain and neurologic symptoms, as well as a normal neurologic examination and full range of cervical spine motion, are required before an athlete with a burner is allowed to return to play. Athletes with prolonged or bilateral symptoms or recurrent episodes should not return to play without further evaluation.

Treatment options for more severe brachial plexus injuries vary, including nonsurgical measures and a variety of surgical repair and reconstruction procedures. Nonsurgical management is aimed at strengthening and stretching exercises and splinting to maintain passive range of motion of the joints affected by muscle paralysis or weakness, protection of anesthetic areas of skin, and pain relief. Referral to a pain clinic is often helpful in this regard.

# ADVERSE OUTCOMES OF TREATMENT

The effectiveness of therapy, splinting, and pain control must be monitored frequently. Although surgical techniques are continuously evolving, the prognosis for severe brachial plexus injuries, especially root avulsions, remains guarded.

# REFERRAL DECISIONS/RED FLAGS

Any injury that is persistent, recurrent, bilateral, or associated with other concomitant injuries requires further evaluation. Cervical spine precautions should be followed if a cervical injury is suspected.

# Fracture of the Clavicle

## Synonym
Collarbone fracture

## Definition
Clavicle fractures are the most common bony injury. The most common location of injury is the middle third of the clavicle (**Figure 1**). Approximately 80% occur in this location, 15% occur in the lateral one third, and 5% involve the medial end.

## Clinical Symptoms
Patients typically report a history of significant injury, such as falling on the shoulder or being struck over the clavicle with a heavy object. The patient cannot lift the arm because of pain at the fracture site.

## Tests

### Physical Examination
Examination typically reveals an obvious deformity, or bump, at the fracture site. Gentle pressure over the fracture site will elicit pain, and a grinding sensation can be felt when the patient attempts to raise the arm. The skin may appear tented over a fracture fragment, but the fragment rarely penetrates the skin to

**ICD-9 Code**

**810.00**
Fracture of clavicle, closed, unspecified part

Section 2 ■ Shoulder

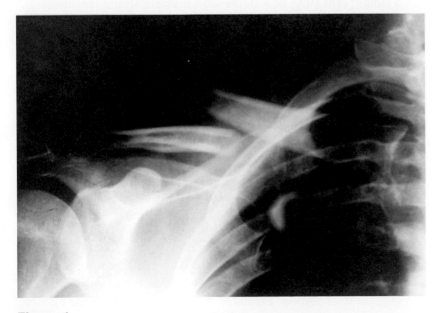

**Figure 1**
Fracture of the middle third of the clavicle.

create an open fracture. Assess neurologic function distal to the fracture, including the axillary, musculocutaneous, median, ulnar, and radial nerves. Check the radial pulse and capillary refill.

### Diagnostic Tests

An AP radiograph of the clavicle will confirm most clavicle fractures (**Figure 1**). Fractures or dislocations at the medial end of the clavicle are uncommon and are often difficult to see on plain radiographs, so if there is a high index of suspicion for a clavicle fracture, CT should be ordered.

# DIFFERENTIAL DIAGNOSIS

Acromioclavicular separation (deformity near the tip of the shoulder)

Sternoclavicular dislocation (deformity at the sternoclavicular junction)

# ADVERSE OUTCOMES OF THE DISEASE

Nonunion is rare, occurring in only 1% to 4% of patients. Some degree of malunion is common, and a visible lump can occur, even when the fracture is well approximated. This lump may be of cosmetic concern to some patients but has little functional significance. Neurovascular complications may occur on an early or delayed basis.

# TREATMENT

Most clavicle fractures can be treated nonsurgically with either a simple arm sling or a figure-of-8 clavicle strap. Treatment with a figure-of-8 strap should be followed closely for possible neurovascular compression or skin breakdown from strap compression overlying the fracture site. Support for 3 to 4 weeks is adequate for a child younger than 12 years, whereas 4 to 6 weeks is usually required for an adult. After 2 to 3 weeks, the patient is encouraged to begin gentle shoulder exercises as pain allows. The most commonly used classification of clavicle fractures is one based on anatomic location (middle third, distal third, proximal third) rather than treatment rationale. Surgical treatment should be considered for open fractures or for fractures associated with neurovascular injury or severe injury to the ipsilateral chest, such as rib fractures or flail chest. Fractures with scapulothoracic dissociation (ipsilateral clavicle and scapular fracture) and malunited or segmental fractures should also be considered for surgical intervention. Fractures of the distal third of the clavicle just medial to the coracoclavicular ligaments in which the medial part of the clavicle is significantly superiorly displaced are associated with a higher rate of nonunion because the proximal fragments buttonhole through the fascia.

# ADVERSE OUTCOMES OF TREATMENT

Pressure over the nerves and vessels in the armpit from a tight clavicle strap may cause numbness and paresthesias in the arm, which are usually transient but may persist.

# REFERRAL DECISIONS/RED FLAGS

Painful nonunion after 4 months of treatment indicates the need for further evaluation. Patients with widely displaced lateral or midshaft clavicle fractures or with segmental fractures have a greater risk of nonunion and should be evaluated for internal fixation.

SECTION 2 ■ SHOULDER

# FRACTURE OF THE HUMERAL SHAFT

**ICD-9 Code**

**812.21**
Fracture of shaft of humerus, closed

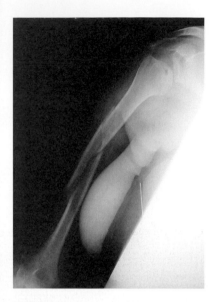

**Figure 1**
Midshaft humeral fracture.

## DEFINITION

Fractures of the humeral shaft often result from a direct blow to the arm, such as occurs in a motor vehicle accident, or from a fall on the outstretched arm (**Figure 1**). These fractures can also occur as a result of sports activities involving a vigorous throwing motion, but these instances are rare. Most of these fractures can be treated nonsurgically, with a rate of union of nearly 100%.

## CLINICAL SYMPTOMS

Severe pain, swelling, and deformity are characteristic of a displaced fracture of the humerus. With gentle palpation and movement of the arm, it is often possible to detect motion at the fracture site. Radial nerve injuries are associated with this fracture. If the radial nerve has been injured, patients are unable to extend the wrist or fingers and may have loss of sensation over the back of the hand. The nerve rarely becomes entrapped within the fracture (**Figure 2**).

## TESTS

### Physical Examination
Examination reveals marked swelling and contusion. Look for puncture wounds in the skin near the fracture site, as these indicate an open (compound) fracture. Assess neurologic function distal to the fracture including the median, radial, and ulnar nerves. Check the radial pulse and record the color and temperature of the hand. The shoulder and elbow should be evaluated for pain, tenderness, and swelling or deformity because concomitant injury proximal or distal to the shaft fracture can be easily missed in the acute setting.

### Diagnostic Tests
AP and lateral radiographs confirm the diagnosis. These views also should include both the shoulder and elbow joints.

## DIFFERENTIAL DIAGNOSIS

Fracture of the distal humerus (evident on radiographs)

Fracture of the proximal humerus (evident on AP and lateral radiographs)

Ruptured biceps tendon (swelling localized to biceps muscle)

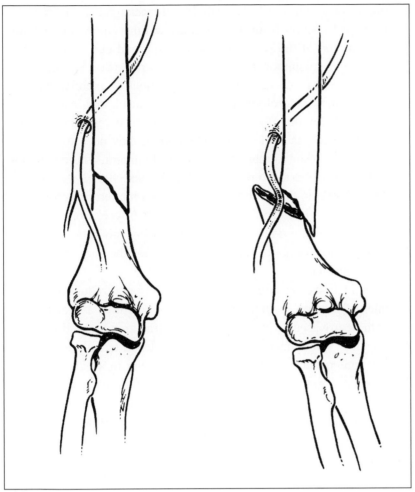

**Figure 2**

Entrapment of the radial nerve at the fracture site.

Reproduced with permission from Rockwood CA, Green DP, Bucholz RW, et al (eds): *Rockwood & Green's Fractures in Adults,* ed 4. Philadelphia, PA, Lippincott/Raven, 1996, p 1044.

## ADVERSE OUTCOMES OF THE DISEASE

Radial nerve injury, indicated by weakness in the wrist or finger extensors and numbness in the first dorsal web space, is possible. Injury to the brachial plexus or vascular system also may occur. Healing of the fracture with angulation is common but results in little functional impairment unless the angulation is severe. Nonunion is possible but uncommon. Persistent stiffness in the shoulder and elbow may be a problem.

## TREATMENT

Most humeral shaft fractures can be treated nonsurgically, with up to 20° of apex anterior or apex lateral angulation being acceptable. Fractures with minimal shortening (2 cm or less) can be treated with a U-shaped coaptation splint for 2 weeks (**Figure 3**), followed by a humeral fracture brace (**Figure 4**). A coaptation splint is applied as follows: place 12 thicknesses of

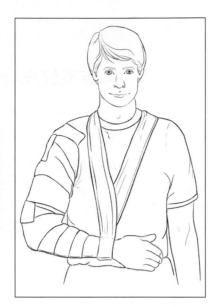

**Figure 3**
Coaptation splint.

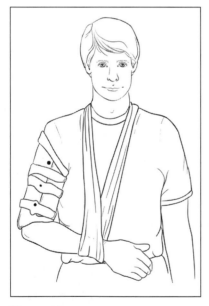

**Figure 4**
Humeral fracture brace.

plaster or a commercially available prepackaged splint in a U-shaped fashion from the axilla around the elbow and extend it to the top of the shoulder. Use a collar and cuff made from stockinette to support the forearm and wrist. (See Splinting Principles, pp 122-128.) Instruct the patient to exercise the fingers, wrist, and elbow at least three times a day. Allow the patient to flex the elbow as tolerated and to extend the elbow to full extension as pain allows. The patient may need to sleep sitting in a chair to maintain fracture alignment. The coaptation splint may need to be reapplied during these first 2 weeks. After 2 weeks, the patient is fitted with a humeral fracture brace, which is worn for at least the next 6 weeks or until there is radiographic evidence of healing. During this time, continue to encourage range-of-motion exercises for the shoulder, elbow, wrist, and hand.

Indications for surgical treatment with open reduction and internal fixation include open fractures, fractures associated with neurovascular injury, pathologic fractures, nonunions, and fractures that cannot be controlled by closed techniques. Ipsilateral forearm and humeral fractures resulting in a "floating elbow" also require surgical treatment. Multiple extremity trauma may also be an indication for open reduction and internal fixation of the humerus because it may allow earlier weight bearing through the extremity, improving patient mobility.

Radial nerve injuries associated with fractures of the humerus should be observed unless they occur after closed reduction of the fracture. Within 6 months, 95% of patients will regain nerve function. During this period of observation, the patient should be fitted with a wrist splint and receive instruction in stretching exercises to avoid flexion contractures of the wrist and fingers. Electromyography is indicated after 3 to 4 months if radial nerve function does not return.

## ADVERSE OUTCOMES OF TREATMENT
Radial nerve injury occurring after manipulation, stiffness of the shoulder and elbow, and discomfort and/or skin irritation from the splint are possible.

## REFERRAL DECISIONS/RED FLAGS
Patients who have one of the following conditions need further evaluation: associated vascular injury; a nerve injury that develops after manipulation; an open fracture; a segmental fracture; a "floating elbow," in which the radius and ulna are fractured along with the humerus; nonunion following 3 months of treatment; an associated head injury, seizure disorder, or multiple injuries; a pathologic fracture; or skin breakdown under the fracture brace.

# FRACTURE OF THE PROXIMAL HUMERUS

## SYNONYMS

Humeral head fracture

Surgical neck fracture

**ICD-9 Code**

**812.00**

Fracture of humerus, upper end, closed

## DEFINITION

Fractures of the proximal humerus commonly occur in elderly patients with osteoporosis, especially women. Most of these fractures are minimally displaced and can be treated with a sling and early motion.

These fractures are generally classified according to which segments of the proximal humerus are fractured and the amount of displacement (**Figure 1**). The four segments are the greater tuberosity (the bony prominence that provides attachment for the supraspinatus, infraspinatus, and teres minor muscles), the lesser tuberosity (attachment site for the subscapularis), the humeral head, and the shaft. The most common two-part fracture occurs at the surgical neck (the region just distal to the tuberosities). Other two-part fractures include fracture at the anatomic neck, isolated fracture of the greater tuberosity, and isolated fractures of the lesser tuberosity. Three-part fractures involve the humeral head, the shaft, and one of the tuberosities. Four-part fractures involve all four components of the proximal humerus. Three- and four-part fractures are severe injuries that are fortunately uncommon. Surgical fixation is indicated if any one of these parts is fractured with greater than 1 cm displacement or greater than 45° angulation to its normal anatomic position.

SECTION 2 ■ SHOULDER

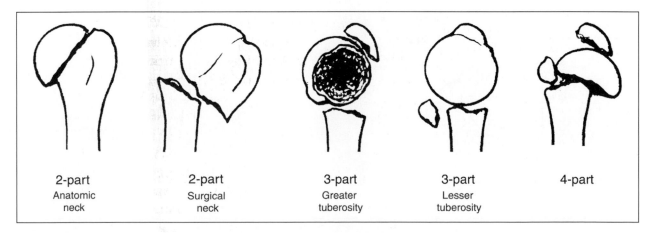

| 2-part | 2-part | 3-part | 3-part | 4-part |
|---|---|---|---|---|
| Anatomic neck | Surgical neck | Greater tuberosity | Lesser tuberosity | |

**Figure 1**

Fracture patterns for displaced fractures of the proximal humerus (Neer classification).

Adapted with permission from Neer CS II: Displaced proximal humeral fractures: I. Classification and evaluation. *J Bone Joint Surg Am* 1970;52:1077-1089.

# CLINICAL SYMPTOMS

Patients typically have severe pain, swelling, and bruising around the upper arm and shoulder following an injury, such as a fall. The pain is worse with even the slightest movement of the arm. If the patient reports a loss of feeling in the arm, a nerve injury is more likely. If the forearm and hand appear pale, the axillary artery may have been injured.

# TESTS

## Physical Examination

Examination reveals swelling and discoloration around the shoulder and upper arm. Assess neurologic function distal to the fracture, including the axillary, musculocutaneous, median, radial, and ulnar nerves. Check the radial pulse and capillary refill as well.

## Diagnostic Tests

A trauma series of plain radiographs of the shoulder should include a true AP and an axillary lateral view to establish the relationship between the humeral head and the glenoid (**Figure 2**). Several techniques are available to obtain an axillary view on a patient with a painful shoulder. If the axillary view is impossible to obtain, a transscapular lateral view (also called the scapular Y view) should be obtained. Great care must be taken in interpreting the AP and the scapular Y views, as errors are easier to make with these views (**Figure 3**). The most common error is misdiagnosis of an associated shoulder dislocation because of inadequate radiographs. AP views alone are insufficient to document an associated shoulder dislocation.

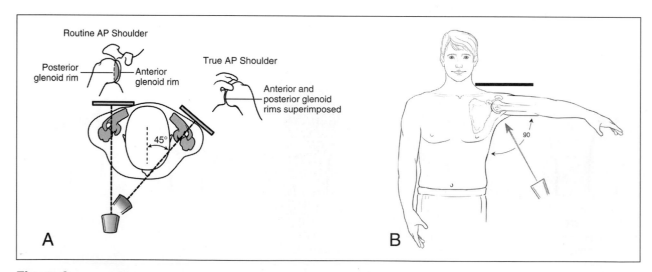

**Figure 2**

Plain radiographs of the shoulder should be obtained in these views: true AP (**A**) and axillary lateral (**B**).

Adapted with permission from Rockwood CA, Szalay EA, Curtis RJ, et al: X-ray evaluation of shoulder problems, in Rockwood CA, Matsen FA III (eds): *The Shoulder*. Philadelphia, PA, WB Saunders, 1990.

## DIFFERENTIAL DIAGNOSIS

Acromioclavicular (AC) separation (pain localized to the AC joint)

Rotator cuff tear (weakness with elevation and external rotation, normal radiographs)

Rupture of the long head of the biceps tendon (asymmetric bulge of arm musculature with biceps contraction)

Shoulder dislocation (evident on AP and lateral radiographs of the glenohumeral joint)

## ADVERSE OUTCOMES OF THE DISEASE

Chronic pain, along with loss of motion, and nerve and vascular injury are possible. Nonunion is also a possibility. Patients may also have posttraumatic arthritis and/or osteonecrosis of the humeral head.

## TREATMENT

Patients with minimally displaced (less than 1 cm) fractures can be treated safely with a sling and, after the first week, can often begin an exercise program consisting of pendulum and circumduction exercises. Isometric exercises of the deltoid and rotator cuff also are encouraged within the first 2 weeks following the injury. Beginning these exercises prior to bony

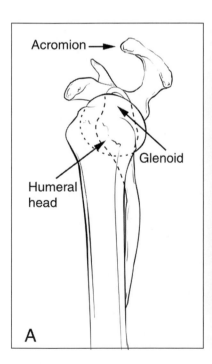
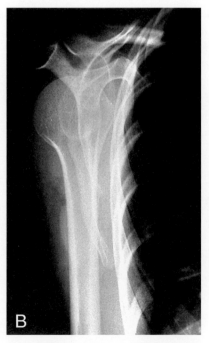

**Figure 3**

Transscapular lateral view of the shoulder. Diagram (**A**) and radiograph (**B**).

Figure B is reproduced from Frymoyer JW (ed): *Orthopaedic Knowledge Update 4*. Rosemont, IL, American Academy of Orthopaedic Surgeons, 1993, p 286.

union is important because disabling stiffness is very common, especially in the elderly. After 3 weeks, the sling can be worn part time, or it can be removed if pain is minimal.

Two-part fractures in which the greater tuberosity is separated more than 1 cm require surgical repair to restore normal function of the rotator cuff muscles. If the patient has a two-part fracture in which the lesser tuberosity is fractured, an associated posterior dislocation is also quite possible. Displaced two-part fractures through the humeral neck and displaced three- and four-part fractures require consideration for surgical treatment. Displaced four-part fractures disrupt the blood supply to the humeral head and in most cases require prosthetic replacement of the proximal humerus rather than internal fixation of the fracture.

# ADVERSE OUTCOMES OF TREATMENT

Nonunion and malunion are both possible. Patients often report persistent stiffness in the shoulder.

Missed shoulder dislocation is also a possibility, especially if insufficient radiographs are obtained.

# REFERRAL DECISIONS/RED FLAGS

Patients with displaced two-part and all three- and four-part fractures need further evaluation. In addition, patients with associated neurovascular symptoms require further evaluation as soon as possible.

# FRACTURE OF THE SCAPULA

## SYNONYMS

Fracture of the acromion
Fracture of the coracoid process
Fracture of the shoulder blade
Glenoid fracture

**ICD-9 Code**

**811.00**
Fracture of scapula, unspecified
part, closed

## DEFINITION

Scapular fractures typically result from high-energy trauma such as motorcycle accidents or falls from a significant height. These fractures may involve the body of the scapula, the glenoid, the acromion, and/or the coracoid process (**Figure 1**). Ninety percent of patients with scapular fractures have associated injuries, including rib fractures, which are the most common; pneumothorax; pulmonary contusion; and head, spinal cord, and brachial plexus injuries. Because of this, scapular fractures are often missed on initial examination.

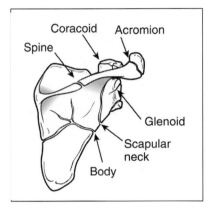

**Figure 1**
Fracture patterns in the scapula.
Reproduced from Zuckerman JD, Koval KJ, Cuomo F: Fractures of the scapula. *Instr Course Lect* 1993;42:271-281.

## CLINICAL SYMPTOMS

Pain and tenderness about the back of the shoulder are the most common complaints. The patient typically holds the arm securely at the side, and any attempts to actively move the extremity result in pain.

## TESTS

### Physical Examination
Skin abrasions, swelling, and ecchymosis over the back of the shoulder are common. Tenderness to gentle palpation over the back of the shoulder or acromion suggests a possible scapular fracture.

### Diagnostic Tests
Radiographic visualization of scapular fractures can be difficult. An AP view of the shoulder and a chest radiograph should be obtained. If the patient is cleared to sit upright, a transscapular lateral or oblique radiograph can be helpful in the diagnosis of a displaced scapular body fracture (**Figure 2**). The axillary view is more useful in revealing acromial and coracoid fractures. Poorly visualized fractures and any fracture involving the glenoid should be further evaluated with CT.

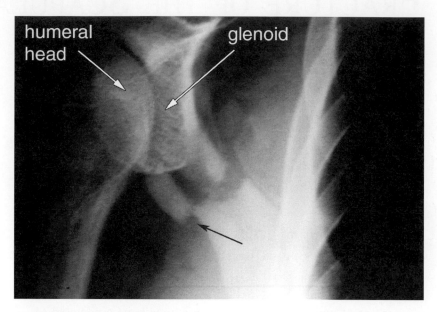

**Figure 2**
Oblique view of the shoulder demonstrating a fracture of the body of the scapula (black arrow).

## DIFFERENTIAL DIAGNOSIS

Acromioclavicular (AC) separation (maximum tenderness over the AC joint)

Fracture of the proximal humerus (radiograph needed to confirm diagnosis)

Fracture of the rib (evident on plain radiographs of the chest)

Os acromiale (nontender, no history of trauma, incidental finding on radiographs)

Shoulder dislocation (deformity of the anterior and lateral shoulder, evident on radiographs)

## ADVERSE OUTCOMES OF THE DISEASE

Persistent loss of motion and chronic pain are possible. Malunion is common but usually asymptomatic. Complications such as suprascapular nerve injury or impingement syndrome are rare.

## TREATMENT

Nonsurgical treatment using a sling is adequate for most patients, followed by early range of motion as tolerated, usually within 1 week of injury. Patients with scapular body fractures should be considered for hospital admission because of the risk of pulmonary contusion.

## ADVERSE OUTCOMES OF TREATMENT

Prolonged immobilization may result in shoulder stiffness.

## REFERRAL DECISIONS/RED FLAGS

Patients with displaced fractures of the glenoid articular surface (greater than 2 mm), fractures of the neck of the scapula with severe angular deformity (greater than 30°), and fractures of the acromion process with impingement syndrome need further evaluation.

SECTION 2 ■ SHOULDER

# FROZEN SHOULDER

**ICD-9 Code**

**726.0**
Adhesive capsulitis of shoulder

**SECTION 2 ■ SHOULDER**

## SYNONYMS
Adhesive capsulitis
Stiff shoulder

## DEFINITION
Adhesive capsulitis of the shoulder, commonly called frozen shoulder, is defined as an idiopathic loss of both active and passive motion. It is considered distinct from posttraumatic shoulder stiffness, a condition that is related to a significant shoulder injury or surgical procedure.

Frozen shoulder most commonly affects patients between the ages of 40 and 60 years, with no clear predisposition based on sex, arm dominance, or occupation. Diabetes mellitus, especially type 1, is the most common risk factor. Patients with diabetes tend to be more refractory to treatment, and 40% to 50% will have bilateral involvement. Other conditions related to frozen shoulder include hypothyroidism, Dupuytren disease, cervical disk herniation, Parkinson's disease, cerebral hemorrhage, and tumors.

## CLINICAL SYMPTOMS
Patients typically progress from an early "freezing" phase of pain and progressive loss of motion to a "thawing" phase of decreasing discomfort associated with a slow but steady improvement in range of motion. The process typically takes 6 months to 2 years or more to resolve, with most patients experiencing minimal long-term pain or functional deficit, although some motion loss may remain.

## TESTS

### Physical Examination
Examination reveals significant (at least 50%) reduction in both active and passive range of motion when compared with the opposite, normal shoulder. Motion is painful, especially at the extremes. Pain and tenderness are common at the deltoid insertion. Diffuse tenderness about the shoulder also may be present.

### Diagnostic Tests
AP and axillary radiographs of the shoulder are indicated to ensure that smooth, concentric joint surfaces with an intact

cartilage space are present and to rule out other pathology such as osteophytes, loose bodies, calcium deposits, or tumors. Other ancillary studies, such as arthrography or MR arthrograms, can substantiate a frozen shoulder diagnosis by demonstrating a contracted capsule and loss of the inferior pouch (**Figure 1**).

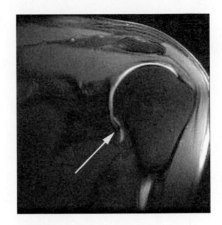

**Figure 1**
MRI scan reveals the contracted capsule, which is the hallmark of a frozen shoulder, and the loss of the inferior pouch (arrow).

## DIFFERENTIAL DIAGNOSIS

Chronic posterior shoulder dislocation (evident on axillary radiographs)

Impingement syndrome (motion preserved and pain primarily with elevation)

Osteoarthritis (evident on radiographs)

Posttraumatic shoulder stiffness (history of clear and significant preceding trauma)

Rotator cuff tear (normal passive range of motion)

Tumor (rare, but evident on shoulder or ipsilateral chest radiograph)

## ADVERSE OUTCOMES OF THE DISEASE

Residual pain and/or stiffness may persist for years in some patients.

## TREATMENT

NSAIDs, nonnarcotic analgesics, and moist heat are indicated, followed by a gentle stretching program. Often ice is used after stretching to control swelling. A transcutaneous electrical nerve stimulation (TENS) unit (applied by a physical therapist) may help control pain. Intra-articular injection of corticosteroid also may be considered. The patient should be instructed in a home stretching program that is to be done within a comfortable range. Advise patients that, on average, a recovery period of 1 to 2 years is to be expected before motion is fully restored and pain completely relieved.

## PHYSICAL THERAPY PRESCRIPTION

The functional goal of rehabilitation for a patient with a frozen shoulder is to reduce pain and increase mobility of the glenohumeral joint and scapula. External rotation in the adducted position tends to be the most restricted range of motion associated with frozen shoulder. Pain in the subscapularis area, localized to the scapular fossa, is also very common.

The home exercise program (see p 187) should include stretching into external rotation with the arm at no greater than 30° to 45° of abduction. A low-load prolonged shoulder

SECTION 2 ■ SHOULDER

stretching device may be ordered for home use to promote passive external rotation. Forced elevation should be avoided. Strengthening exercises are initiated after the inflammation and painful period of frozen shoulder has subsided and should include strengthening of the glenohumeral joint and scapula rotators.

The formal physical therapy prescription should include evaluation of the mobility of the glenohumeral joint and scapula mobility and posture. Aggressive mobilization is very effective in increasing the range of motion.

## ADVERSE OUTCOMES OF TREATMENT

Therapy that is too aggressive may aggravate symptoms and/or cause a fracture of the humerus.

## REFERRAL DECISIONS/RED FLAGS

Patients who fail to show significant improvement in pain and motion after 3 months of consistent rehabilitation need further evaluation.

# HOME EXERCISE PROGRAM FOR FROZEN SHOULDER

Perform the exercises in the order listed. Apply moist or dry heat to the shoulder for 5 or 10 minutes before the exercises and during the external rotation passive stretch. If you experience pain during or after the exercises, call your doctor.

| Exercise Type | Muscle Group | Number of Repetitions/Sets | Number of Days per Week | Number of Weeks |
|---|---|---|---|---|
| External rotation passive stretch | Anterior capsule | 4 repetitions/3 sets | Daily | 3 to 4 |
| Bent over rowing | Posterior deltoid Middle trapezius | 8 to 10 repetitions/2 sets, progressing to 15 repetitions/3 sets | 3 | 3 to 4 |

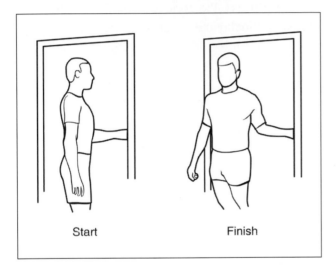

Start        Finish

## External Rotation Passive Stretch

Stand in a doorway, facing the doorjamb. With the affected arm held next to your side and the elbow bent 90°, grasp the edge of the doorjamb. Keeping the hand in place, rotate your upper body as shown in the illustration. Hold the stretch for 30 seconds; then return to the starting position for 30 seconds. Perform 3 sets of 4 repetitions daily, continuing for 3 to 4 weeks.

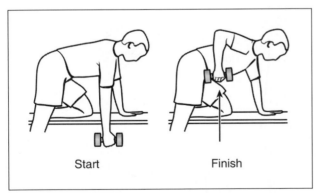

Start        Finish

## Bent Over Rowing

Stand next to a bench or chair with your knee and hand resting on the bench and your free hand grasping a weight. Lift the weight while you count to 3 slowly by bending the elbow, squeezing the shoulder blade across the back. Lower the weight slowly to a count of 3. Begin with a weight that allows 2 sets of 8 to 10 repetitions without pain. Progress to 3 sets of 15 repetitions. Add weight in increments up to 5 pounds, returning to 8 to 10 repetitions and 2 sets each time weight is added. Perform the exercise 3 days a week, continuing for 3 to 4 weeks.

SECTION 2 ■ SHOULDER

# IMPINGEMENT SYNDROME

**ICD-9 Code**

**726.10**
Rotator cuff syndrome NOS

## SYNONYMS
Rotator cuff tendinitis
Shoulder bursitis

## DEFINITION
Four muscles come together to form the rotator cuff that covers the anterior, superior, and posterior aspects of the humeral head. As these muscles assist in elevation of the arm, the rotator cuff, primarily the supraspinatus tendon, is pulled repetitively under the coracoacromial arch (**Figure 1**). The coracoacromial arch includes the coracoid process, the coracoacromial ligament, the acromion, and the acromioclavicular joint capsule.

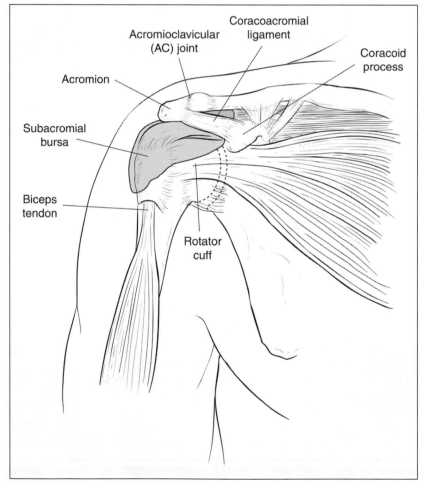

**Figure 1**
Anatomy of the front of the shoulder.

Reproduced from Sullivan JA, Anderson SJ (eds): *Care of the Young Athlete*. Rosemont, IL, American Academy of Orthopaedic Surgeons, 2000, p 326.

Inflammation of the subacromial bursa and underlying rotator cuff tendons is a common cause of shoulder pain in middle-aged patients. Rotator cuff pathology spans a continuum from edema and hemorrhage to chronic inflammation and fibrosis to microscopic tendon fiber failure progressing to full-thickness rotator cuff tears. The etiology is likely a combination of factors, including loss of microvascular blood supply to the tendon and repeated mechanical insult as the tendon passes under the coracoacromial arch.

## CLINICAL SYMPTOMS

Gradual onset of anterior and lateral shoulder pain exacerbated by overhead activity is characteristic. Night pain and difficulty sleeping on the affected side are also common. Atrophy of the muscles about the top and back of the shoulder may be apparent if the patient has had symptoms for several months.

## TESTS

### Physical Examination

Palpation over the greater tuberosity and subacromial bursa commonly elicits tenderness and crepitus with shoulder motion. Pain will be elicited by having the patient slowly lower the abducted arm against resistance. Patients with impingement generally have positive Neer and Hawkins signs. (See Physical Examination—Shoulder: Special Tests, p 155.) After completing these tests, 10 mL of 1% plain local anesthetic can be injected into the subacromial space (see Subacromial Bursa Injection, p 194), followed by impingement testing. Complete pain relief supports a diagnosis of impingement syndrome.

To demonstrate weakness of the supraspinatus tendon, position the arm in 90° of elevation and internal rotation (thumb turned down). Ask the patient to resist while you push the arm down (**Figure 2**). Compare the result with that of the opposite shoulder. If the shoulder initially demonstrates weakness but is strong following subacromial injection, pain inhibition from inflammation and fibrosis rather than a full-thickness rotator cuff tear is the likely cause of the weakness. Muscle atrophy about the top and back of the shoulder usually indicates a rotator cuff tear (**Figure 3**).

### Diagnostic Tests

AP and axillary radiographs of the shoulder are usually normal. Narrowing of the space between the head of the humerus and the undersurface of the acromion (normally greater than 7 mm) suggests a long-standing rotator cuff tear.

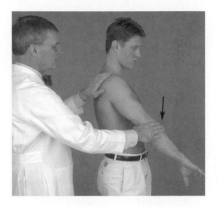

**Figure 2**
Testing the strength of the supraspinatus.

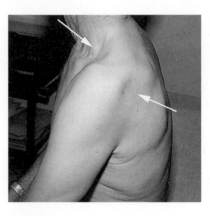

**Figure 3**
Visible muscle atrophy (arrows) indicative of a rotator cuff tear.

SECTION 2 ■ SHOULDER

# DIFFERENTIAL DIAGNOSIS

Acromioclavicular (AC) arthritis (tenderness over the AC joint)

Frozen shoulder (active and passive motion loss)

Glenohumeral arthritis (pain with any motion, evident on radiographs)

Herniated cervical disk (associated neck stiffness, deltoid weakness with absent biceps reflex, possible sensory loss)

Rotator cuff tear (weakness of the supraspinatus that does not improve following subacromial injection of local anesthetic)

Suprascapular nerve entrapment (atrophy of the supraspinatus and infraspinatus muscles, negative impingement sign)

# ADVERSE OUTCOMES OF THE DISEASE

Pain may be persistent or recurrent. Rotator cuff tendinitis may progress to a full-thickness tear.

# TREATMENT

NSAIDs and rest from the offending activity may relieve an acute exacerbation of pain. The patient should begin a stretching program (see Appendix A—Musculoskeletal Conditioning, pp 959-992) with emphasis on posterior capsule stretching. If a home therapy program performed three to four times a day for 6 weeks does not result in any improvement, a subacromial corticosteroid injection can be considered, followed by continued stretching. Steroid injections should not be repeated if the previous injection did not produce significant and sustained (4 to 6 weeks) relief. Rotator cuff weakness with impingement is often the result of subacromial bursitis, rotator cuff tendinitis, or even calcific tendinitis.

A rotator cuff strengthening program should be added to the stretching program once the shoulder is supple and pain is improved. Avoidance of repetitive overhead activities is also recommended.

# PHYSICAL THERAPY PRESCRIPTION

The functional goal of rehabilitation for a patient with shoulder impingement should be to perform overhead activities without pain. Patients with shoulder impingement typically have a restricted glenohumeral joint capsule and weakness of the glenohumeral and scapulothoracic rotators.

A home exercise program (see pp 192-193) may be initiated that includes stretching and very basic strengthening exercises. The home program should not cause more pain, although patients may report muscle soreness and a stretching sensation that may be considered uncomfortable. Ice may be used after exercise to prevent inflammation.

Formal physical therapy should be started within 3 to 4 weeks if the home exercise program has not increased the ability of the patient to perform overhead activities of daily living without pain. The prescription should include an evaluation of the strength of the glenohumeral and scapulothoracic rotator muscles as well as an appropriate strengthening program. In addition, mobilization of the glenohumeral and scapulothoracic joints may be very effective.

## ADVERSE OUTCOMES OF TREATMENT

NSAIDs may cause gastric, renal, or hepatic complications. Tearing of the rotator cuff and rupture of the long head of the biceps tendon may occur after repeated corticosteroid injections. The latter is more likely with more than three injections.

## REFERRAL DECISIONS/RED FLAGS

Significant weakness of the rotator cuff or failure of 2 to 3 months of rehabilitation (with or without subacromial steroid injection) is an indication for further evaluation and surgical consideration.

SECTION 2 ■ SHOULDER

# HOME EXERCISE PROGRAM FOR SHOULDER IMPINGEMENT

Perform the exercises in the order listed. Apply a bag of crushed ice or frozen peas to the shoulder for 20 minutes after performing the exercises to prevent inflammation. These exercises should not increase the pain in your shoulder, although you may experience muscle soreness and a stretching sensation. Call your doctor if you experience increased pain or if you do not see improvement in your ability to perform overhead activities without pain after performing the exercises for 3 or 4 weeks.

| Exercise Type | Muscle Group | Number of Repetitions/Sets | Number of Days per Week | Number of Weeks |
|---|---|---|---|---|
| Sleeper stretch | Posterior rotator cuff Posterior inferior capsule/glenohumeral ligament | 4 repetitions/3 to 4 sets | Daily | 3 to 4 |
| External rotation | Infraspinatus Teres minor | 8 repetitions/2 sets, progressing to 15 repetitions/3 sets | 3 to 4 | 6 to 8 |
| Internal rotation | Subscapularis Teres major | 8 repetitions/2 sets, progressing to 15 repetitions/3 sets | 3 to 4 | 6 to 8 |

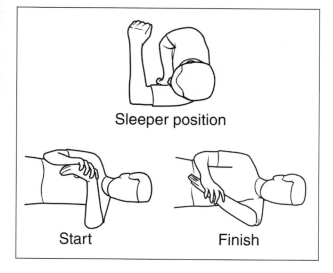

Sleeper position

Start          Finish

## *Sleeper Stretch*

Lie on your side on a firm, flat surface with the affected shoulder under you and the arm positioned as shown, keeping your back perpendicular to the surface. With the unaffected arm, push the other wrist down, toward the surface. Stop when you feel a stretching sensation in the back of the affected shoulder. Hold this position for 30 seconds, then relax the arm for 30 seconds. Perform 3 or 4 sets of 4 repetitions daily, continuing for 3 to 4 weeks.

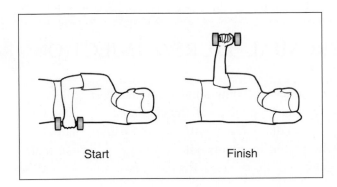

Start          Finish

## External Rotation

Lie on your side on a firm, flat surface with the unaffected arm under you, cradling your head. Hold the affected arm against your side as shown, with the elbow bent at a 90° angle. Slowly rotate the arm at the shoulder, keeping the elbow bent and against your side, to raise the weight to a vertical position, and then slowly lower the weight to the starting position to a count of 5. Begin with weights that allow 2 sets of 8 repetitions (approximately 1 to 2 pounds), progressing to 3 sets of 15 repetitions. Add weight in 1-pound increments, starting over at each new weight level with 2 sets of 8 repetitions up to a maximum of 3 to 6 pounds, depending on your size and fitness level. Perform the exercise 3 or 4 days a week, continuing for 6 to 8 weeks.

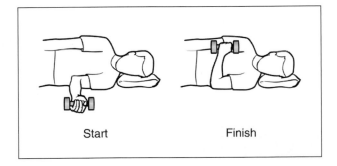

Start          Finish

## Internal Rotation

Lie on your side on a firm, flat surface with the affected arm under you and with a pillow or folded cloth under your head to keep your spine straight. Hold the affected arm against your side as shown, with the elbow bent at a 90° angle. Slowly rotate the arm at the shoulder, keeping the elbow bent and against your torso, to raise the weight to a vertical position, and then slowly lower the weight to the starting position. Begin with weights that allow 2 sets of 8 repetitions, progressing to 3 sets of 15 repetitions. Add weight in 1-pound increments, starting over at each new weight level with 2 sets of 8 repetitions up to a maximum of 3 to 6 pounds, depending on your size and fitness level. Perform the exercise 3 or 4 days a week, continuing for 6 to 8 weeks.

SECTION 2 ■ SHOULDER

# PROCEDURE

## SUBACROMIAL BURSA INJECTION

### CPT Code

**20610**

Arthrocentesis, aspiration and/or injection; major joint or bursa (eg, shoulder, hip, knee joint, subacromial bursa)

*Current Procedural Terminology* © 2004 American Medical Association. All Rights Reserved

### MATERIALS

Sterile gloves

Bactericidal skin prep solution

1% lidocaine solution without epinephrine

2 mL of betamethasone 40 mg/mL or similar steroid

10-mL syringe with a 22-gauge, 1¼″ needle

3-mL syringe with a 25-gauge, ¾″ needle

Adhesive bandage

**Note:** Opinions differ regarding single- versus two-needle injection techniques. Proponents of the single-needle technique believe that one needle is less painful for the patient than two. Physicians who prefer the two-needle technique point out that the smaller gauge needle is easier for patients to tolerate and that the pain of the second injection is dulled by the anesthetic. A two-syringe, two-needle technique is described on the DVD.

### STEP 1

Wear protective gloves at all times during this procedure and use sterile technique.

### STEP 2

Seat the patient with the arm hanging down to distract the subacromial space. The injection site can be anterior, anterolateral, or straight posterior into the subacromial space (**Figure 1**).

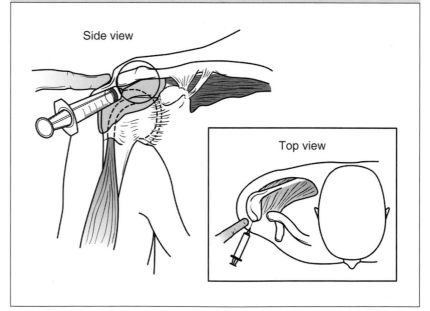

**Figure 1**

Location for needle insertion for subacromial bursa injection.

# Subacromial Bursa Injection (continued)

## Step 3

Palpate the acromion both anteriorly and laterally until the anterolateral corner is located.

## Step 4

Cleanse this area with a bactericidal solution.

## Step 5

With an index finger on the lateral acromion, insert the 25-gauge needle about 1 cm below the palpating finger and raise a wheal with the local anesthetic.

## Step 6

Insert the syringe with the 22-gauge needle. Angle the needle superiorly approximately 20° to 30° to access the subacromial space. Inject 8 to 10 mL of the 1% lidocaine solution. If resistance is encountered while attempting to inject the solution, partially withdraw the needle and reinsert. If the needle is in the proper place, there is little resistance to injection. If you feel the needle hit bone, redirect it superiorly if the bony obstruction is thought to be the humerus, or inferiorly if the bone is thought to be the acromion.

## Step 7

Detach the syringe from the needle hub, leaving the needle in the correct location. Attach the second syringe with 2 mL of corticosteroid preparation and inject it into the subacromial space. The syringe can again be exchanged and local anesthetic injected as the needle is withdrawn to avoid steroid deposition subcutaneously. This reduces the risk of fat atrophy or depigmentation in dark-skinned patients.

## Step 8

Dress the puncture wound with a sterile adhesive bandage.

## Adverse Outcomes

Temporarily increased pain is possible, and, although rare, infection can occur. Subcutaneous atrophy and depigmentation also may occur.

# Subacromial Bursa Injection (continued)

## Aftercare/Patient Instructions

One third of patients will experience a temporary increase in pain for 24 to 48 hours from the corticosteroid injection. Advise the patient to apply ice bags to the shoulder and take an NSAID or acetaminophen if increased pain occurs the night following the injection. Instruct the patient to resume usual activities as soon as tolerated, but no later than 24 to 48 hours after the injection.

# OVERHEAD THROWING SHOULDER

## SYNONYMS
Rotator cuff tendinitis (syndrome)

## DEFINITION
The unique anatomy of the glenohumeral joint provides multiple and extreme degrees of functional motion. All overhead athletic motions (eg, throwing a baseball) require the repeated systematic and sequential delivery of kinetic energy to the four rotator cuff muscle/tendon units (**Figure 1**). The primary function of these relatively small muscle/tendon units is to precisely seat and center the humeral head in the shallow fossa of the glenoid (**Figure 2**). This working relationship between the rotator cuff and the humeral head must be operational in order for the larger power muscles such as the deltoid and pectoralis to function effectively, resulting in the desired fluid shoulder motion. When the relationship between the rotator cuff and the humeral head malfunctions, the humeral head translocates forcefully, causing damage to surrounding structures.

Repetitive overhead throwing produces very significant dynamic stress forces on the rotator cuff–glenohumeral complex. Of the five primary phases of the optimal overhead throwing motion (**Figure 3**), late cocking, early acceleration, and follow-through are the most violent and are chiefly responsible for the inflammatory tissue response. Compression forces are experienced where the humeral head contacts the glenoid and soft tissues. Tensile forces tend to stretch, irritate, and cause plastic deformation of ligaments, tendons, and capsular tissues. As a result, with repetitive throwing, excessive wear (abuse), subacute stress accumulation (overuse), and obsessive sport participation (wearout) will invariably damage the rotator cuff–glenohumeral complex. This damage leads to malfunctioning of the rotator cuff–humeral head relationship so that the humeral head is no longer firmly seated. Given the complex anatomy and mechanism of the shoulder, combining all thrower's shoulder symptoms under rotator cuff tendinitis fails to appreciate the broad spectrum of rotator cuff–glenohumeral pathology. A clearer understanding of the mechanism, treatment, and prevention of these debilitating injuries is important to guide treatment.

Rotator cuff tendinitis develops initially as a result of the throwing arm being abducted and placed in extreme external rotation. As a consequence, the suprapinatus and infraspinatus

**ICD-9 Codes**

**353.0**
Thoracic outlet syndrome

**718.81**
Anterior instability

**723.4**
Suprascapular nerve entrapment

**726.1**
Biceps tendinitis
Rotator cuff tendinitis (syndrome)
Internal impingement

**726.19**
External impingement (subacromial bursitis)

**727.61**
Rotator cuff tear, nontraumatic

**840.4**
Rotator cuff sprain

**840.7**
SLAP lesion

**953.4**
Brachial plexus compression

**955.0**
Axillary nerve involvement

SECTION 2 ■ SHOULDER

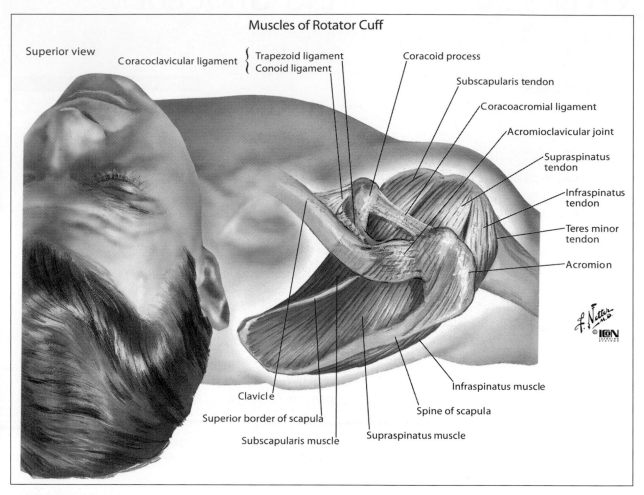

**Muscles of Rotator Cuff**

Superior view

Coracoclavicular ligament { Trapezoid ligament
Conoid ligament

Coracoid process

Subscapularis tendon

Coracoacromial ligament

Acromioclavicular joint

Supraspinatus tendon

Infraspinatus tendon

Teres minor tendon

Acromion

Infraspinatus muscle

Spine of scapula

Supraspinatus muscle

Subscapularis muscle

Superior border of scapula

Clavicle

**Figure 1**

Superior view of the muscles of the rotator cuff.

Reproduced with permission from Icon Learning Systems, Inc.

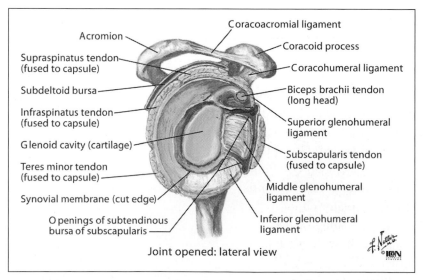

Coracoacromial ligament

Acromion

Coracoid process

Supraspinatus tendon (fused to capsule)

Coracohumeral ligament

Subdeltoid bursa

Biceps brachii tendon (long head)

Infraspinatus tendon (fused to capsule)

Superior glenohumeral ligament

Glenoid cavity (cartilage)

Subscapularis tendon (fused to capsule)

Teres minor tendon (fused to capsule)

Middle glenohumeral ligament

Synovial membrane (cut edge)

Openings of subtendinous bursa of subscapularis

Inferior glenohumeral ligament

Joint opened: lateral view

**Figure 2**

Lateral view of the glenohumeral (shoulder) joint, opened.

Reproduced with permission from Icon Learning Systems, Inc.

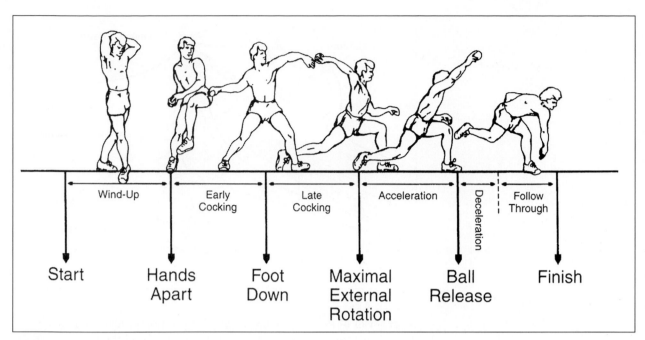

**Figure 3**

Phases of throwing.

Reproduced with permission from DiGiovine NM, Jobe FW, Pink M, et al: An electromyographic analysis of the upper extremity in pitching. *J Shoulder Elbow Surg* 1992;1:15-25.

muscles and their tendons are compressed between the posterosuperior glenoid rim, the posterior humeral head, and the greater tuberosity. This compression is termed internal impingement (**Figure 4**). External impingement occurs with excessive superior translation of the humeral head in the glenoid fossa. Such translation decreases the space available in the subacromial area, resulting in impingement of the structures that occupy this space, most notably the subacromial bursa and the tendons of the rotator cuff.

In throwers, repetitive hyperextension together with internal impingement (abnormal positioning of the humeral head) causes fraying of the deep layers of the infraspinatus, ultimately establishing a partial-thickness tear. A similar situation is seen on the articular surface of the supraspinatus. With continued throwing, partial-thickness tears may proceed to full-thickness tears, but full-thickness tearing is usually the result of a nonthrowing injury.

If the athlete with a dysfunctional rotator cuff–glenohumeral complex continues to pitch without resting the shoulder, the relatively unrestrained humeral head will translate (migrate) and abut the glenoid labrum, and compression and shear forces will cause roughening, fraying, and tearing of the fibrocartilaginous labrum. More significant forces may result in superior labrum anterior-to-posterior lesions (SLAP) detachment with or without the biceps tendon remaining intact. The exact etiology is

SECTION 2 ■ SHOULDER

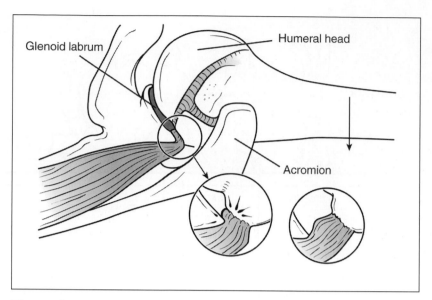

**Figure 4**

Mechanism of internal impingement. The position of abduction and extreme external rotation that occurs during overhead throwing compresses the supraspinatus and infraspinatus muscles and their tendons between the posterosuperior glenoid rim, the posterior humeral head, and the greater tuberosity, causing fraying of the deep layers of the infraspinatus.

controversial, but some authors believe SLAP lesions develop from traction of the biceps. Others believe that the extreme external rotation that occurs during overhead throwing causes the lesion; ie, the labrum is "peeled back" by the rotating humeral head. Loss of the anchoring function of the biceps results in increased stress on the inferior glenohumeral ligament. The anterior band of the inferior glenohumeral ligament and the anterior capsule serve as static restraints to anterior translation of the humeral head. When the static restraints become dysfunctional and the dynamic muscle restraints are insufficient, anterior instability results.

Biceps tendinitis may present in the throwing athlete as anterior shoulder pain that increases with activity. Palpation of the biceps tendon in its groove on the front of the humerus typically reproduces the patient's discomfort.

Brachial plexus compression, thoracic outlet syndrome, and axillary nerve involvement should be considered when a thrower has atypical shoulder symptoms.

In a patient with significant atrophy of the infraspinatus muscle, consider the possibility of suprascapular nerve entrapment. Electromyographic and nerve conduction studies are diagnostic.

# CLINICAL SYMPTOMS

## Stage I–Sore Shoulder Syndrome

Initially, the athlete reports aching and soreness deep in the anterior shoulder when throwing certain pitches (usually sliders and curve balls) or after pitching a few innings. The athlete also reports a decrease in pitch velocity and accuracy and difficulties with activities of daily living. The situation improves with rest, and the athlete is able to continue to pitch.

## Stage II–Profound Pathologic Pain

In this stage, the aching and soreness of stage I has gradually progressed to pain, predominantly located in the posterior shoulder, that prevents full abduction and external rotation (the throwing motion). A period of rest no longer is effective. Sleeping on the affected shoulder produces night pain, and pain medication is requested.

# TESTS

## Physical Examination

Inspect the fully exposed trunk for muscle asymmetry, atrophy, and obvious deformity. Examine the skin for abrasion, rashes, and boils, and especially note ecchymosis or swelling. Dominant arm hypertrophy may be evident.

Palpate the shoulder area systematically, searching for tenderness in the scapular support muscles as well as the supraspinatus and infraspinatus area, posterior capsule, quadrilateral space, and posterior deltoid. Anteriorly, palpate the muscles about the humeral head, the rotator cuff attachment to the greater and lesser tuberosity, the bicipital groove, and the deltoid and pectoralis muscles. Note any tenderness of the acromioclavicular and sternoclavicular joints, clavicle, and adjacent neck structures. Similarly palpate the upper arm, elbow, forearm, wrist, and hand.

Evaluate full range of passive motion of the shoulder in forward flexion, abduction, external rotation with the arm at the side, and internal rotation (hitchhiking thumb up the back). (For these and other tests, see Physical Examination—Shoulder, pp 150-156). Repeat the examination, providing active resistance, and compare the results with the opposite extremity. Active resistance to full range of motion should also be evaluated in the biceps, triceps, forearm muscles, and intrinsic muscles of the hand.

Generalized musculoskeletal laxity is indicated by the ability to actively hyperextend the elbows, wrist, and fingers. Inferior shoulder laxity is exhibited as the sulcus, or sag, sign. Perform the lift-off test bilaterally to compare subscapularis strength. With the patient supine and with the elbow flexed 90°, measure external rotation at 30°, 90°, and at full overhead, also comparing with the opposite extremity. Also perform the cross-chest maneuver. To evaluate anterior instability, the shoulder is abducted to about 150°, and pressure is applied anteriorly and then posteriorly to the humeral head in order to estimate the amount of translation and firmness of resistance.

Pain that limits motion, especially in forward flexion, is an indication of impingement. If application of anterior pressure to the humeral head relieves the pain, internal impingement may be suspected.

With the patient in the prone position, scapular protraction, tilt, and retraction are assessed. Winging may be tested by having the patient perform a push-up. (A better method for assessing winging is to have the patient perform a seated press. For the seated press, the patient, who is seated in a chair without arms, grips the seat of the chair on either side and, by extending the arms at the elbows, attempts to lift his or her body up off the chair.) Axillary nerve irritation on deep palpation of the quadrilateral space indicates compression by the posterior capsule and pectoralis minor. Likewise, if pressure on the posterior capsule produces localized discomfort, capsulitis should be suspected. Also with the patient in the prone position, allow the arm to hang freely over the edge of the table and then forward flex it to 90°; pain in the anterior shoulder is indicative of rotator cuff tendinitis.

With the patient seated and the elbow flexed 90°, abduct the arm to 90°. While one hand of the examiner stabilizes the scapula, rotate the arm forcefully posteriorly (exteriorly). If the pain of throwing is reproduced, the pathology may be subacromial bursitis. With the arm in the same position, apply internal rotation pressure. If this maneuver produces pain, rotator cuff tendinitis should be suspected. Crepitus noted in the subacromial space with rotation of the arm in abduction is a probable indication of subacromial bursitis.

Provocative testing to produce pain at a specific shoulder location is very sensitive but is not specific. Impingement is indicated by positive Hawkins and Neer impingement tests (see Physical Examination—Shoulder: Special Tests, pp 155-157).

## Diagnostic Tests

Radiographs provide additional information. Evidence of sclerosis on AP internal and external rotation views represents contact erosive areas on the greater tuberosity of the humeral head and the posterior glenoid rim.

An additional diagnostic tool is the subacromial injection (9 mL lidocaine/1 mL dexamethasone). Alleviation of the patient's pain supports a diagnosis of subacromial bursitis. In addition, gadolinium-saline enhanced MRI may be helpful to establish a working diagnosis.

## DIFFERENTIAL DIAGNOSIS

Acromial abnormalities (radiographic findings)

Anterior instability (apprehension with abduction and external rotation of the shoulder)

External impingement (positive impingement test)

Internal impingement (pain with the cocking motion of throwing)

Labral pathology (labral defect apparent on MRI)

Rotator cuff tendinitis (pathology) (weakness on testing, positive MRI)

SLAP lesion (may be seen on MRI with contrast; arthroscopy is diagnostic)

## ADVERSE OUTCOMES OF THE DISEASE

Effective pitching requires an intact rotator cuff/glenohumeral complex and pain-free motion. Therefore, athletes with the shoulder symptoms described in this chapter are usually unable to participate effectively in their sport.

## TREATMENT

### Stage I

Initially, the athlete with stage I disease, or "sore shoulder syndrome," is placed on active rest (activity modification). No overhead weight training or throwing of any object is allowed, but daily core stability work, leg work, and running for cardiovascular endurance is encouraged. Dynamic stabilization of the humeral head by rehabilitation of the rotator cuff muscles is undertaken. Stabilization is followed by strengthening of the rotator cuff muscles with isometric exercises. Basic rehabilitation includes internal and external rotation of the shoulder with the elbow at the side, using elasticized bands of increasing stiffness. Riding a stationary bicycle or an elliptical trainer with arms that move alternately also is advised. A rope-and-pulley system to increase range of motion can be used at home. Ice bags may be applied locally for pain, and trainers and physical therapists may apply electrical modalities. Initial time away from throwing is about 10 days, or until the shoulder is free from soreness. Then a published protocol of interval throwing, which must be supervised and followed closely, is begun.

SECTION 2 ■ SHOULDER

## Stage II

In the overhead thrower with stage II disease (ie, unable to compete because of pain), rehabilitation must be instituted in a very precise, scientific, but individualized manner. This is necessary because pain is an indication that tissue injury (inflammation) is already established.

First, upper body activity is controlled and modified to reestablish dynamic stability and muscle balance and to improve flexibility. Trainers and physical therapists, using hands-on methods, initiate the basic rotator cuff protocols as outlined previously. They also use electrical stimulation and ultrasound modalities and proprioception techniques. As pain permits, isotonic muscle strengthening and neuromuscular control exercises are begun. Core stabilization, which includes leg work, is coupled with a well-structured shoulder exercise program such as the Thrower's Ten Program (see Thrower's Ten Exercise Program on the DVD that accompanies this book).

# ADVERSE OUTCOMES OF TREATMENT

Rehabilitation, even when consistently and adequately performed, is often unsuccessful in returning the overhead thrower to the preinjury level of participation.

# REFERRAL DECISIONS/RED FLAGS

Referral to an orthopaedic surgeon specializing in sports medicine, especially if labral pathology is suspected, is indicated if painful overhead motion persists after an initial trial of rehabilitation exercises.

# ROTATOR CUFF TEAR

## SYNONYMS
Musculotendinous cuff rupture
Rotator cuff rupture
Rotator cuff tendinitis

## DEFINITION
The rotator cuff is composed of four muscles: the supraspinatus, the infraspinatus, the subscapularis, and the teres minor (see the illustration on p 198). These muscles form a cover around the head of the humerus and function to rotate the arm and stabilize the humeral head against the glenoid.

Rotator cuff tears sometimes occur with acute injury, but most are the result of age-related degeneration, chronic mechanical impingement, and altered blood supply to the tendons. Tears generally originate in the supraspinatus tendon and may progress posteriorly and anteriorly (**Figure 1**). Full-thickness tears are uncommon in individuals younger than age 40 years but are present in 25% of individuals over age 60 years. Most older people with rotator cuff tears are asymptomatic or have only mild, nondisabling symptoms.

## CLINICAL SYMPTOMS
Patients often report recurrent shoulder pain for several months and a specific injury that triggered the onset of the pain. Night pain and difficulty sleeping on the affected side are characteristic. Weakness, catching, and grating are common symptoms, especially when lifting the arm overhead.

## TESTS

### Physical Examination
The back of the shoulder may appear sunken, indicating atrophy of the supraspinatus and infraspinatus muscles following a long-standing cuff tear. Passive range of motion is near normal, but active range of motion may be limited. With large tears, the patient can only shrug, or "hike," the shoulder when asked to lift the arm (**Figure 2**) and cannot hold the arm elevated when it is lifted parallel to the floor. Some patients, however, maintain remarkably good active motion despite large cuff tears. As the patient lifts the arm, a grating sensation about the tip of the shoulder can be felt. Tenderness to palpation over the greater tuberosity is usually present as well.

**ICD-9 Codes**

**726.10**
Rotator cuff syndrome NOS

**727.61**
Nontraumatic complete rupture of rotator cuff

**840.4**
Rotator cuff sprain

SECTION 2 ■ SHOULDER

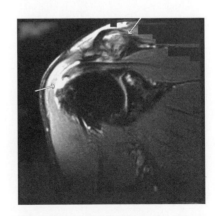

**Figure 1**
Coronal oblique MRI scan of the shoulder demonstrating a rotator cuff tear (arrows).

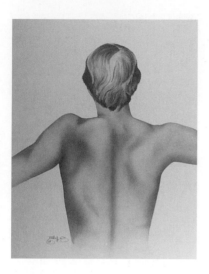

**Figure 2**

Atrophy of the supraspinatus and infraspinatus muscles and shoulder shrug with attempted abduction.

Reproduced with permission from Rockwood CA Jr: Subluxations and dislocations about the shoulder, in Rockwood CA Jr, Green DP (eds): *Rockwood and Green's Fractures in Adults, ed 2.* Philadelphia, PA, JB Lippincott, 1984, pp 722-805.

## *Diagnostic Tests*

A 30° caudal tilt view will often show a spur projecting down from the inferior surface of the acromion (**Figure 3**). To complete the diagnosis, often a coracoacromial arch view (outlet view) should be taken to show a hooked acromion, indicative of this spur (**Figure 4**). With large, long-standing tears, AP radiographs may reveal a high-riding humerus relative to the glenoid, indicative of rotator cuff arthropathy (**Figure 5**).

If the diagnosis is equivocal or if surgical treatment is being considered, MRI is the imaging study of choice because it can provide additional information on the status of the muscle and on the size of full-thickness and some partial-thickness tears.

# DIFFERENTIAL DIAGNOSIS

Acromioclavicular joint arthritis (localized pain and tenderness and preserved motion)

Cervical spondylosis (neck stiffness, absent biceps reflex, sensory changes)

Frozen shoulder (restricted active and passive motion)

Glenohumeral joint arthritis (evidence of arthritis on radiographs)

Impingement syndrome/cuff tendinitis (similar pain, but preserved active motion)

Pancoast tumor (venous distention, pulmonary changes, or bony metastases)

Thoracic outlet syndrome (ulnar nerve paresthesias, worse with "military brace" position)

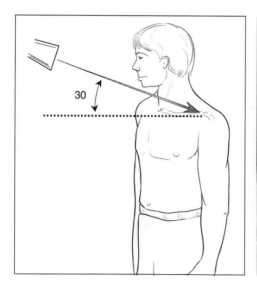
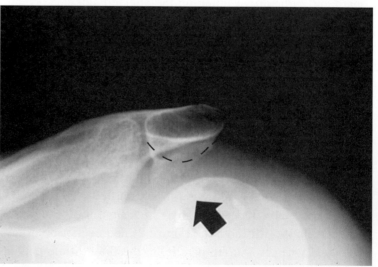

**Figure 3**

**A,** Positioning of x-ray beam for 30° caudal tilt view. **B,** Radiograph showing a bone spur of the inferior acromion.

Figure A is adapted with permission from Rockwood CA, Matsen FA (eds): *The Shoulder.* Philadelphia, PA, WB Saunders, 1990.

## ADVERSE OUTCOMES OF THE DISEASE

Loss of shoulder motion, especially the ability to lift the arm overhead; chronic pain; and/or weakness in the affected arm are possible. Long-standing large tears sometimes lead to joint degeneration.

## TREATMENT

Nonsurgical treatment includes NSAIDs, physical therapy with stretching and strengthening exercises (see Appendix A— Musculoskeletal Conditioning, pp 959-992), and avoiding overhead activities. Corticosteroid injections should be used judiciously. The steroid injection may decrease inflammation of an associated subacromial bursitis and provide short-term pain relief, but the steroid injection also weakens the tendon. Repeated injections may ultimately accelerate propagation of the rotator cuff tear. Therefore, patients should never receive more than three or four subacromial injections per year.

Only patients with significant symptoms and failed rehabilitation over 3 to 6 months should be considered candidates for surgery. The exception to this rule is the patient who has an acute traumatic cuff tear, in which case rotator cuff repair is best done acutely or no later than within 6 weeks of injury. If an acute tear is neglected longer than this, it may propagate and become retracted and much harder to repair.

## PHYSICAL THERAPY PRESCRIPTION

The functional goal of rehabilitation for a patient with a rotator cuff tear is to reduce pain, increase strength, and increase the range of motion of the involved shoulder. Stiffness of the glenohumeral joint and poor scapulothoracic mobility may be present, secondary to a period of immobilization. Rehabilitation should not involve forcing the shoulder into passive or active elevation. It is very important to avoid further damage to the rotator cuff. Instructions to the patient regarding a home exercise program should emphasize that the patient should experience no pain during or after the exercises. The home exercise program (see pp 209-210) begins with light weights and high repetitions to increase range of motion and progresses to heavier weights and fewer repetitions to strengthen the rotator cuff and the scapula rotators. Active elevation should be avoided.

Formal physical therapy should be prescribed immediately for athletes or if the patient does not progress on the home program. Poor progress would include the presence of pain and/or stiffness during or after the exercises. In addition, formal physical therapy is indicated when, upon reevaluation by the

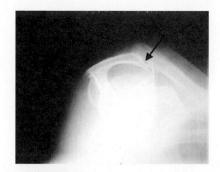

**Figure 4**
Outlet view demonstrating a hooked acromion (arrow).

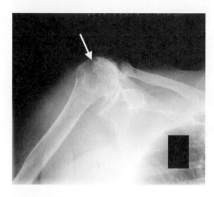

**Figure 5**
AP view of shoulder shows high-riding humeral head (arrow), indicative of rotator cuff arthropathy.

SECTION 2 ■ SHOULDER

physician in 3 to 4 weeks, muscle strength or range of motion has not improved. The prescription should include an evaluation of glenohumeral and scapula rotator muscle strength and initiation of an appropriate strengthening program. Pain-relieving modalities such as interferential current, ultrasound, or heat also may help to prepare the soft tissues for mobilization and strengthening.

## Adverse Outcomes of Treatment

NSAIDs may cause gastric, renal, or hepatic complications. Corticosteroid injections may result in a transient increase in pain because of the injection itself and degeneration of cuff tissue. Repair of large rotator cuff tears has a high incidence of failure, though the débridement alone may relieve persistent pain.

## Referral Decisions/Red Flags

Failure of 6 weeks of nonsurgical treatment is indication for further evaluation.

# HOME EXERCISE PROGRAM FOR ROTATOR CUFF TEAR

Perform the exercises in the order listed. Apply a bag of crushed ice or frozen peas to the shoulder for 20 minutes after performing both exercises to prevent any further inflammation or pain. You should not experience pain with any of the exercises. If pain or stiffness occurs that prevents you from performing any of the exercises correctly, call your doctor.

| Exercise Type | Muscle Group | Number of Repetitions/Sets | Number of Days per Week | Number of Weeks |
|---|---|---|---|---|
| Trapezius strengthening | Middle and posterior deltoid<br>Supraspinatus<br>Middle trapezius | 20 repetitions/3 to 4 sets, decreasing to 8 to 10 repetitions/ 3 to 4 sets as weight is added, then progressing to 15 repetitions/3 sets | 3 to 5 | 3 to 4 |
| Internal and external rotation at 90° or 45° elevation | *Internal rotation:*<br>Anterior deltoid<br>Pectoralis<br>Subscapularis<br>Latissimus<br>*External rotation:*<br>Posterior deltoid<br>Infraspinatus<br>Teres minor | 20 repetitions/3 to 4 sets, decreasing to 8 to 10 repetitions/ 3 to 4 sets as weight is added, then progressing to 15 repetitions/3 sets | 3 to 5 | 3 to 4 |

SECTION 2 ■ SHOULDER

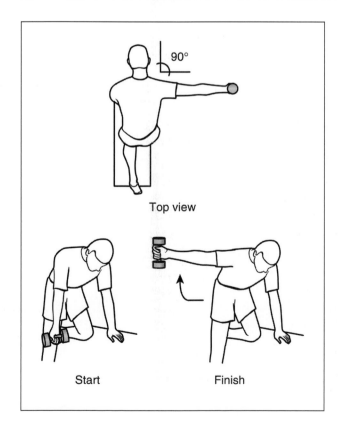

90°

Top view

Start                    Finish

## *Trapezius Strengthening*

Stand next to a bench or chair with your knee and hand (on the unaffected side) resting on the bench. The other hand should be at your side, palm facing the body. As you lift the arm slowly, rotate the hand to the thumb-up position, stopping when the arm is parallel to the floor. Slowly lower the arm to the original position to a count of 5. Begin with a light enough weight to allow 3 to 4 sets of 20 repetitions without pain. Decrease the repetitions to 8 to 10 and add no more than 2 to 3 pounds of weight so that the last few repetitions are difficult but pain free. Progress to 3 sets of 15 repetitions at each weight increment. Perform the exercise 3 to 5 times a week, continuing for 3 to 4 weeks.

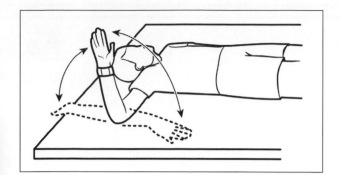

## Internal and External Rotation

Lie on your back on the floor or a bed. Extend your arm straight out from the shoulder and bend the elbow 90°. Keeping your elbow bent, slowly move your arm in the arc shown in the illustration. Change the angle of the arm to 45° if you experience pain at 90°. Begin with a light enough weight to allow 3 to 4 sets of 20 repetitions without pain. Decrease the repetitions to 8 to 10 and add no more than 2 to 3 pounds of weight so that the last few repetitions are difficult but pain free. Progress to 3 sets of 15 repetitions at each weight increment up to a maximum of approximately 5 to 7 pounds. Perform the exercises 3 to 5 times a week, continuing for 3 to 4 weeks.

# RUPTURE OF THE PROXIMAL BICEPS TENDON

## DEFINITION

Rupture of the biceps tendon usually involves the proximal long head of the biceps. Most often, ruptures occur in older adults who have a long history of shoulder pain secondary to an impingement syndrome. The tendon of the long head of the biceps, by its position in the intertubercular groove, has an active role in depressing the humeral head. This position, however, also predisposes the tendon to attritional changes, and the tendon ultimately ruptures, often as a result of a trivial event.

Rupture of the proximal biceps tendon is uncommon in young adults but may occur in athletic individuals involved in weight lifting or throwing sports. Rupture of the distal biceps tendon also may occur but is less common. (See Rupture of the Distal Biceps Tendon, p 279.)

## CLINICAL SYMPTOMS

Sudden pain in the upper arm, often accompanied by an audible snap, is often reported. Subsequently, patients notice a bulge in the lower arm. Pain in the acute stage is often mild.

## TESTS

### Physical Examination

Examination reveals a bulge in the lower arm, which results from the muscle belly of the biceps retracting into the lower arm after the long head ruptures (**Figure 1**). A defect can also be palpated proximally. Acutely, ecchymosis can be seen tracking down the middle and lower arm.

The bulge can be accentuated by having the patient contract the biceps against resistance with the elbow flexed or by doing the Ludington test (the patient puts his or her hands behind the head and flexes the biceps muscle). Gentle pressure over the bicipital groove of the humerus with the arm in 10° of internal rotation will elicit pain (**Figure 2**).

### Diagnostic Tests

AP and axillary radiographs of the shoulder are useful to rule out a fracture but are not helpful in confirming a diagnosis of a ruptured biceps tendon. For patients with a previous history of disabling shoulder pain, a shoulder arthrogram or MRI should be considered to rule out a rotator cuff tear.

**ICD-9 Code**

**840.8**
Sprain of other specified site of shoulder and upper arm

SECTION 2 ■ SHOULDER

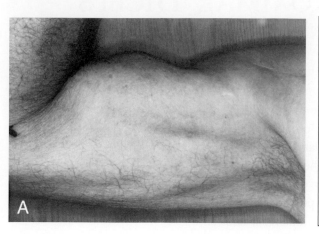

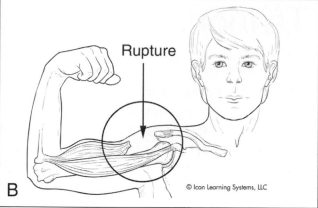

## Figure 1

Rupture of the proximal biceps tendon made more obvious by attempted contraction. **A,** Clinical photograph. **B,** Drawing showing the underlying anatomy.

Figure B is adapted with permission from Netter FH: *The CIBA Collection of Medical Illustrations.* Copyright © Icon Learning Systems, Inc.

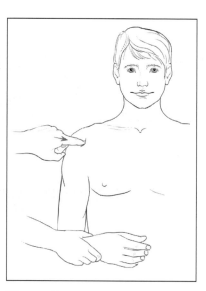

## Figure 2

Palpation of the bicipital groove.

# DIFFERENTIAL DIAGNOSIS

Dislocated biceps tendon (tenderness over the bicipital groove, but no distal muscle bulge)

Distal biceps rupture (pain and ecchymosis distally with high-riding muscle belly, often missed until late)

Glenohumeral arthritis (pain in the joint exacerbated with motion, evident on radiographs)

Impingement syndrome (can coexist with biceps tendon rupture)

Rotator cuff tear (often coexists with biceps tendon rupture)

Rupture of the pectoralis major muscle (abnormal muscle contour apparent in anterior axillary fold)

# ADVERSE OUTCOMES OF THE DISEASE

Patients can lose approximately 10% of elbow flexion and forearm supination strength (the motion required to use a manual screwdriver). Cosmetic deformity of the arm in the form of a bulge in the lower arm may also be of concern to the patient.

# TREATMENT

Nonsurgical treatment is effective for most patients, resulting in little loss of function and acceptable cosmetic deformity. Most patients regain full range of motion and normal elbow flexion strength with an exercise program consisting of range of motion and strengthening as pain allows. Patients with persistent shoulder pain and young athletes need evaluation for a concomitant rotator cuff tear.

In young athletes and in adults younger than 40 years who work as heavy laborers and need the extra strength for lifting, surgical repair of the biceps tendon should be considered.

## Adverse Outcomes of Treatment

Functional improvement from surgery is often modest, and postoperative stiffness is a potential concern. Bodybuilders may trade a distal muscle bulge for a surgical scar with little subjective cosmetic improvement.

## Referral Decisions/Red Flags

Young patients who are heavy laborers and older patients with a concomitant rotator cuff tear and persistent symptoms need further evaluation.

Section 2 ■ Shoulder

# SHOULDER INSTABILITY

**ICD-9 Codes**

**718.81**
Instability of shoulder joint NOS

**831.00**
Closed dislocation shoulder,
unspecified

## SYNONYMS

Dislocation
Multidirectional instability
Recurrent dislocation
Subluxation

## DEFINITION

With its shallow glenoid and loose capsule, the shoulder joint has great mobility. As a corollary, instability is also most common at the shoulder. Patients with shoulder instability have recurrent episodes of subluxation (humeral head partially slips out of the socket) and/or dislocation (**Figure 1**). Instability can be anterior, posterior, inferior, or multidirectional, with anterior and multidirectional being the most common (**Figure 2**). It is important to determine where an instability lies along the pathologic spectrum, from Traumatic Unidirectional instability with a Bankart lesion (a tear of the anterior glenoid labrum) best treated with Surgery (TUBS) (**Figure 3**) to Atraumatic, Multidirectional, Bilateral signs of laxity, Rehabilitation as the preferred treatment, and Inferior capsular shift as the indicated procedure if surgery becomes necessary (AMBRI). Posterior dislocations result from a posteriorly directed force when the arm is in adduction and internal rotation. This uncommon injury is associated with seizures or electric shock injuries.

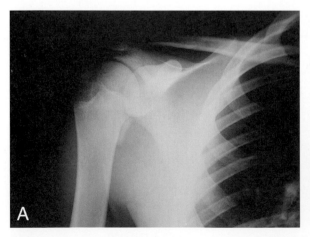
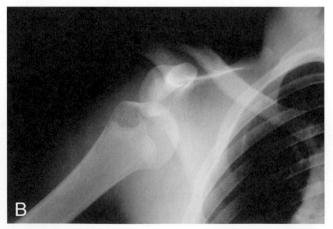

**Figure 1**
AP views of shoulder. **A,** Nondislocated shoulder. **B,** Dislocated shoulder.

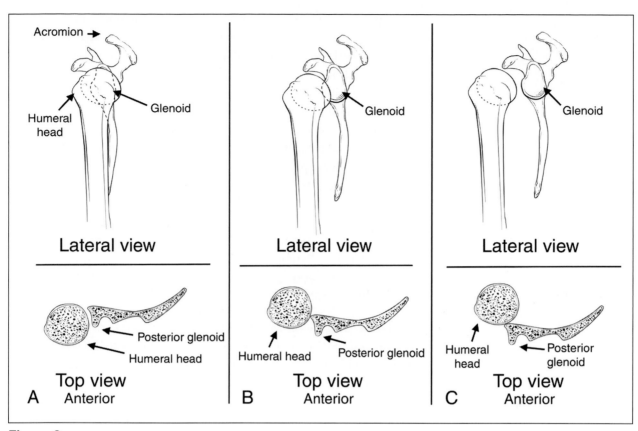

**Figure 2**
Relative positions of the humeral head and the glenoid with the humeral head reduced (**A**), subluxated anteriorly (**B**), and dislocated anteriorly (**C**).

# CLINICAL SYMPTOMS

Patients with anterior instability typically describe the sensation of the shoulder slipping out of joint when the arm is abducted and externally rotated. The initial anterior shoulder dislocation is associated with significant trauma from a fall or forceful throwing motion, but with recurrent dislocations, the patient may experience instability by simply positioning the arm overhead. With multidirectional instability, symptoms may be vague but tend to be activity related. Ask the patient whether he or she can voluntarily dislocate the shoulder, as this is an important clue. The ability to voluntarily dislocate the shoulder is quite frequently associated with a multidirectional instability component and may indicate a poor prognosis for surgical treatment or the presence of a personality disorder.

# TESTS

## Physical Examination
With an acute dislocation, any movement of the shoulder is associated with considerable pain. With an anterior dislocation, the patient supports the arm in a neutral position. Patients with

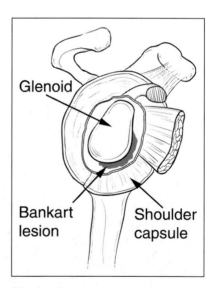

**Figure 3**
Detachment of the labrum—
Bankart lesion.

Adapted with permission from Matsen F III (ed): *Practical Evaluation and Management of the Shoulder.* Philadelphia, PA, WB Saunders, 1994, p 103.

a posterior dislocation hold the arm in adduction and internal rotation; external rotation is impossible. Neurovascular function, particularly that of the axillary nerve, should be carefully assessed before and after reduction.

Assessment of a patient believed to have recurrent instability should include the apprehension test for anterior instability, the sulcus sign test for inferior laxity (**Figure 4**), and the jerk test for posterior instability. (See Physical Examination—Shoulder: Special Tests, p 156.) The patient also should be assessed for generalized ligamentous laxity. Ask the patient to touch the thumb against the volar (flexor) surface of the forearm . Bend the fingers back at the metacarpophalangeal joint to determine how far they extend past neutral with the finger and hand in a straight line. Patients with ligamentous laxity are more likely to have multidirectional instability, but other types of instability are still possible.

## Diagnostic Tests

AP and axillary radiographs of the shoulder should be obtained. The axillary view may show a bony defect at the anterior edge of the glenoid rim (**Figure 5**). A compression fracture of the posterior humeral head (a Hill-Sachs lesion) is created when the head is pressed against the anterior edge of the glenoid. A Hill-Sachs lesion is clear evidence of an anterior dislocation. Patients older than 40 years with a history of traumatic dislocation are also prone to tear the rotator cuff at the time of dislocation. A shoulder arthrogram or MRI may be indicated in these cases.

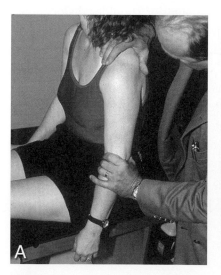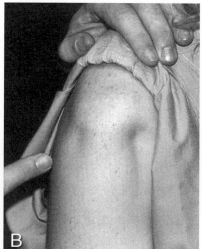

**Figure 4**
Sulcus sign. **A,** With the patient's arm relaxed at the side, the examiner applies traction in an inferior direction. **B,** Positive sulcus sign, indicative of inferior shoulder laxity.

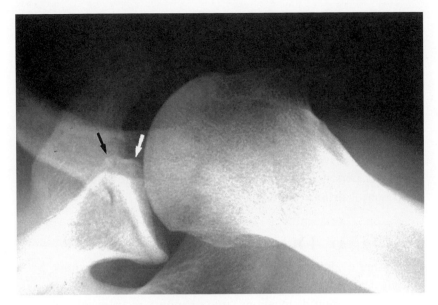

**Figure 5**
Axillary view showing erosion of the glenoid rim (arrows) associated with anterior glenohumeral instability.
Reproduced from Bigliani LU (ed): *The Unstable Shoulder.* Rosemont, IL, American Academy of Orthopaedic Surgeons, 1996.

Posterior dislocation of the shoulder is easily missed if only an AP radiograph is obtained. If an axillary view cannot be obtained, request a transscapular lateral view.

## DIFFERENTIAL DIAGNOSIS

Glenohumeral arthritis (confirm with radiographs)
Impingement syndrome (pain but no apprehension of instability)
Rotator cuff tear (pain and weakness without apprehension)

## ADVERSE OUTCOMES OF THE DISEASE

Axillary nerve injury (deltoid dysfunction and numbness over lateral arm) is not uncommon but usually resolves. The risk of recurrent instability is greater in younger patients and in those with multiple episodes.

## TREATMENT

Most acute shoulder dislocations can be reduced in the emergency department. There are several ways to reduce a shoulder, but only two are described here. (See Reduction of Anterior Shoulder Dislocation, pp 219-221.) Patients with a first-time dislocation can be treated with a physical therapy program that emphasizes strengthening the rotator cuff muscles, especially the subscapularis muscle. (See Appendix A— Musculoskeletal Conditioning, pp 959-992.)

Patients with atraumatic or voluntary instability (AMBRI) should be treated nonsurgically with the shoulder exercise program described in Appendix A. Educating patients to avoid voluntarily dislocating the shoulder and to avoid positions of known instability is an important part of the treatment plan.

## Adverse Outcomes of Treatment

Axillary nerve injury, osteoarthritis of the glenohumeral joint, and/or persistent dislocation is possible. Failure to recognize a posterior dislocation can also occur.

## Referral Decisions/Red Flags

Further evaluation is warranted in the following situations: when closed manipulation fails to reduce an acute dislocation; when recurrent dislocations (two or more) occur despite a 3-month trial of shoulder rehabilitation exercises; and in patients with multidirectional instability whose symptoms are intolerable and do not respond to a rehabilitation program.

# PROCEDURE
## REDUCTION OF ANTERIOR SHOULDER DISLOCATION

Prior to reduction, a neurovascular examination should be performed. Assess function of the axillary, musculocutaneous, median, radial, and ulnar nerves, with emphasis on evaluating the axillary nerve through voluntary isometric contraction of the deltoid and sensation over the lateral deltoid region. Obtain AP and axillary radiographs to document the dislocation and rule out any fractures that may displace during the reduction maneuver. Reducing a first-time dislocation is most safely done in the emergency department with a resuscitation cart available.

Establish an intravenous line, ensure that naloxone is available, and initiate pulse oximetry and cardiac monitoring if narcotics are used for anesthesia. Apply oxygen by mask or nasal cannula throughout the procedure. Fentanyl in a dose of 100 µg is given IV over 1 minute, and then repeated every 3 to 5 minutes until adequate sedation is achieved. The usual total dose of fentanyl is 3 µg/kg. Patients with recurrent dislocations may not require anesthesia.

## STIMSON TECHNIQUE (GRAVITY-ASSISTED REDUCTION)

### STEP 1
Place the patient prone on a stretcher with the dislocated arm hanging off the cart. Secure the patient to the stretcher with a sheet.

### STEP 2
Either have an assistant sit on the floor and provide downward traction, or attach 5 to 15 lb of weight to the patient's arm (**Figure 1**). The weights should not touch the floor.

### STEP 3
For reduction of the left shoulder, place your left thumb on the patient's acromion and the fingers of your left hand over the front of the humeral head.

### STEP 4
As the muscles relax, gently push the humeral head caudally until it reduces.

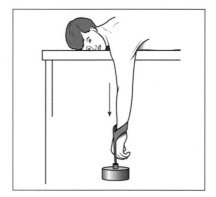

**Figure 1**
Stimson technique (gravity-assisted reduction with patient lying on stomach).

# REDUCTION OF ANTERIOR SHOULDER DISLOCATION (CONTINUED)

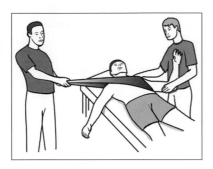

**Figure 2**
Longitudinal traction technique for shoulder reduction.

## LONGITUDINAL TRACTION

### STEP 1

Place the patient supine on a stretcher with a sheet folded into a band 4″ to 5″ wide around the patient's chest (**Figure 2**). Stand next to the patient on the same side as the injured shoulder, at or below the patient's waist.

### STEP 2

Position the patient's elbow in 90° of flexion to relax the biceps muscle. An assistant applies traction to the sheet that is wrapped around the patient's thorax while you apply a steady traction to the arm.

### STEP 3

Reduction may be aided if you gently rotate the arm while the longitudinal traction is applied. You usually can feel and see the shoulder reduce. Occasionally, especially in large patients, the reduction may be subtle, and you may neither feel nor see it.

## ADVERSE OUTCOMES

Axillary nerve palsy may develop with reduction. Be sure to test axillary nerve function (motor and sensory) before and after the reduction. General anesthesia may be required to reduce the shoulder.

The administration of opioids such as fentanyl carries the risk of overdose. Fentanyl overdose is treated with naloxone. Initially, give 0.2 to 0.4 mg IV, and if there is no response, administer repeated doses of up to 4 to 5 mg; doses as high as 15 to 20 mg may be administered with resistant opioids such as fentanyl. First-time dislocation in a patient older than 40 years may be associated with a rotator cuff tear, so examine these patients with a high index of suspicion for a tear.

## AFTERCARE/PATIENT INSTRUCTIONS

Obtain postreduction AP and axillary radiographs to confirm the reduction. Immobilize the arm in a sling, but have the patient remove the sling and extend the elbow several times daily to prevent elbow stiffness. Begin isometric exercises for the rotator cuff. Have the patient externally rotate the arm to 0° (palm facing straight ahead) and flex the shoulder to 90° (humerus parallel with the floor) at least 10 times each day for 2 weeks.

# REDUCTION OF ANTERIOR SHOULDER DISLOCATION (CONTINUED)

Begin strengthening exercises for the subscapularis and infraspinatus muscles at 2 to 3 weeks postreduction in the older patient and at 6 weeks in the younger patient.

Increase shoulder external rotation to 30° or 40° and shoulder flexion to 140°. This occurs at 6 weeks postreduction in patients younger than 30 years and at 3 weeks in patients older than 30 years.

Begin vigorous shoulder motion at 6 weeks postreduction in patients older than 30 years, but delay this step to 3 months for patients younger than 30 years.

The propensity for shoulder stiffness in patients older than 30 years is an advantage in regaining stability; however, these patients are more likely to sustain a rotator cuff tear at the time of the dislocation.

In the athlete, allow return to sports activities once near-full flexion and rotation of the arm and near-normal strength of the cuff have been regained.

# SUPERIOR LABRUM ANTERIOR-TO-POSTERIOR LESIONS

## ICD-9 Codes

**718.01**
Articular cartilage disorder, shoulder region (for chronic SLAP lesion)

**840.7**
Superior glenoid labrum lesion (for acute SLAP lesion)

## SYNONYMS

Biceps labral complex injuries
SLAP lesions
Superior glenoid labrum tears

## DEFINITION

Superior labrum anterior-to-posterior (SLAP) lesions involve an injury to the superior glenoid labrum and the biceps anchor complex. The long head of the biceps tendon originates from the superior aspect of the glenoid labrum and is confluent with the labrum in this region, also called the biceps anchor. The glenoid labrum itself, which has been likened to the shoulder equivalent of the meniscus of the knee, consists of a cartilaginous lining of the glenoid, which serves to deepen the glenoid, thereby providing increased stability of the shoulder. Injuries to the labrum involve either fraying (usually degenerative in nature) or frank tears (associated with acute and chronic symptoms). Injuries that involve the superior labrum are termed SLAP lesions.

## CLINICAL SYMPTOMS

SLAP lesions are difficult to diagnose and are often a diagnosis of exclusion, confirmed only at the time of surgery. Symptoms may include painful popping or catching in the shoulder as well as pain with overhead activities. In a throwing athlete, symptoms may be present only with maximal effort throwing, but a thorough history may reveal an insidious onset of pain while performing overhead sports that limits performance and eventually leads to a persistent aching in the shoulder. The aching is often described as being "deep inside" the shoulder.

## TESTS

### Physical Examination

Several tests are used to detect SLAP lesions, but they have poor sensitivity and specificity. They include the active compression test (the O'Brien test), the crank test, the resisted supination/external rotation test, and the clunk test. They are designed to elicit pain as the lesion is compressed

For the active compression test, the arm is positioned in 20° of adduction and 90° of forward elevation. The examiner applies a downward force, first with the wrist fully supinated and then again with the wrist fully pronated. The test is considered positive if the patient experiences more pain with the wrist pronated.

For the crank test, the arm is elevated to 160° in the scapular plane and is then loaded axially by the examiner. Maximal internal and external rotation of the arm is applied while still axially loading the shoulder. A positive test is pain and/or a clicking produced by the maneuver.

For the resisted supination/external rotation test, the patient is placed supine with the shoulder at 90° of abduction. The elbow is flexed to 70° with the wrist in neutral rotation. The patient actively supinates against the examiner's resistance as the shoulder is slowly externally rotated to maximum external rotation. Supination is resisted throughout the motion. Pain at or just before maximal external rotation is a positive test. This test attempts to mimic the "peel-back" position in an overhead thrower.

For the clunk test, the patient is placed supine with the shoulder flexed to 180°, the elbow flexed to 90°, and the hand pointing to the floor. With the elbow held in place, the hand is grasped by the examiner and used to internally rotate the shoulder. The test is considered positive if the patient experiences a sharp pain with the internal rotation.

### Diagnostic Tests

Plain radiographs should be obtained because they are part of a thorough workup of any shoulder disorder, but they cannot confirm a diagnosis of a SLAP lesion. MR arthrography (injection of contrast medium into the shoulder before the MRI is done) is the gold standard to evaluate for a SLAP lesion, although its sensitivity and specificity for the condition is no greater than 90%. MRI without contrast has a sensitivity of less than 50%.

## DIFFERENTIAL DIAGNOSIS

Acromioclavicular (AC) joint arthritis (tenderness over AC joint, positive cross-body adduction test, AC pain on bench pressing)

Biceps tendinitis (tender anteriorly over biceps tendon)

Rotator cuff disease (pain referred to lateral deltoid)

Shoulder instability (history of shoulder "slipping out of place," positive apprehension test)

Subacromial impingement (positive clinical impingement signs, palpable crepitus, local tenderness over rotator cuff insertion)

Suprascapular nerve entrapment (possible wasting of infraspinatus on exam, diagnosed with electromyography)

SECTION 2 ■ SHOULDER

## Adverse Outcomes of the Disease

Continued shoulder pain and some disability with activities are possible.

## Treatment

Nonsurgical care should be attempted initially. This includes NSAIDs as well as physical therapy directed at rotator cuff and periscapular stabilization, posterior capsule stretching, and strengthening with gradual return to activities. In a throwing athlete, gradual return to activities would include the use of an interval throwing program after at least 6 weeks of rest to return the athlete to a competitive level of play in a controlled fashion. If nonsurgical care fails and symptoms persist, diagnostic shoulder arthroscopy is the only other alternative. At the time of surgery, all intra-articular pathology can be delineated and addressed.

## Physical Therapy Prescription

The functional goal of rehabilitation for a patient with a SLAP lesion is to reduce pain and protect the joint from further damage. Unfortunately, many SLAP lesions do not respond well to nonsurgical treatment. The home exercise program (see pp 225-226) should include stretching of the posterior structures. In addition, deep bench presses, overhead presses, and biceps curls should be prohibited. Reaching behind and overhead activities should be limited to pain-free movement. If the patient does not respond to the home program of exercises, stretching, and activity modification, referral to a physical therapist is indicated. The physical therapist should evaluate the muscle strength and posterior capsule mobility and determine the appropriate exercises for the patient's condition.

## Adverse Outcomes of Treatment

NSAIDs may cause gastric, renal, and hepatic complications. Physical therapy may not lead to improvements in symptoms but has no other adverse effect. The most common adverse effect following surgical repair of a SLAP lesion is shoulder stiffness.

## Referral Decisions/Red Flags

Patients with continued shoulder pain despite negative findings from a thorough workup and clinical examination may have a SLAP lesion and warrant further evaluation.

# HOME EXERCISE PROGRAM FOR SLAP LESIONS

Perform the exercises in the order listed. Apply dry or moist heat to the shoulder prior to the exercises and during the sleeper stretch. To reduce inflammation, apply a bag of crushed ice or frozen peas to the shoulder for 15 to 20 minutes after performing both exercises. You should not experience pain during or after the exercises. If the exercises cause pain, call your doctor. Avoid activities that may cause additional damage to the labral tear, such as arm curls while lifting heavy objects (heavier than 5 pounds), overhead sports activities (a tennis serve or throwing a baseball), and reaching overhead or behind your body.

| Exercise Type | Muscle Group | Number of Repetitions/Sets | Number of Days per Week | Number of Weeks |
|---|---|---|---|---|
| Sleeper stretch | Infraspinatus<br>Teres minor<br>Posterior capsule | 4 repetitions/2 to 3 sets | Daily | 2 to 3 |
| External rotation | Infraspinatus<br>Teres minor<br>Posterior deltoid | 8 to 10 repetitions/2 sets, progressing to 15 repetitions/3 sets | 3 | 2 to 3 |

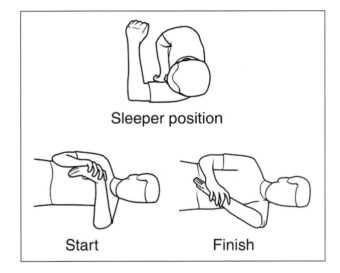

Sleeper position

Start          Finish

## Sleeper Stretch

Lie on your side on a firm, flat surface with the affected shoulder under you and the arm positioned as shown, keeping your back perpendicular to the surface. With the unaffected arm, push the other wrist down, toward the surface. Stop when you feel a stretching sensation in the back of the affected shoulder. Hold this position for 30 seconds, then relax the arm for 30 seconds. Perform 2 to 3 sets of 4 repetitions daily. Continue for a total of 2 to 3 weeks.

**SECTION 2 ■ SHOULDER**

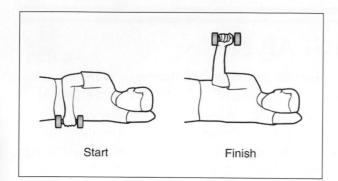

Start Finish

## External Rotation

Lie on your side on a firm, flat surface with the unaffected arm under you, cradling your head. Hold the injured arm against your side as shown, with the elbow bent at a 90° angle. Slowly rotate the arm at the shoulder, keeping the elbow bent and against your side, to raise the weight to a vertical position, and then slowly lower the weight to the starting position to a count of 5. Begin with weights that allow 2 sets of 8 to 10 repetitions and progress to 3 sets of 15 repetitions. Add weight in 1-pound increments, starting over with 8 to 10 repetitions each time weight is added. Perform the exercise 3 days a week. Continue for a total of 2 to 3 weeks.

SECTION 2 ■ SHOULDER

# THORACIC OUTLET SYNDROME

## DEFINITION

Thoracic outlet syndrome (TOS) is compression of the brachial plexus and/or subclavian vessels as they exit the narrow space between the superior shoulder girdle and the first rib (**Figure 1**). These structures may be affected individually or in combination. Women between the ages of 20 and 50 years are most commonly affected.

The etiology of TOS may be secondary to congenital anomalies such as a cervical rib or abnormally long transverse process of C7, or an anomalous fibromuscular band in the thoracic outlet. Posttraumatic fibrosis of the scalene muscles also is a possibility.

## CLINICAL SYMPTOMS

Symptoms are often vague and variable. Compression of the brachial plexus accounts for most presenting symptoms and may mimic distal nerve entrapment, especially of the ulnar nerve, with little and ring finger paresthesias. Aching pain and

**ICD-9 Code**
**353.0**
Brachial plexus lesions

SECTION 2 ■ SHOULDER

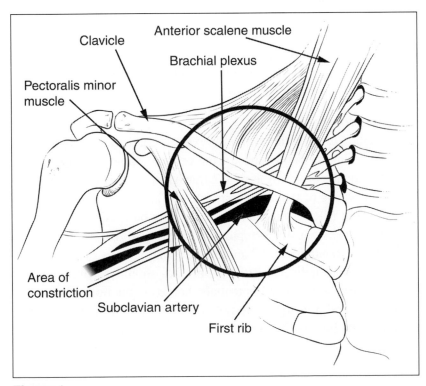

**Figure 1**

Anatomy of the thoracic outlet.

Adapted with permission from Rockwood CA Jr: Subluxation and dislocations about the shoulder, in Rockwood CA Jr, Green DP (eds): *Rockwood and Green's Fractures in Adults,* ed 3. Philadelphia, PA, JB Lippincott, 1988, pp 722-985.

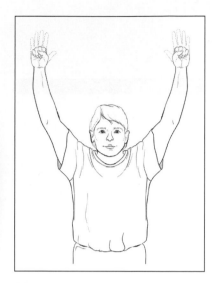

**Figure 2**
Elevated arm stress test (EAST).

paresthesias can extend from the neck into the shoulder, arm, medial forearm, and the fingers. Symptoms from vascular compression include intermittent swelling and discoloration of the arm. The aching fatigue and weakness are worse when the arm is in an overhead position. Psychological disturbances such as depression are seen with TOS, but whether they contribute to the causation or are the result of a chronically painful condition is unclear.

# TESTS

## Physical Examination

Inspect for swelling or discoloration of the arm and palpate the supraclavicular fossa to rule out a mass lesion. Auscultation over this area may reveal the presence of a bruit, especially while doing the provocative maneuvers described below. Compare distal pulses with those on the opposite side. Assess sensory and motor function of the axillary, musculocutaneous, medial antebrachial cutaneous, median, radial, and, most important, ulnar nerve.

Several clinical tests have been described to diagnose TOS. Perhaps the simplest and most reproducible provocative maneuver is the elevated arm stress test (EAST) (**Figure 2**). With both shoulders abducted at least 90° and braced somewhat posteriorly, the patient opens and closes his or her fists at a moderate speed for 3 minutes. Reproduction of neurologic and/or vascular symptoms is a positive test. A sense of fatigue without neurologic or vascular symptoms is considered a negative or inconclusive test.

## Diagnostic Tests

No laboratory studies currently exist to confirm the diagnosis. AP and lateral radiographs of the cervical spine identify cervical ribs or overly long C7 transverse processes. PA and lateral views of the chest help rule out an apical lung tumor or infection. MRI of the cervical spine may be needed if the patient has signs and symptoms of a cervical disk rupture or a cervical spondylosis. AP and axillary radiographs of the shoulder are indicated if the patient has shoulder symptoms. Somatosensory evoked potentials, nerve conduction velocity studies, and ultrasound are not reliable in confirming the diagnosis but can be useful in ruling out alternative diagnoses (eg, ulnar nerve entrapment).

# DIFFERENTIAL DIAGNOSIS

Brachial plexus neuritis (sudden onset, severe pain, proximal muscle weakness)

Carpal tunnel syndrome (numbness on the radial side of the hand, positive Phalen maneuver)

Herniated cervical disk (neck pain and stiffness with unilateral or bilateral pain and neurologic findings in a radicular pattern)

Impingement syndrome (localized shoulder pain with positive impingement signs)

Pancoast tumor (venous congestion, lesion on apical lordotic chest radiograph)

Ulnar nerve entrapment (Tinel sign at elbow, abnormal nerve conduction velocity studies, no symptoms above the elbow)

# ADVERSE OUTCOMES OF THE DISEASE

Weakness and loss of coordination of the upper extremity, chronic headaches, and the inability to work with the arm overhead are possible. Ulcerations on the arm and hand and the Raynaud phenomenon are rare. Serious problems such as venous thrombosis and aneurysm of the subclavian artery are uncommon but can develop.

# TREATMENT

Most patients can be treated nonsurgically with 3 months of a home exercise program that emphasizes muscle strengthening and postural education exercises. Strenuous activities, such as carrying heavy objects, should be avoided, as should placing straps over the affected shoulder, including bras, purses, and seat belts. Activities that aggravate symptoms, such as prolonged overhead activities, strenuous aerobic exercises, and sleeping on the affected shoulder, should be discouraged as well.

Maintaining proper posture is important. The patient should be taught to stand up straight with the shoulders back, not slumped forward. The use of NSAIDs, muscle relaxants, and transcutaneous electrical nerve stimulation (TENS) units can help decrease the severity of the symptoms. Weight reduction, when indicated, should be encouraged as well. A multidisciplinary approach, including physical therapists, occupational therapists, and physiatrists, may be beneficial.

Because the success rate from surgery is variable and the complication rate is significant, every effort should be made to treat these patients nonsurgically.

## ADVERSE OUTCOMES OF TREATMENT

The following conditions may develop following or as a result of treatment: complex regional pain syndrome, intercostal neuroma, frozen shoulder, brachial plexus injury, or pneumothorax.

## REFERRAL DECISIONS/RED FLAGS

Vascular compromise with swelling and/or ulceration necessitates early consultation. Similarly, patients with TOS and a cervical rib or extra-long transverse process need early specialty evaluation when these findings are associated with loss of sensation, muscle atrophy, and weakness. Finally, failure of a well-supervised exercise program in a patient with disabling symptoms is an indication for further evaluation.

# HOME EXERCISE PROGRAM FOR THORACIC OUTLET SYNDROME

The following exercises are designed to stretch the soft-tissue structures that may be compressing the neurovascular bundle. Perform the exercises in the order listed. If any of the exercises causes an increase in your symptoms, discontinue the exercises and call your doctor.

| Exercise Type | Number of Repetitions/Sets | Number of Days per Week | Number of Weeks |
|---|---|---|---|
| Corner stretches | 10 repetitions/2 sets | Daily | 12 |
| Neck stretches | 10 repetitions/2 sets | Daily | 12 |
| Shoulder rolls | 10 repetitions/2 sets | Daily | 12 |
| Neck retractions | 10 repetitions/2 sets | Daily | 12 |

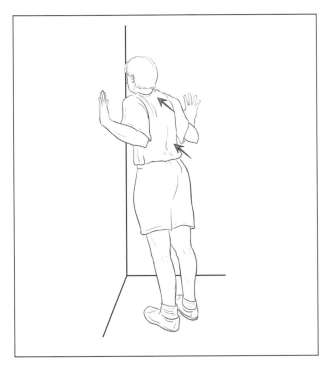

Adapted with permission from Visual Health Information, Tacoma, WA.

## *Corner Stretches*

Stand in a corner with your hands against the walls at shoulder height. Lean into the corner until you feel a gentle stretch. Hold for 5 seconds.

SECTION 2 ■ SHOULDER

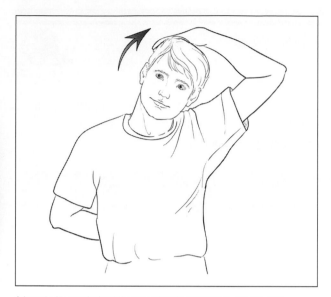

Adapted with permission from Visual Health Information, Tacoma, WA.

## Neck Stretches

Place your left hand on the far side of your head and your right hand behind your back. Pull your head toward your shoulder until you feel a gentle stretch. Hold for 5 seconds. Switch hand positions and repeat the exercise in the opposite direction.

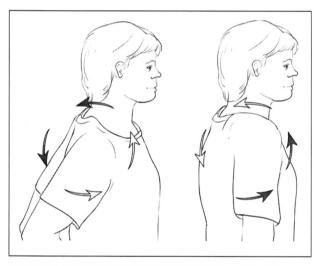

Adapted with permission from Visual Health Information, Tacoma, WA.

## Shoulder Rolls

Roll your shoulders up, back, and then down in a circular motion.

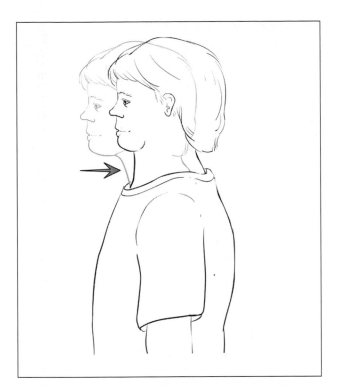

Adapted with permission from Visual Health Information, Tacoma, WA.

## Neck Retractions

Pull your head straight back, keeping your jaw level. Hold in the retracted position for 5 seconds.

SECTION 2 ■ SHOULDER

# PAIN DIAGRAM—ELBOW AND FOREARM

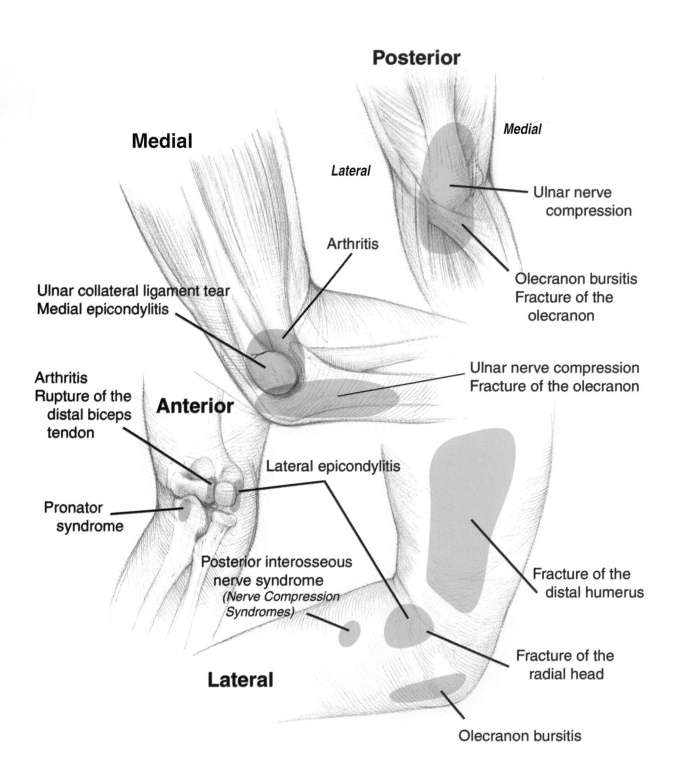

**Posterior**

*Medial*

*Lateral*

**Medial**

Ulnar nerve
compression

Arthritis

Ulnar collateral ligament tear
Medial epicondylitis

Olecranon bursitis
Fracture of the
olecranon

Arthritis
Rupture of the
distal biceps
tendon

**Anterior**

Ulnar nerve compression
Fracture of the olecranon

Lateral epicondylitis

Pronator
syndrome

Posterior interosseous
nerve syndrome
*(Nerve Compression
Syndromes)*

Fracture of the
distal humerus

Fracture of the
radial head

**Lateral**

Olecranon bursitis

# ELBOW AND FOREARM

**Section Editor**
Joseph B. Chandler, MD
Director of Medical Services
Atlanta Braves
Resurgens Orthopaedics
Atlanta, Georgia

Robert Donatelli, PhD, PT, OCS
National Director of Sports Rehabilitation
Physiotherapy Associates
Las Vegas, Nevada

Dawn D. Hassinger, MD, PhD
Atlanta, Georgia

Gary M. Lourie, MD
Hand Consultant
Atlanta Braves
The Hand Treatment Center
Atlanta, Georgia

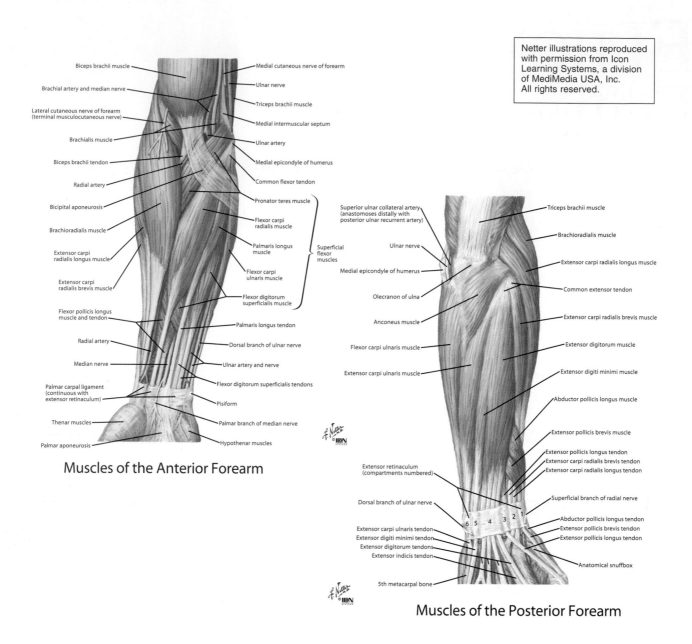

**Muscles of the Anterior Forearm**

- Biceps brachii muscle
- Brachial artery and median nerve
- Lateral cutaneous nerve of forearm (terminal musculocutaneous nerve)
- Brachialis muscle
- Biceps brachii tendon
- Radial artery
- Bicipital aponeurosis
- Brachioradialis muscle
- Extensor carpi radialis longus muscle
- Extensor carpi radialis brevis muscle
- Flexor pollicis longus muscle and tendon
- Radial artery
- Median nerve
- Palmar carpal ligament (continuous with extensor retinaculum)
- Thenar muscles
- Palmar aponeurosis
- Medial cutaneous nerve of forearm
- Ulnar nerve
- Triceps brachii muscle
- Medial intermuscular septum
- Ulnar artery
- Medial epicondyle of humerus
- Common flexor tendon
- Pronator teres muscle
- Flexor carpi radialis muscle
- Palmaris longus muscle
- Flexor carpi ulnaris muscle
- Flexor digitorum superficialis muscle
- Superficial flexor muscles
- Palmaris longus tendon
- Dorsal branch of ulnar nerve
- Ulnar artery and nerve
- Flexor digitorum superficialis tendons
- Pisiform
- Palmar branch of median nerve
- Hypothenar muscles

**Muscles of the Posterior Forearm**

- Superior ulnar collateral artery (anastomoses distally with posterior ulnar recurrent artery)
- Ulnar nerve
- Medial epicondyle of humerus
- Olecranon of ulna
- Anconeus muscle
- Flexor carpi ulnaris muscle
- Extensor carpi ulnaris muscle
- Extensor retinaculum (compartments numbered)
- Dorsal branch of ulnar nerve
- Extensor carpi ulnaris tendon
- Extensor digiti minimi tendon
- Extensor digitorum tendons
- Extensor indicis tendon
- 5th metacarpal bone
- Triceps brachii muscle
- Brachioradialis muscle
- Extensor carpi radialis longus muscle
- Common extensor tendon
- Extensor carpi radialis brevis muscle
- Extensor digitorum muscle
- Extensor digiti minimi muscle
- Abductor pollicis longus muscle
- Extensor pollicis brevis muscle
- Extensor pollicis longus tendon
- Extensor carpi radialis brevis tendon
- Extensor carpi radialis longus tendon
- Superficial branch of radial nerve
- Abductor pollicis longus tendon
- Extensor pollicis brevis tendon
- Extensor pollicis longus tendon
- Anatomical snuffbox

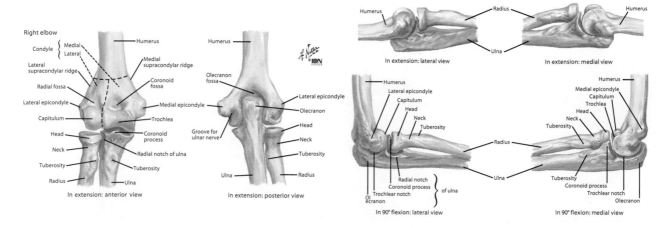

**Bones of the Elbow Joint**

- Right elbow
- Condyle { Medial / Lateral }
- Lateral supracondylar ridge
- Radial fossa
- Lateral epicondyle
- Capitulum
- Head
- Neck
- Tuberosity
- Radius
- Humerus
- Medial supracondylar ridge
- Coronoid fossa
- Medial epicondyle
- Trochlea
- Coronoid process
- Radial notch of ulna
- Tuberosity
- Ulna

In extension: anterior view

- Humerus
- Olecranon fossa
- Groove for ulnar nerve
- Ulna
- Lateral epicondyle
- Olecranon
- Head
- Neck
- Tuberosity
- Radius

In extension: posterior view

- Humerus
- Radius
- Ulna

In extension: lateral view

- Radius
- Humerus
- Ulna

In extension: medial view

- Humerus
- Lateral epicondyle
- Capitulum
- Head
- Neck
- Tuberosity
- Radial notch
- Coronoid process
- Trochlear notch
- Olecranon
- Radius
- Ulna

In 90° flexion: lateral view

- Humerus
- Medial epicondyle
- Capitulum
- Trochlea
- Head
- Neck
- Tuberosity
- Radius
- Ulna
- Tuberosity
- Coronoid process
- Trochlear notch
- Olecranon

In 90° flexion: medial view

# ELBOW AND FOREARM—OVERVIEW

This section of *Essentials of Musculoskeletal Care* focuses on the more common and important conditions encountered in the elbow and forearm. Making a correct diagnosis of a condition in the elbow or forearm begins with clearly defining the nature and the anatomic location of the patient's chief symptom, which usually is related to pain, stiffness, swelling, or a combination of the three. Unlike the shoulder, the elbow has considerable articular congruency, and elbow instability is a much less common problem than shoulder instability.

The elbow joint comprises three distinct articulations: the ulnohumeral, radiocapitellar, and proximal radioulnar joints. The ulnohumeral and radiocapitellar joints provide flexion/extension of the elbow and pronation/supination of the forearm, and the proximal radioulnar joint works in conjunction with the distal radioulnar joint at the wrist to achieve forearm pronation and supination. Basic radiographic assessment consists of an AP view of the extended elbow and a lateral view with the elbow flexed 90° and with the forearm supinated. Oblique views can be helpful in identifying subtle fractures and when the elbow cannot be extended enough to obtain an AP view. The basic evaluation should include not only assessment of the bony anatomy but also attention to soft tissue; for example, the presence of a posterior fat pad may herald an intra-articular fracture.

## ACUTE PAIN

Acute pain and swelling after an injury can be caused by a fracture, dislocation, or tendon/ligament rupture. The location of the pain, tenderness, deformity, and ecchymosis are important physical findings. Pain with elbow flexion/extension suggests involvement of the ulnohumeral articulation, whereas pain with forearm pronation/supination should direct attention to the radiocapitellar and proximal radioulnar joints.

Radiographs will confirm a fracture or dislocation, although some radial head or other articular surface fractures can be easily missed. Subtle radiographic signs such as bony avulsions or soft-tissue swelling seen with a fat pad sign can signal important bony injury. When radiographs are normal, a tendon or ligament rupture, such as of the distal biceps or triceps, is possible.

Acute pain or swelling over the tip of the elbow may indicate an acute olecranon bursitis. Intra-articular conditions, which may produce acute synovitis of the elbow, include septic arthritis (especially in intravenous drug abusers), rheumatoid arthritis, or other inflammatory conditions, such as crystalline deposition diseases (gout, pseudogout). A thorough evaluation of all body systems is helpful as the elbow may be only one of many joints that are involved in an inflammatory condition.

# CHRONIC PAIN

Most elbow and forearm conditions are chronic in nature (greater than 2 weeks' duration) and represent overuse injuries from work or sport. Very often a change in training habits or a change in sports equipment, for example, a tennis racket, can be identified in the patient's history. Localization of the pain and tenderness, as well as identifying the movement or position that provokes pain, is important.

Chronic pain resulting from elbow arthritis may be diffuse and poorly defined. Arthritis of the elbow includes posttraumatic arthritis, inflammatory (rheumatoid or crystalline) arthritis, osteoarthritis, and septic arthritis (though this typically presents acutely). The pain may be localized based on the area of greatest involvement. For example, lateral elbow pain that is exacerbated by forearm rotation is probably caused by arthritis in the radiocapitellar articulation. These lateral symptoms are often the initial presentation of rheumatoid arthritis involving the elbow, or of posttraumatic arthritis after a radial head fracture. Early morning pain and stiffness and pain with weather changes are frequent findings in patients with osteoarthritis. Loose bodies often develop in arthritic elbows and may produce catching or locking.

## Localization of Pain

### Lateral elbow

Pain and tenderness localized to the lateral epicondyle and the common extensor origin of the forearm muscles extending from it indicate lateral epicondylitis. This condition is commonly referred to as tennis elbow, although many patients with lateral epicondylitis have no history of playing tennis. The pain of lateral epicondylitis is exacerbated by forearm supination and wrist extension against resistance. Asking the patient with lateral epicondylitis to pick up a chair with the forearm pronated (the chair test) will usually elicit pain, whereas the same maneuver in the supinated position will not. When the pain and tenderness is localized about 5 cm distal to the lateral epicondyle, entrapment of the posterior interosseous branch of the radial nerve (radial tunnel syndrome) might be present. Because this nerve compression syndrome typically produces pain without distal motor or sensory deficits, distinguishing it from tennis elbow sometimes is difficult. In fact, some authors think the two conditions coexist in 5% of patients.

### Medial elbow

Pain over the medial aspect of the elbow is most commonly the result of one of two conditions: ulnar nerve entrapment or medial epicondylitis (golfer's elbow). Ulnar nerve entrapment is associated with localized pain at the elbow, usually accompanied by numbness and tingling in the little finger and ulnar half of the ring finger that is exacerbated by tapping over the nerve in the ulnar groove. Patients with medial epicondylitis have pain and tenderness over and just lateral and distal to the medial epicondyle. This pain increases with wrist flexion or forearm pronation against resistance. Ulnar neuritis may complicate medial epicondylitis in up to 20% of patients. In the overhead throwing athlete with medial elbow pain, injury to the ulnar collateral ligament must be considered.

### Posterior elbow

Posterior elbow pain usually is associated with chronic olecranon bursitis. Overhead throwing athletes may develop painful spurs on the posteromedial olecranon secondary to repetitive valgus strain on the elbow during the throwing motion. Tendinitis or even frank rupture of the triceps tendon sometimes develops in weightlifters.

### Anterior elbow

Anterior elbow pain occurring acutely and associated with tenderness, ecchymosis, and change in the contour of the biceps muscle indicates a distal biceps tendon rupture. Exceedingly rare in females, this rupture typically occurs in middle-aged men who also report weak supination (screwdriver motion) following a sudden jerking movement or heavy lifting. Chronic anterior elbow discomfort may represent chronic degeneration of the biceps tendon, arthritis, synovitis, or compression of the median nerve at the elbow (pronator syndrome).

# STIFFNESS

The normal elbow has a range of motion from 0° (arm out straight) to 140° to 150° of flexion. Normal forearm rotation is from 80° of pronation to 80° of supination. The elbow has a particular predisposition to develop stiffness with arthritis, trauma, or immobilization; however, mild loss of motion causes no significant disability because most daily activities, including reaching one's mouth and performing other aspects of personal hygiene, are performed in an arc of motion from 30° to 130° of flexion and 50° each of pronation and supination.

SECTION 3 ■ ELBOW AND FOREARM

# Physical Examination Elbow and Forearm

## Inspection/Palpation

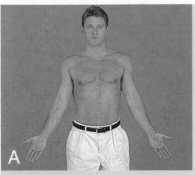

### Anterior view

Inspect the elbow for swelling and ecchymosis. Measure the "carrying angle" (the angle made by the axis of the humerus and the forearm) with the elbow extended and the forearm supinated (**A**). Note that the normal carrying angle is a cubitus valgus of 5° to 8°. Cubitus varus (reversed carrying angle) usually results from a malunion of a supracondylar fracture of the humerus.

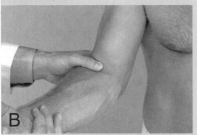

The biceps tendon can be easily palpated in the middle of the antecubital fossa, especially when the patient flexes the elbow against resistance with the forearm supinated (**B**). Absence of this normally palpable tendon with associated tenderness and ecchymosis suggests a complete biceps tendon rupture. A partial rupture also can occur. The brachial artery is deep and medial to the biceps tendon. The median nerve is medial to the brachial artery.

### Lateral view

Check for an effusion by inspecting and palpating the area in the center of a triangle bounded by the lateral epicondyle of the humerus, the tip of the olecranon, and the radial head. Confirm the position of the radial head by feeling it move with forearm pronation/supination.

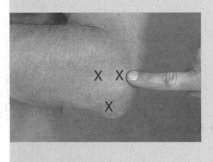

Palpate the area over the radial head to check for pain and crepitus. These findings, along with limited forearm rotation, suggest a radial head fracture (if acute) or arthritis (if chronic). Tenderness to palpation just distal to the lateral epicondyle indicates lateral epicondylitis (tennis elbow). Tenderness 5 cm distal to the lateral epicondyle that is localized deep to the extensor muscles suggests entrapment of the posterior interosseous branch of the radial nerve.

### Medial view

Pain and tenderness immediately distal to the medial epicondyle suggest medial epicondylitis. The ulnar nerve passes in the ulnar groove just posterior to the medial epicondyle. Palpation and light percussion in this area may produce local pain and paresthesias in the forearm and ulnar two fingers in association with ulnar nerve entrapment.

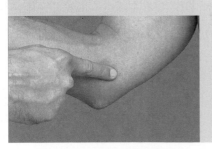

# INSPECTION/PALPATION

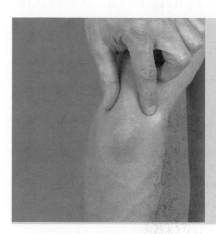

### *Posterior view*

Inspect the area over the olecranon for focal swelling and palpate for tenderness to confirm the presence of olecranon bursitis. An olecranon fracture produces a broader area of swelling with ecchymosis and a possible skin abrasion at the point of impact. Palpate just above the olecranon (as shown in figure) to identify elbow effusion. A palpable defect may indicate a triceps tear.

# RANGE OF MOTION

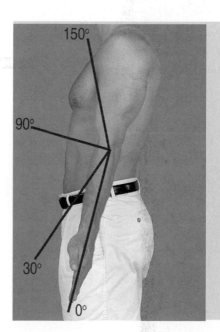

### *Flexion/Extension: Zero Starting Position*

Use the Zero Starting Position (with the extremity straight) to measure elbow flexion/extension. Young children commonly hyperextend the elbow by 10° to 15°, but adults show minimal, if any, elbow hyperextension. Normal elbow range of motion is from 0° to 140° to 150° of flexion. Mild flexion contractures are of little functional consequence, as most activities of daily living are accomplished in an arc of elbow flexion from 30° to 130°.

Limitation of motion may be expressed as in the following examples: (1) the elbow flexes from 30° to 90°; (2) the elbow has a flexion contracture of 30° with further flexion to 90°.

SECTION 3 ■ ELBOW AND FOREARM

# RANGE OF MOTION

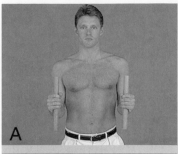

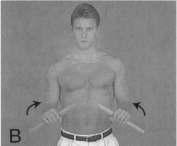

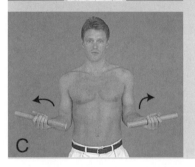

## *Forearm rotation*

Forearm rotation (pronation/supination) is a composite motion occurring at the proximal and distal radioulnar joints, as well as the radiohumeral joint. Measure forearm rotation by stabilizing the arm against the chest wall and flexing the elbow to 90°. The Zero Starting Position is with the extended thumb aligned with the humerus (**A**). Palpate the radial and ulnar styloid as the forearm is rotated to estimate pronation and supination. Ask the patient to grasp a pencil or similar object to facilitate visual estimation of forearm rotation.

Pronation is the position in which the palm is turned down (**B**), and supination is the position in which the palm is turned up (**C**). Normal pronation and supination is approximately 80° in each direction. Many activities of daily living are accomplished in an arc of motion between 50° pronation to 50° supination. A very restricted arc of forearm rotation may be of limited consequence if shoulder mobility is normal and if the forearm is ankylosed in a neutral position.

# MUSCLE TESTING

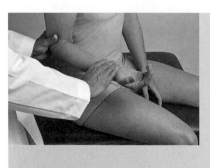

## *Resisted flexion*

Test the strength of the flexors of the elbow, primarily the biceps muscle, by resisting the patient's maximum effort to flex the supinated forearm. Weakness will be present with biceps tendinitis or rupture, dysfunction of the musculocutaneous nerve, or a lesion involving the C5 and C6 nerve roots.

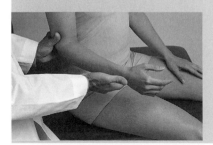

## *Resisted extension*

Test the strength of the extensors of the elbow, primarily the triceps muscle, by resisting the patient's maximum effort to extend the elbow with the forearm in neutral position. Weakness will be present with triceps tendinitis or rupture, or a lesion involving the C7 or C8 nerve roots.

# MUSCLE TESTING

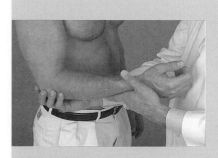

### Resisted supination

Test the strength of the forearm supinators, the most powerful of which is the biceps muscle, by grasping the patient's distal forearm and resisting the patient's maximum effort to turn the palm up. Weakness will be evident with rupture or tendinitis of the biceps tendon at the elbow, subluxation of the biceps tendon at the shoulder, a lesion of the musculocutaneous nerve, or a lesion involving the C5 and C6 nerve roots. Patients with lateral epicondylitis also may experience pain with this maneuver.

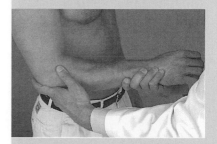

### Resisted pronation

Test the strength of the forearm pronators, the most powerful of which is the pronator teres muscle, by grasping the patient's distal forearm and resisting the patient's maximum effort to turn the palm down. Weakness will be evident with rupture of the pronator origin from the medial epicondyle, fracture of the medial elbow, or lesions involving the median nerve or the C6 and C7 nerve roots. Patients with medial epicondylitis also may experience pain with this maneuver.

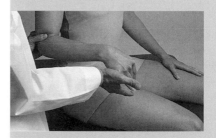

### Resisted wrist flexion

Test the strength of the wrist flexors by positioning the wrist in flexion and the fingers in extension. (This eliminates wrist flexion activity by the finger flexors.) Ask the patient to keep the wrist flexed while you push the wrist into extension. Weakness will be evident with rupture of the muscle origin, fracture of the medial elbow, medial epicondylitis, or lesions involving the ulnar nerve (C8 and T1 nerve roots) or median nerve (C6 and C7 nerve roots).

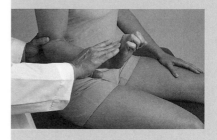

### Resisted wrist extension

Test the strength of the wrist extensors, the most powerful of which are the extensor carpi ulnaris and extensor carpi radialis brevis muscles, by positioning the wrist in extension and the fingers in flexion. (This eliminates wrist extension activity by the finger extensors.) Ask the patient to hold the wrist in extension as you push the wrist into flexion. Weakness will be evident with rupture of the extensor origin, fracture of the lateral elbow, lateral epicondylitis, or lesions involving the radial nerve or C6 to C8 nerve roots.

SECTION 3 ■ ELBOW AND FOREARM

# STABILITY TESTING

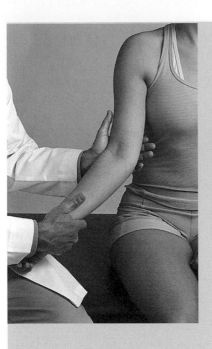

### *Valgus stress test*

To test the stability of the medial ligamentous structures, primarily the ulnar collateral ligament, apply valgus stress, which involves applying pressure on the lateral side of the elbow while the forearm is stabilized in a supinated position, attempting to "open" the medial joint line of the elbow. The elbow should be held in approximately 20° of flexion to disengage the olecranon tip from the olecranon fossa of the distal humerus.

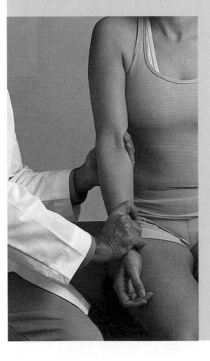

### *Varus stress test*

To test the stability of the lateral collateral ligament and lateral capsule, apply varus stress, which involves applying pressure on the medial side of the elbow while the forearm is stabilized in a pronated position, attempting to "open" the lateral joint line of the elbow. The elbow should be held in approximately 20° of flexion to disengage the olecranon tip from the olecranon fossa of the distal humerus.

# ARTHRITIS OF THE ELBOW

## DEFINITION

Arthritis of the elbow may result from numerous pathologic conditions. These include rheumatoid arthritis (RA), nonrheumatoid inflammatory arthritis (including gout and "pseudogout"), posttraumatic arthritis, osteoarthritis (OA) (**Figure 1**), and septic arthritis. Rheumatoid arthritis is the most common cause of elbow joint destruction, which nearly always develops in patients with multiple joint involvement by RA. Concomitant wrist and hand involvement occurs in 90% and shoulder involvement in 80% of patients with RA. Similar to other joints, an active synovitis of the elbow causes periarticular erosions and symmetric joint narrowing. Further progression causes gross destruction of the bone and soft-tissue constraints. The end result is a grossly unstable elbow.

Nonrheumatoid inflammatory arthritis of the elbow generally presents as an acute crystalline synovitis (gout or pseudogout) with acute pain, swelling, stiffness, and warmth. This is often difficult to distinguish from septic arthritis. Long-standing degenerative changes of the elbow joint are unusual in these conditions.

Posttraumatic arthritis results from primary injury to the articular cartilage at the time of trauma, as well as fracture malunion. The end result is incongruity of the articular cartilage and progressive arthritis. Because posttraumatic arthritis often presents as an isolated joint impairment in an otherwise young and active patient, treatment options and the patient's expectations are often quite different from those of patients with RA.

Because the elbow is not a weight-bearing joint, OA is not nearly as common in the elbow as it is in the hip, knee, or even the shoulder and may not be as symptomatic. Elbow OA most often is seen in manual laborers and weightlifters, suggesting repetitive overuse as an underlying cause. Repetitive overuse of the elbow also commonly causes intra-articular loose bodies that can act as gravel and promote joint degeneration.

Septic arthritis results from infection (bacterial and nonbacterial) within the elbow joint producing acute pain, swelling, loss of motion, and warmth. Septic arthritis is more common in patients with RA, HIV, and other immuno-compromised states, as well as in intravenous drug abusers. Septic arthritis may lead to articular cartilage destruction and ultimately to joint degeneration.

**ICD-9 Codes**

**274.02**
Gouty arthropathy of the elbow

**711.02**
Pyogenic arthritis of the elbow

**712.12**
Chondrocalcinosis due to dicalcium phosphate crystals, elbow

**714.02**
Rheumatoid arthritis of the elbow

**715.12.1**
Osteoarthrosis, localized, primary, of the elbow

**715.22**
Osteoarthrosis, localized, secondary, of the elbow

**716.12**
Traumatic arthropathy of the elbow

**719.22**
Villonodular synovitis, elbow

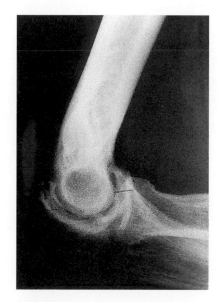

**Figure 1**

Lateral radiograph of an arthritic elbow.

Reproduced with permission from Norberg FB, Savoie FH III, Field LD: Arthroscopic treatment of arthritis of the elbow. *Instr Course Lect* 2000;49:248.

# CLINICAL SYMPTOMS

RA of the elbow causes pain and swelling, as it does in other joints. In the early stages, the pain may be primarily localized to the lateral side of the joint and exacerbated by forearm rotation. Advanced disease causes diffuse pain and often gross instability that makes even light household tasks impossible.

Symptoms of nonrheumatiod inflammatory arthritis include acute pain, swelling, effusion, loss of motion, and warmth, mimicking septic arthritis.

The primary symptom reported by patients with posttraumatic arthritis is either pain or stiffness, depending on the type of injury. With malunion of a radial head fracture, the pain may be isolated to the lateral side of the joint and exacerbated by forearm rotation.

OA is characterized by pain and restricted motion. Intra-articular loose bodies are associated with symptoms of catching and locking. Posterior osteophytes typically cause limited extension and pain on terminal extension. Less commonly, anterior osteophytes can cause pain and limited flexion. Pain during midrange motion and at rest are symptoms of late disease. Osteophytes on the medial side of the elbow can cause ulnar nerve irritation.

Septic arthritis generally produces acute and severe pain, stiffness, warmth, swelling, and effusion, as well as constitutional symptoms of fever, chills, and malaise.

# TESTS

## Physical Examination

Inspection of the rheumatoid elbow demonstrates joint swelling, best seen laterally, and occasionally rheumatoid nodules over the olecranon and extensor surface of the forearm. Tenderness may occur primarily over the radial head or may be diffuse. Range of motion and varus/valgus stability also should be assessed.

Elbows with posttraumatic arthritis or OA typically do not have an effusion. The joint lines should be palpated for tenderness, and range of motion should be measured. Gently "jogging" the joint in full extension and then full flexion will elicit impingement pain from posterior and anterior osteophytes, respectively.

Synovitis resulting from nonrheumatoid inflammatory arthritis and septic arthritis typically produces severely painful range of motion, which is restricted. A significant effusion and warmth are usually present.

## *Diagnostic Tests*

AP and lateral radiographs of the elbow often are sufficient for diagnosis. RA produces the typical picture of osteopenia, symmetric joint narrowing, and periarticular erosions, or may show gross joint destruction. Malunion, nonunion, and joint space narrowing are possible findings in posttraumatic arthritis. With OA, radiographs reveal osteophytes and narrowing of the joint space. Loose bodies may be multiple and present in the anterior and posterior portion of the elbow. Radiographs of nonrheumatoid inflammatory arthritis and septic arthritis are usually normal acutely.

If an effusion is present, aspiration of the joint fluid may be helpful. Fluid should be examined for WBC (to differentiate between inflammatory and noninflammatory arthritis), crystals (present with nonrheumatoid inflammatory arthritis), Gram stain, and culture.

# DIFFERENTIAL DIAGNOSIS

Fracture of the distal humerus (evident on radiographs)

Fracture of the radial head (evident on radiographs)

Osteochondritis dissecans of the elbow (typically affects adolescent boys, capitellum usually involved, seen with repetitive overuse, may produce loose bodies)

# ADVERSE OUTCOMES OF THE DISEASE

Progressive pain and stiffness are common to all arthritic conditions. RA can lead to an unstable, essentially flail elbow. Septic arthritis, left untreated, may lead to rapid joint destruction and even osteomyelitis.

# TREATMENT

Mild limitation of elbow motion does not interfere with daily activities and is well tolerated, often making treatment unnecessary. Modification of job or sports activities can be very helpful when symptoms warrant.

For RA, medical management should be optimized (see Rheumatoid Arthritis, Treatment, p 114). Intra-articular corticosteroid injection and gentle physical therapy may be of benefit. Static and hinged splints may be helpful for some patients. Synovectomy with or without radial head excision can provide pain relief in early stages of RA that is resistant to nonsurgical management. Total elbow arthroplasty is the best option for patients with RA who have advanced joint destruction.

SECTION 3 ■ ELBOW AND FOREARM

Nonrheumatoid inflammatory arthritis is treated medically to address the underlying pathology (ie, gout or pseudogout). Intra-articular steroid injections may be helpful in episodes of acute nonrheumatoid inflammatory synovitis.

For posttraumatic arthritis and OA, nonsurgical measures are limited to analgesics and gentle stretching to preserve motion. Arthroscopic débridement and removal of loose bodies can be quite helpful. Unless the patient is elderly with a very limited activity level, total elbow replacement generally is not considered beneficial because of concern for prosthesis loosening and breakage.

Prompt treatment of septic arthritis is critical and should specifically address the causal agent. Therapy generally involves a combination of appropriate antibiotics and surgical drainage.

## ADVERSE OUTCOMES OF TREATMENT

Patients with RA require regular monitoring for side effects from NSAIDs and disease-modifying agents. Nerve injury and infection are possible with surgery. Joint replacements can loosen or fracture with time.

## REFERRAL DECISIONS/RED FLAGS

Patients with persistent pain or significant loss of motion require further evaluation. Septic arthritis usually requires a combined medical/surgical approach.

# DISLOCATION OF THE ELBOW

## DEFINITION

The elbow is the most common joint to dislocate during childhood, and is second only to the shoulder and finger in adults. Typically, a dislocated elbow is the result of a fall on an outstretched hand. More than 80% of elbow dislocations are posterior (**Figure 1**) unless associated with an olecranon fracture. A dislocation may be complete or perched (subluxation, with the trochlea resting "perched" on top of the coronoid process). The ulnar collateral ligament usually is disrupted, and other soft-tissue restraints commonly are injured as well. Concomitant fractures of the radial head (in adults) or medial epicondyle (in children) may be present. Neurovascular structures such as the brachial artery, median nerve, and ulnar nerve may also be injured.

### ICD-9 Code

**832.0**
Dislocation of elbow, closed

## CLINICAL SYMPTOMS

Extreme pain, swelling, and inability to bend the elbow after a fall on the outstretched hand are characteristic of a dislocated elbow.

## TESTS

### Physical Examination
Note areas of abnormal prominence and tenderness. The most important part of the examination is the neurovascular evaluation.

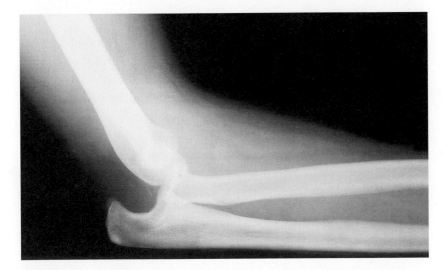

**Figure 1**
Posterior dislocation of the elbow.

Reproduced with permission from Crosby LA, Lewallen DG (eds): *Emergency Care and Transportation of the Sick and Injured*, ed 6 revised. Rosemont, IL, American Academy of Orthopaedic Surgeons, 1997, p 544.

SECTION 3 ■ ELBOW AND FOREARM

Check the radial pulse and capillary refill. Assess motor and sensory function of the median, radial, and ulnar nerves.

## Diagnostic Tests

AP and lateral radiographs of the elbow are adequate to make a diagnosis. Look carefully for associated fractures and bony fragments incarcerated in the joint, as these may cause widening of the joint space. In the pediatric patient, a comparison radiograph of the contralateral elbow may help secure the diagnosis.

## DIFFERENTIAL DIAGNOSIS

Fracture-dislocation of the elbow (same deformity, evident on radiographs)

Fracture of the distal humerus (evident on radiographs)

Fracture of the olecranon process of the ulna (evident on radiographs)

Hemarthrosis (positive fat pad sign)

Occult fractures (positive fat pad sign)

Synovitis (normal radiographs, no deformity)

## ADVERSE OUTCOMES OF THE DISEASE

Persistent loss of motion is common, especially in extension. Although most simple dislocations (that is, without fractures) are stable after reduction, persistent or recurrent instability is possible and should be specifically addressed rather than treated with prolonged immobilization. Heterotopic bone formation and the development of arthritis of the elbow joint also are possible.

## TREATMENT

Reduction of an elbow dislocation should be performed as soon as possible after the injury. Because of the possibility of occult fractures and the potential for neurovascular complications, reduction of elbow dislocations ideally should be performed by an orthopaedic surgeon unless this would result in an unacceptable delay in treatment. The reduction usually can be accomplished in the emergency department with the patient under conscious sedation. The sedation may be supplemented by aspirating the hemarthrosis and injecting 10 mL of 1% lidocaine into the joint from a lateral approach (**Figure 2**). If muscle spasm or marked swelling precludes reduction with the patient under conscious sedation, general anesthesia may be required.

Flexing the elbow tenses the triceps attachment to the olecranon and makes the reduction more difficult. The reduction should be performed by holding the elbow relatively extended

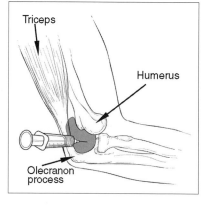

**Figure 2**

Site of aspiration of hemarthrosis and injection of local anesthetic.

(flexed about 45°) and applying slow, steady, downward traction on the forearm in line with the long axis of the humerus. The reduction usually is easily felt (a "clunk"), and once achieved, is most stable with the elbow flexed and forearm pronated. The stability of the reduction should be tested by slowly extending the elbow until the beginning of some subluxation is felt. The arm should be splinted in its stable range but avoiding more than 100° of flexion, which may contribute to vascular compromise as swelling develops.

After completing the reduction, the neurovascular examination must be repeated. After applying the splint, obtain AP, lateral, and oblique radiographs to confirm the reduction. Failure to obtain a perfectly concentric reduction suggests the possibility of a bony or cartilaginous intra-articular loose body or extensive soft-tissue injury, either of which may require surgical treatment.

Motion should begin 5 to 7 days later and gradually progress during the next 3 to 4 weeks. A brace that blocks terminal extension may be required during this time if some instability persists. NSAIDs can be useful during this period and may decrease the incidence of heterotopic bone formation.

## ADVERSE OUTCOMES OF TREATMENT

Fracture and neurovascular injury are possible during the reduction maneuver. The median nerve, because of its close proximity, may become entrapped in the elbow joint. Subsequent vascular problems may result from compressive bandages or splinting in more than 100° of elbow flexion. Prolonged immobilization leads to elbow contracture and pain, and at the same time may not correct the underlying instability. Failure to identify and address persistent instability may lead to the difficult situation of chronic instability. Chronic instability (especially chronic posterolateral rotatory instability of the elbow) is unusual, but may require surgical reconstruction.

## REFERRAL DECISIONS/RED FLAGS

Patients with associated neurovascular or bony injury require further evaluation, although a gentle reduction may be attempted to avoid lengthy delays. Incomplete reduction, as shown on radiographs, should never be accepted. Patients with a flexion contracture greater than 45° or persistent instability 3 weeks after injury also require further evaluation.

SECTION 3 ■ ELBOW AND FOREARM

# FRACTURE OF THE DISTAL HUMERUS

**ICD-9 Code**

**812.40**
Fracture of humerus, lower end, closed, unspecified part

SECTION 3 ■ ELBOW AND FOREARM

## FRACTURE PATTERNS
Supracondylar fracture
Transcondylar fracture
Intercondylar fracture
T condylar fracture
Lateral/medial condylar fracture

## DEFINITION
Fractures of the distal humerus are relatively uncommon, accounting for only 2% of fractures in adults. Because these fractures are often comminuted and intra-articular, the potential morbidity is high. Classification schemes used for these fractures can be quite complex, but the most important factors to consider in deciding the best course for initial treatment are whether the fracture is displaced (**Figures 1** and **2**), whether the fracture involves the joint surface, and whether the skin and neurovascular structures are involved.

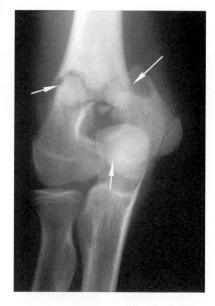

**Figure 1**
AP radiograph of elbow demonstrating displaced supracondylar fracture.

Reproduced with permission from Beaty JH, Kasser JR: Fractures about the elbow. *Instr Course Lect* 1995;44:199–215.

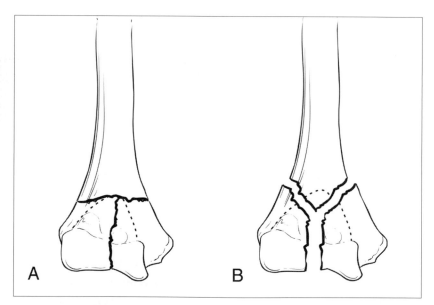

**Figure 2**
**A,** Nondisplaced T condylar fracture of the distal humerus. **B,** Displaced intercondylar fracture of the distal humerus.

Part B is adapted from Mehne DK, Jupiter JB: Fractures of the distal humerus, in Browner BD, Jupiter JB, Levine AM, et al (eds): *Skeletal Trauma: Fractures, Dislocations, Ligamentous Injuries*. Philadelphia, PA, WB Saunders, 1992, pp 1146–1176.

# CLINICAL SYMPTOMS

Marked swelling, ecchymosis, deformity, and pain about the elbow after an injury are common. Patients report increased pain with attempted flexion of the elbow.

# TESTS

## Physical Examination

Swelling and deformity usually are clearly visible with any displaced fracture. Inspect the skin around the site to identify any open wounds. Palpation around the joint may reveal an effusion, and crepitus may be felt with gentle flexion. Palpate the radial pulse and check capillary refill. Assess median, radial, and ulnar nerve function. All peripheral nerves crossing the fracture may be injured, but ulnar nerve dysfunction is most common. Brachial artery occlusion is less common but requires early diagnosis and treatment to avoid devastating complications. Check the wrist and shoulder on the affected side for associated injuries.

## Diagnostic Tests

AP and lateral radiographs of the elbow, as well as other radiographic views as clinically indicated, are adequate in most patients. Without radiographic evidence of fracture, look carefully for a fat pad sign indicative of bleeding into the joint, often from an occult fracture (**Figure 3**). In the pediatric patient, comparison views may help differentiate a true fracture from a growth plate. CT may be necessary to fully define the extent of fracture.

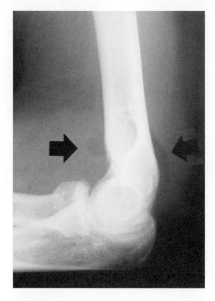

**Figure 3**
Lateral radiograph of elbow. Note the anterior and posterior fat pad signs (arrows).

# DIFFERENTIAL DIAGNOSIS

Elbow dislocation (evident on radiographs)

Olecranon fracture (evident on radiographs)

Radial head fracture (evident on radiographs)

Rupture of the distal biceps tendon (radiographs negative)

# ADVERSE OUTCOMES OF THE DISEASE

Unfortunately, some degree of residual pain and stiffness is common. Other complications include deformity with malunion, nonunion, and ulnar neuropathy. Vascular injury may lead to ischemia in the forearm and hand, or to compartment syndrome of the forearm muscle compartments (see Compartment Syndrome, pp 30-33). Prompt treatment is required to salvage function.

SECTION 3 ■ ELBOW AND FOREARM

# TREATMENT

The goal of treatment is to achieve and maintain a stable reduction that permits early motion. Stable, nondisplaced fractures may be treated with splinting for 10 days, followed by protected range of motion. Unfortunately, most distal humeral fractures are displaced to some degree, requiring open reduction and internal fixation. Other techniques, such as hinged external fixation or primary total elbow replacement, might be considered under circumstances such as severe osteoporosis and/or fracture communution.

# ADVERSE OUTCOMES OF TREATMENT

Pain and stiffness may persist after treatment. Deformity, nonunion, arthritis, and ulnar neuropathy may develop, as well as symptoms related to the prominent implants used for internal fixation. Infection, nerve damage, or hardware failure may complicate surgery.

# REFERRAL DECISIONS/RED FLAGS

Patients with displaced fractures of the distal humerus need further evaluation to determine whether surgical stabilization of the fracture is necessary. Likewise, patients with associated neurovascular injury need further evaluation.

Patients treated nonsurgically require close follow-up for complications such as fracture displacement and joint stiffness. Delayed vascular compromise may occur because of progressive swelling and/or tight splinting. Failure to regain motion is also an indication for referral.

# FRACTURE OF THE OLECRANON

**ICD-9 Code**

**813.01**
Fracture of olecranon process of ulna

## DEFINITION

The olecranon is the portion of the ulna that constitutes the bony prominence of the posterior elbow. Because of its subcutaneous location, the olecranon is easily fractured as a result of a direct blow to the elbow or a fall on an outstretched arm with the elbow flexed. As with other fractures, the most important consideration is determining whether the fracture is displaced or nondisplaced. Most of these fractures are displaced and can be further classified as noncomminuted or comminuted fractures of the olecranon or fracture-dislocations of the elbow **(Figure 1)**.

## CLINICAL SYMPTOMS

A history of trauma followed by marked swelling and ecchymosis is typical. When an associated dislocation is present, the elbow will appear deformed as well. Because of the close proximity of the ulnar nerve, the trauma itself or the resultant swelling may compress the nerve and cause numbness in the little and ring fingers.

## TESTS

### Physical Examination
Examination usually reveals marked swelling of the entire elbow joint. Superficial abrasions at the site of impact are

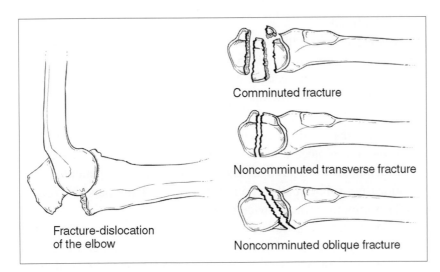

Comminuted fracture

Noncomminuted transverse fracture

Fracture-dislocation of the elbow

Noncomminuted oblique fracture

**Figure 1**
Types of olecranon fractures.

Adapted with permission from Jupiter JB, Mehne DK: Trauma to the adult elbow and fractures of the distal humerus, in Browner BD, Jupiter JB, Levine AM, et al (eds): *Skeletal Trauma: Fractures, Dislocations, Ligamentous Injuries.* Philadelphia, PA, WB Saunders, 1992, vol 2, pp 1125–1175.

SECTION 3 ■ ELBOW AND FOREARM

common and must be distinguished from deep wounds, which would make the injury an open fracture. Gentle palpation may reveal a defect if the fracture is displaced. Flexion of the elbow produces pain and is met with resistance. Median, radial, and ulnar nerve function should be assessed; of these, ulnar nerve injury is most common. Radial and ulnar pulses and capillary refill should be assessed, but significant vascular injury is uncommon with this fracture.

## Diagnostic Tests

AP and lateral radiographs usually are adequate to confirm the diagnosis.

# DIFFERENTIAL DIAGNOSIS

Dislocation of the elbow (more grotesque deformity, evident on radiographs)

Fracture of the coronoid process of the olecranon (nearly always associated with an elbow dislocation)

Fracture of the distal humerus (more proximal area of pain, evident on radiographs)

Fracture of the radial head (lateral elbow pain increases with forearm rotation, fracture may be difficult to see on radiographs)

# ADVERSE OUTCOMES OF THE DISEASE

Loss of motion and/or stability in the elbow is possible. Because the triceps inserts on the tip of the olecranon, active elbow extension may be lost with displaced fractures. Arthritis of the elbow may develop.

# TREATMENT

Nondisplaced fractures of the olecranon may be treated with a posterior splint. To avoid excessive pull on the triceps and possible loss of reduction, position the elbow in approximately 45° of flexion. Follow-up radiographs should be obtained 7 to 10 days after the injury to ensure that the fracture has not become displaced. In order to avoid significant permanent loss of motion, protected motion should begin within 2 to 3 weeks. To maintain hand strength and flexibility, instruct patients to squeeze a rubber ball or commercially available hand exerciser for 5 minutes at least twice each day.

Most olecranon fractures are displaced and are best treated surgically. Occasionally, a displaced fracture in a debilitated elderly patient who is a poor risk for surgery may be treated with a sling and early range-of-motion exercises, as pain allows.

## Adverse Outcomes of Treatment

Elbow stiffness, loss of motion, or arthritis may develop despite treatment. Nonunion or displacement of the fracture due to hardware failure is possible. After surgical treatment, irritation from the implants used to fix the fracture commonly occurs, necessitating a second procedure for implant removal.

## Referral Decisions/Red Flags

Patients with displaced fractures or open fractures need further evaluation for possible surgical treatment.

Section 3 ■ Elbow and Forearm

# FRACTURE OF THE RADIAL HEAD

**ICD-9 Codes**

**813.05**
Fracture of head of radius

**813.06**
Fracture of neck of radius

## DEFINITION

Fractures of the radial head and neck result from falls on the outstretched arm. The most commonly used classification system (modified Mason classification) separates these fractures into three types (**Figure 1**). Type I is a nondisplaced or minimally displaced fracture. Type II includes radial head fractures that are displaced more than 2 mm at the articular surface or angulated neck fractures that produce articular incongruity or a mechanical block. Type III fractures are severely comminuted fractures of the radial head and neck.

## CLINICAL SYMPTOMS

Following a fall on the outstretched arm, pain and swelling develop over the lateral aspect of the elbow. Loss of elbow motion may be related to pain inhibition and joint effusion, but a mechanical block to full forearm pronation and supination may be present in type II and III injuries. Radial head fractures also may be present in the context of an elbow dislocation. The radial head fracture may rarely be associated with an injury of the forearm (called an Essex-Lopresti fracture), and the forearm and wrist should be assessed.

## TESTS

### Physical Examination

Tenderness to palpation is localized to the lateral aspect of the joint, and a joint effusion can often be palpated. Passive forearm rotation is limited and may be associated with palpable crepitus. Elbow flexion and extension also may be limited by pain.

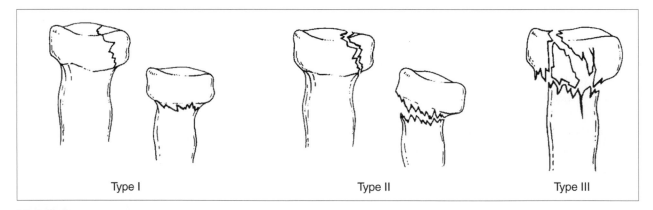

| Type I | Type II | Type III |

**Figure 1**

Modified Mason classification of radial head fractures.

Adapted with permission from Jupiter JB, Mehne DK: Trauma to the adult elbow and fractures of the distal humerus, in Browner BD, Jupiter JB, Levine AM, et al (eds): *Skeletal Trauma: Fractures, Dislocations, Ligamentous Injuries.* Philadelphia, PA, WB Saunders, 1992, vol 2, pp 1125–1175.

Tenderness over the forearm and/or wrist may signify a more extensive soft-tissue injury involving the radioulnar interosseous membrane and the distal radioulnar joint. Presence of this type of injury makes treatment more difficult.

### Diagnostic Tests

Type I fractures may be difficult to visualize radiographically but should be suspected based on positive clinical findings. Type II and III fractures are usually obvious on AP and lateral radiographs. CT is occasionally necessary to define the extent of the fracture.

# DIFFERENTIAL DIAGNOSIS

Elbow dislocation (clinical deformity and diffuse pain)

Hemarthrosis of the elbow (present with radial head fracture or with other bony or soft-tissue injury)

Olecranon fracture (pain and tenderness over the posterior tip of the elbow)

Supracondylar fracture of the humerus (location of pain, tenderness, and deformity)

# ADVERSE OUTCOMES OF THE DISEASE

Loss of motion, especially the last 10° to 15° of extension, is common, even with type I injuries. Posttraumatic arthritis of the radiocapitellar joint also may develop.

# TREATMENT

Type I fractures should be treated with a sling or splint for comfort and early active motion as soon as pain allows. Because early motion is the key to a successful outcome, aspiration of the associated elbow hemarthrosis should be considered.

Aspiration with local anesthetic injection is useful diagnostically in type II fractures to determine whether a mechanical block to forearm rotation is present. When the fracture involves displacement of less than 30% of the head and no block is present, treatment should consist of early range of motion, as in type I fractures. Otherwise, open reduction and internal fixation is preferred.

Type III fractures usually are best treated by early excision of the bone fragments. If the patient has associated injuries of the ulnar collateral ligament or interosseous membrane, other treatment considerations are required because elbow stability is a concern.

SECTION 3 ■ ELBOW AND FOREARM

## ADVERSE OUTCOMES OF TREATMENT

Loss of motion, instability, and wrist pain caused by proximal radial migration after radial head excision can all occur. Infection, nerve damage, hardware failure, malunion, loss of motion, and arthritis are possible following surgical intervention.

## REFERRAL DECISIONS/RED FLAGS

Type II fractures that block rotation or involve more than 30% of the head, type III fractures, and any fracture associated with elbow dislocation or instability should be referred for surgical consideration. Failure of nonsurgical treatment, manifested by persistent pain or limited motion, also indicates the need for further evaluation.

# MEDIAL AND LATERAL EPICONDYLITIS

## SYNONYMS

Medial epicondylitis:
   Golfer's or bowler's elbow
   Medial tendinosis of the elbow
Lateral epicondylitis:
   Lateral tendinosis of the elbow
   Tennis elbow

**ICD-9 Codes**
**726.31**
Medial epicondylitis
**726.32**
Lateral epicondylitis

## DEFINITION

Lateral epicondylitis and tennis elbow are the most commonly used terms to describe a condition that produces pain and tenderness at the site of origin of the extensor carpi radialis brevis muscle (lateral epicondyle of the humerus). Although the term epicondylitis is commonly used, the pathology and point of maximal pain are in the tendon substance just distal to the epicondyle (**Figure 1**). The term elbow tendinitis also is inaccurate because it implies an inflammatory origin. In fact, the histologic pattern of lateral epicondylitis is one of tissue degeneration with fibroblast and microvascular hyperplasia and the absence of inflammation. The term lateral tendinosis of the elbow is probably the most accurate but rarely is used.

Medial epicondylitis (also called golfer's or bowler's elbow) is similar to lateral epicondylitis in etiology and pathology and occurs in the common tendinous origin of the flexor/pronator muscles just distal to the medial epicondyle. Medial epicondylitis is much less commonly encountered than lateral epicondylitis.

## CLINICAL SYMPTOMS

The typical patient with lateral epicondylitis is between 35 and 50 years of age and reports a gradual onset of pain in the lateral elbow and forearm during activities involving wrist extension, such as lifting, turning a screwdriver, or hitting a backhand in tennis. With time, the pain may become more severe and may occur at rest or during activities as minimal as holding a cup of coffee or using a key. Less commonly, the patient may relate the onset of symptoms to an acute event, such as a direct blow to the elbow or a sudden maximal muscle contraction.

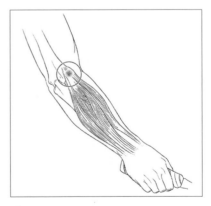

**Figure 1**
Location of pain in lateral epicondylitis.

The pain of medial epicondylitis typically occurs with active wrist flexion and forearm pronation, such as takes place in a golf swing, baseball pitching, the pull-through strokes of swimming, weightlifting, bowling, and many forms of manual labor.

## TESTS

### Physical Examination

The most consistent finding in lateral epicondylitis is localized tenderness over the common extensor origin 1 cm distal to the lateral epicondyle (**Figure 2**). During the examination, it is best to have the patient's elbow flexed to 90° and the forearm pronated. Tapping lightly on the lateral epicondyle may be painful. Pain in the region also may be produced with resisted extension of the wrist when the elbow is in extension. Ask the patient to lift a stool or chair with the palm up (using the wrist flexors) and then the palm down (using the wrist extensors) to help differentiate lateral epicondylitis from other painful elbow conditions. Patients with lateral epicondylitis will have pain when lifting with the palm down.

With medial epicondylitis, the area of tenderness is just distal to the medial epicondyle, and the pain is exacerbated by pronating the forearm and flexing the wrist against resistance. These patients also may have pain when lifting a chair with the palm up.

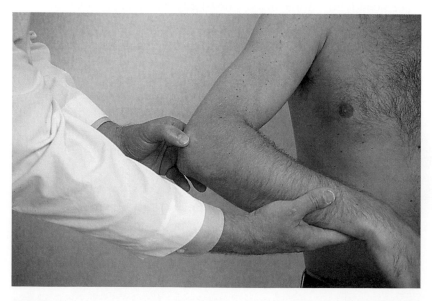

**Figure 2**
Palpating the point of maximum tenderness.

### Diagnostic Tests

AP and lateral radiographs of the elbow are necessary to rule out arthritis or osteochondral loose bodies. Rarely, an area of calcification may be seen at the attachment of the extensor muscles to the lateral epicondyle or the flexor/pronator mass to the medial epicondyle of the humerus. MRI is helpful in confirming the diagnosis and severity, but it is rarely helpful in predicting treatment outcome.

## DIFFERENTIAL DIAGNOSIS

Cubital tunnel syndrome (compression of the ulnar nerve, paresthesias in little and ring fingers)

Fracture of the radial head (radiographs should differentiate; pain and tenderness over the radial head that is exacerbated by passive pronation and supination)

Osteoarthritis of the radiocapitellar portion of the elbow joint (radiographs should differentiate; similar examination to radial head fracture but without a history of acute trauma)

Osteochondral loose body (medial or lateral joint line pain, symptoms of locking)

Radial tunnel syndrome (compression of the posterior interosseous nerve, tenderness typically approximately 5 cm distal to lateral epicondyle)

Synovitis of the elbow (swelling, palpable effusion)

Triceps tendinitis (tenderness above the olecranon)

## ADVERSE OUTCOMES OF THE DISEASE

Persistent pain is the most common problem. Weakness or poor endurance with motions that involve forceful wrist flexion/extension or forearm pronation/supination, such as heavy or repetitive lifting, also is common. Inability to optimally participate in sport is common. Rupture of the flexor/pronator mass or the extensor mass from the respective epicondyle is occasionally seen.

## TREATMENT

Modifying or eliminating the activities that cause symptoms is the most important step in treatment. In the case of tennis-related epicondylitis, this may include changing to a lighter weight tennis racket, changing the tension of the racket strings, or overwrapping the handle to make it slightly larger or using a racket with a larger grip. For patients with severe and long-standing conditions, this activity modification may have to be permanent. NSAIDs and rub-in anti-inflammatory creams may be helpful during acute exacerbations. Use of a commercial tennis elbow strap worn just below the elbow during heavy-lifting activities may be helpful as well. Application of heat or ice may relieve pain and inflammation. Once the pain has decreased, gentle stretching and forearm-strengthening exercises can be initiated and are the key to successful treatment.

If symptoms persist, corticosteroid injection into the area of maximum tenderness may be helpful in lateral or medial epicondylitis (see Tennis Elbow Injection, pp 267-268). Advise patients that they might experience an increase in pain for 1 to 2 days after the injection. No more than three injections should be given. If the pain recurs and symptoms are severe, surgery (typically involving débridement of the area of tendinosis) can be considered. More than 95% of patients with lateral epicondylitis and 85% of patients with medial epicondylitis will heal with nonsurgical treatment.

## PHYSICAL THERAPY PRESCRIPTION

Treatment of the patient with humeral epicondylitis has four stages: (1) reduction of overload, pain, and inflammation; (2) promotion of total arm strength; (3) return to limited activites (those that are pain free); and (4) maintenance.

A home exercise program includes the use of ice following early attempts at exercise or unavoidable daily activities. Early submaximal exercise is begun as signs and symptoms allow; for example, patient tolerance to a firm handshake is a criterion for determining whether a patient is ready for early exercise. Early use of submaximal isometrics such as squeezing a ball and manual resistive exercises for the wrist flexors, extensors, pronators, and supinators is advocated (see p 266). The early goal of the home program is to promote muscle endurance and improve resistance to repetitive stress. To accomplish this goal, high repetitions per set with extremely low or no resistance are used. This promotes local muscle endurance and provides a vascular response to the exercising tissues.

If the pain persists after the patient has been on the home program for 3 to 4 weeks, formal physical therapy may be initiated. The orders should include a thorough evaluation of muscle strength, pain, and joint mobility. No single pain-relieving modality has been found to be most effective for all patients. The physical therapist should determine the most effective modality for the individual patient based on patient tolerance and response.

## ADVERSE OUTCOMES OF TREATMENT

NSAIDs may cause gastric, renal, or hepatic complications. Although surgery always carries a small risk of complications such as wound infection or nerve injury, the most common adverse outcome is incomplete pain relief despite adequate surgical release. Surgical failure may result from misdiagnosis, especially in cases involving nerve entrapment syndromes (with lateral epicondylitis, the posterior interosseous nerve; with medial epicondylitis, the ulnar nerve). Return to a workplace that was related to the onset of symptoms may be difficult to achieve due to recurrence of symptoms or issues of secondary gain.

# REFERRAL DECISIONS/RED FLAGS
Failure of nonsurgical management indicates the need for further evaluation.

SECTION 3 ■ ELBOW AND FOREARM

# HOME EXERCISE PROGRAM FOR EPICONDYLITIS AND RADIAL TUNNEL SYNDROME

Perform the exercises in the order listed. To prevent inflammation, apply ice, such as a bag of crushed ice or frozen peas, to the painful area of the elbow for 20 minutes after performing both exercises. If you are unable to add weight or perform the indicated number of repetitions because of pain, call your doctor.

| Exercise Type | Muscle Group | Number of Repetitions/Sets | Number of Days per Week | Number of Weeks |
|---|---|---|---|---|
| Wrist flexion and extension | Flexor and extensor muscle groups | 25 repetitions/3 sets, progressing to 45 repetitions/4 sets | 5 to 7 | 3 to 4 |
| Forearm pronation and supination | Pronator teres Supinator | 25 repetitions/3 sets, progressing to 45 repetitions/4 sets | 5 to 7 | 3 to 4 |

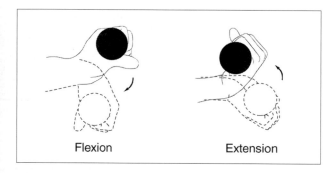

Flexion          Extension

## Wrist Flexion and Extension

To exercise the wrist flexors, rest the forearm on a hard surface with the palm up. Flex the wrist as shown. Perform 3 sets of 25 repetitions, progressing to 4 sets of 45 repetitions. To exercise the wrist extensors, rest the forearm on a hard surface with the hand extending over the side. Extend the wrist as shown. Perform 3 sets of 25 repetitions, progressing to 4 sets of 45 repetitions. Use no weight initially; add weight in 1-pound increments to a maximum of 5 pounds. Perform the exercises 5 to 7 days a week for 3 to 4 weeks.

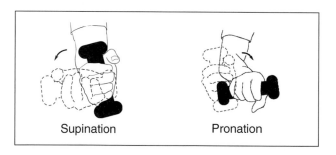

Supination          Pronation

## Forearm Supination and Pronation

Hold the forearm parallel to the ground, with the elbow bent 90°. For the forearm supination exercise, supinate the forearm and then return to vertical as shown. Perform 3 sets of 25 repetitions, progressing to 4 sets of 45 repetitions. For forearm pronation, pronate the forearm and then return to vertical as shown. Perform 3 sets of 25 repetitions, progressing to 4 sets of 45 repetitions. Use no weight initially; add weight in 1-pound increments to a maximum of 5 pounds. Perform the exercises 5 to 7 days a week for 3 to 4 weeks.

# PROCEDURE
## TENNIS ELBOW INJECTION

The classic tender spot in lateral epicondylitis of the elbow (tennis elbow) is just distal to the lateral epicondyle of the humerus with the elbow in 90° of flexion.

**Note:** Opinions differ regarding single- versus two-needle injection techniques. A two-needle technique is shown on the DVD.

### STEP 1
Wear protective gloves at all times during this procedure and use sterile technique.

### STEP 2
Place the patient's arm against the chest or abdomen, with the elbow flexed at least 90° and the forearm fully pronated.

### STEP 3
Prep the skin with a bactericidal solution.

### STEP 4
Palpate just distal to the lateral epicondyle and locate the point of maximal tenderness. At this point, insert the 25-gauge needle, make a subcutaneous skin wheal with the local anesthetic, and advance through the tendon of the extensor carpi radialis brevis muscle to inject the remaining 2 to 3 mL of local anesthetic (**Figure 1**).

### CPT Code
**20550**
Injection(s); single tendon sheath, or ligament, aponeurosis (eg, plantar "fascia")

**20551**
Injection(s); single tendon origin/ insertion

*Current Procedural Terminology* © 2004 American Medical Association. All Rights Reserved.

### MATERIALS
Sterile gloves

Bactericidal skin preparation solution

5-mL syringe with a 25-gauge, 1¼″ needle

3 to 4 mL of a 1% lidocaine solution without epinephrine

2-mL syringe

1 mL of a corticosteroid preparation

Adhesive bandage

SECTION 3 ■ ELBOW AND FOREARM

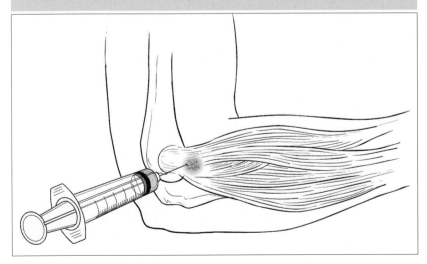

**Figure 1**
Location for needle insertion for tennis elbow injection.

# Tennis Elbow Injection (continued)

## Step 5

Exchange syringes on the needle and inject the corticosteroid preparation. The syringe can again be exchanged and local anesthetic injected as the needle is withdrawn to avoid steroid deposition subcutaneously. This reduces the risk of depigmentation in dark-skinned patients or fat atrophy.

## Step 6

Dress the puncture wound with a sterile adhesive bandage.

## Adverse Outcomes

Subcutaneous infiltration of the corticosteroid preparation may cause subcutaneous fat atrophy, leading to a waxy-appearing depression in the skin, and may cause depigmentation in dark-skinned patients. Although rare, infection is possible. Between 25% and 33% of patients will experience a "flare," characterized by increased pain at the injection site.

## Aftercare/Patient Instruction

Advise the patient that pain may increase for 24 to 48 hours after the injection. Pain often improves with the application of ice. Acetaminophen or an NSAID also is beneficial.

# OLECRANON BURSITIS

## DEFINITION

Because of its superficial location on the extensor side of the elbow, the olecranon bursa is easily irritated and inflamed **(Figure 1)**. Olecranon bursitis may be secondary to trauma, inflammation, or infection. Falls or direct blows may cause an acute inflammatory bursitis. Prolonged irritation from excessive leaning on the elbow, often associated with certain occupations and avocations, may result in chronic inflammation. Olecranon bursitis may also develop in patients with chronic lung disease who lean on their elbows to aid breathing. The condition may be caused by systemic inflammatory processes, such as rheumatoid arthritis, gout, chondrocalcinosis, or hydroxyapatite crystal deposition. Infection of the olecranon bursa (septic bursitis) may occur primarily or develop as a secondary complication of an aseptic bursitis.

## CLINICAL SYMPTOMS

The swelling associated with bursitis may develop either gradually (chronic) or suddenly (infection or trauma). Pain is variable but may be intense, and may limit motion after an acute injury or when infection is present. Such severe swelling of the bursa may occur that patients report difficulty putting on long-sleeved shirts. As the mass diminishes in size, patients may feel firm "lumps" that are tender when the elbow is bumped. These lumps or nodules are scar tissue left as the fluid recedes.

Olecranon bursitis also occurs in patients with gout or rheumatoid arthritis. Gouty tophi (masses of monosodium urate crystals) may form in the olecranon bursa as well as along the ulnar border of the forearm, in the synovium of the elbow joint, and in numerous distant locations. Tophi are found only in patients with fairly advanced gout. As with gout, rheumatoid nodules may appear in several subcutaneous locations, such as over the olecranon and the ulnar border of the forearm. With time, these nodules may spontaneously shrink or disappear.

## TESTS

### Physical Examination

Examination may reveal a large mass, up to 6 cm in diameter, over the tip of the elbow. The skin might be abraded or even lacerated if related to trauma. Redness and heat are not uncommon with acute bursitis and could indicate infection.

**ICD-9 Code**
**726.33**
Olecranon bursitis

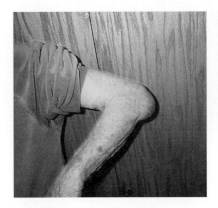

**Figure 1**
Swollen olecranon bursa.

Adapted with permission from Jupiter JB, Mehne DK: Trauma to the adult elbow and fractures of the distal humerus, in Browner BD, Jupiter JB, Levine AM, et al (eds): *Skeletal Trauma: Fractures, Dislocations, Ligamentous Injuries.* Philadelphia, PA, WB Saunders, 1992, vol 2, pp 1125–1175.

SECTION 3 ■ ELBOW AND FOREARM

Exquisite tenderness usually results from an infectious or traumatic origin. Chronic, recurrent swelling usually is less tender. The dimensions of the bursa should be measured periodically to monitor progress.

### Diagnostic Tests

When the mass is large and symptomatic, aspiration may be both diagnostic and therapeutic (see Olecranon Bursa Aspiration, pp 272-273). After an acute injury, bloody fluid may be found. Fluid aspirated from the bursa should be analyzed for WBC, crystals, Gram stain, and culture. The index of suspicion for infection should be high because about 20% of cases of acute bursitis have a septic cause, involving either primary or secondary infection. When the origin is traumatic, radiographs should be obtained to rule out a fracture of the olecranon process of the ulna.

## DIFFERENTIAL DIAGNOSIS

Fracture of the olecranon process of the ulna (evident on radiographs)

Gouty tophus or rheumatoid nodule (generally a tophus or nodule will be smaller and more discrete than an inflamed olecranon bursa)

## ADVERSE OUTCOMES OF THE DISEASE

Secondary infection, chronic recurrence or drainage, and swelling or limited motion may develop.

## TREATMENT

If the mass is small and symptoms are mild, the bursitis should be left alone or treated symptomatically with activity modifications and possibly NSAIDs. Wearing an elbow pad and avoiding hyperflexion against hard surfaces may improve symptoms. Patients with more symptomatic bursitis should undergo aspiration of the bursa, followed by Gram stain and culture of any suspicious fluid. If there is no indication of septic bursitis, a compression bandage consisting of a circular piece of foam, 8 cm in diameter, and an elastic wrap should be applied. Reassess the patient in 2 to 7 days. If cultures are negative and fluid has reaccumulated in the bursa, repeat the aspiration and, if the fluid remains sterile, inject 1 mL of a corticosteroid preparation into the sac. The bursal sac may have to be aspirated two or more times. If the elbow is at risk for repeated trauma, recommend an elbow protector.

Septic olecranon bursitis requires organism-specific antibiotic coverage based on the culture and sensitivity of the aspirate (frequently involving coverage for penicillin-resistant *Staphylococcus aureus*) and decompression by either surgical drainage or daily aspiration. Oral antibiotics may be administered if the septic bursitis is treated early and the patient is not immunocompromised. Hospitalization with intravenous antibiotics and surgical drainage and irrigation is indicated if the patient does not respond to oral antibiotics or if the patient has a more serious infection.

Excision of chronically inflamed aseptic bursitis is not commonly necessary and should be avoided because a chronically draining or infected sinus may develop.

# ADVERSE OUTCOMES OF TREATMENT

Secondary infection, chronic drainage, or recurrence is possible.

# REFERRAL DECISIONS/RED FLAGS

Recurrence of fluid despite repeated (three or more) aspirations or septic bursitis needs further evaluation.

# PROCEDURE

**CPT Code**

**20605**

Arthrocentesis, aspiration and/or injection; intermediate joint or bursa (eg, temporomandibular, acromioclavicular, wrist, elbow or ankle, olecranon bursa)

*Current Procedural Terminology* © 2004 American Medical Association. All Rights Reserved.

## MATERIALS

Sterile gloves

Bactericidal skin preparation solution

2 1-mL syringes

27-gauge, ¾″ needle

1 mL of 1% lidocaine without epinephrine

10-mL syringe

18-gauge needle

1 mL of a 40 mg/mL corticosteroid preparation (optional)

Adhesive bandage

## OLECRANON BURSA ASPIRATION

The olecranon bursa lies on the extensor aspect of the elbow, over the olecranon process of the ulna. The ulnar nerve lies adjacent to the medial face of the olecranon, behind the ulnar groove of the distal humerus. For this reason, aspiration is best done from the lateral side.

### STEP 1
Wear protective gloves at all times during this procedure and use sterile technique. This is important in aspirating an olecranon bursa because secondary infection may develop.

### STEP 2
Prepare the skin with a bactericidal solution.

### STEP 3
Use a 27-gauge needle to infiltrate the skin over the lateral aspect of the bursa with 1 mL of 1% lidocaine.

### STEP 4
Through the skin wheal, insert the 18-gauge needle attached to the 10-mL syringe into the enlarged bursa (**Figure 1**). Aspirate

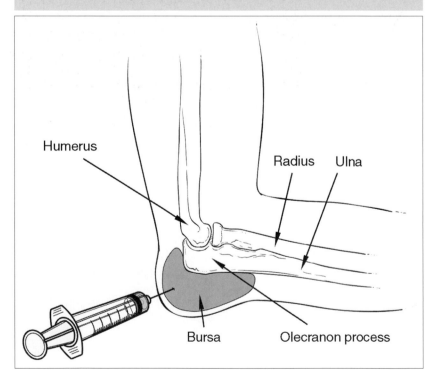

**Figure 1**
Location for needle insertion for olecranon bursa aspiration.

# OLECRANON BURSA ASPIRATION (CONTINUED)

the contents until the bursa is flat. If there is any concern about infection, send the fluid for culture and sensitivity and do not inject the corticosteroid preparation into the cavity.

## Step 5
If infection does not seem probable, a corticosteroid injection may be helpful. Remove the aspirating syringe and attach a 1-mL syringe containing 1 mL of a 40 mg/mL corticosteroid preparation. Inject this into the bursal cavity.

## Step 6
Dress the puncture wound with a sterile adhesive bandage.

## Step 7
Lightly wrap the elbow with an elastic dressing.

## ADVERSE OUTCOMES
Secondary infection is possible, though not likely if sterile technique is used. Recurrence of the bursal effusion is common but can be minimized by a compressive dressing and having the patient avoid direct trauma to the elbow such as resting the elbow on tabletops.

## AFTERCARE/PATIENT INSTRUCTIONS
Advise the patient to limit elbow motion for 1 or 2 days after the aspiration. If the patient has a recurrent bursitis, use a posterior plaster splint to limit elbow motion for 1 to 2 weeks after the aspiration.

SECTION 3 ■ ELBOW AND FOREARM

# NERVE COMPRESSION SYNDROMES

**ICD-9 Codes**

**354.1**
Mononeuritis of upper limb and
nononeuritis multiplex, other lesion
of median nerve

**354.2**
Mononeuritis of upper limb and
nononeuritis multiplex, lesion of
ulnar nerve

**354.3**
Mononeuritis of upper limb and
nononeuritis multiplex, lesion of
radial nerve

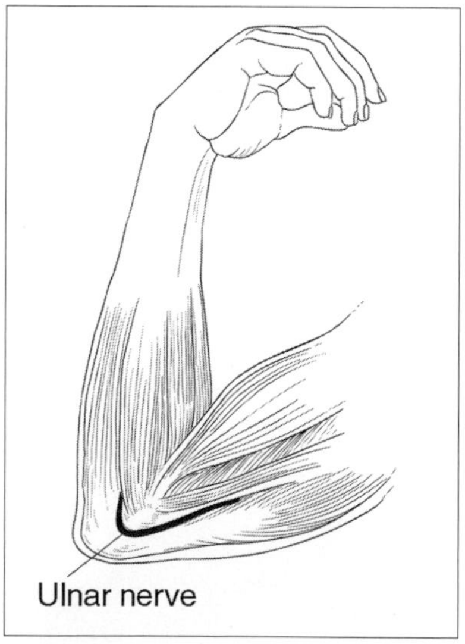

**Figure 1**
Compression of ulnar nerve during
elbow flexion.

Adapted with permission from Mackinnon SE,
Dellon AL: *Surgery of the Peripheral Nerve*. New
York, NY, Thieme Medical Publishers, 1988.

## SYNONYMS
Cubital tunnel syndrome
Median nerve compression at the elbow
Posterior interosseous nerve compression
Pronator syndrome
Radial tunnel syndrome
Tardy ulnar palsy
Ulnar nerve neuritis

## DEFINITION
Compression of the ulnar nerve at the elbow is second only to
carpal tunnel syndrome as a source of nerve entrapment in the
upper extremity. The nerve can be compressed at a number of
sites, from 10 cm proximal to the elbow to 5 cm below the
joint. The most common sites are where the ulnar nerve passes
in the groove on the posterior aspect of the medial epicondyle
(in the so-called "cubital tunnel") and where it passes between
the humeral and ulnar heads of the flexor carpi ulnaris muscle.

Ulnar nerve compression can develop acutely after a direct
blow. Chronic symptoms occur in individuals who put
prolonged pressure on the nerve by continuously leaning on the
elbow or who keep the nerve on stretch by holding the elbows
flexed for long periods during work or recreation (**Figure 1**).
Ulnar nerve compression also can occur after trauma that
results in osteophytes or scar tissue that encroach upon the
nerve. Cubitus valgus (a carrying angle greater than 10°) places
the nerve on stretch and over time also may cause ulnar
neuritis. Instability of the ulnar nerve with repetitive
subluxation or dislocation of the ulnar nerve on elbow flexion
also can cause ulnar palsy.

Compression of the posterior interosseous nerve (a deep
branch of the radial nerve), or radial tunnel syndrome, is a
cause of lateral elbow pain and is commonly misdiagnosed as
lateral epicondylitis. The posterior interosseous nerve has no
sensory distribution but innervates the thumb and finger
extensors and the extensor carpi ulnaris. The posterior
interosseous nerve is most commonly compressed by fibrous
bands between the two heads of the supinator muscle in a
region termed the radial tunnel.

Pronator syndrome refers to muscular compression of the
median nerve in the proximal forearm. Diagnosis is often
difficult and delayed because of the vague symptoms, lack of

easily observed findings, and the frequent association with workers' compensation.

# CLINICAL SYMPTOMS

Symptoms vary depending on the duration and severity of the nerve compression. Early symptoms of ulnar nerve compression include aching pain at the medial aspect of the elbow, and numbness and tingling in the ring and little fingers. The paresthesias occasionally radiate proximally into the shoulder and neck. Weakness of the intrinsic muscles is a late finding and can interfere with activities of daily living, such as opening jars or turning a key in a door. Visible muscle wasting implies ulnar nerve compression of several months' to years' duration.

Patients with radial tunnel syndrome present with symptoms similar to lateral epicondylitis, but with pain that is 4 to 5 cm more distal than that of lateral epicondylitis. Because the posterior interosseous nerve contains only motor fibers, there is no numbness or tingling. Obvious muscular weakness is rarely encountered until late in the disease process.

Symptoms of pronator syndrome are often vague, consisting of discomfort in the forearm with occasional proximal radiation into the arm. Repetitive strenuous motions, such as industrial activities, weight training, or driving, often provoke the symptoms. Numbness may affect all or a part of the median nerve distribution. Women seem to be at greater risk than men for this syndrome, especially in the industrial setting.

# TESTS

## Physical Examination

Inspect the elbow for deformity and measure the carrying angle. The nerve should be palpated for any masses or localized tenderness. Lightly tapping on the nerve can cause pain and paresthesias over the ulnar border of the hand and the ring and little fingers (Tinel sign).

Palpate the ulnar groove as the elbow is flexed and extended to determine if the nerve slips out of the groove. The elbow flexion test is a provocative maneuver. The patient should flex the elbow as far as possible, reporting any tingling or numbness in the hand as soon as it is felt (elbow flexion test). Record how quickly symptoms appear; if the symptoms do not develop within 60 seconds, the test is considered negative.

Assess sensation and muscle function of the ulnar nerve. Vibration and light touch perception are the first to be affected, and the little finger and the ulnar half of the ring finger are most likely to be involved. Two-point discrimination is affected when nerve compression has progressed to axonal degeneration.

SECTION 3 ■ ELBOW AND FOREARM

Weakness is assessed by testing abduction and adduction of the little and index fingers, the ability to cross the index and middle fingers, and thumb-to-index pinch. The ulnarly innervated extrinsic muscles are less commonly involved. Wasting of the intrinsic muscles is a late finding and produces a hollowed-out appearance between the metacarpals on the dorsal aspect of the hand.

With posterior interosseous nerve compression, the area of tenderness is directly over the radial tunnel, which lies 4 to 5 cm distal and slightly anterior to the lateral epicondyle. With radial tunnel syndrome, pain in the proximal forearm may be noted by extending the middle finger against resistance (middle finger test).

With pronator syndrome, physical examination findings are often subtle. The most reliable test is reproduction of pain with direct pressure over the proximal portion of the pronator teres approximately 4 cm distal to the antebrachial crease while exerting moderate resistance to pronation. Resisted pronation for 60 seconds may initiate the symptoms by contracting the flexor-pronator muscle.

## Diagnostic Tests

EMG/NCV (electromyographic/nerve conduction velocity) studies provide an objective measurement of ulnar nerve compression. A reduction in velocity of 30% or more suggests significant compression of the ulnar nerve. EMG/NCV studies are usually normal in cases of radial tunnel and pronator syndromes. Plain radiographs of the elbow are indicated when previous elbow trauma has occurred.

# DIFFERENTIAL DIAGNOSIS

Carpal tunnel syndrome (numbness in thumb, index, and middle fingers; thenar muscle wasting)

Herniated cervical disk or cervical radiculopathy (history, physical examination, and EMG/NCV should differentiate, though MRI may sometimes be necessary)

Lateral epicondylitis (tenderness over lateral epicondyle/ extensor attachment, no neurogenic symptoms)

Medial epicondylitis (tenderness over the medial epicondyle; no distal weakness, paresthesias, or numbness)

Thoracic outlet syndrome (normal NCV studies at the elbow; rarely, wasting in the hand)

Ulnar nerve entrapment at the wrist (strong wrist flexors and ulnar deviators, sensation intact over the dorsomedial hand and the dorsum of the little and ring fingers)

## ADVERSE OUTCOMES OF THE DISEASE

Loss of strength and sensation can be progressive and permanent in long-standing cases. Pain, tenderness, and stiffness at the elbow also can persist.

## TREATMENT

For ulnar nerve compression, modifying activities in the workplace to limit elbow flexion and direct pressure on the ulnar nerve is the most important step in treatment. At night, an elbow splint that keeps the elbow from flexing to 90° can be worn. (A towel wrapped around the elbow is sufficient if a commercial splint is not available.) A sports elbow protector can be used at work to keep from bumping the elbow. NSAIDs may be of benefit for an acute, severe episode. Corticosteroid injections are not recommended.

Surgical decompression and transposition of the ulnar nerve should be considered for patients with bothersome symptoms or mild weakness that persists despite 3 to 4 months of nonsurgical management, or for patients with significant or progressive weakness. There are several different methods of surgical decompression, but all involve inspecting the nerve and removing all compressive etiologies.

Decompression of the radial tunnel is indicated for patients with radial tunnel syndrome who have significant discomfort that has not responded to prolonged nonsurgical care over a period of at least 3 to 6 months.

Likewise, surgical decompression is indicated for pronator syndrome if all measures of nonsurgical treatment (including activity/job modification, anti-inflammatory medications, physical therapy, and steroid injection) have not resulted in adequate pain relief over a period of at least 3 to 6 months.

## ADVERSE OUTCOMES OF TREATMENT

Care should be taken that any splint applied does not have straps across the medial elbow because this could increase nerve compression. NSAIDs can cause gastric, renal, or hepatic complications. Surgery may be complicated by infection and/or nerve damage. Symptoms are not always improved after surgery. The importance of nonsurgical care and careful selection of surgical candidates cannot be overemphasized, due to the fact these nerve compressive injuries are often work-related and are complicated by issues of secondary gain.

SECTION 3 ■ ELBOW AND FOREARM

# REFERRAL DECISIONS/RED FLAGS

Significant or progressive weakness or atrophy of the intrinsic muscles, increasing numbness despite nonsurgical treatment, or persistent symptoms that interfere with activities or work and have failed to respond to prolonged nonsurgical care indicate the need for further evaluation.

# RUPTURE OF THE DISTAL BICEPS TENDON

## DEFINITION

Rupture of the distal biceps brachii tendon is uncommon, accounting for less than 5% of biceps tendon ruptures. However, complete tears of the distal biceps tendon cause significantly greater weakness than do tears of the proximal biceps tendon. If the lesion is not recognized and repaired in a timely fashion, strength of elbow flexion and forearm supination is decreased by 30% to 50%. Most often, ruptures occur in men older than 40 years of age who have preexisting degenerative changes in the biceps tendon.

These ruptures typically are located at the insertion of the biceps tendon into the radius (radial tuberosity). The rupture may be incomplete or complete. With complete ruptures, the biceps aponeurosis may remain intact initially.

## CLINICAL SYMPTOMS

Patients often report a history of sudden, sharp pain in the anterior elbow that followed an excessive extension force on the flexed elbow. The pain typically is severe for a few hours (acute inflammatory response) and then is followed by a chronic, dull ache in the anterior elbow region that is made worse by lifting activities.

## TESTS

### Physical Examination

Examination reveals tenderness and a defect in the antecubital fossa due to the absence of the usually prominent biceps tendon. Early on, ecchymosis will be present in the antecubital fossa and proximal forearm. With flexion of the elbow against resistance, the muscle belly retracts proximally **(Figure 1)**.

If the rupture is incomplete, the defect will not be apparent, but the patient will exhibit pain and weakness on flexion and supination of the elbow against resistance. If the rupture is complete but the bicipital aponeurosis is intact, the defect is not as obvious; however, comparison with the opposite side helps to confirm the diagnosis.

### Diagnostic Tests

AP and lateral radiographs of the elbow usually are normal, but they may reveal an avulsion fracture of the bicipital tuberosity. MRI is usually necessary to confirm the diagnosis.

**ICD-9 Code**

**841.9**
Sprains and strains of elbow and forearm, unspecified site

SECTION 3 ■ ELBOW AND FOREARM

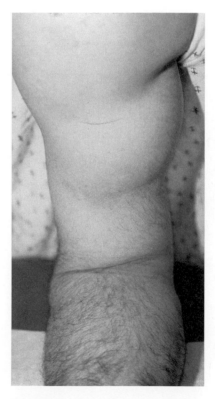

**Figure 1**

Clinical appearance of distal biceps tendon rupture.

Reproduced with permission from Ramsey ML: Distal biceps tendon injuries: Diagnosis and management. *J Am Acad Orthop Surg* 1999;7:199-207.

# DIFFERENTIAL DIAGNOSIS

Bicipital tendinosis (tendon degenerative changes without rupture)

Cubital bursitis (enlargement of the bursa between the biceps tendon and the radial tuberosity; may occur primarily or secondary to other conditions)

Entrapment of the lateral antebrachial cutaneous nerve (pain and dysesthesia at the lateral aspect of the proximal forearm)

Pronator syndrome (no weakness or defect)

# ADVERSE OUTCOMES OF THE DISEASE

Loss of elbow flexion strength is significant, particularly with the forearm in supination. Loss of forearm supination power (eg, turning a screwdriver) also occurs. With time, the muscle retracts and becomes fibrotic. In this situation, surgical repair either is not possible or the results are compromised, with less predictable return of muscle strength.

# TREATMENT

Most patients with complete ruptures do better with surgical repair of the tendon. Partial ruptures may be managed nonsurgically with activity modification and intermittent splinting, but if this treatment fails, surgical repair is indicated. Nonsurgical management is used with older patients who are sedentary and do not require normal elbow flexor strength and endurance. Nonsurgical treatment may also be appropriate for the nondominant arm in selected patients and in cases of delayed diagnosis.

# ADVERSE OUTCOMES OF TREATMENT

Full return of muscle strength may not occur. Injury to the radial nerve is possible. Infection, ectopic ossification, and chronic pain may ensue.

# REFERRAL DECISIONS/RED FLAGS

Because of the adverse and progressive effect on muscle strength, patients with rupture of the distal tendon of the biceps should be evaluated for possible surgical repair.

# ULNAR COLLATERAL LIGAMENT TEAR

## DEFINITION

The ulnar collateral ligament (UCL) is the primary structure resisting valgus stress at the elbow. Trauma to this ligament (including strains and tears) is relatively uncommon, and should rarely lead to symptomatic instability or disability. However, the overhead-throwing athlete (particularly in baseball and javelin) places repetitive valgus stress across the medial elbow and the UCL (**Figure 1**). This may result in injury to the ligament, leading to instability and disability that may require treatment in these throwing athletes.

## CLINICAL SYMPTOMS

Onset may be acute, with the athlete experiencing a "pop" while throwing, followed by medial elbow pain. Most commonly, patients have a gradual onset of symptoms with progressive medial elbow pain with throwing. Paresthesias along the ulnar nerve distribution while throwing is a commonly associated symptom. Swelling and ecchymosis are usually minimal. This injury is being seen with increasing frequency at younger ages, especially high school–aged athletes. A history of abuse to the arm (excessive numbers of pitches per game, excessive innings per year, year-round baseball, use of "breaking" pitches—curve or slider—at a young age) is common.

## TESTS

### Physical Examination

Examination generally demonstrates tenderness over the UCL, and there may be some loss of terminal extension. Swelling and ecchymosis are generally absent. There is usually pain over the UCL with valgus stress testing, though gross opening of the joint is uncommon. Tenderness over the ulnar nerve and a positive Tinel sign are common, often leading to an inaccurate diagnosis of primary ulnar neuritis.

### Diagnostic Tests

AP and lateral radiographs are necessary to rule out fracture. Ossification within the UCL may be seen in chronic cases. Posteromedial olecranon osteophytes, loose bodies, and marginal spurring may also be seen in chronic cases. MRI with intra-articular contrast is the gold standard to image and diagnose pathology of the UCL.

**ICD-9 Code**

**841.1**
Sprains and strains of elbow and forearm, ulnar collateral ligament

SECTION 3 ■ ELBOW AND FOREARM

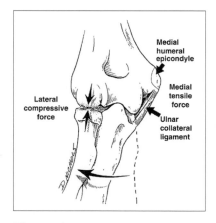

**Figure 1**
Forces resulting in valgus sprain of the UCL in the throwing athlete.

Reproduced with permission from Andrews JR, Zarins B, Wilk KE (eds): *Injuries in Baseball.* Philadelphia, PA Lippincott-Raven, 1998.

## DIFFERENTIAL DIAGNOSIS

Cubital tunnel syndrome (stability examination, history; frequently coexists with UCL injury)

Medial epicondyle avulsion (evident on radiographs, adolescent age group)

Medial epicondylitis (history and stability examination; typically, older age group)

## ADVERSE OUTCOMES OF THE DISEASE

Persistent pain and disability in throwing sports are most common. Rarely are problems encountered with activities of daily living or in nonthrowing sports. Chronic stiffness and loss of motion may be encountered.

## TREATMENT

Nonsurgical care, including rest, NSAIDs, physical therapy, stretching and strengthening exercises, and activity modification, is appropriate following such an injury. Steroid injections in the UCL may cause weakening and attenuation of the ligament, and should be avoided. A very slow return to sport (involving a detailed progressive throwing program) should be stressed. If pain relief is the main goal of the patient, nonsurgical care is likely to be successful. If a return to a highly competitive level of a throwing sport is the main goal, surgery may be necessary. If an athlete has failed to respond to an appropriate course of nonsurgical care within 3 months, surgical reconstruction (the so-called "Tommy John surgery") should be considered. The patient must realize that postoperative rehabilitation is critical and lengthy, requiring approximately 12 months before return to competition. In the properly selected athlete, surgery is over 90% successful in returning the athlete to the preinjury level of competition. With the alarming trend of younger baseball players injuring the UCL, emphasis should be placed on education and prevention in youth sports (ie, following pitch counts, limiting number of innings pitched per season or per year, avoiding year-round baseball, and delaying throwing breaking pitches until the young athlete's body matures).

## ADVERSE OUTCOMES OF TREATMENT

Surgical risks include stiffness, nerve injury, infection, and persistent pain.

## REFERRAL DECISIONS/RED FLAGS

Failure of nonsurgical management in the high-level thrower who wishes to continue to compete at this level indicates the need for further evaluation.

SECTION 3 ■ ELBOW AND FOREARM

# PAIN DIAGRAM—HAND AND WRIST

de Quervain tenosynovitis

Fracture of the scaphoid

Arthritis of the wrist

Arthritis of the thumb CMC joint

Fracture of the base of the thumb metacarpal

Boutonnière deformity

Paronychia *(Fingertip Infection)*

Glomus tumor *(Tumors of the Hand and Wrist)*

Mucous cyst *(Tumors of the Hand and Wrist)*

Osteoarthritis (fingers) *(Arthritis of the Hand)*

Mallet finger

Epidermal inclusion cyst *(Tumors of the Hand and Wrist)*

Felon *(Fingertip Infections)*

Flexor tendon sheath ganglion *(Ganglia of the Wrist and Hand)*

Ulnar collateral ligament tear

Sprained collateral ligament *(Sprains and Dislocations of the Hand)*

Fracture of the phalanges

Rheumatoid arthritis *(Arthritis of the Hand)*

Trigger finger

Arthritis of the thumb CMC joint

Fracture of the metacarpals

Flexor tendon sheath infection

Dupuytren disease

Arthritis of the wrist

Ulnar nerve entrapment at the wrist

Carpal tunnel syndrome

Volar ganglion *(Ganglia of the Wrist and Hand)*

Fracture of the scaphoid

Ganglia of the wrist and hand

Kienböck disease

Osteoarthritis *(Arthritis of the Wrist)*

Rheumatoid arthritis

Fracture of the distal radius

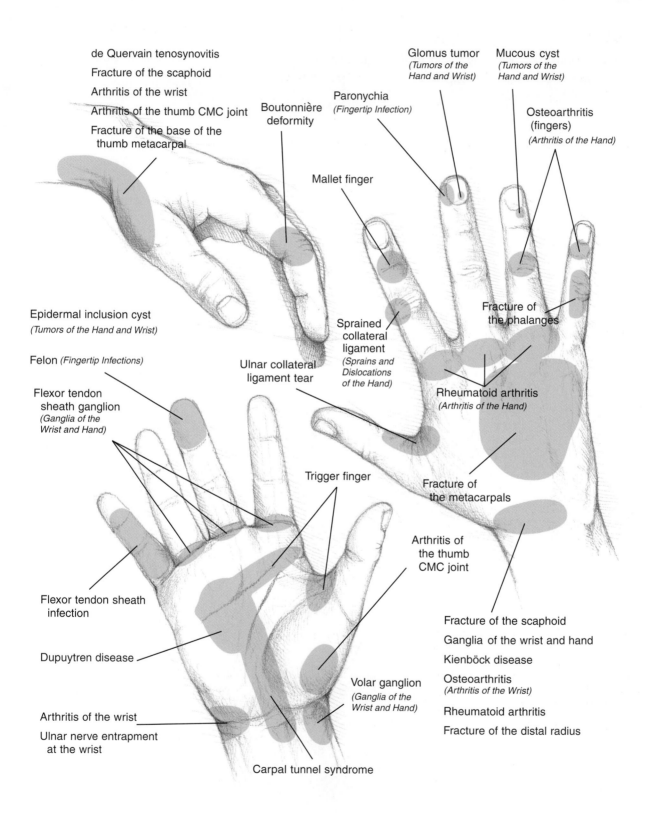

# HAND AND WRIST

**Section Editor**
John Gray Seiler III, MD
Clinical Associate Professor
Department of Orthopaedic Surgery
Georgia Hand and Microsurgery
Emory University
Atlanta, Georgia

John F. Dalton IV, MD
Department of Orthopaedic Surgery
Emory University
Atlanta, Georgia

Robert Donatelli, PhD, PT, OCS
National Director of Sports Rehabilitation
Physiotherapy Associates
Las Vegas, Nevada

Alexandra Louthan, OTR/L, CHT
Physiotherapy Associates
Atlanta, Georgia

Scott Olvey, MD
Department of Hand Surgery/
Upper Extremity
Center for Orthopedic Surgery
and Sports Medicine
Indianapolis, Indiana

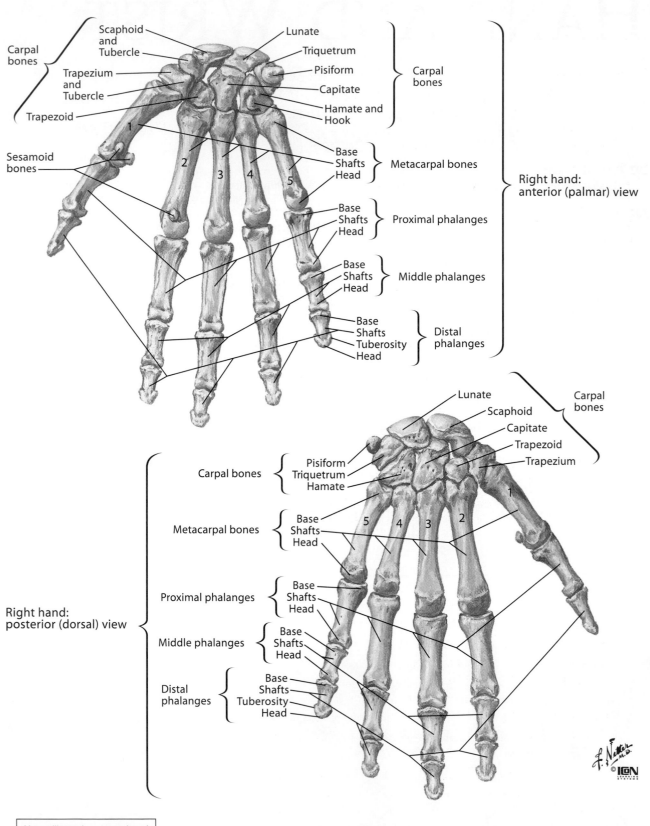

Carpal bones

Scaphoid and Tubercle — Lunate — Triquetrum

Trapezium and Tubercle — Pisiform — Capitate

Trapezoid — Hamate and Hook

Carpal bones

1

Sesamoid bones

2

3  4  5

Base
Shafts
Head — Metacarpal bones

Base
Shafts
Head — Proximal phalanges

Base
Shafts
Head — Middle phalanges

Base
Shafts
Tuberosity
Head — Distal phalanges

Right hand: anterior (palmar) view

Lunate — Scaphoid — Capitate — Trapezoid — Trapezium

Carpal bones

Pisiform
Triquetrum — Carpal bones
Hamate

1

Base
Shafts
Head — Metacarpal bones

5  4  3  2

Base
Shafts
Head — Proximal phalanges

Base
Shafts
Head — Middle phalanges

Base
Shafts
Tuberosity
Head — Distal phalanges

Right hand: posterior (dorsal) view

Bones of the Wrist and Hand

# Hand and Wrist—Overview

Carpal tunnel syndrome, trigger finger, ganglion formation, carpometacarpal (CMC) arthritis of the thumb, and radiocarpal arthritis are among the more common hand and wrist problems that bring patients to a primary care physician. Patients with chronic hand and wrist problems typically have one or more of the following symptoms: (1) pain, (2) instability, (3) stiffness, (4) swelling, (5) weakness, (6) numbness, or (7) a mass.

To begin the evaluation, obtain a complete history from the patient, including a statement of the chief symptom, a thorough history of the present condition, and a general medical history. The history of the present condition should include the duration of symptoms, the specific type and location of symptoms, factors that improve or worsen the symptoms, and previous treatments. After obtaining the history, a complete physical examination should be done. With these two pieces of information, a working diagnosis can be established in a high percentage of patients. Diagnostic testing, which often includes plain radiographs, should be done to help confirm the working hypothesis that has been synthesized from the history and physical examination.

## Location of Pain

The best method of localizing the pain is to have the patient use one finger to identify the point of maximum tenderness. Categorize the pain as being in one of the following four areas: radial, ulnar, volar, or dorsal. This localization of pain by anatomic region will help narrow the field of probable diagnoses (**Figure 1**).

### Radial Pain

Wrist pain in patients younger than 30 years most commonly results from trauma. Posttraumatic tenderness and pain over the radial aspect of the wrist may suggest a fracture of the scaphoid, which is the most commonly missed fracture in the wrist and hand. In the absence of trauma, pain associated with tenderness over the radial styloid is most likely de Quervain (wrist) tenosynovitis. Pain that is dorsal and slightly more proximal may be caused by intersection syndrome (tenosynovitis of the radial wrist extensors) or superficial radial neuritis. Pain that occurs without numbness in patients older than 40 years is likely to be caused by posttraumatic arthritis or osteoarthritis. Pain at the base of the thumb in women in this age group is likely to be caused by CMC arthritis.

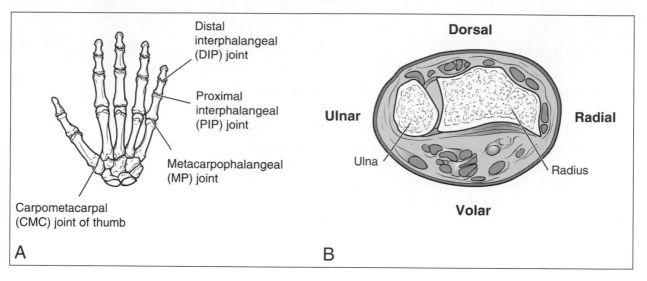

**Figure 1**

**A,** Joints of the hand: dorsal view. **B,** Localizing symptoms to one of the four quadrants of the wrist can be helpful in guiding the physical examination and for establishing a differential diagnosis.

Part A adapted with permission from Anderson JE: *Grant's Atlas of Anatomy*, ed 8. Baltimore, MD, Williams & Wilkins, 1983.

## Dorsal Pain

Generalized dorsal wrist discomfort may be associated with radiocarpal arthritis. Pain in this region associated with a well-defined mass over the dorsoradial aspect of the wrist is usually a ganglion cyst. Pain and loss of motion in the wrist can also be caused by ligamentous injury to the wrist or by Kienböck disease (osteonecrosis of the lunate). Plain radiographs are valuable in the initial assessment of these patients.

## Ulnar Pain

Pain in this region after trauma can be caused by a tear of the triangular fibrocartilage complex, which is located distal to the ulnar styloid. Swelling and tenderness over the dorsoulnar or volar aspects of the wrist are likely to be caused by a tendinitis of the ulnar wrist extensor or flexor tendons.

## Volar Pain

Carpal tunnel syndrome, ganglion cyst formation, and tenosynovitis are by far the most common causes of volar wrist pain. Carpal tunnel syndrome is commonly associated with numbness and tingling in the radial three digits (thumb plus index and long fingers) and, often, half of the ring finger. Other causes of discomfort include a volar ganglion cyst formation, which should be easily palpable on the volar radial aspect of the wrist, or wrist tendinitis. Swelling over the volar region suggests inflammation of the finger flexor tendons. Patients with radiocarpal arthritis might have pain over both the dorsal and volar aspects of the wrist. Volar wrist pain also can be caused by arthritis between the pisiform and the triquetrum bones.

# CHRONIC WRIST AND FINGER INSTABILITY

Diagnosis of wrist instability is often complex, requiring considerable experience in history taking, physical examination, and interpretation of radiographs. Typical symptoms are sensations of slipping, snapping, or clunking with certain wrist motions after an injury. The unstable structure might be a joint (following a tear of the supporting and stabilizing ligaments that hold together the carpal bones) or a subluxating tendon (following a tear of the restraining ligaments, or retinaculum, that contain the tendon). Plain PA radiographs of the wrist might show separation between the scaphoid and the lunate (Terry Thomas sign), indicating a tear of the intrinsic ligament binding the scaphoid and the lunate (scapholunate dissociation). Chronic ligamentous instability commonly occurs in the metacarpophalangeal (MP) joint of the thumb and can occur in any of the proximal interphalangeal (PIP) joints or MP joints.

# STIFFNESS

Morning stiffness is a common symptom of arthritis or tenosynovitis and may be associated with carpal tunnel syndrome or trigger finger. Patients with trigger finger often have pain, and they commonly (and erroneously) localize the problem to the PIP joint when it locks or "jumps" as the finger is flexed. In fact, the source of the problem is in the palm, where the thickened flexor tendon catches under the proximal (A1) tendon pulley at the distal palmar crease. Tenderness and palpable catching just distal to this crease confirm the diagnosis.

# SWELLING

Swelling in the joints of the hand and wrist is caused by synovitis, which can be secondary to osteoarthritis, infection, or a systemic inflammatory disease (such as rheumatoid arthritis or gout). A history of penetrating trauma or immunocompromise in patients who present for evaluation of swelling should suggest infection as opposed to inflammatory disease. Plain radiographs are useful in diagnosing osteoarthritis and rheumatoid arthritis. Swelling around the tendons can occur in association with rheumatoid arthritis and/or overuse syndromes such as de Quervain tenosynovitis. Pain and swelling around the wrist flexor or extensor tendons suggest tendinitis; plain radiographs may show a calcific deposit close to the involved tendon in patients who develop calcific tendinitis.

SECTION 4 ■ HAND AND WRIST

# WEAKNESS

Weakness in the hand may be secondary to pain, as with CMC or radiocarpal arthritis or intrinsic muscle disease. Weakness without pain suggests possible peripheral nerve entrapment. Ulnar nerve entrapment at the elbow will result in decreased grip and pinch strength in addition to loss of sensation in the little and ring fingers. Wasting of the intrinsic muscles is seen on physical examination in advanced cases.

# NUMBNESS

Dysesthesias, paresthesias, and hand-based numbness and tingling are commonly caused by entrapment neuropathy. **Figure 2** shows the typical sensory distribution of the median, ulnar, and radial nerves; however, variations from this pattern can occur. Positive provocative signs (Tinel sign, Phalen maneuver, Durkan carpal compression test) and abnormal sensory testing should be considered indicative of carpal tunnel syndrome. With carpal tunnel syndrome, the numbness characteristically occurs in the thumb, the index and long

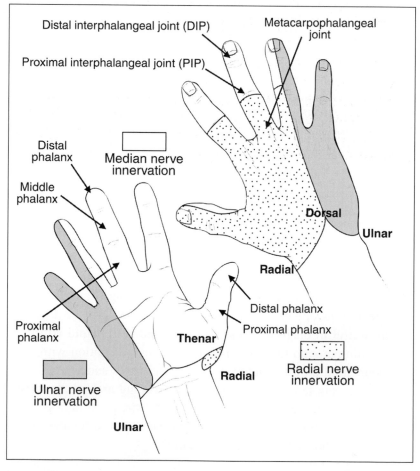

**Figure 2**
Regions of and sensory distribution in the hand.

fingers, and, often, the radial half of the ring finger; some patients report that the entire hand is numb.

Loss of sensation in the little and ring fingers usually is caused by entrapment of the ulnar nerve at the elbow or the wrist. Patients with thoracic outlet syndrome often report symptoms at the ulnar side of the hand and forearm, but this condition is much less common than ulnar nerve entrapment at the elbow. Both the Tinel sign and elbow flexion tests should be negative with thoracic outlet syndrome.

Neck pain associated with a positive Spurling test and with loss of sensation in the thumb and index finger suggests a common cervical radiculopathy. Electrophysiologic testing is commonly used to confirm the clinical diagnosis in patients who present for evaluation of numbness.

# MASSES

The most common mass in the hand and wrist is a ganglion cyst. These cysts most often occur in four locations: the dorsoradial and volar radial aspects of the wrist; the proximal finger flexor crease; and the distal interphalangeal joint. Multilobulated masses along the sides of the finger are most likely giant cell tumors. Nontender nodules in the palm and cords that cross both the MP and PIP joints are consistent with Dupuytren disease. A hard mass at the dorsal base of the index metacarpal is usually a carpal boss—a bony mass consisting of spurs from the second and third metacarpals, the trapezoid, and the capitate. A serpiginous mass that follows the path of the tendon sheaths is often tenosynovitis. Masses with bluish discoloration or masses that have a pulsation are usually vascular in origin.

SECTION 4 ■ HAND AND WRIST

# PHYSICAL EXAMINATION HAND AND WRIST

## INSPECTION/PALPATION

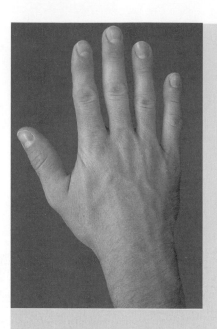

### Dorsum

Observe the alignment of the fingers. Inspect the nails for pitting and other evidence of systemic disorders. Look for swelling and synovitis of the finger and wrist joints. Note any osteophytes or bony prominences associated with degenerative arthritis. Muscle atrophy between the metacarpals is caused by weakness of the intrinsic muscles.

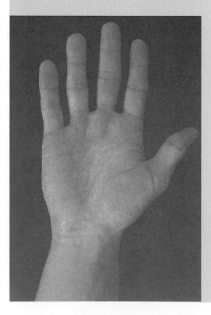

### Palm

Look for atrophy of the thenar muscles (median nerve–innervated) and hypothenar muscles (ulnar nerve–innervated). Note any thickening of the palmar fascia associated with Dupuytren contracture. Pain elicited by pressure over the thumb metacarpophalangeal (MP) joint suggests arthritis or instability of this joint.

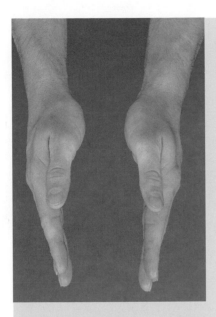

## Side view

Position the patient's hands with the palms facing each other to best visualize atrophy of the thenar muscles. Swelling in the joints of the thumb also is prominent in this position.

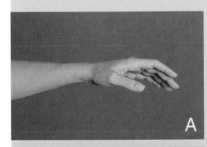

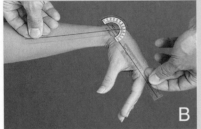

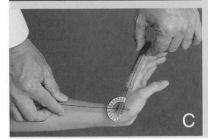

## Wrist flexion/extension: Zero Starting Position

To measure flexion and extension, place the patient's forearm in the Zero Starting Position (**A**) with the forearm in pronation and the carpus aligned with the plane of the forearm. Place the goniometer on the dorsum of the wrist or on the radial side of the forearm. Aligning the goniometer on the ulnar side may falsely elevate the measurement because of the mobility of the fifth metacarpal. Wrist motion occurs at the radiocarpal and midcarpal joints. Normal wrist palmar flexion (**B**) is 75° to 80°, and normal dorsal extension (**C**) is 75° to 85°.

SECTION 4 ■ HAND AND WRIST

SECTION 4 ■ HAND AND WRIST

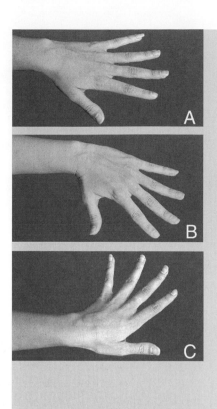

## Wrist radial/ulnar deviation

To measure radial and ulnar deviation, place the patient's forearm in the Zero Starting Position (**A**) with the forearm in pronation and the carpus aligned with the plane of the forearm. Align the goniometer with the third metacarpal and the axis of the forearm. In radial and ulnar deviation, the carpal rows move as linked segments. The buttress of the radial styloid limits radial deviation so that its arc of motion is significantly less. Normal radial deviation (**B**) is 20° to 25°, and normal ulnar deviation (**C**) is 35° to 40°.

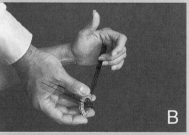

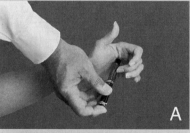

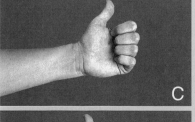

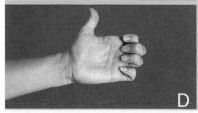

## Finger flexion/extension

Finger joint motion occurs primarily in the flexion-extension plane, with flexion accounting for most finger joint motion. From a functional perspective, finger flexion is a composite movement of motion of the MP, PIP, and distal interphalangeal (DIP) joints. To estimate the loss of digital flexion, measure the distance from the maximally flexed fingertip to the distal palmar crease using a pen (**A**) or goniometer (**B**). In young and middle-aged adults, the fingertip should touch the distal palmar crease (**C**). Flexion and extension also can be measured individually at the MP, PIP, and DIP joints (**D**). The wrist should be in neutral when measuring finger flexion. If the wrist is flexed, the extensor digitorum longus will be effectively tethered, thereby limiting finger flexion. Finally, active motion should be compared with passive motion.

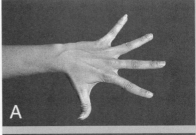
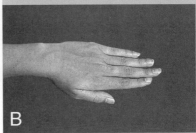

## Finger abduction/adduction

Abduction and adduction occur in the plane of the palm, primarily at the MP joints and centered on the long finger. Abduction (**A**) is movement of the fingers away from the long finger; adduction (**B**) is movement of the other fingers toward the long finger.

# RANGE OF MOTION

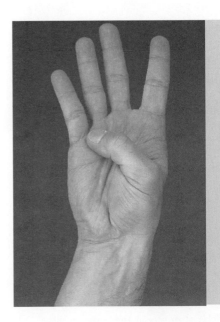

## Thumb opposition

Thumb motions are complex and reflect the overall importance of the thumb to the function of the hand. The principal thumb motions are abduction, adduction, flexion, extension, and opposition. Opposition is a composite motion created by movement at the CMC, MP, and IP joints and is valued as 50% to 60% of thumb function.

Measure composite thumb flexion by asking the patient to touch the tip of the thumb to the base of the little finger. The amount of impairment can be assessed by measuring the distance from the tip of the thumb to the base of the little finger.

SECTION 4 ■ HAND AND WRIST

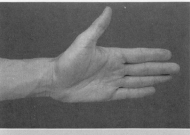

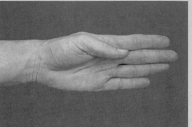

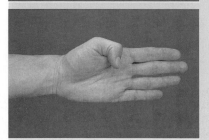

### Thumb flexion/extension

All thumb joints move in the plane of flexion-extension, but this movement is difficult to quantify at the CMC joint. Flexion at the thumb MP joint is typically 50° to 60°, but normal measurements are highly variable. Flexion at the IP joint ranges from 55° to 75° and depends on age and gender. Extension beyond 0° is not often observed at the MP joint and is only 5° to 10° at the IP joint.

Measure thumb motion with the wrist in a neutral position. If the wrist is flexed, the extensor pollicis longus may be tethered, limiting flexion at the MP and IP joints.

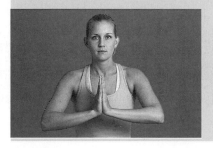

### Wrist extension

To assess loss of wrist motion, compare the extension of the right and left wrists when held in similar positions, as shown. Take care to position the elbows in flexion.

## MUSCLE TESTING

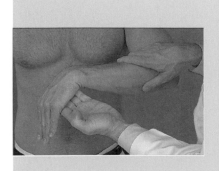

### Wrist flexion

In general, manual motor testing should be done by first asking the patient to demonstrate the primary function of a muscle and then, when possible, asking the patient to show resistance (provided by the examiner) to the opposition of that function. Responses to testing should be graded objectively. To test the strength of the wrist flexors (the most powerful of which is the flexor carpi ulnaris), stabilize the patient's elbow at 90°. With the fingers extended to eliminate action of the finger flexors, resist the patient's attempt to flex the wrist. Weakness will be evident with fracture of the medial humeral condyle, tendinitis of the medial elbow, or lesions involving the median or ulnar nerve.

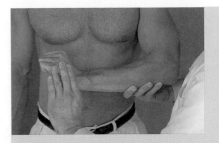

### Wrist extension

To test the strength of the wrist extensors (the most powerful of which are the extensor carpi ulnaris and extensor carpi radialis brevis), resist the patient's attempt to extend the wrist. Weakness will be evident with rupture of the extensor origin, fracture of the lateral humeral condyle, epicondylitis, lesions involving the radial nerve or C6-C7 nerve roots, or distal rupture of the tendon insertion.

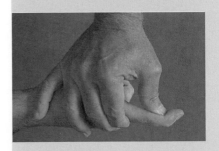

### Flexor digitorum profundus

Position the patient's hand palm up on the examining table, with the fingers extended. Hold the PIP joint in extension and ask the patient to bend the distal finger joint. Inability to flex the DIP joint indicates an injury to the profundus tendon, injury to the median nerve or its anterior interosseous branch (innervates the flexor digitorum profundus to the index and, often, the long finger), or to the ulnar nerve (innervates the ring and little finger DIP joint).

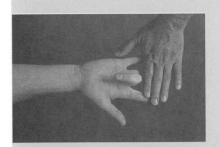

### Flexor digitorum sublimis

Position the patient's hand palm up on the examining table, with the fingers extended. Hold all the fingers in full extension except for the finger being tested. Ask the patient to bend the finger. The flexor digitorum profundus cannot independently flex the finger when it is tethered by the other fingers being kept in extension. However, the flexor digitorum sublimis of each finger can work independently. A normal response is flexion at the PIP joint. Inability to flex this finger indicates an injury to the sublimis tendon to that finger or injury to the median nerve.

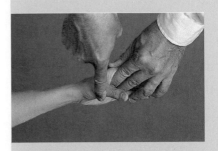

### Thumb abduction strength

With the patient's hand on the examining surface, ask the patient to abduct the thumb (place it straight up) and resist your attempt to push it down onto the table (abduction and extension). Weakness indicates damage to the motor branch of the median nerve, most commonly related to carpal tunnel syndrome.

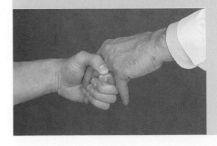

### Grip strength

A decrease in total grip strength reflects weakness of the finger flexors and/or intrinsic muscles of the hand. Grip strength testing can be easily quantified using grip meters. This objective measurement can be used to follow a patient's progress in strengthening.

SECTION 4 ■ HAND AND WRIST

# SENSORY TESTING

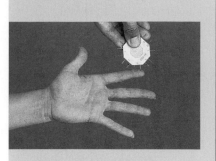

## Median, ulnar, and radial nerves

Assess median nerve sensation at the tip of the thumb, ulnar nerve sensation at the tip of the little finger, and radial nerve sensation at the dorsum of the thumb metacarpal. Check light touch and, for a more complete evaluation, assess two-point discrimination as follows.
Ask the patient to close both eyes as you lightly touch two points to the fingertip. (Apply just enough pressure to blanch the skin.) Determine whether the patient is able to distinguish the two points as separate points or perceives them as a single point. Two-point discrimination of 5 mm is generally considered to be normal. Inability to discriminate the two points indicates a sensory abnormality. The wider the distance required for the patient to discern two distinct points, the poorer the sensory discrimination.

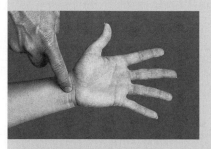

## Tinel sign

Lightly percuss the median nerve at the wrist flexion crease in line with the metacarpal of the long finger. Reproduction of paresthesias into the median nerve distribution is a positive Tinel sign.

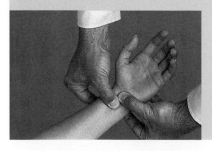

## Durkan carpal compression test

Compress the median nerve at the wrist. Reproduction of paresthesias or numbness into the median nerve distribution is a positive sign.

# SPECIAL TESTS

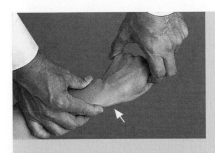

## *Finkelstein test—de Quervain tenosynovitis*

Have the patient make a fist with the thumb inside the fingers. Push the fist into ulnar deviation. Pain at the dorsoradial aspect of the wrist (arrow) indicates tenosynovitis of the first dorsal compartment (abductor pollicis longus and extensor brevis) tendons.

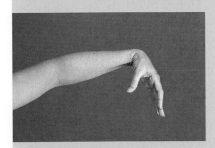

## *Phalen maneuver—Carpal tunnel syndrome*

Ask the seated patient to position the elbows in relaxed extension and then allow gravity flexion of the wrists. Numbness or tingling in the distribution of the median nerve within 60 seconds is a positive result.

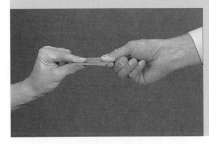

## *Froment sign*

Ask the patient to pinch a piece of paper between the thumb and index fingertip while you apply tension to the other end of the paper. If the adductor pollicis muscle is weak (ulnar nerve paralysis), the thumb IP joint will flex. (The figure shows normal muscle function.) Compare function with that of the opposite, normal thumb.

SECTION 4 ■ HAND AND WRIST

# THUMB CMC ARTHRITIS TESTS

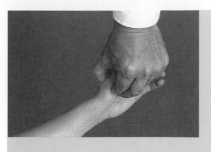

## Grind test

The grind test for thumb CMC arthritis is done as follows: With the patient's hand resting palm up on the examining surface and with the thumb in palmar abduction, grasp the metacarpal base and rotate the thumb CMC joint. This motion applied to the CMC joint is painful in patients with CMC arthritis.

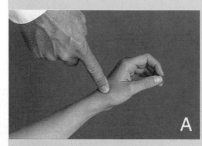

## CMC joint relocation test

In **A**, the examiner is pointing to the thumb CMC joint. In the CMC joint relocation test, the examiner places dorsal pressure on the thumb metacarpal (**B**), relocating the CMC joint. This is commonly painful in patients with CMC joint arthritis.

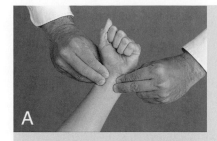

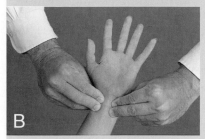

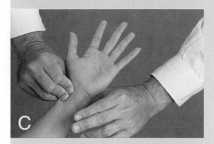

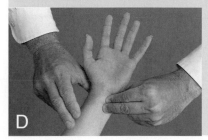

## *Allen test–Arterial circulation to the hand*

Ask the patient to open and close the hand three times, making a tight fist to exsanguinate the hand. Compress the radial and ulnar arteries at the wrist with the fingers clenched (**A**) and then ask the patient to open the fingers (**B**). Release the ulnar artery while keeping the radial artery compressed (**C**). If the fingers and palm fill with blood (typically within 5 seconds), the ulnar artery is patent. Repeat these steps keeping the ulnar artery compressed but releasing the radial artery (**D**). Note the time for refilling of the hand. Commonly, one artery is dominant in supplying circulation to the hand.

SECTION 4 ■ HAND AND WRIST

# ANIMAL BITES

**ICD-9 Codes**

**882.0**
Open wound of hand, except fingers, without mention of complications

**883.0**
Open wound of finger(s) without mention of complication

**883.1**
Open wound of finger(s), complicated

**E906.0**
Dog bite

**E906.3**
Bite of other animal except arthropod

## DEFINITION

As many as 3 million people in the United States sustain animal bites each year. Animal bites most commonly occur on the fingers of the dominant hand of children. Dog bites account for up to 90% of animal bites; cat bites are second most common, constituting 5% of animal bites.

The risk of infection from a dog bite is 5% to 10%; the risk of infection from a cat bite is much higher (30% to 50%) because a cat's sharp teeth create deeper puncture wounds that often seal quickly at the surface. The causative organism varies. *Pasteurella multocida* is a bacterium commonly associated with dog and cat bite wounds. Other bacteria isolated in dog bite wounds include α-hemolytic streptococci and *Staphylococcus aureus*, and anaerobic organisms such as *Bacteroides* and *Fusobacterium.*

Because rabies is a concern with animal bites, it is important to be familiar with the status of rabies in your area. In the United States, more than 90% of rabies comes from wild animals, especially bats, skunks, raccoons, and foxes. However, outside the United States, the dog is the most common vector for rabies transmission to humans. Approximately 50% of rabies cases reported to the Centers for Disease Control and Prevention in 1985 were from dog bites that occurred in countries other than the United States.

## CLINICAL SYMPTOMS

Pain, swelling, and redness around the puncture suggest an infection secondary to the bite. Loss of sensation and motion distal to the bite may indicate that a nerve or tendon is severed. Determine whether the bite was provoked by a sudden movement toward the animal because an animal that initiates an unprovoked attack is more likely to be rabid. The animal should be found, if possible, and observed for 10 days for signs of rabies. If necessary, consult with an infectious disease specialist regarding the risk of rabies.

## TESTS

### Physical Examination

Examination may reveal an irregular, jagged wound with devitalized tissue at the margins and swelling and redness around the wound. The depth and age of the wound should be determined. Purulent drainage may be present if the wound is more than 10 to 12 hours old. Sensation and tendon function should be tested in the affected hand or finger. Inspect the forearm for the presence of red streaks that indicate lymphangitis. The inner aspect of the elbow and the axilla should be palpated for the presence of enlarged lymph nodes. The patient's temperature should be checked.

### Diagnostic Tests

AP and lateral radiographs of the affected part are necessary to rule out a fracture or presence of a foreign body. These views also may reveal gas in the soft tissues. Routine laboratory studies are not needed for wounds seen shortly after injury. However, if an infection is suspected, a swab of the wound should be sent for a Gram stain and aerobic and anaerobic cultures.

## DIFFERENTIAL DIAGNOSIS

Foreign body with secondary infection (foreign body apparent on radiograph, ultrasound, or CT)

## ADVERSE OUTCOMES OF THE DISEASE

Any of the following conditions could develop as a result of an untreated animal bite: sepsis in the joint, deep space infection, septic tenosynovitis, osteomyelitis, and/or rabies. Patients also may lose sensation and motion, and possibly the affected fingers, following an animal bite. Chronic lymphedema with hand and finger stiffness is also possible.

## TREATMENT

Débridement, wound irrigation with 500 to 1,000 mL of saline solution or an antibiotic irrigation solution, and outpatient antibiotics are appropriate for superficial wounds that do not have a nerve, tendon, or bony injury. Use of an anesthetic block will facilitate débridement of bite wounds on the finger. When the bite wound is on the back of the hand, 3 to 10 mL of local anesthetic should be infiltrated around the wound. Oral amoxicillin-clavulanate, 875 mg twice a day for 5 days, is one standard antibiotic regimen for the treatment of early infection.

Primary suturing of animal bite wounds is controversial and can be hazardous. Some dog bite wounds may be sutured primarily as long as all necrotic tissue is débrided and the closure is loose over a Penrose drain. Because of the higher rate of infection associated with cat bites, these wounds should not be sutured. In general, it is safest to leave animal bites open.

SECTION 4 ■ HAND AND WRIST

## Table 1 Guide to Tetanus Prophylaxis in Wound Management

| History of Tetanus Toxoid (Doses) | Clean, Minor Wound | | Contaminated Wound | |
|---|---|---|---|---|
| | Td | TIG | Td | TIG |
| Unknown | Yes | No | Yes | Yes* |
| Fewer than 3 doses | Yes | No | Yes | Yes* |
| 3 or more | Yes, if more than 10 years since last dose | No | Yes, if more than 5 years since last dose | No |

Td = combined tetanus and diphtheria toxoid adsorbed (dose = 0.5 mL IM). TIG = tetanus immune globulin (dose = 250 IU IM).
*Td and TIG should be administered at different sites.
Adapted with permission from the Centers for Disease Control and Prevention.

When there is sign of active infection, closure should be delayed or the wound allowed to close by secondary intention. Intravenous antibiotics are indicated in this situation. Empiric therapy can be started with intravenous ampicillin-sulbactam, 1.5 to 3.0 g every 6 hours, pending culture results and sensitivities. Tetracycline can be used in patients with a penicillin allergy. Antibiotic therapy should be organism-specific whenever possible. The patient may be switched to oral antibiotics in 48 hours if the wound is healing satisfactorily. Tetanus prophylaxis should be given as outlined in **Table 1**.

If the animal is believed to be rabid, contact local or state public health officials regarding the need for rabies prophylaxis.

## Adverse Outcomes of Treatment

Infection secondary to primary wound closure can occur. Patients also may have allergic reactions to antibiotics.

## Referral Decisions/Red Flags

Any patient with an animal bite that involves the tendon, nerve, joint capsule, or an underlying fracture requires further evaluation.

# ARTHRITIS OF THE HAND

## SYNONYMS

Degenerative joint disease
Osteoarthritis
Rheumatoid arthritis

## DEFINITION

Osteoarthritis and secondary degenerative joint disease are the most common causes of arthritis of the hand and wrist. These conditions are characterized by progressive loss of articular cartilage, reactive bony changes at the joint margins, and subchondral cyst formation. The cause of primary osteoarthritis is unknown. Secondary osteoarthritis develops in joints affected by trauma, mechanical problems, or preexisting lesions.

Rheumatoid arthritis is a systemic condition that affects synovial tissue (**Figure 1**). All deformities, joint destruction, and pathologic anatomy that occur in patients with rheumatoid arthritis are a result of synovial hypertrophy and inflammation. The boggy synovium stretches the joint capsule and ligaments, causing deformity and joint instability. The articular cartilage also may be destroyed. Rheumatoid synovitis may also involve the tenosynovium and invade the flexor and extensor tendons, disrupting their motion and function.

SECTION 4 ■ HAND AND WRIST

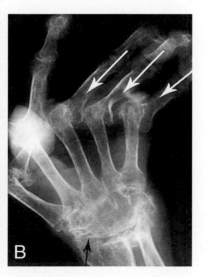

**Figure 1**
Advanced rheumatoid arthritis. **A,** Clinical appearance. Note the severe ulnar drift of the MP joint and limited finger extension. **B,** PA radiograph demonstrating the severe ulnar drift of the MP joints (white arrows) and the destruction of the wrist (black arrow).

## Clinical Symptoms

In osteoarthritis, the distal interphalangeal (DIP) and proximal interphalangeal (PIP) joints are most often involved. Patients report stiffness and loss of motion in the fingers. In rheumatoid arthritis, the wrist and metacarpophalangeal (MP) joints are most often involved. Extensor or flexor tenosynovitis (inflammation of the tendon sheath) also is common, resulting in pain that is caused by activation, whereas patients with osteoarthritis have more pain with joint palpation. Patients with rheumatoid arthritis have increased pain in the morning and after extended activities.

## Tests

### Physical Examination
Patients with rheumatoid arthritis involving the hands have fusiform swelling of multiple joints, with some joints swollen more than others. Rheumatoid arthritis commonly involves the MP joint and the wrist joint. A boggy mass over the dorsum of the hand and crepitus with movement is also common. Flexor tenosynovitis with crepitus at the wrist or in the fingers also is characteristic. Ulnar drift of the fingers may exist at the level of the MP joint. Other findings include contractures of the fingers at the PIP joints (boutonnière deformity) or hyperextension at the PIP joints with flexion at the DIP joints (swan-neck deformity).

Patients with osteoarthritis of the hand have bony nodules at the DIP joint (Heberden nodes). These nodules may be painful at first, but the pain usually resolves. Nodules also may occur at the PIP joints (Bouchard nodes). Involvement of the MP joints is much less common with osteoarthritis, and when it occurs at this location it is often the result of previous trauma.

### Diagnostic Tests
PA, oblique, and lateral views with the fingers positioned in different degrees of flexion, allowing each finger to be examined in detail, are necessary. When a single digit is involved, isolated PA and true lateral views of the digit also are appropriate. Serologic studies should be ordered for patients who have the characteristic changes of inflammatory arthritis but for whom the diagnosis has not been established.

## Differential Diagnosis

Pyogenic arthritis (may resemble the swollen joints of rheumatoid arthritis) (bacteria in joint aspirate, markedly elevated white blood cell count)

## ADVERSE OUTCOMES OF THE DISEASE

Rheumatoid arthritis can be slowly progressive, resulting in the typical rheumatoid hand deformity (Figure 1). Progressive osteoarthritis can cause joint destruction, particularly at the DIP, PIP, and wrist joints, with decreased mobility and function.

## TREATMENT

Rheumatoid arthritis has no cure. NSAIDs and other anti-inflammatory medications should be optimized. Newer medications such as etanercept (Enbrel) or infliximab (Remicade) may be more effective in limiting symptoms but may be associated with other medical complications. Cortisone injections can be extremely helpful for a severely inflamed joint or tendon sheath (see Metacarpophalangeal or Proximal Interphalangeal Joint Injection, pp 308-309). Nonsurgical treatment may include referral to an experienced occupational therapist to assist with splinting and the use of modalities. Occupational therapy and splinting can reduce deformity and limit symptoms but may not alter the natural history of the disease.

Treatment of osteoarthritis typically includes NSAIDs and, occasionally, temporary splinting of an involved joint for pain relief. Occupational therapy can be useful to facilitate hand splinting and the use of externally applied modalities such as home paraffin treatments and externally applied rub-in creams. Surgery for pain relief or stabilization may be necessary.

## ADVERSE OUTCOMES OF TREATMENT

NSAIDs may cause gastric, hepatic, and renal complications. Corticosteroids may adversely affect the immune system. Cortisone injections should be used very judiciously because tendon rupture may occur. Infection also is a risk but can be minimized by careful use of sterile technique.

## REFERRAL DECISIONS/RED FLAGS

When a cortisone injection for extensor tenosynovitis is not effective, surgery to excise the inflamed synovium can prevent rupture of the tendon. Patients who cannot extend their fingers, especially the little finger, ring finger, or the thumb, may have ruptured the extensor tendon, and further evaluation is needed immediately.

Patients with rheumatoid arthritis who report increasing deformity and increasing pain in the hand may need reconstructive surgery.

Further evaluation is needed for patients with osteoarthritis whose pain is no longer controlled with splinting and NSAIDs and who show radiographic evidence of joint destruction.

# PROCEDURE

# METACARPOPHALANGEAL OR PROXIMAL INTERPHALANGEAL JOINT INJECTION

## MATERIALS

Sterile gloves

Bactericidal skin preparation solution

Two 3-mL syringes with a 25-gauge needle

0.5 mL of a 1% local anesthetic solution without epinephrine

0.5 to 1 mL corticosteroid preparation

Adhesive dressing

**Note:** Opinions differ regarding single- versus two-needle injection techniques. Proponents of the single-needle technique believe that one needle is less painful for the patient than two. Because the corticosteroid preparation is thicker than the local anesthetic, however, a slightly larger gauge needle is required at the outset. A two-syringe, two-needle technique is described on the DVD.

Injections are performed on the extensor aspect of either the metacarpophalangeal (MP) or proximal interphalangeal (PIP) joint.

The entry site for the MP joint is the small sulcus just below the prominent metacarpal head that is most obvious with the finger flexed 20°. Identify this sulcus while moving the joint through a small amount of flexion and extension. Applying axial traction to the finger can facilitate the localization of the joint.

Identify the PIP joint in the same manner. Be aware, however, that the dorsal rim of the middle phalanx often is more easily palpated with this joint in extension.

### STEP 1

Wear protective gloves at all times during this procedure and use sterile technique.

### STEP 2

Cleanse the skin with a bactericidal skin preparation solution.

### STEP 3

Insert the 25-gauge needle at the joint level on the dorsolateral side of the joint (**Figure 1**). Inject 0.5 mL of a 1% local anesthetic preparation into the joint, change syringes, and then, with the new syringe, inject 0.5 to 1.0 mL of corticosteroid preparation. Slight pressure against the syringe plunger should make the joint bulge slightly on either side.

### STEP 4

Dress the puncture wound with a sterile adhesive bandage.

SECTION 4 ■ HAND AND WRIST

# METACARPOPHALANGEAL OR PROXIMAL INTERPHALANGEAL JOINT INJECTION (CONTINUED)

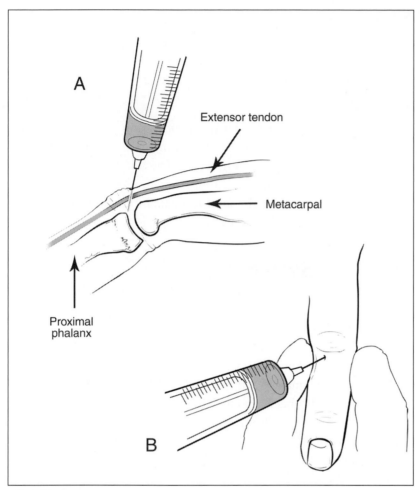

**Figure 1**
Location for needle insertion for MP joint injection (**A**) and PIP joint injection (**B**).

## ADVERSE OUTCOMES

Although rare, infection is possible. Subcutaneous fat atrophy may occur if the corticosteroid preparation is injected external to the joint. This may produce a depressed area of thin, tender, and unsightly skin. Some patients experience changes in skin pigmentation following injection. Occasionally, these changes in coloration of the skin are permanent.

## AFTERCARE/PATIENT INSTRUCTIONS

The joint might be sore for 24 to 48 hours after injection. Instruct the patient to return to your office if undue swelling, pain, or redness occurs.

# ARTHRITIS OF THE THUMB CARPOMETACARPAL JOINT

## ICD-9 Codes

**714.0**
Rheumatoid arthritis

**715.14**
Osteoarthritis, primary, localized to the hand

**715.24**
Osteoarthritis, secondary, localized to the hand

**715.94**
Osteoarthritis, unspecified, localized to the hand

**716.44**
Traumatic arthropathy of the hand

**716.94**
Arthropathy, unspecified, hand

## SYNONYMS

Carpometacarpal degenerative arthritis
Degenerative arthritis of the basal joint

## DEFINITION

Idiopathic degenerative arthritis of the thumb carpometacarpal (CMC) joint most commonly occurs in women between the ages of 40 and 70 years (**Figure 1**). The idiopathic variety is caused by anatomic factors (joint configuration and ligamentous laxity) that predispose the joint to instability, shear forces, and subsequent degenerative change.

## CLINICAL SYMPTOMS

The most common symptom is pain at the base of the thumb that occurs with grip and pinch activities. The pain may radiate proximally into the wrist and forearm. Decreased pinch strength is a common complaint. Patients also may note instability, "catching," or "clicking" with certain movements. Late manifestations include stiffness of the CMC joint in adduction with secondary metacarpophalangeal (MP) hyperextension.

Carpal tunnel syndrome may coexist with or mimic the symptoms of CMC arthritis.

## TESTS

### Physical Examination

The hallmark of this condition is tenderness over the palmar and radial aspects of the joint in the region of the base of the thumb. Manipulation of the CMC joint with simultaneous longitudinal loading (compression) causes pain and often some crepitus or instability. The grind test for thumb CMC arthritis readily reproduces the pain of CMC arthritis (see Physical Examination—Hand and Wrist, Grind test, p 300). With the palm facing up and the back of the hand resting on the table, the thumb is pushed down toward the table with the MP and PIP joints extended. The CMC joint relocation test, in which dorsal pressure is placed on the thumb metacarpal and the CMC joint is relocated by applying pressure in a palmar direction, is also useful in localizing the point of maximum discomfort (see Physical Examination—Hand and Wrist, CMC joint relocation test, p 300).

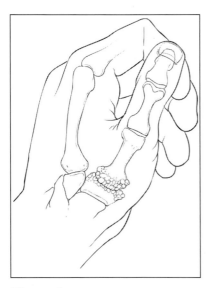

**Figure 1**
CMC arthritis of the thumb.

*Diagnostic Tests*

PA and lateral radiographs of the thumb show joint space narrowing, subchondral sclerosis, and varying degrees of subluxation or dislocation at the CMC joint (**Figure 2**).

# DIFFERENTIAL DIAGNOSIS

Arthritis of the wrist (evident on radiographs)

Carpal tunnel syndrome (positive Phalen maneuver, decreased sensation in median nerve distribution)

de Quervain tenosynovitis (positive Finkelstein test)

Flexor carpi radialis tendinitis (pain with resisted wrist flexion, swelling over flexor carpi radialis tendon)

Fracture of the scaphoid (tenderness over the anatomic snuffbox)

Scaphoid-trapezium-trapezoid arthritis (tenderness over the scaphoid-trapezium-trapezoid joint)

Volar radial ganglion (palpable mass over the palmar surface of the wrist)

# ADVERSE OUTCOMES OF THE DISEASE

Chronic pain, loss of pinch and grip strength, adduction contracture of the thumb (thumb held against the index finger), and chronic MP joint instability can occur.

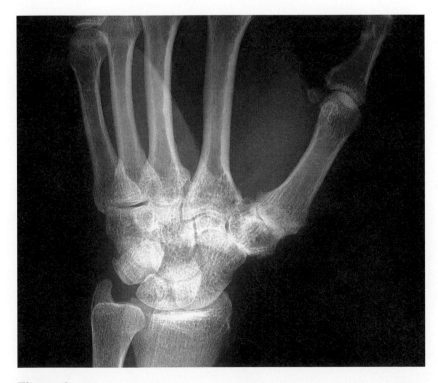

**Figure 2**
Radiographic appearance of CMC arthritis of the thumb.

SECTION 4 ■ HAND AND WRIST

# TREATMENT

Initial treatment should consist of placing the thumb in a thumb spica splint for 3 weeks, with NSAIDs for pain relief. If symptoms recur, intermittent splinting that immobilizes the entire thumb should be continued. If splinting fails, a corticosteroid preparation may be injected into the joint (see Thumb Carpometacarpal Joint Injection, pp 313-314). Although injections do not alter the natural history of the disease, many patients report pain relief that lasts a few months with each injection. At least three injections can be given. Occupational therapy consultation is appropriate to assist with splinting and the use of externally applied modalities such as ice, heat, or rub-in creams.

# ADVERSE OUTCOMES OF TREATMENT

NSAIDs can cause gastric, renal, or hepatic complications. Infection can develop after corticosteroid injection. Rapid progression of arthritis is possible as a result of multiple corticosteroid injections.

# REFERRAL DECISIONS/RED FLAGS

Failure of nonsurgical treatment indicates the need for further evaluation.

# PROCEDURE
## THUMB CARPOMETACARPAL JOINT INJECTION

VIDEO

**Note:** Opinions differ regarding single- and two-needle injection techniques. Proponents of the single-needle technique believe that one needle is less painful for the patient than two. Because the corticosteroid preparation is thicker than the local anesthetic, however, a slightly larger gauge needle is required at the outset.

### STEP 1
Wear protective gloves at all times during this procedure and use sterile technique.

### STEP 2
Before putting on the gloves, mark the level of the carpometacarpal (CMC) joint on the dorsum of the hand with your thumbnail by gently indenting the skin at the interval between the base of the thumb metacarpal and the trapezium.

### STEP 3
Cleanse the skin over the CMC joint at the marked site with a bactericidal skin preparation solution.

### STEP 4
Insert the 25-gauge needle, attached to the syringe with the anesthetic solution, at the mark on the back of the CMC joint. Inject 0.5 mL of the 1% anesthetic subcutaneously.

### STEP 5
Next, pull on the end of the thumb to open the joint space. Advance the needle into the joint and inject 0.5 to 1 mL of the anesthetic solution (**Figure 1**). If resistance is encountered, redirect the needle and reinsert. After the anesthetic solution is injected, leave the needle in place and change syringes.

### STEP 6
Inject 0.5 mL of the corticosteroid preparation through the same needle tract. The injection of fluid should meet little resistance if the needle is in the CMC joint.

### STEP 7
Dress the puncture wound with a sterile adhesive bandage.

**CPT Code**

**20600**
Arthrocentesis, aspiration and/or injection; small joint or bursa (eg, fingers, toes)

*Current Procedural Terminology* © 2004 American Medical Association. All Rights Reserved.

### MATERIALS

Sterile gloves

Bactericidal skin preparation solution

Two 3-mL syringes with a 25-gauge needle

0.5 mL corticosteroid preparation

2 mL of a 1% local anesthetic without epinephrine

Adhesive bandage

SECTION 4 ■ HAND AND WRIST

# THUMB CARPOMETACARPAL JOINT INJECTION (CONTINUED)

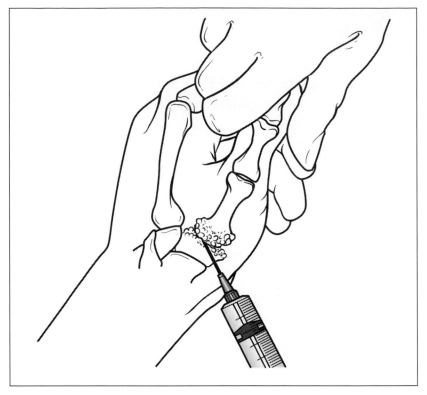

**Figure 1**
Injecting the CMC joint of the thumb.

## ADVERSE OUTCOMES

Depigmentation and/or fat atrophy at the site of injection, injury to sensory branches of the radial nerve, and joint space infection are possible.

## AFTERCARE/PATIENT INSTRUCTIONS

Advise the patient that 33% of patients may experience a flare of discomfort, manifested by increased joint pain, for 1 to 2 days. NSAIDs or an analgesic may be given to alleviate this pain. Ice also can be helpful during the first 24 hours to decrease the pain. Also, the patient can wear a thumb spica splint for 2 or 3 days after the injection. The patient should experience relief within 5 to 7 days after the injection.

# ARTHRITIS OF THE WRIST

## SYNONYM
Synovitis

## DEFINITION
Arthritis in the wrist is most commonly secondary to previous trauma (eg, fractures of the distal radius) or rheumatoid arthritis. Pseudogout and primary osteoarthritis may also affect the wrist.

## CLINICAL SYMPTOMS
Patients with rheumatoid arthritis typically report generalized swelling, tenderness, and limited motion. Hand function is often impaired by the synovitis and resultant instability of the carpal bones. The result is radial deviation of the wrist, ulnar deviation of the fingers, inefficient wrist and finger tendon function, decreased grip strength, and pain with daily activities.

Degenerative arthritis of the wrist is associated with swelling, pain, and limited motion of the wrist.

## TESTS

### Physical Examination
Examination reveals swelling, increased warmth, and limited motion and pain to palpation of the radiocarpal joint. Patients with rheumatoid arthritis often have associated involvement of the MP joints and deformity at the wrist and fingers. The ulna may appear prominent (caput ulnae).

In posttraumatic degenerative arthritis, the finger joints usually appear normal.

### Diagnostic Tests
PA and lateral radiographs are helpful in distinguishing the various types of arthritis. Generalized thinning of bone structure (osteopenia) with erosions in the area of the joint surface is characteristic of rheumatoid arthritis. Subchondral sclerosis, joint space narrowing, spur formation, and, in some cases, erosion characterize primary or secondary osteoarthritis (**Figure 1**). Early calcification of the triangular fibrocartilage complex may indicate pseudogout, which can be confirmed by the presence of calcium pyrophosphate crystals in synovial fluid aspirate.

### ICD-9 Codes
**712.23**
Pseudogout of the wrist

**714.0**
Rheumatoid arthritis

**715.13**
Osteoarthritis of the wrist, primary

**715.23**
Osteoarthritis of the wrist, secondary

**715.93**
Osteoarthritis of the wrist, unspecified

**716.13**
Traumatic arthropathy of the wrist

SECTION 4 ■ HAND AND WRIST

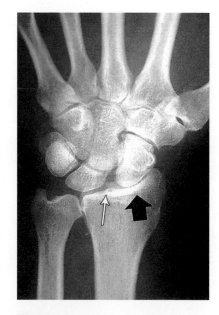

**Figure 1**
PA radiograph showing osteoarthritis of the wrist. Note the subchondral sclerosis of the radius and the loss of radiocarpal joint space (black arrow). The scapholunate interval is also widened (white arrow).

Laboratory studies, including erythrocyte sedimentation rate and tests for rheumatoid factor, antinuclear antibodies, and uric acid, may help confirm the diagnosis.

## DIFFERENTIAL DIAGNOSIS

Septic arthritis of the wrist (acute onset, severe pain and restriction of wrist motion, systemic signs of infection)

Tenosynovitis (normal radiographs, swelling over the involved tendon)

## ADVERSE OUTCOMES OF THE DISEASE

Pain, loss of motion and/or strength, and impaired function in the wrist and fingers are possible.

## TREATMENT

Medical management depends on the type of arthritis present. Temporary immobilization in a splint can help relieve pain and swelling. In the absence of infection, injection of a corticosteroid may provide temporary pain relief (see Wrist Aspiration/Injection, p 317). Surgery usually is necessary when hand function decreases, when the joint becomes unstable, or when nonsurgical treatment fails to relieve pain. Surgical treatment usually focuses on improving stability and limiting discomfort.

## ADVERSE OUTCOMES OF TREATMENT

Loss of motion and persistent pain can develop. NSAIDs can cause gastric, renal, or hepatic complications.

## REFERRAL DECISIONS/RED FLAGS

Patients with a possible wrist infection require immediate evaluation. Those with radiographic evidence of advanced disease from degenerative or rheumatoid arthritis and those who do not respond to splinting and NSAIDs also are candidates for further evaluation.

# PROCEDURE

## WRIST ASPIRATION/INJECTION

### STEP 1

Wear protective gloves at all times during this procedure and use sterile technique.

### STEP 2

Cleanse the area with a bactericidal skin preparation solution.

### STEP 3

Palpate the distal edge of the radius between the extensor carpi radialis brevis and extensor digitorum communis tendons. The depression just distal to the distal edge of the radius indicates the radiocarpal joint.

### STEP 4

Inject 1% local anesthetic in the subcutaneous tissue and joint capsule with the 25-gauge needle and then remove the needle.

### STEP 5

Insert the 22-gauge needle into the same site to aspirate the joint fluid. The joint fluid should be submitted for crystal analysis, cell count, smear Gram stain, and culture.

### STEP 6

If infection is not apparent, change the syringe and inject 0.5 to 1 mL of the corticosteroid preparation. The corticosteroid preparation may be mixed with an equal amount of 2% local anesthetic for pain relief.

### STEP 7

Dress the puncture wound with a sterile adhesive bandage.

## MATERIALS

Sterile gloves

Bactericidal skin preparation solution

3-mL syringe with a 25-gauge needle

3-mL syringe with a 22-gauge needle

1-mL syringe

0.5 to 1 mL of 1% local anesthetic without epinephrine

0.5 to 1 mL corticosteroid preparation (optional)

## ADVERSE OUTCOMES

Infection is possible. The infection may progress because corticosteroids can mask the usual signs of infection.

## AFTERCARE/PATIENT INSTRUCTIONS

Instruct the patient to watch for signs of infection, such as increasing pain, swelling, heat, or redness, and to call your office if any of these signs occur.

**SECTION 4 ■ HAND AND WRIST**

# BOUTONNIÈRE DEFORMITY

**ICD-9 Code**
**736.21**
Boutonnière deformity

## SYNONYMS
Central slip extensor tendon injury
Jammed finger

## DEFINITION
Boutonnière deformity is caused by a rupture of the central portion of the extensor tendon at its insertion onto the middle phalanx (**Figure 1**). The proximal interphalangeal (PIP) joint flexes from the unopposed pull of the flexor tendon. The head of the proximal phalanx "buttonholes" between the lateral bands of the extensor tendon mechanism. As a result, the lateral bands are displaced below the axis of rotation of the PIP joint, causing it to flex further. More distally, the lateral bands are displaced dorsal to the axis of the distal interphalangeal (DIP) joint, causing it to extend or hyperextend.

## CLINICAL SYMPTOMS
Patients typically report a history of trauma. The finger is held partially flexed at the PIP joint and extended or hyperextended at the DIP joint. With a recent injury, the PIP joint is painful and tender. Initially, the boutonnière deformity may not be apparent, but can develop over 7 to 21 days as the intact lateral bands of the extensor tendon slip inferiorly.

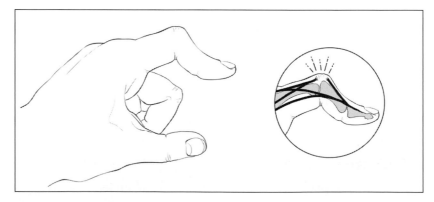

**Figure 1**
Boutonnière deformity.
Adapted with permission from Steinberg GG, Akins CM, Baran DT: *Ramamurti's Orthopaedics in Primary Care,* ed 2. Philadelphia, PA, Williams & Wilkins, 1992, p 112.

# TESTS

## Physical Examination

Ask the patient to extend the injured finger and observe the position of the PIP and DIP joints. The PIP joint will be flexed more than 30° and the DIP joint will be extended or hyperextended. To demonstrate less severe deformities, hold the metacarpophalangeal and wrist joints in flexion and ask the patient to extend the PIP joint. Patients who lack 15° to 20° of extension at the PIP joint probably have a rupture of the central slip of the extensor tendon.

## Diagnostic Tests

AP and lateral radiographs will rule out a fracture or a pseudo-boutonnière deformity, in which the PIP joint is fixed in flexion and radiographs show calcification at the lateral aspect of the PIP joint.

# DIFFERENTIAL DIAGNOSIS

Dislocation of the PIP joint (painful, locked joint following surgery)

Fracture around the PIP joint (radiographs required to confirm)

Pseudo-boutonnière deformity (PIP joint fixed in flexion, radiographs show calcification at the lateral aspect of the PIP joint)

Rupture of the flexor tendon sheath (annular pulley) (painful flexor tendon sheath following injury)

Sprain of the PIP joint (may be difficult to differentiate on initial examination; sprains have isolated collateral ligament tenderness and/or instability)

# ADVERSE OUTCOMES OF THE DISEASE

Flexion contracture of the PIP joint and extension contracture of the DIP joint are both possible.

# TREATMENT

Nonsurgical treatment is usually preferable. The PIP joint should be splinted in extension for 6 weeks in a young patient and for 3 weeks in an elderly patient (**Figure 2**). The DIP joint is left free. Active and passive motion should be initiated at the DIP joint.

If the injury is more than 1 or 2 weeks old at presentation, it may not be possible to achieve full extension at the first visit. Use of a dynamic extension splint (Figure 2, C) until full extension is achieved is required, followed by a static splinting program. Surgical treatment is occasionally necessary if the deformity does not correct with splinting.

SECTION 4 ■ HAND AND WRIST

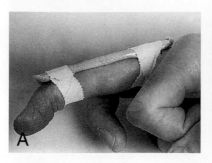 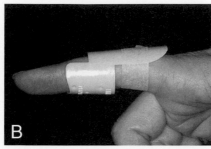 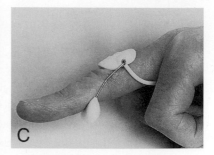

**Figure 2**

Static extension splint **(A),** a commercial static splint **(B),** and a dynamic extension splint **(C)** for the PIP joint.

Reproduced from Culver JE: Office management of athletic injuries of the hand and wrist. *Instr Course Lect* 1989;38:473-486.

## ADVERSE OUTCOMES OF TREATMENT

Failure to achieve full extension, residual PIP flexion deformity, or both are possible.

## REFERRAL DECISIONS/RED FLAGS

Failure to achieve full extension, residual deformity, or both are indications for further evaluation.

SECTION 4 ■ HAND AND WRIST

# CARPAL TUNNEL SYNDROME

## SYNONYMS

Median nerve compression
Median nerve entrapment at the wrist

ICD-9 Code

**354.0**
Carpal tunnel syndrome

## DEFINITION

Carpal tunnel syndrome (entrapment of the median nerve at the wrist) is the most common compression neuropathy in the upper extremity. It most commonly affects middle-aged or pregnant women.

   Any condition that reduces the size or space of the carpal tunnel can cause compression of the median nerve, resulting in paresthesias, pain, and sometimes paralysis (**Figure 1**). Common precipitating conditions include tenosynovitis of the adjacent flexor tendons (repetitive overuse trauma or rheumatoid arthritis), tumors, and medical conditions such as pregnancy, diabetes mellitus, and thyroid dysfunction.

## CLINICAL SYMPTOMS

Patients typically report a vague aching that radiates into the thenar area. Aching also may be perceived in the proximal forearm, and occasionally the pain can extend to the shoulder.

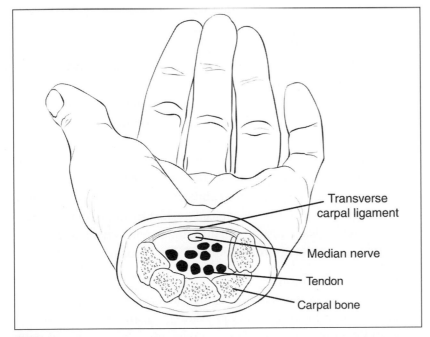

**Figure 1**
Cross-section of the carpal tunnel.

Adapted from Szabo RM, Steinberg DR: Nerve entrapment syndromes in the wrist. *J Am Acad Orthop Surg* 1994;2:116.

SECTION 4 ■ HAND AND WRIST

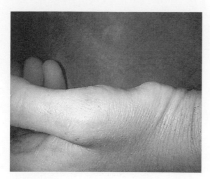

**Figure 2**
Thenar atrophy.

The pain is typically accompanied by paresthesias or numbness in the median distribution (thumb and index finger, long finger, and radial half of the ring finger, or some combination thereof). Often the symptoms are worse at night.

Patients report that they frequently drop objects, or that they cannot open jars or twist off lids. Pain or numbness sometimes is made worse by activities that require repetitive motion of the hand, repetitive activities, or stationary tasks done with the wrist held flexed or extended for long periods, such as when driving or reading. Patients often awaken at night with pain or numbness and typically report the need to rub or shake the hand to "get the circulation back." When the compression is severe and long-standing, persistent numbness and thenar atrophy can occur (**Figure 2**).

# TESTS

## Physical Examination

Inspect the hand for thenar atrophy. Testing thumb opposition against resistance may reveal weakness of the thenar muscles (see Physical Examination—Hand and Wrist, Special Tests: Thumb abduction strength, p 297). Evaluate the sensation in the fingers.

The Phalen maneuver is the most useful clinical test and is performed by placing the wrists in flexion (see Physical Examination—Hand and Wrist, Special Tests: Phalen maneuver, p 299). Avoid excessive elbow flexion when performing this test. Aching and numbness in the distribution of the median nerve within 60 seconds (often within 15 seconds or less) is a positive test for carpal tunnel syndrome. Tapping over the median nerve at the wrist may produce tingling in some or all of the digits in the median nerve distribution (see Physical Examination—Hand and Wrist, Special Tests: Tinel sign, p 298). Thumb pressure (see Physical Examination—Hand and Wrist, Special Tests: Durkan carpal compression test, p 298) over the median nerve at the wrist for up to 30 seconds may elicit pain or paresthesias in the median distribution.

Patients with carpal tunnel syndrome may be unable to distinguish the two points of a caliper as separate points when they are closer than 5 mm together (see Physical Examination—Hand and Wrist, Sensory Testing: Median, ulnar, and radial nerves, p 298). Two-point discrimination of 5 mm is considered normal.

## Diagnostic Tests

Radiographs of the wrist should be obtained if the patient has limited wrist motion. Electrophysiologic testing is the most useful confirmatory test. These studies must be interpreted with caution, however. Some patients have no clinical signs or symptoms yet have abnormal nerve conduction velocity studies.

Conversely, as many as 5% to 10% of patients with carpal tunnel syndrome have normal results. In general, the diagnosis of carpal tunnel syndrome is made based on history and physical examination, with electrophysiologic tests used to confirm the diagnosis.

## Differential Diagnosis
Arthritis of the carpometacarpal joint of the thumb (painful motion)

Cervical radiculopathy affecting C6 nerve (neck pain, numbness in the thumb and index fingers only)

Diabetes mellitus with neuropathy (history)

Flexor carpi radialis tenosynovitis (tenderness near the base of the thumb)

Hypothyroidism (abnormal results on thyroid function tests)

Median nerve compression at the elbow (tenderness at the proximal forearm)

Ulnar neuropathy (first dorsal interosseous weakness, numbness of the ring and little fingers)

Volar radial ganglion (mass near the base of the thumb above the wrist flexion crease)

Wrist arthritis (limited motion, evident on radiographs)

## Adverse Outcomes of the Disease
Permanent loss of sensation, hand strength, and fine motor skills are possible.

## Treatment
For mild cases, splinting the wrist (in a neutral position wrist splint) and a short-term course of NSAIDs are suggested. The splint should be worn at night (at a minimum) and can be worn during the day if doing so does not interfere with the patient's work or daily activities. If these measures fail, consider injecting a corticosteroid into the carpal canal (see Carpal Tunnel Injection, pp 326-327). Injection has diagnostic as well as therapeutic benefits, but improvement may be only temporary. Care must be taken to avoid direct injection into the median nerve, which may cause severe pain.

Work-related carpal tunnel syndrome may be improved with ergonomic modifications, such as using keyboard or forearm supports, adjusting the height of computer keyboards, and avoiding holding the wrist in a flexed position (as with dental hygienists).

Carpal tunnel syndrome that occurs during pregnancy usually resolves when the pregnancy terminates; therefore, treatment should consist of splinting and other nonsurgical measures, such as injection of corticosteroid.

Surgical management is often necessary for patients who have fixed sensory loss or weakness of the thenar muscles and for those who have intolerable symptoms despite a course of nonsurgical treatment.

## Physical Therapy Prescription

The purpose of nonsurgical management of carpal tunnel syndrome is to reduce compressive forces on the median nerve, to decrease demands on the wrist and hand, and to reduce inflammation and fibrosis. In the early stages, the use of a night splint with the wrist in neutral position (0° of extension) is advocated. The wrist splint is worn for 3 to 4 weeks, during the day as well as at night. To reduce inflammation and pain, ice is used in the early stages. Heat is used to increase circulation and to promote tendon gliding. Exercises to promote tendon gliding are very important in the early stages of treatment (see p 325).

If the symptoms do not respond to the home program, the patient should be referred to a certified hand therapist. The therapist should evaluate range of motion, muscle strength, and sensory changes to determine the next stage of treatment. Strengthening exercises, continued use of a night splint, and ergonomic evaluation of the patient's job station should be part of the management of this condition.

## Adverse Outcomes of Treatment

NSAIDs can cause gastric, renal, or hepatic complications. Fluid retention, flushing of the skin, and shakiness can result from taking oral corticosteroids. Injecting corticosteroids is associated with the risk of an intraneural injection, which can have long-term adverse consequences. Prolonged nonsurgical treatment in patients with persistent sensory loss or motor weakness can result in loss of sensation and thenar atrophy.

## Referral Decisions/Red Flags

Failure of nonsurgical treatment after 3 months warrants further evaluation. Persistent numbness, weakness, atrophy of the thenar muscles, or any combination of these are indications for further evaluation.

# HOME PHYSICAL THERAPY PROGRAM FOR CARPAL TUNNEL SYNDROME

Apply heat to the hand for 15 minutes before performing the exercises, and apply ice (a bag of crushed ice or frozen peas) to the hand for 20 minutes after each exercise session to prevent inflammation. If numbness steadily worsens, if the exercises increase the pain, or if the pain does not improve after you have performed the exercises for 3 to 4 weeks, call your doctor.

| Exercise Type | Targeted Structure | Number of Repetitions/Sets | Number of Days per Week | Number of Weeks |
|---|---|---|---|---|
| Nerve gliding | Median nerve | 10 to 15 repetitions | 6 to 7 | 3 to 4 |

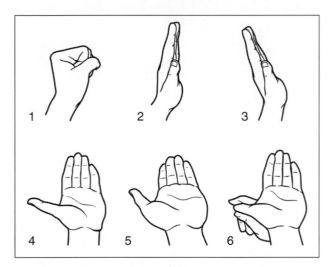

(Adapted with permission from Donatelli R, Wooden M (eds): *Orthopaedic Physical Therapy*. Philadelphia, PA, Elsevier.)

## Nerve Gliding

Begin with the affected hand raised. (1) Make a fist, with the thumb outside the fingers. (2) Extend the fingers, keeping the thumb close to the side of the hand. (3) Extend the hand at the wrist (bend it backward, toward the forearm), keeping the fingers straight. (4) With the wrist straight, extend the thumb as shown. (5) Keeping the thumb extended, extend the hand at the wrist. (6) Reach behind your hand and grasp the thumb with the thumb and forefinger of the opposite hand. Pull the thumb downward, away from the palm of your hand.

SECTION 4 ■ HAND AND WRIST

# PROCEDURE

# CARPAL TUNNEL INJECTION

## CPT Code

**20526**

Injection, therapeutic (eg, local anesthetic, corticosteroid), carpal tunnel

*Current Procedural Terminology* © 2004 American Medical Association. All Rights Reserved.

## MATERIALS

Sterile gloves

Bactericidal skin preparation solution

Two 3-mL syringes with a 25-gauge needle

2 to 5 mL of a 1% local anesthetic without epinephrine

1 to 2 mL of a corticosteroid preparation

Adhesive bandage

**Note:** Opinions differ regarding single- and two-needle injection techniques. Proponents of the single-needle technique believe that one needle is less painful for the patient than two. Because the corticosteroid preparation is thicker than the local anesthetic, however, a slightly larger gauge needle is required at the outset.

### STEP 1

Wear protective gloves at all times during this procedure and use sterile technique.

### STEP 2

Cleanse the volar aspect of the wrist with a bactericidal skin preparation solution.

### STEP 3

Insert the needle 1 cm proximal to the wrist flexion crease and in line with the ring finger metacarpal. Direct the needle toward the hand at an angle of 30° to 45° (**Figure 1**). Have the patient flex the fingers fully into the palm, then advance the needle approximately 1 to 1.5 cm until resistance is felt. If the patient reports paresthesias, redirect the needle.

### STEP 4

Instruct the patient to slightly wiggle the tips of the ring and little fingers. If this causes slight movement of the tip of the needle, the needle is safely positioned.

### STEP 5

Ask the patient to extend the fingers as gentle pressure is applied to the syringe. The distal excursion of the flexor tendons of the ring and little fingers will carry the point of the needle into the carpal canal.

### STEP 6

If the patient reports any tingling, the needle has entered the nerve. If this occurs, do not continue with the injection. Otherwise, inject 1 to 2 mL of local anesthetic into the carpal canal. If resistance is encountered on attempting to inject the local anesthetic, the tip of the needle is embedded in the flexor tendons. Maintain some pressure on the syringe while slowly withdrawing the needle, until the anesthetic flows freely. Leave the needle in place and change syringes. Inject 1 to 2 mL of corticosteroid into the carpal canal, and then remove the needle.

### STEP 7

Dress the puncture wound with a sterile adhesive bandage.

SECTION 4 ■ HAND AND WRIST

# CARPAL TUNNEL INJECTION (CONTINUED)

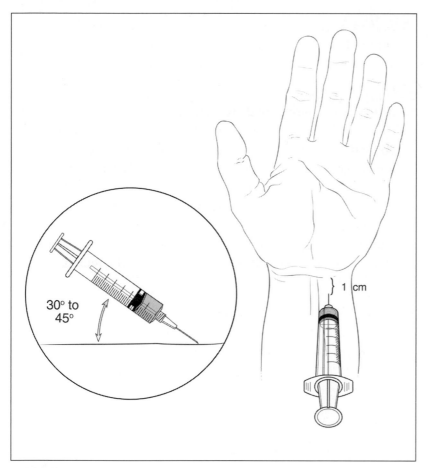

**Figure 1**
Location for needle insertion.

## ADVERSE OUTCOMES

Infection or intraneural injection is possible.

## AFTERCARE/PATIENT INSTRUCTIONS

Advise the patient that occasional mild soreness may develop, that the hand and fingers may be numb for 1 to 2 hours following the injection, and that the injection could require 24 to 48 hours to take effect.

# DE QUERVAIN TENOSYNOVITIS

**ICD-9 Code**

**727.04**
de Quervain tenosynovitis

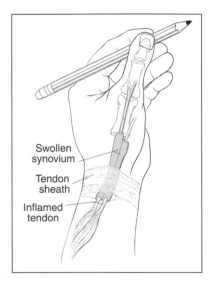

**Figure 1**
de Quervain tenosynovitis of the
first extensor compartment.

*Labels in figure:*
Swollen synovium
Tendon sheath
Inflamed tendon

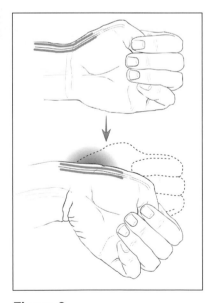

**Figure 2**
Finkelstein test. Arrow indicates
location of pain when test is
positive.

**Adapted with permission from the American
Society for Surgery of the Hand: Brochure: de
Quervain's Stenosing Tenosynovitis. Engelwood,
CO, 1995.**

## SYNONYM
Stenosing tenosynovitis

## DEFINITION
de Quervain tenosynovitis is swelling or stenosis of the sheath
that surrounds the abductor pollicus longus and extensor
pollicus brevis tendons at the wrist (**Figure 1**). The
inflammation thickens the tendon sheath (tenosynovium) and
constricts the tendon as it glides in the sheath. This can cause
pain, swelling, and a triggering phenomenon, resulting in
locking or sticking of the tendon as the patient moves the
thumb. The disorder is more common in middle-aged women
and is often precipitated by repetitive use of the thumb.

## CLINICAL SYMPTOMS
Patients report swelling over the radial styloid and pain that is
aggravated by attempts to move the thumb or make a fist. They
also may notice creaking as the tendon moves.

## TESTS

### Physical Examination
Examination reveals swelling and tenderness over the tendons
of the first dorsal compartment in the region of the distal
radius. Crepitus may be palpable as the patient flexes and
extends the thumb. Full flexion of the thumb into the palm,
followed by ulnar deviation of the wrist (Finkelstein test;
**Figure 2** and p 299), will produce pain and is diagnostic for
de Quervain tenosynovitis.

### Diagnostic Tests
Even though this is largely a clinical diagnosis, PA and lateral
radiographs of the wrist should be considered to rule out any
bony abnormality, such as a deformed radial styloid process
resulting from trauma, that might be a precipitating cause.
Calcification associated with tendinitis occasionally can be seen
on radiographs.

# DIFFERENTIAL DIAGNOSIS

Carpometacarpal arthritis of the thumb (swelling over the joint, pain with joint compression)

Dorsal wrist ganglion (palpable mass)

Flexor carpi radialis tendinitis (pain and swelling over the tendon)

Fracture of the scaphoid (tenderness over the anatomic snuffbox)

Intersection syndrome

Superficial radial neuritis

Wrist arthritis (pain with movement, evident on radiographs)

# ADVERSE OUTCOMES OF THE DISEASE

Chronic pain, loss of strength, and loss of thumb motion can occur; tendon rupture is possible but is rare.

# TREATMENT

Initial treatment should consist of a thumb spica splint that immobilizes both the wrist and thumb as well as a 2-week course of NSAIDs. If this initial treatment fails, the tendon sheath may be injected with a corticosteroid preparation, taking care not to inject the steroid into the tendon (see de Quervain Tenosynovitis Injection, p 330). After injection, immobilize the thumb in a long opponens splint for 48 hours. The patient should have no more than three injections.

Surgical treatment should be considered if corticosteroid injections are not successful.

# ADVERSE OUTCOMES OF TREATMENT

NSAIDs may cause gastric, renal, or hepatic complications. The patient may experience some discomfort from wearing the splint and will stop using it. Corticosteroids can sometimes cause subcutaneous atrophy and unslightly loss of pigmentation. Infection after corticosteroid injection also is a risk but largely can be avoided by careful use of sterile technique. Injury to the radial sensory nerve or incomplete release is possible with surgical treatment.

# REFERRAL DECISIONS/RED FLAGS

Failure to respond to splinting and corticosteroid injections indicates the need for further evaluation.

SECTION 4 ■ HAND AND WRIST

# PROCEDURE

## DE QUERVAIN TENOSYNOVITIS INJECTION

**CPT Code**

**20500**

Injection(s); single tendon sheath, or ligament, aponeurosis (eg, plantar "fascia")

*Current Procedural Terminology* © 2004 American Medical Association. All Rights Reserved.

### MATERIALS

Sterile gloves

Bactericidal skin preparation solution

Two 3-mL syringes with a 27-gauge, 7/8″ needle

2 mL of corticosteroid preparation

2 mL of a 1% local anesthetic without epinephrine

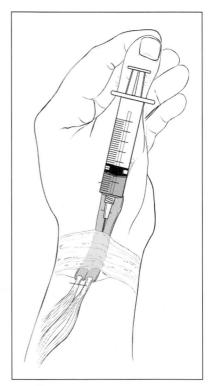

**Figure 1**

Location for needle insertion for de Quervain injection.

**Note:** Opinions differ regarding single- and two-needle injection techniques. Proponents of the single-needle technique believe that one needle is less painful for the patient than two. Because the corticosteroid preparation is thicker than the local anesthetic, however, a slightly larger gauge needle is required at the outset.

### STEP 1

Wear protective gloves at all times during this procedure and use sterile technique.

### STEP 2

Cleanse the skin with a bactericidal skin preparation solution.

### STEP 3

Insert the 27-gauge needle at a 45° angle to the skin in line with the two tendons (**Figure 1**). If the patient reports paresthesia into the thumb, the needle has depolarized the sensory branch of the radial nerve. Reposition the needle 2 to 3 mm dorsal or volar, to a position that does not cause paresthesia.

### STEP 4

Create a skin wheal with 0.5 mL of 1% local anesthetic and advance the needle until it strikes one of the underlying tendons. Inject the remaining anesthetic while slowly withdrawing the needle, until the anesthetic flows freely. Leave the needle in place and change syringes.

### STEP 5

Inject 2 mL of corticosteroid preparation into the tendon sheath. Palpation of the tendon sheath proximal to the point of injection should reveal swelling as the corticosteroid is injected.

### STEP 6

Dress the puncture wound with a sterile adhesive bandage.

## ADVERSE OUTCOMES

Subcutaneous fat atrophy can follow subcutaneous infiltration of the corticosteroid preparation, leading to a waxy-appearing depression in the skin. In addition, although rare, infection is possible.

## AFTERCARE/PATIENT INSTRUCTIONS

Increased pain is not uncommon after the injection, especially in the first 24 to 48 hours. At least one third of patients will experience increased discomfort during this time.

# DUPUYTREN DISEASE

## SYNONYMS

Palmar fibromatosis
Viking disease

ICD-9 Code
728.6
Dupuytren contracture

## DEFINITION

Dupuytren disease is a nodular thickening and contraction of the palmar fascia (**Figure 1**). The disease has a dominant genetic component, particularly involving people of northern European descent (hence the name Viking disease). Dupuytren disease most commonly affects men older than 50 years. Associated factors include epilepsy, diabetes mellitus, pulmonary disease, alcoholism, smoking, and repetitive trauma (vibrational).

## CLINICAL SYMPTOMS

Patients initially notice one or more painless nodules near the distal palmar crease that are moderately sensitive to pressure. The nodule or nodules may gradually thicken and contract, causing the finger to flex at the metacarpophalangeal (MP) joint and, occasionally as the disease progresses, the proximal interphalangeal (PIP) joint. The ring finger is most commonly involved, followed by the little, long, thumb, and index fingers. Although extension is limited, finger flexion is often normal. The condition is usually painless in its later stages, but as the contractures increase, patients have trouble grasping objects, pulling on gloves, and putting the hand into a pocket. Sensation in the affected fingers usually is normal unless the patient has concomitant carpal tunnel syndrome.

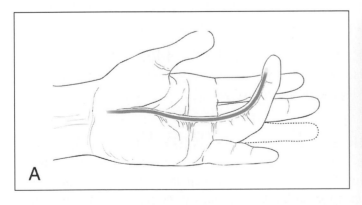
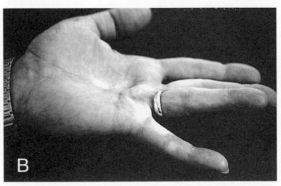

**Figure 1**
Dupuytren contracture of the ring finger. **A,** Drawing showing affected palmar fascial cord. **B,** Clinical appearance.
**Adapted with permission from the American Society for Surgery of the Hand: Brochure: *Dupuytren's Disease*. Englewood, CO, 1995.**

SECTION 4 ■ HAND AND WRIST

# TESTS

## *Physical Examination*

Examination reveals a palmar skin nodule that in the early stages may resemble a callus. As the disease progresses, the abnormal cords extend distally and sometimes proximally to the nodule. These bands may cross the PIP joint and commonly cross the MP joint, holding the finger in a contracted position. The bands are seldom tender unless the patient is in the early stages of the disease.

## *Diagnostic Tests*

Diagnosis is made upon clinical examination. Radiographs are not needed.

# DIFFERENTIAL DIAGNOSIS

Flexion contracture secondary to joint or tendon injury (no cords or bands)

Locked trigger finger (no associated nodules)

# ADVERSE OUTCOMES OF THE DISEASE

Progressive flexion contracture of the fingers and limited function are possible.

# TREATMENT

Splinting or other nonsurgical treatment is not curative, but night splints may slow the progression of the contractures. Surgery involves excising the thick soft-tissue bands and release of the joint contractures. Surgery is considered when there is a 30° fixed flexion deformity of the MP joint or a 10° deformity of the PIP joint. More severe contractures are more difficult to correct, have a higher incidence of recurrent contracture, and require a longer course of postoperative occupational therapy.

# ADVERSE OUTCOMES OF TREATMENT

Patients may experience nerve injury, skin loss, and recurrence of the disease postoperatively.

# REFERRAL DECISIONS/RED FLAGS

Patients with significant contractures (greater than 30°) of the MP joints who are troubled by their lack of extension are candidates for further evaluation. Likewise, patients with involvement of the PIP joint in association with Dupuytren disease require close follow-up.

# FINGERTIP INFECTIONS

## SYNONYMS
Felon
Paronychia

## DEFINITION

Infections of the fingertip typically occur in two locations: in the pulp or palmar tip of the finger (felon) and in the soft tissues directly surrounding the fingernail (paronychia). *Staphylococcus aureus* is the most common causative organism in both conditions.

Felons usually are caused by a puncture wound and most commonly occur in the thumb and index finger (**Figure 1**). Herpetic whitlow, a virally mediated hand infection that is characterized by the formation of vesicles filled with clear fluid, can also occur in and around the fingertip (**Figure 2**). Differentiating a felon from herpetic whitlow is important, as incision and drainage of a felon usually is indicated, whereas incision of a whitlow is contraindicated and observation is sufficient. Health care workers who are frequently exposed to the herpes simplex virus from human saliva (eg, respiratory therapists, dental hygienists) are at increased risk for herpetic whitlow. Paronychial infections often occur after a manicure or the development of a nail deformity, such as a hangnail or an ingrown nail.

## CLINICAL SYMPTOMS

A felon is characterized by severe pain and swelling in the pad of the fingertip. With a felon, the entire pulp of the fingertip is swollen, tense, red, and very tender. Also, a puncture wound may be visible.

Paronychial infection is characterized by swelling of the tissues about the fingernail, usually along one side and about the base of the nail. Occasionally, the swelling extends completely around the nail and is then referred to as a "runaround abscess." The pain associated with a paronychia is not as intense as that with a felon.

Swelling associated with a felon or paronychia should not extend proximal to the distal flexion crease. Any such extension suggests a deeper, more complex process, such as an infection in the flexor tendon sheath. Significantly increased pain with passive motion also may indicate flexor tendon sheath infection.

**ICD-9 Codes**
**054.6**
Herpetic whitlow
**681.01**
Felon
**681.02**
Paronychia of finger

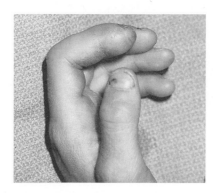

**Figure 1**
Felon of the index finger.
Reproduced from Stern PJ: Selected acute infections. *Instr Course Lect* 1990;39:539-546.

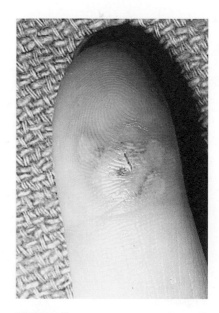

**Figure 2**
Herpetic whitlow.
Reproduced from Stern PJ: Selected acute infections. *Instr Course Lect* 1990;39:539-546.

SECTION 4 ■ HAND AND WRIST

# TESTS

## Physical Examination

The fingertip should be examined for the location and extent of the swelling. The presence of small vesicles suggests herpetic whitlow. Tenderness, redness and fluctuance are more characteristic of a bacterial abscess (paronychia or felon).

## Diagnostic Tests

Plain radiographs show soft-tissue swelling. Late in the course of infection, osteomyelitis of the distal phalanx may occur and is evident on radiographs as partial or complete resorption of the distal tuft of the phalanx. More aggressive surgical débridement is required in these cases.

# DIFFERENTIAL DIAGNOSIS

Chronic fungal infection (not responsive to antibiotics)

Epidermal inclusion cyst (dorsal swelling proximal to the nail, usually not very painful)

Septic tenosynovitis (increased pain with active and passive motion of finger)

# ADVERSE OUTCOMES OF THE DISEASE

Untreated felons may lead to osteomyelitis of the distal phalanx. Nail deformities and progressive infection involving the distal joint and/or the flexor tendon sheath also may develop late in the course of these infections. Untreated felons may occasionally rupture into the flexor tendon sheath and cause septic flexor tenosynovitis.

# TREATMENT

Most felons require surgical drainage under digital block anesthesia (see Digital Anesthetic Block (Hand), pp 336-337) and tourniquet control. Either of two different incisions can be used: a central volar longitudinal incision or a dorsal midaxial incision.

When a collection of pus can be seen under the skin on the pad side of the finger, use a central longitudinal incision, extending from the flexion crease to the fingertip (**Figure 3**). Culture the drainage for aerobic and anaerobic organisms. It is most important to use a curved hemostat to break up the septae of the digital pulp to ensure that the abscess is completely evacuated. To allow drainage, keep the wound open, using a gauze packing strip, and remove it in 2 to 3 days. Allow the wound to close by secondary intention; never suture the wound.

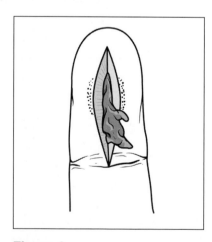

**Figure 3**

Central volar longitudinal incision of the pulp.

Reproduced from Stern PJ: Selected acute infections. *Instr Course Lect* 1990;39:539-546.

When no collection of pus is readily visible under the skin, use a dorsal midaxial incision (**Figure 4**). For the thumb, make the incision on the radial (noncontact) side, and for the fingers, on the ulnar (noncontact) side. Extend the incision to the fingertip but do not wrap it around the tip. Make the incision down to the bone where the soft-tissue attachments to the bone can be separated by blunt dissection with a small hemostat. Use open packing gauze and then remove it in 2 to 3 days.

Treatment of an early-stage paronychia should be nonsurgical. Application of warm, moist soaks for 10 minutes four times a day, combined with an oral antibiotic for 5 days, is usually adequate. Because *Staphylococcus aureus* is the most likely causative organism, an oral cephalosporin such as cephalexin, 250 mg four times a day, or dicloxacillin, 250 mg four times a day, is a good initial choice.

In later stages, when a purulent collection is noted at the nail bed margin or under the nail, drainage can be done by elevating the skin fold at the margin of the nail. More severe infections require partial or complete removal of the nail (**Figure 5**). Under digital or metacarpal block anesthesia, the nail can be carefully elevated from the underlying sterile matrix using a hemostat or blunt metal probe. The nail can be completely removed by freeing the overlying cuticle, and the nail bed protected by a nonadherent gauze (Xeroform or Adaptic) carefully tucked underneath the cuticle and extending to the tip of the finger. The wound should be checked in 3 to 4 days, and the patient advised that the nail should grow out within several months.

## ADVERSE OUTCOMES OF TREATMENT

A painful scar may develop as a result of a misplaced incision, or a nail deformity can develop from injury to the germinal matrix. Inadequate drainage with persistent or recurrent infection may occur.

## REFERRAL DECISIONS/RED FLAGS

Persistent or progressive swelling or any evidence of an ascending infection, despite adequate antibiotic treatment and surgical decompression, is an indication for further evaluation.

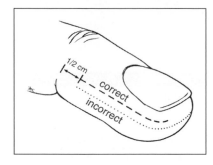

**Figure 4**
Midaxial incision for drainage of a felon.
Reproduced from Stern PJ: Selected acute infections. *Instr Course Lect* 1990;39:539-546.

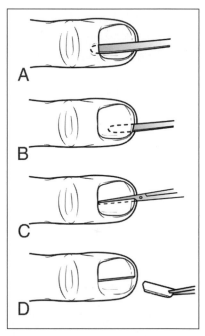

**Figure 5**
Removing a portion of a nail for paronychia. **A,** Use an elevator to separate the nail from the dorsal skin. **B,** Use an elevator to separate the nail from the underlying nail bed. **C,** With straight scissors, divide the nail itself. **D,** Remove the nail segment with a hemostat by application of gentle traction.
Reproduced with permission from the American Society for Surgery of the Hand: *Regional Review Course Manual*. Rosemont, IL, American Society for Surgery of the Hand, 1998, pp 7/8-7/9.

SECTION 4 ■ HAND AND WRIST

# PROCEDURE

# DIGITAL ANESTHETIC BLOCK (HAND)

**CPT Code**

**64450**

Injection, anesthetic agent; other peripheral nerve or branch

*Current Procedural Terminology* © 2004 American Medical Association. All Rights Reserved.

## MATERIALS

Sterile gloves

Bactericidal skin preparation solution

5-mL syringe with a 27-gauge needle

5 mL of 1% local anesthetic without epinephrine

Sterile dressing

### STEP 1

Wear protective gloves at all times during this procedure and use sterile technique.

### STEP 2

Cleanse all surfaces of the base of the finger with a bactericidal skin preparation solution.

### STEP 3

Draw 5 mL of the local anesthetic into the syringe.

### STEP 4

Insert the 27-gauge needle into the palmar midline of the digit near the distal palmar crease. The first injection (approximately one third of the anesthetic) should be made at the midline. The needle should then be repositioned and another one third of the anesthetic injected toward the radial digital nerve. Reposition the needle again and inject the remainder of the anesthetic toward the ulnar digital nerve (**Figure 1**).

### STEP 5

Dress the injection site with a sterile dressing.

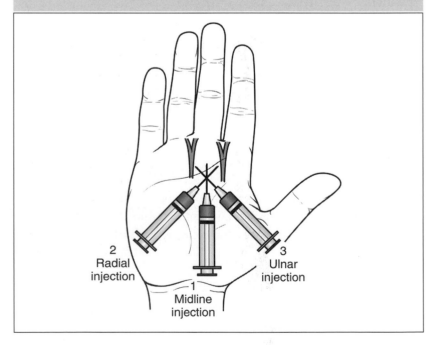

**Figure 1**

Injection technique for digital anesthetic block for the long finger.

# Digital Anesthetic Block (Hand) (continued)

## Adverse outcomes

Although rare, infection is possible. Necrosis of a digit is possible if epinephrine is used in the anesthetic solution. Never inject circumferentially around the base of a digit.

## Aftercare/Patient Instructions

Advise the patient that local swelling at the site of the block should resolve in a few hours. Instruct the patient to call your office if the finger becomes dusky or completely white and to avoid touching hot surfaces or using sharp objects until all sensation has returned.

# FINGERTIP INJURIES/AMPUTATIONS

**ICD-9 Codes**

**883.0**
Open wound of finger(s) without mention of complication

**885.0**
Traumatic amputation of thumb without mention of complication

**886.0**
Traumatic amputation of finger(s) without mention of complication

**927.3**
Crushing injury of finger(s)

## DEFINITION

Fingertip injuries and amputations are common. Some apparent amputations are actually crush injuries or lacerations. In addition to the soft tissue of the pulp, the distal phalanx and nail may be involved.

## CLINICAL SYMPTOMS

Patients report a history of a crush injury or knife injury to the fingertip. The latter usually involves a finger in the nondominant hand.

## TESTS

### Physical Examination

The fingertip should be inspected carefully to determine the vascularity and sensation of the skin flaps and if bone is exposed. The orientation of the amputation also should be noted (**Figure 1**) because the level and angle of amputation may determine appropriate treatment. The nail bed should be carefully examined for a painful subungual hematoma that should be drained and for lacerations of the nail bed that should be repaired. The vascularity of the tip, as well as the sensation, should be noted.

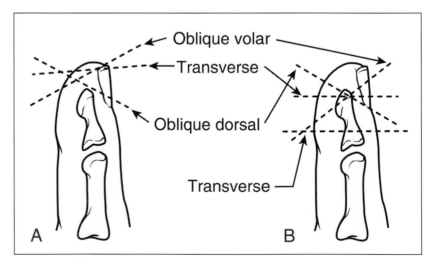

**Figure 1**
**A,** Levels of soft-tissue amputations that can be treated open and allowed to close by secondary intention. **B,** Levels of amputation that require shortening of the bone.

## *Diagnostic Tests*

If bone is exposed or if the finger is markedly swollen, AP and lateral radiographs of the finger should be obtained.

# DIFFERENTIAL DIAGNOSIS

Amputation with injury to the nail matrix (evident on clinical examination)

Amputation with open fracture (evident on radiographs)

# ADVERSE OUTCOMES OF THE DISEASE

A painful amputation stump, dystrophic nail, loss of motion in the finger, and loss of grip and pinch strength are possible. Cold sensitivity/Raynaud phenomenon, a painful neuroma, or epidermal inclusion cyst also can develop. Complex regional pain syndrome also is possible.

# TREATMENT

The goals of treatment are to provide the fingertip with good soft-tissue coverage and adequate sensation, and to preserve as much length as is consistent with good function. Whether or not bone is exposed and the angle of the amputation relative to the long axis of the finger often dictate the appropriate treatment options (Figure 1).

If no bone is exposed, the physician must decide if the skin can be closed without excess tension. If not, the wound should be allowed to close by secondary intention. Initial treatment consists of thorough débridement and irrigation of the finger under a digital block and application of sterile dressings and a distal splint for comfort and contact protection. The initial dressings should be changed after 24 to 72 hours. Wet to dry dressings using normal saline solution twice a day are then applied. The patient should be taught how to apply these dressings and the removable splint at home. The dressing changes are continued until the tip has healed. Finger range-of-motion exercises should begin after 48 hours. Once the wound has healed, tip desensitization techniques can be started in occupational therapy. In most cases, allowing the wound to heal by secondary intention provides good function and acceptable cosmetic results while retaining maximum length of the finger. Almost all fingertip injuries involving an area less than 1 cm square can be treated with débridement and the application of a dressing.

If bone is exposed, a decision must be made whether to shorten the bone or to provide skin coverage by a reconstructive flap procedure. As a general guide, the exposed phalanx of any of the fingers can be shortened sufficiently to provide soft-tissue coverage without sacrificing function. Shortening the thumb is more controversial. Associated nail bed injuries require special attention (see Nail Bed Injuries, pp 376-378).

Treatment of amputation in children under age 6 years differs somewhat from the treatment in adults. Most children heal rapidly and can be treated with local care and serial dressings. For some patients, "composite" grafting, or reapplication of the amputated fingertip as a full-thickness skin graft, is desirable. After thorough débridement and defatting, the skin of a child's amputated fingertip can be sutured to the finger as a composite graft. Even if this tip does not survive (approximately 50% do survive), it serves as a biologic dressing until reepithelialization of the tip occurs.

The tetanus immunization status of the patient must be checked and updated if necessary. If the wound is grossly contaminated and/or crushed, or if the patient has diabetes mellitus, antibiotics may be used.

Replantation should be considered if the thumb is amputated at or proximal to the interphalangeal (IP) joint, if a finger is amputated proximal to the middle of the middle phalanx, or when multiple fingers are amputated. A replantation center should be contacted for specific instructions. The amputated part is wrapped in a sterile gauze soaked in normal saline solution and placed in a plastic bag, and then the bag is placed on ice. The replantation team will usually make the determination if replantation is possible.

Most patients, however, function quite well with single finger amputations. Some patients are concerned with cosmesis, in which case cosmetic finger prostheses can be fitted.

## ADVERSE OUTCOMES OF TREATMENT

Necrosis of the fingertip and infection can develop. Cold sensitivity/Raynaud phenomenon, a painful neuroma, or epidermal inclusion cyst also can develop. Complex regional pain syndrome also is possible.

## REFERRAL DECISIONS/RED FLAGS

Patients with thumb amputations proximal to the IP joint and multiple finger amputations are suitable candidates for specialty evaluation. Patients with single finger amputations who desire replantation also should be referred to a replantation center.

# FLEXOR TENDON INJURIES

## SYNONYMS
Jersey finger
Tendon laceration or rupture

## DEFINITION
The flexor tendons of the hand are vulnerable to laceration or rupture. Complete lacerations of both the flexor digitorum sublimis (FDS) and flexor digitorum profundus (FDP) cause immediate loss of flexion at the proximal interphalangeal (PIP) and distal interphalangeal (DIP) joints. Incomplete or partial lacerations can be missed on initial examination, only to present several days later as a spontaneous rupture in the weakened tendon.

Ruptures of flexor tendons can be spontaneous, as in patients with rheumatoid arthritis and other inflammatory arthritis conditions, or traumatic. The latter type usually occurs during athletics (eg, football, wrestling, or rugby) when a player grabs another's jersey (thus the name jersey finger). When the fingers flex, the ring finger is most prominent and, therefore, the profundus tendon of the ring finger is most commonly ruptured during this activity.

## CLINICAL SYMPTOMS
Each finger is supplied with two flexor tendons: the FDP inserts onto the distal phalanx, and the FDS inserts onto the middle phalanx (**Figure 1**). Therefore, if the FDP is cut but the FDS is intact, patients can flex the PIP and metacarpophalangeal (MP) joints but not the DIP joint. If the FDS is cut but the FDP is intact, patients can flex the DIP, PIP, and MP joints (**Figure 2**).

**ICD-9 Codes**
**727.64**
Rupture of flexor tendons of hand and wrist, nontraumatic

**842.1**
Tendon injuries of the wrist and hand, unspecified site

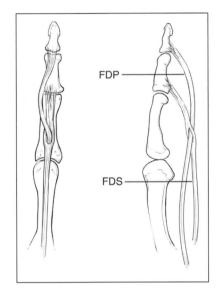

**Figure 1**
Extrinsic flexor tendons of the finger.
Adapted with permission from Green DP (ed): *Operative Hand Surgery*, ed 2. New York, NY, Churchill Livingstone, 1988, p 1971.

| Level of cut tendon | Tendon(s) cut | Loss of flexion joint(s) | Retained flexion joint(s) |
|---|---|---|---|
| (1) | FDP | DIP | MP & PIP |
| (2) | FDP & FDS | PIP & DIP | MP |
| (3) | FDS | NONE | MP, PIP, & DIP |

FDP = Flexor digitorum profundus tendon
FDS = Flexor digitorum sublimus tendon
DIP = Distal interphalangeal joint
PIP = Proximal interphalangeal joint
MP = Metacarpophalangeal joint

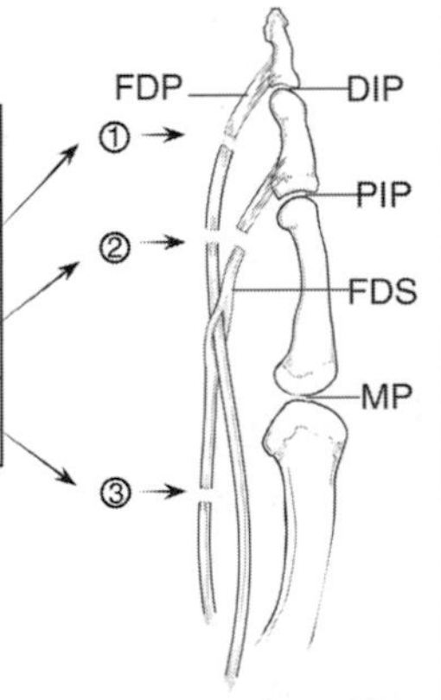

**Figure 2**
Effects of flexor tendon injuries on flexion of the finger joint.
Adapted with permission from Green DP (ed): *Operative Hand Surgery*, ed 2. New York, NY, Churchill Livingstone, 1988, p 1971.

Because of the close proximity of the digital nerves to the flexor tendons, open injuries to the flexor tendons are commonly associated with injuries to the digital nerves as well. In this situation, patients will report numbness on one or both sides of the finger.

With traumatic rupture of the FDP, the ring finger becomes caught, as in a sports jersey (**Figure 3**), and the profundus tendon is avulsed from its insertion, possibly accompanied by a bony fragment. This injury can be missed or diagnosed late because it is often considered to be a jammed finger. In patients with rheumatoid arthritis, ruptures usually are "silent," meaning that the patient notices that the finger will not bend but does not remember when the function was lost.

# Tests

## Physical Examination

First, test for active flexion, then for strength of flexion. If the peritendinous structures are intact, the patient may retain flexion even in the presence of a complete laceration; however, flexion will be weak. Test flexion strength at both the DIP and PIP joints by asking the patient to flex the injured finger against your finger as you apply resistance.

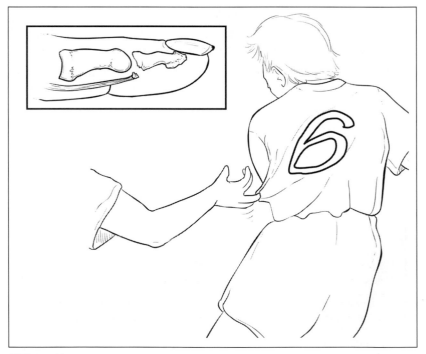

**Figure 3**

Typical mechanism of injury in rupture of the flexor digitorum profundus tendon (jersey finger).

Check flexion of the FDP by asking the patient to flex the fingertip at the DIP joint while the PIP joint is held in extension (see Physical Examination—Hand and Wrist, Muscle Testing: Flexor digitorum profundus, p 297). To test the integrity of the FDS, hold the fingers straight, then have the patient flex each finger individually at the PIP joint (see Physical Examination—Hand and Wrist, Muscle Testing: Flexor digitorum sublimis, p 297). With a lacerated FDS but an intact FDP, PIP flexion will not occur when the other fingers are held extended. This is because the FDP tendons cannot function independently. This test is not reliable at the little finger because 20% to 30% of the population has a band connecting the ring and little fingers that prevents independent function of the sublimis to the little finger. In addition, in some patients, the FDP of the index finger can weakly flex the finger with the other fingers held extended.

Partial lacerations may pose a diagnostic challenge. Patients typically have full range of motion, but they have more *pain* with active flexion than would be expected. When the diagnosis is unclear, evaluation for possible surgical exploration should be considered.

Patients with a tendon rupture may have mild swelling over the flexion surface of the DIP joint and tenderness along the palmar surface of the finger. Test the strength of flexion at the DIP joint. When flexion is weak, rupture of the FDP must be considered a possibility. Patients with rheumatoid arthritis may not remember the point at which the tendon ruptured; they usually report only that the finger will not flex.

Sensation in the finger also should be evaluated because open tendon injuries are often accompanied by injuries to the nearby digital nerves. The vascular status of injured fingers should be checked and documented as well.

*Diagnostic Tests*
PA and lateral radiographs of the involved finger may show a small avulsed fragment from the distal phalanx in an FDP rupture. These views also may identify a fracture.

# DIFFERENTIAL DIAGNOSIS

Anterior interosseous nerve paralysis (no laceration)
Partial tendon laceration (full flexion with pain and weakness)
Stenosing tenosynovitis ("trigger finger") with the finger locked in extension (no visible wound, tenderness over the proximal flexor pulley)

# ADVERSE OUTCOMES OF THE DISEASE

Loss of flexion and of grip and pinch strength in the involved and adjacent fingers is possible.

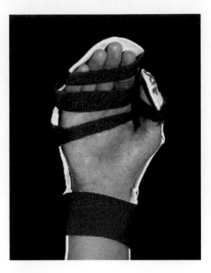

**Figure 4**
Flexor tendon splint.

## TREATMENT

The principal goal of initial treatment is to correctly identify the condition and ensure that the patient is evaluated for surgical repair. Flexor tendon injuries need surgical repair; initial treatment consists of cleaning and repairing superficial wounds and splinting the hand in the position shown in **Figure 4**. Surgical exploration and repair should be done within a few days after injury.

## ADVERSE OUTCOMES OF TREATMENT

Postoperative infection or failure of the repair is possible.

## REFERRAL DECISIONS/RED FLAGS

Patients with any type of suspected flexor tendon injury (rupture or laceration) require further evaluation for surgical repair.

# FLEXOR TENDON SHEATH INFECTIONS

## SYNONYM
Septic tenosynovitis

**ICD-9 Code**

**727.89**
Abscess of bursa or tendon

## DEFINITION
The flexor tendons of the fingers and thumb are enclosed in a specialized tenosynovial sheath that extends from the distal palm to the distal joint (**Figure 1**). Infections within this space can develop from a puncture wound or can spread to the sheath from more superficial infection. These infections are a type of abscess and are rapidly progressive, requiring prompt diagnosis and treatment.

## CLINICAL SYMPTOMS
Patients typically present with a history of a recent puncture wound to the flexor surface of the finger or thumb. Progressive swelling of the entire digit and significant pain develop 24 to 48 hours after injury (**Figure 2**).

## TESTS

### Physical Examination
Signs of a well-established septic flexor tenosynovitis include (1) fusiform swelling of the finger, (2) significant tenderness along the course of the tendon sheath, (3) a marked increase in pain on passive extension, and (4) a flexed position of the finger at rest (**Figure 3**).

### Diagnostic Tests
Plain radiographs may show soft-tissue swelling or, rarely, a foreign body or subcutaneous air.

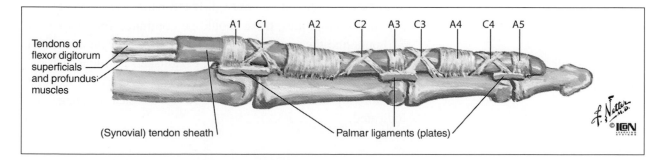

**Figure 1**
Oblique palmar view of a finger showing the tendons lying in their sheath.
**(Reproduced with permission from Icon Learning Systems.)**

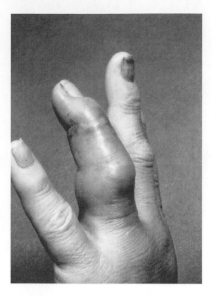

**Figure 2**

Septic tenosynovitis of the ring finger.

Reproduced from Stern PJ: Selected acute infections. *Instr Course Lect* 1990;39:539-546.

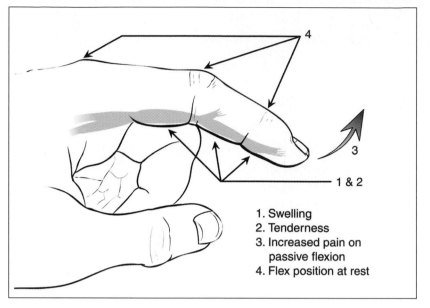

1. Swelling
2. Tenderness
3. Increased pain on passive flexion
4. Flex position at rest

**Figure 3**

Signs of septic tenosynovitis.

Adapted with permission from Carter PR: *Common Hand Injuries and Infections: A Practical Approach to Early Treatment*. Philadelphia, PA, WB Saunders, 1983, p 220.

## DIFFERENTIAL DIAGNOSIS

Aseptic flexor synovitis (negative bacterial cultures)

Cellulitis (little or no pain with active motion of the finger)

## ADVERSE OUTCOMES OF THE DISEASE

These infections progress rapidly; therefore, complications such as skin loss or loss of the entire finger are possible. Other problems include significant stiffness from adhesions and ascending infection or involvement of the bone and joint.

## TREATMENT

If septic tenosynovitis is suspected but the swelling is not severe, parenteral antibiotics should be initiated and the patient reevaluated in 12 to 24 hours. Both *Staphylococcus* and *Streptococcus* should be covered. If the patient responds to parenteral antibiotics, these should be continued for 24 to 72 hours and then switched to oral antibiotics for an additional 7 to 14 days. If the patient has an established purulent flexor tenosynovitis or if the infection progresses or does not respond to antibiotic treatment, urgent referral for surgical drainage is indicated.

## ADVERSE OUTCOMES OF TREATMENT

Finger stiffness can persist, despite successful treatment of septic tenosynovitis.

## REFERRAL DECISIONS/RED FLAGS

Patients with well-established septic tenosynovitis and those who do not respond to antibiotic treatment require evaluation for possible surgery.

SECTION 4 ■ HAND AND WRIST

# Fracture of the Base of the Thumb Metacarpal

**ICD-9 Code**

**816.00**
Fracture of one or more phalanges
of hand, site unspecified, closed

## Synonyms
Bennett fracture
Rolando fracture

## Definition
A Bennett fracture is an oblique fracture of the base of the thumb metacarpal that enters the carpometacarpal (CMC) joint. This fracture has two pieces, one large, the other small. The small volar fragment remains attached to the carpus, and the major metacarpal fragment subluxates at the CMC joint (**Figure 1**).

A Rolando fracture, which is less common than a Bennett fracture, is a Y-shaped intra-articular fracture at the base of the thumb metacarpal. A comminuted intra-articular fracture at the base of the thumb metacarpal also occurs.

## Clinical Symptoms
Patients report pain and limited motion. Swelling and ecchymosis about the base of the thumb are common and are indicative of a metacarpal fracture or CMC dislocation.

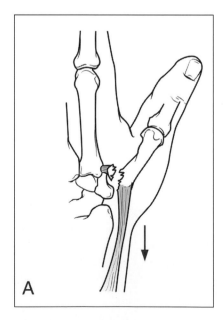
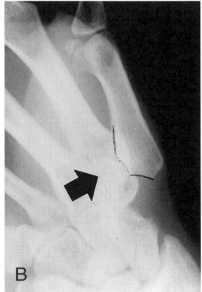

**Figure 1**
Fracture-subluxation of the base of the thumb metacarpal (Bennett fracture). **A,** Drawing showing the mechanism of injury. The medial fragment of the thumb metacarpal is stabilized by the intact volar oblique ligament. The arrow indicates the proximal pull of the abductor pollicis longus tendon. **B,** Radiograph showing a Bennett fracture.

# TESTS

## Physical Examination

Examination reveals that, when the tip of the thumb is held into the palm, the base of the thumb metacarpal is displaced radially and posteriorly. The patient cannot move the thumb without pain.

## Diagnostic Tests

AP and lateral radiographs of the thumb will show these fractures.

# DIFFERENTIAL DIAGNOSIS

Arthritis of the CMC joint (narrow joint space evident on radiographs)

Dislocation of the CMC joint (evident on radiographs)

Fracture of the scaphoid (evident on radiographs)

Synovitis of the CMC joint (swollen joint, normal radiographs)

# ADVERSE OUTCOMES OF THE DISEASE

Posttraumatic arthritis of the CMC joint is possible, resulting in pain at the base of the thumb, along with loss of motion and pinch strength.

# TREATMENT

The goal of treatment is to restore the axial length of the thumb and to replace the metacarpal shaft fragment against the smaller volar lip fragment. Although anatomic reduction of the fracture is the goal, even with some offset a good functional outcome is possible. A Bennett fracture almost always requires some form of surgical fixation to achieve stability in the joint.

Nondisplaced two-part fractures of the base of the thumb metacarpal can be treated in a thumb spica cast for 4 weeks.

# ADVERSE OUTCOMES OF TREATMENT

After surgery, pin tract irritation and infection can occur, as can tenderness around the surgical plates and screws. Displacement of the fracture (loss of position) and posttraumatic arthritis also are possible.

# REFERRAL DECISIONS/RED FLAGS

Intra-articular base of the thumb metacarpal fractures often require surgical treatment. These patients should be considered for early referral.

SECTION 4 ■ HAND AND WRIST

# FRACTURE OF THE DISTAL RADIUS

**ICD-9 Codes**

**813.41**
Colles fracture, Smith fracture

**813.42**
Other fractures of distal end of
radius (alone)

## SYNONYMS

Barton fracture
Chauffeur's fracture
Colles fracture
Die-punch fracture
Smith fracture

## DEFINITION

Fractures involving the distal radius are the most frequently occurring fractures in adults (**Figure 1**). The most common type is the Colles fracture, in which the distal radius fracture fragment is tilted upward, or dorsally. The articular surface of the radius may or may not be involved, and the ulnar styloid could be fractured. A Smith fracture is the opposite of a Colles fracture: the distal fragment is tilted downward, or volarly. A Barton fracture is an intra-articular fracture associated with subluxation of the carpus, either dorsally or volarly, along with the displaced articular fragment of the radius. A chauffeur's fracture is an oblique fracture through the base of the radial styloid. A die-punch fracture is a depressed fracture of the articular surface opposite the lunate or scaphoid bone.

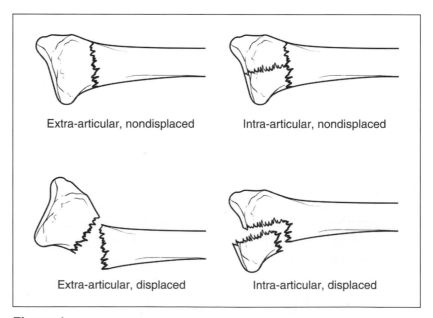

Extra-articular, nondisplaced

Intra-articular, nondisplaced

Extra-articular, displaced

Intra-articular, displaced

**Figure 1**

Types of fractures of the distal radius. Illustration shows a lateral view of the radius.

# ESSENTIALS OF MUSCULOSKELETAL CARE, 3RD EDITION
**Letha Yurko Griffin, MD, PhD**
**Editor**

# MEASURING JOINT MOTION—UPPER EXTREMITY

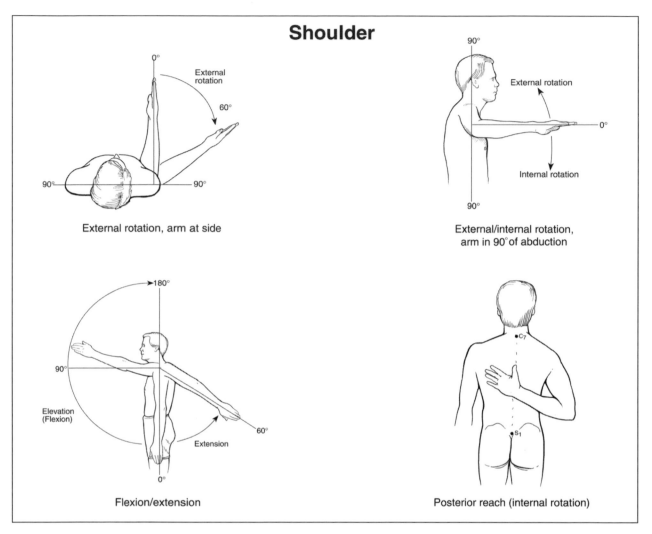

## Shoulder

External rotation, arm at side

External/internal rotation, arm in 90° of abduction

Flexion/extension

Posterior reach (internal rotation)

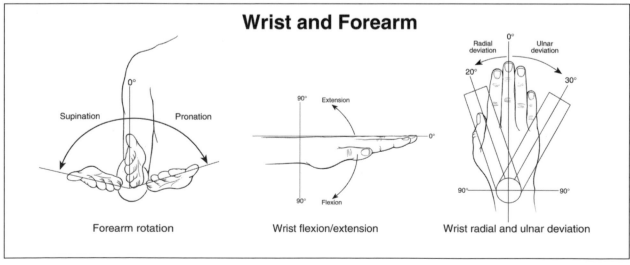

## Wrist and Forearm

Forearm rotation

Wrist flexion/extension

Wrist radial and ulnar deviation

# MEASURING JOINT MOTION—LOWER EXTREMITY

## Hip

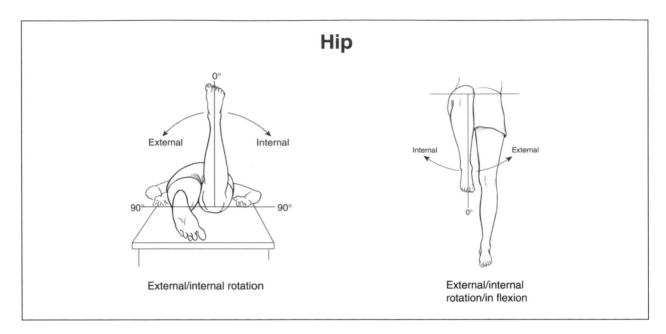

External/internal rotation

External/internal
rotation/in flexion

## Knee

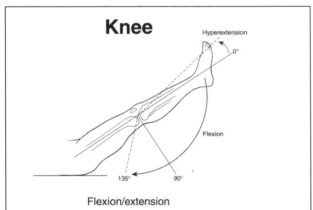

Flexion/extension

## Ankle

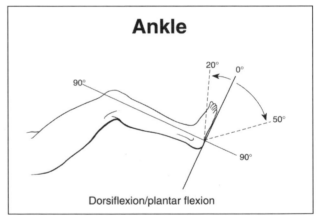

Dorsiflexion/plantar flexion

## Foot

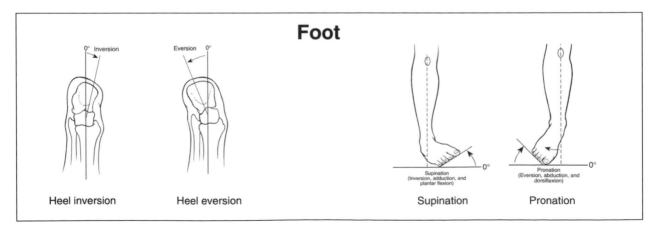

Heel inversion

Heel eversion

Supination

Pronation

## CLINICAL SYMPTOMS

Patients have acute pain, tenderness, swelling, and deformity of the wrist, as well as a history of falling onto an outstretched arm.

## TESTS

### Physical Examination

Look for swelling, deformity, and discoloration around the wrist and distal radius. Observe for skin injury and bleeding (usually with fat droplets in the blood) that would suggest an open fracture. Test for sensation in the hand over the median, radial, and ulnar nerve distribution. Also check the circulation to the fingertips. Examine the elbow for swelling and tenderness.

### Diagnostic Tests

AP and lateral radiographs of the forearm, including the wrist, are necessary. Radiographs of the elbow should be obtained when elbow swelling and tenderness are present because some patients will have combined injuries to the distal end of the radius, the forearm, and the elbow.

## DIFFERENTIAL DIAGNOSIS

Carpal fracture-dislocation (evident on radiographs)

Fracture of the scaphoid (tenderness over anatomic snuffbox, possibly evident on radiographs)

Tenosynovitis of the wrist (normal radiographs)

## ADVERSE OUTCOMES OF THE DISEASE

Malunion, loss of wrist motion, loss of finger motion, complex regional pain syndrome, decreased grip strength, posttraumatic arthritis, or (uncommonly) compartment syndrome can occur when a fracture of the distal radius is not treated.

## TREATMENT

Open fractures need irrigation and débridement and antibiotics. Initial treatment usually focuses on reduction and splinting of the fracture. For most fractures, a sugar tong splint is appropriate. Anatomic reduction is ideal, but less-than-perfect bone alignment can be associated with a good functional outcome. Older, less active persons are more tolerant of residual deformity than are younger individuals. There is significant controversy in the orthopaedic literature as to what constitutes an acceptable reduction.

SECTION 4 ■ HAND AND WRIST

General guidelines for acceptable radiographic alignment after reduction of distal radius fractures are as follows (**Figure 2**): (1) On the lateral view, no more than 5° of dorsal angulation is acceptable. (2) On the AP view, no less than 15° of radial inclination is acceptable. (3) A step-off in the articular surface greater than 2 mm should be reduced. If these parameters are not met, early referral to an orthopaedic surgeon should be considered.

AP and lateral radiographs of the fracture should be repeated each week for 2 weeks after the fracture.

For nondisplaced and minimally displaced extra-articular fractures, a sugar tong splint should be applied for 2 to 3 weeks and a short arm cast for an additional 2 to 3 weeks. (Two weeks in a sugar tong splint plus 2 weeks in a short arm cast is adequate full-time immobilization for some older, less active patients.) After the short arm cast is removed, the patient should wear a removable splint for 3 weeks to allow removal for bathing and gentle exercise. The patient should be encouraged to move the shoulder and elbow of the injured arm through a full range of motion twice a day to prevent shoulder stiffness. Likewise, active and passive finger motion done in five sets four times a day should be encouraged.

Displaced fractures often are unstable and require additional internal and/or external fixation techniques.

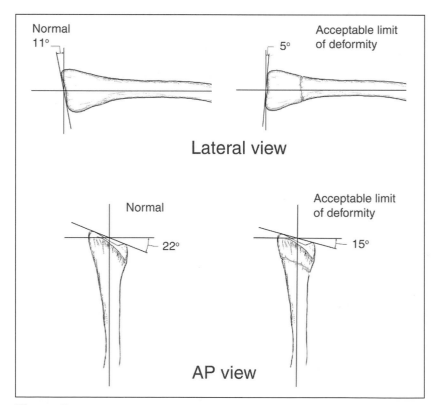

**Figure 2**
General guidelines for alignment of distal radius fractures following reduction.

## ADVERSE OUTCOMES OF TREATMENT

Recurrence of deformity, malunion, loss of wrist motion (flexion, extension, pronation, and supination), posttraumatic wrist arthritis, carpal tunnel syndrome, loss of finger motion, compartment syndrome, or paresthesias of the radial sensory nerve all can result following treatment.

## REFERRAL DECISIONS/RED FLAGS

Displaced fractures that exceed the parameters outlined above and intra-articular fractures require further evaluation. Fractures that initially are nondisplaced but that show progressive collapse on radiographic follow-up require further evaluation.

SECTION 4 ■ HAND AND WRIST

# FRACTURE OF THE METACARPALS AND PHALANGES

## ICD-9 Codes

**815.00**
Fracture of metacarpal bone(s), site unspecified, closed

**816.00**
Fracture of one or more phalanges of hand, site unspecified, closed

## SYNONYMS

Boxer's fracture
Fighter's fracture

## DEFINITION

Metacarpal fractures are most common in adults (**Figure 1**). The most common fracture in the hand is a boxer's fracture, an injury of the distal metaphysis of the fifth metacarpal that results from a closed fist striking an object (**Figure 2**). In phalangeal fractures in adults, the distal phalanx is the most commonly injured (**Figure 3**), followed by the proximal and the middle phalanges. Approximately 20% of these fractures are intra-articular.

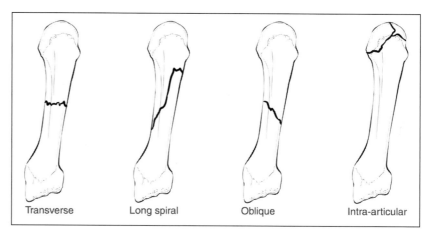

Transverse    Long spiral    Oblique    Intra-articular

**Figure 1**

Types of metacarpal fractures.

Adapted with permission from Dabezies EJ, Schutte JP: Fixation of metacarpal and phalangeal fractures with miniature plates and screws. *J Hand Surg* 1986;11A:283 288.

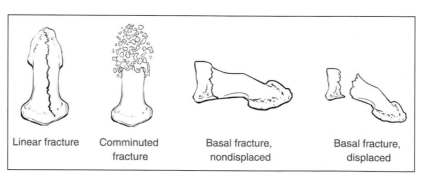

Linear fracture    Comminuted fracture    Basal fracture, nondisplaced    Basal fracture, displaced

**Figure 3**

Types of distal phalanx fractures.

Adapted with permission from Rockwood CA, Green DP, Bucholz RW, et al (eds): *Rockwood and Green's Fractures in Adults*, ed 4. Philadelphia, PA, Lippincott-Raven, 1996, vol 2, pp 614, 627.

**Figure 2**

Fracture of the distal metaphysis of the little finger metacarpal (boxer's fracture).

Adapted with permission from Green DP (ed): *Operative Hand Surgery*, ed 3. New York, NY, Churchill Livingstone, 1993.

Phalangeal fractures are more common in children. The most common fracture involves the physis of the little finger. Growth disturbances from physeal injuries of the phalanges are rare.

# CLINICAL SYMPTOMS

Patients typically have a history of trauma. Local tenderness, swelling, deformity, or decreased range of motion are common findings.

# TESTS

## Physical Examination

Examination reveals swelling over the fracture site. The involved finger may appear shortened, or the knuckle may be depressed. The distal fragment may be rotated in relation to the proximal fragment. This is not easy to see with the fingers extended; however, when the patient makes a partial fist, the rotated fragments cause the involved finger to overlap onto its neighbor (**Figure 4**). In general, assess the bones of the involved finger for angulation, rotation, and the potential for digital crossover in flexion. Assess sensory function of the digital nerves.

## Diagnostic Tests

Radiographs are always indicated for suspected fractures. For fractures of the phalanges, PA and true lateral views of the individual digits should be obtained. For metacarpal fractures, PA, lateral, and oblique views of the hand are indicated.

# DIFFERENTIAL DIAGNOSIS

Metacarpophalangeal (MP) and interphalangeal (IP) joint sprains (instability and joint tenderness)

MP and IP joint dislocations (evident on clinical examination)

# ADVERSE OUTCOMES OF THE DISEASE

Malunion, nonunion, posttraumatic arthritis, and loss of finger motion are all possible.

# TREATMENT

## Metacarpal Neck Fracture

For a boxer's fracture, in patients with 10° to 15° of angulation, apply an ulnar gutter splint for 2 to 3 weeks. This treatment also is appropriate with more than 15° of angulation but no extensor lag (the patient can fully extend the finger). Advise the patient that although this fracture will not result in any functional deficit, there could be a loss of the prominence of

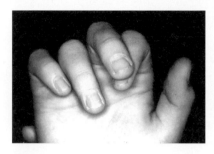

**Figure 4**

Malrotation of a finger associated with a phalangeal fracture is more apparent with the fingers in flexion. In normal alignment, the nail plates of the fingers would be parallel, with no crossover of the fingers. Note the malrotation of the index finger.

Reproduced with permission from Breen TF: Sport-related injuries of the hand, in Pappas AM, Walzer J (eds): *Upper Extremity Injuries in the Athlete.* New York, NY, Churchill Livingstone, 1995, pp 451-496.

SECTION 4 ■ HAND AND WRIST

the metacarpal head dorsally. If this is unsatisfactory to the patient, further evaluation is indicated.

With an extensor lag, or with more than 40° of angulation, referral for reduction is appropriate. Similar guidelines are appropriate for fractures of the metacarpal neck of the ring finger, although slightly less angulation is accepted because of prominence of the metacarpal head. The second and third metacarpals have less mobility, and therefore less angulation is acceptable in these injuries. Use of a radial gutter splint is appropriate with less than 10° of angulation, but with greater angulation, functional loss could result, and referral for reduction is appropriate.

## Nondisplaced Fractures of the Metacarpal and Phalangeal Shafts

Casting or splint immobilization for 3 weeks is indicated for phalangeal fractures and for 4 weeks for metacarpal fractures. When casting or splinting, always include the joint above and below the fracture and the adjacent digits. To avoid fixed contracture formation, the safe position of immobilization is with the MP joints held in approximately 70° of flexion and the proximal interphalangeal (PIP) and distal interphalangeal (DIP) joints held in extension (0° to 10° of flexion). When loss of position is a possible problem, radiographs should be repeated 1 week after the injury.

Immobilization of phalangeal fractures for more than 3 to 4 weeks will result in stiffness. Do not wait for radiographic evidence of healing to begin exercises because full healing may not be apparent for 2 to 5 months. If the fracture seems clinically stable after cast removal, motion should be started.

## Displaced Fractures of the Metacarpal and Phalangeal Shafts

Because of pull by the flexor tendons, displaced transverse fractures of the metacarpals and phalanges tend to angulate (**Figure 5**), spiral fractures tend to rotate, and oblique fractures tend to shorten. Patients with these types of fractures need further evaluation upon initial presentation.

## Intra-articular Fractures

Splint nondisplaced intra-articular fractures with the MP joints in flexion and the PIP and DIP joints in extension. Repeat radiographs in 1 week to assess for continued articular congruity, then initiate active range of motion at 3 weeks. Displacement of intra-articular fractures greater than 1 mm is unacceptable because of loss of joint congruity; therefore, patients with displaced intra-articular fractures need further evaluation.

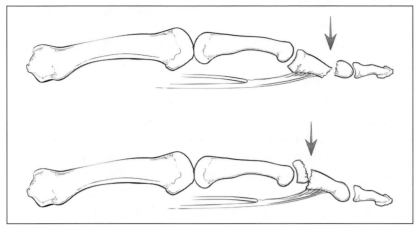

**Figure 5**
Phalangeal fractures angulate because of pull by the flexor tendons.
Adapted with permission from Rockwood CA, Green DP, Bucholz RW, et al (eds): *Rockwood and Green's Fractures in Adults*, ed 4. Philadelphia, PA, Lippincott-Raven, 1996, vol 2, pp 614, 627.

## ADVERSE OUTCOMES OF TREATMENT

Joint stiffness is the most common problem with hand fractures and is directly related to prolonged immobilization. Malunion caused by inadequate reduction also is possible.

## REFERRAL DECISIONS/RED FLAGS

Displaced fractures and intra-articular fractures often require surgical treatment. Patients with these types of fractures should be considered for early referral.

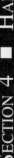

SECTION 4 ■ HAND AND WRIST

# FRACTURE OF THE SCAPHOID

**ICD-9 Code**

**814.01**
Fracture of carpal bone, closed, navicular (scaphoid) of wrist

## DEFINITION

The scaphoid spans the distal and proximal rows of the carpus and in that position is vulnerable to falls on the outstretched hand. The scaphoid is the most commonly fractured carpal bone. Young male adults are most commonly affected. These fractures are not common in children and older adults because the distal radius is the weak link in patients in these age groups. Of all scaphoid fractures, approximately 20% occur in the proximal pole, 60% in the middle or waist, and 20% in the distal pole (**Figure 1**).

Fractures of the scaphoid are important both because of their frequency and because their diagnosis is often delayed or missed. Patients may think they have a simple sprain and fail to seek medical attention. At the time of initial injury, routine radiographs may not demonstrate the fracture and, as a result, the fracture is inadequately immobilized.

Scaphoid fractures also have a high incidence of nonunion and osteonecrosis. The blood supply to this bone is limited because articular cartilage covers 80% of the scaphoid, and the major blood supply, which enters the bone in the distal third at the dorsal ridge, might be disrupted by the injury. Because of these anatomic features, displaced fractures of the scaphoid (more than 1 mm) have a relatively high rate of nonunion (up to 90%). Fractures of the middle third are vulnerable to osteonecrosis, and fractures of the proximal third are most susceptible to the development of osteonecrosis.

## CLINICAL SYMPTOMS

Pain and tenderness about the radial (thumb) side of the wrist are characteristic. Any type of wrist motion, such as gripping, is

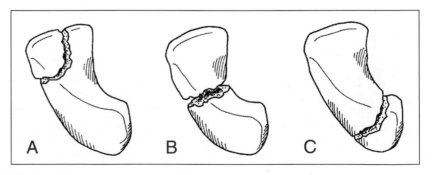

**Figure 1**
Types of scaphoid fractures. **A,** Distal tubercle fracture. **B,** Waist fracture. **C,** Proximal-pole fracture.

Reproduced with permission from Trumble TE (ed): *Principles of Hand Surgery and Therapy.* Philadelphia, PA, WB Saunders, 2000, p 93.

painful. Swelling about the back and radial side of the wrist is also common. If the patient reports a history of a high-energy injury, such as a car accident, ligamentous injuries and resultant carpal instability (perilunar instability) are possible in addition to the scaphoid fracture.

# TESTS

## Physical Examination

Palpation over the anatomic snuffbox, defined by the abductor and long thumb extensor tendons just distal to the radial styloid, reveals marked tenderness (**Figure 2**). Likewise, pressure over the scaphoid tubercle on the underside of the wrist will produce pain. In addition, the patient may have decreased motion and grip strength. An intra-articular effusion is not uncommon for patients who present with an acute scaphoid fracture. Assess function of the median, ulnar, and radial nerves, as well as circulatory status.

## Diagnostic Tests

At the time of initial injury, scaphoid fractures may not be visible on PA and lateral radiographs of the wrist. Therefore, if these radiographs appear normal, obtain a PA view with the wrist in ulnar deviation and an oblique view to help visualize the fracture (**Figure 3**). If this series of initial radiographs is normal but the pain persists for 2 to 3 weeks, the PA and

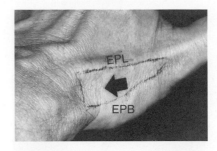

**Figure 2**
The triangular area outlined on this hand is the anatomic snuffbox. EPL = extensor pollicis longus; EPB = extensor pollicis brevis.

SECTION 4 ■ HAND AND WRIST

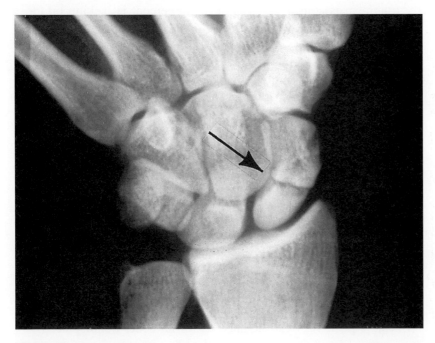

**Figure 3**
PA view with the wrist in ulnar deviation demonstrating a scaphoid fracture (arrow).

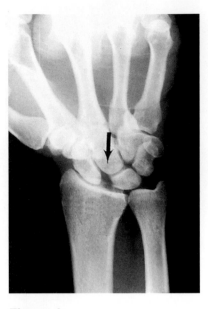

**Figure 4**

Clenched fist view showing scapholunate dissociation (arrow) with increased gap between the scaphoid and lunate.

oblique views should be repeated. If the radiographs are still normal, a bone scan or MRI can be considered.

## DIFFERENTIAL DIAGNOSIS

de Quervain tenosynovitis (positive Finkelstein test)

Fracture of the distal radius (evident on plain radiographs)

Scapholunate dissociation (increased gap between scaphoid and lunate [**Figure 4**])

Wrist arthritis (narrowing of joint space, evident on radiographs)

## ADVERSE OUTCOMES OF THE DISEASE

Nonunion, decreased grip strength and range of motion, and osteoarthritis of the radiocarpal joint are possible.

## TREATMENT

Patients with significant snuffbox tenderness (even with normal radiographs) should be treated initially as though they have a scaphoid fracture and placed in a thumb spica splint. Close follow-up with additional radiographs or MRI will identify occult scaphoid fractures. Because the interval to treatment can be important in minimizing the risk of nonunion, patients should be immobilized at the time of initial presentation until a definitive diagnosis can be reached. Once the diagnosis of an acute nondisplaced fracture of the scaphoid has been confirmed, treatment is controversial because agreement is lacking on the optimal type of immobilization for these fractures. Data are conflicting regarding the optimal position of the wrist, whether the elbow should be immobilized, and whether the thumb should be included in the cast. Immobilization for 6 weeks in a long arm thumb spica cast with the wrist in a neutral position can be necessary. If radiographs obtained after this time show that the fracture is healing, apply a short arm thumb spica cast. However, if the fracture line appears to be getting wider, indicating resorption at the fracture site, or if the fracture shows any displacement, then further evaluation for possible surgery is indicated.

If the patient has pain over the region of the snuffbox but the initial radiographs are normal, place the hand and wrist in a thumb spica splint for 2 to 3 weeks, then repeat the radiographs. If the radiographs are still normal but tenderness over the scaphoid persists, order a bone scan or MRI. If the scan is positive, treat the hand as for an acute nondisplaced scaphoid fracture.

It may be difficult to determine from routine radiographs whether a scaphoid fracture has healed, and immobilization may be discontinued too soon. As a general rule, the closer the fracture line is to the proximal pole, the longer the time for healing. For fractures of the distal pole, the average time for healing is 6 to 8 weeks. Fractures of the middle third require 8 to 12 weeks to heal, and fractures of the proximal pole can take 12 to 24 weeks or longer. If plain radiographs do not clearly reveal that the fracture has healed, a computerized axial tomogram can be ordered to better visualize the fracture site.

## ADVERSE OUTCOMES OF TREATMENT

Loss of motion from prolonged immobilization, and/or loss of grip strength can result.

## REFERRAL DECISIONS/RED FLAGS

All patients with displaced fractures of the scaphoid need early further evaluation for possible surgical treatment. All patients with scaphoid fractures in association with other wrist ligament injuries (perilunar instability) need urgent referral to a hand surgeon. Patients who show cystic absorption at the fracture site or displacement of the fracture after immobilization, or those with nondisplaced fractures that have not healed after 2 months of immobilization, need further evaluation for possible surgical treatment.

SECTION 4 ■ HAND AND WRIST

# GANGLIA OF THE WRIST AND HAND

**ICD-9 Codes**
**727.41**
Ganglion of joint
**727.42**
Ganglion of tendon sheath

## SYNONYMS

Flexor tendon sheath ganglion
Mucous cyst
Synovial cyst
Volar retinacular ganglion

## DEFINITION

A ganglion is a cystic structure that arises from the capsule of a joint or a tendon synovial sheath (**Figure 1**). The cyst contains a thick, clear, mucinous fluid identical in composition to joint fluid. Through degeneration or tearing of the joint capsule or tendon sheath, a connection to the joint or tendon sheath with a one-way valve is established. Thus, synovial fluid can enter the cyst but cannot flow freely back into the synovial cavity. Ganglia vary in size, and significant symptoms may result from increased pressure on surrounding structures.

Ganglia are the most common soft-tissue tumors of the hand, generally affecting individuals between the ages of 15 and 40 years. These benign tumors typically develop, and sometimes disappear, spontaneously. Common locations include the dorsum of the wrist, the volar radial aspect of the wrist, and the base of the finger. The latter typically arises from the proximal annular ligament (A1 pulley) of the flexor tendon sheath. These also are known as volar retinacular ganglia.

Mucous cysts are a type of ganglion that develops from an arthritic distal interphalangeal (DIP) joint, most commonly in women between the ages of 40 and 70 years.

## CLINICAL SYMPTOMS

### Wrist

Patients typically have a lump, which may or may not be painful (**Figure 2**). The pain is described as aching and is aggravated by activities that require frequent movement of the wrist. Ganglia in the wrist often vary in size, with an increase in size associated with times of increased activity. A history of variation in size is a key factor to distinguish a ganglion from other soft-tissue tumors.

Occasionally, a ganglion will occur in an area of the wrist where it may result in compression of the median or ulnar nerve. In this situation, sensory symptoms in the fingers and/or weakness of the intrinsic muscle may develop.

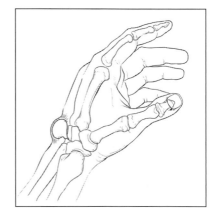

**Figure 1**
Wrist ganglion.

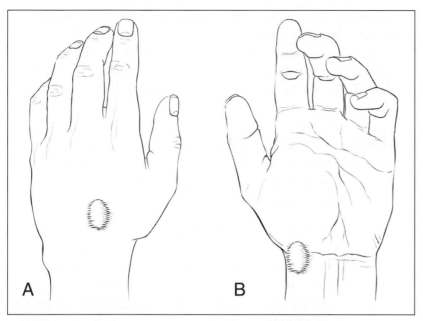

**Figure 2**
Clinical appearance of dorsal (**A**) and volar (**B**) wrist ganglia.
Adapted with permission from the American Society for Surgery of the Hand: Brochure: *Ganglion Cysts.* Englewood, CO, 1995.

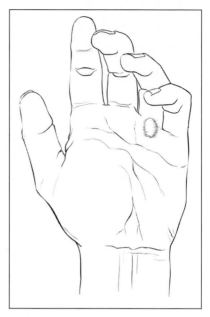

**Figure 3**
Flexor tendon sheath ganglion.
Adapted with permission from the American Society for Surgery of the Hand: Brochure: *Ganglion Cysts.* Englewood, CO, 1995.

### Hand and Finger

Patients with flexor tendon sheath cysts report tenderness when grasping and have a bump at the base of the finger (usually at the level of the proximal flexion crease) (**Figure 3**). A tender mass in this area usually is a flexor tendon sheath ganglion.

Patients with mucous cysts have swelling on the dorsum of the finger distal to the DIP joint (**Figure 4**). They also may report a cycle of the cyst breaking open, draining a clear, jelly-like fluid, and healing. Treatment often is sought when the cyst becomes painful, ulcerated, or infected, or is cosmetically displeasing. Patients also may have furrowing of the fingernail because of pressure of the cyst on the nail matrix.

## TESTS

### Physical Examination–Wrist

A dorsal ganglion is typically a smooth, round or multilobulated structure on the dorsoradial aspect of the wrist that becomes more prominent with flexion. It usually is positioned directly over the scapholunate joint but can occur more distally even though its stalk usually emanates from the scapholunate joint.

A volar radial ganglion usually is a less well-defined mass situated between the flexor carpi radialis tendon and the radial styloid. It may extend underneath the radial artery and, in some cases, may adhere to the radial artery. On palpation, the ganglion may appear to pulsate and can be confused with an

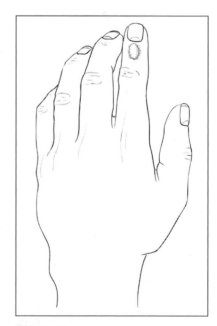

**Figure 4**
Mucous cyst.
Adapted with permission from the American Society for Surgery of the Hand: Brochure: *Ganglion Cysts.* Englewood, CO, 1995.

SECTION 4  ■  HAND AND WRIST

aneurysm. Symptoms also become more pronounced with extreme flexion or extension.

Ganglia are mildly tender with pressure. A prominent ganglion often will transilluminate when a penlight is shined through it from the side. Solid tumors will not transilluminate.

If a definite mass is not visible, the possibility of an occult ganglion, which is characterized by more subtle swelling, should be considered. Palpation must be more thorough and careful in order to identify a small tender mass that is different from what is felt on the opposite wrist. MRI may be necessary to determine if an occult ganglion is present.

### Physical Examination–Hand and Finger

A volar retinacular ganglion of the flexor tendon sheath is characterized by a small, firm, tender mass at the base of the finger in the area of the metacarpophalangeal flexion crease, most often at the long or ring fingers (Figure 3). These ganglia are sometimes difficult to detect because of their small size. They rarely affect motion and do not move with excursion of the tendon.

Mucous cysts usually lie to one side of the extensor tendon at the DIP joint (Figure 4). Initial clinical findings include a mass or a blister. Periarticular arthritic nodules may contain mucous cysts.

### Diagnostic Tests

PA, lateral, and oblique radiographs of the hand or PA and lateral radiographs of the wrist or the involved finger should be obtained to rule out bony pathology. In most cases, ganglia are not associated with radiographic changes. With a mucous cyst, degenerative changes and a small bony spur usually are seen rising from the dorsum of the distal phalanx at the DIP joint.

## DIFFERENTIAL DIAGNOSIS

### Wrist

Arthritis (evident on radiographs)

Bone tumor (evident on radiographs)

Intraosseous ganglion (evident on radiographs)

Kienböck disease (collapse of the lunate)

Soft-tissue tumor, benign or malignant (solid mass on palpation, rare)

### Hand and Finger

Dupuytren disease (presence of cords or bands)

Epidermal inclusion cyst (history of laceration and repair)

Giant cell tumors (different locations, but usually about the phalanges)

Lipoma (larger in size, often in the palm)

Soft-tissue tumor, benign or malignant (solid mass on palpation, rare)

# ADVERSE OUTCOMES OF THE DISEASE

## Wrist

Patients may experience a decrease in grip strength and painful wrist motion; they also may complain about the unsightly bump. On rare occasions, ganglia will cause significant compression on the median nerve.

## Hand and Finger

Patients often have pain in the hand and finger and an obvious deformity at the fingernail. Infection also can occur in association with a mucous cyst.

# TREATMENT

## Wrist

If the wrist ganglion is typical in presentation and physical findings, reassurance usually is adequate. When the patient has acute, severe symptoms, immobilizing the wrist will relieve symptoms and may cause the ganglion to decrease in size. However, immobilization is rarely a permanent solution. Occasionally, aspiration of a dorsal wrist ganglion will lead to resolution (see Dorsal Wrist Ganglion Aspiration, p 367). Because of the proximity of the radial artery, volar wrist ganglia should be aspirated with great care.

When the patient has significant symptoms or is seriously bothered by the appearance of the wrist ganglion, then surgical excision is indicated.

## Hand and Finger

Treatment of a ganglion of the tendon sheath consists of needle rupture followed by massage to disperse the contents of the cyst, or injection with 1% or 2% local anesthetic until the cyst pops. Exercise caution when performing a needle rupture because of the proximity of the neurovascular bundle. Surgical management is occasionally required for painful flexor sheath ganglia.

Aspiration and/or rupture of a mucous cyst is not recommended because of the danger of introducing an infection into the DIP joint. If infection occurs, the patient should be started on a first generation cephalosporin (unless allergic), tetanus immunization status should be updated if necessary, and a specialist should be consulted promptly.

## ADVERSE OUTCOMES OF TREATMENT

### Wrist

Recurrence of wrist ganglia occurs in 5% to 10% of patients after surgical excision, and in up to 90% after needle aspiration. Injury to the radial artery can occur as a result of aspiration of a volar wrist ganglion.

### Hand and Finger

Recurrence of hand and finger ganglia is quite common. Skin loss is possible, as is injury to the digital nerve.

## REFERRAL DECISION/RED FLAGS

### Wrist

Any mass with atypical findings should be evaluated with additional diagnostic tests or excisional biopsy. Recurrence after aspiration also is an indication for further evaluation.

### Hand and Finger

Persistence of a painful or bothersome cyst after one or two attempts at needle rupture or aspiration indicates that surgical excision should be considered. Increased erythema and pain in a mucous cyst suggests infection that may require surgical treatment.

# PROCEDURE
## DORSAL WRIST GANGLION
### ASPIRATION

### STEP 1
Wear protective gloves at all times during this procedure and use sterile technique.

### STEP 2
Cleanse the area with a bactericidal skin preparation solution.

### STEP 3
Use a syringe with a 27-gauge needle to infiltrate 1% local anesthetic into the area immediately proximal to and surrounding the ganglion. Remove the 27-gauge needle and change to the 18-gauge needle.

### STEP 4
Penetrate the ganglion with the 18-gauge needle and attempt to withdraw as much fluid as possible (**Figure 1**). With your free hand, compress the ganglion and displace the thick fluid toward the needle. As you compress the mass, you may need to move the needle to the right or left slightly to break small cavities within the ganglion. Injecting corticosteroid has not been shown to influence the recurrence rate and is not recommended.

### STEP 5
Apply a sterile dressing.

## ADVERSE OUTCOMES
Infection and recurrence of the ganglion are possible. Injury to the radial artery also can occur following attempts to aspirate volar wrist ganglia.

## AFTERCARE/PATIENT INSTRUCTIONS
Instruct the patient to wear the elastic bandage for 1 week, removing it only for bathing.

## CPT Code
**20612**
Aspiration and/or injection of ganglion cyst(s) any location
*Current Procedural Terminology* © 2004 American Medical Association. All Rights Reserved.

## MATERIALS
Sterile gloves

Bactericidal skin preparation solution

3-mL syringe with a 27-gauge, ¾" needle

18-gauge needle

3 mL of a 1% local anesthetic without epinephrine

Elastic bandage

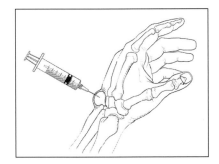

**Figure 1**
Location for needle insertion for dorsal wrist ganglion aspiration.

**SECTION 4 ■ HAND AND WRIST**

# HUMAN BITES

ICD-9 Codes

**882.0**
Open wound of hand except finger(s) alone, without mention of complication

**883.0**
Open wound of finger(s) without mention of complication

## SYNONYMS
Clenched fist injury
Fight bite

## DEFINITION
Human bite wounds to the hand occur either directly, from a bite (usually to the fingers), or indirectly, when the hand strikes a tooth (clenched fist injury) (**Figure 1**). Few infections of the hand can progress more quickly or result in more significant complications. Early recognition and appropriate treatment are important.

Human bite wounds contain greater concentrations of bacteria than animal bite wounds, especially anaerobic species. *Eikenella corrodens* is associated with human bite wounds, but the most common organisms causing these infections are α-hemolytic streptococci and *Staphylococcus aureus*.

## CLINICAL SYMPTOMS
The history of the injury and a laceration is diagnostic but may be difficult to elicit. Warmth, swelling, pain, and a purulent discharge are often present (**Figure 2**). Examination may reveal evidence of damage to underlying structures, including lack of extension or flexion due to tendon damage or a loss of sensation over the tip of the finger due to nerve injury.

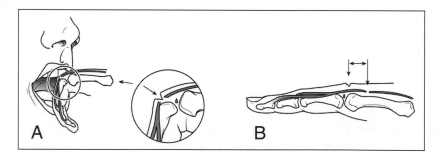

**Figure 1**
**A,** Mechanism of tendon laceration and intra-articular contamination by saliva in human bite. **B,** An injury to a tendon that is cut in flexion will retract as the joint extends.

Adapted with permission from Carter PR: *Common Hand Injuries and Infections: A Practical Approach to Early Treatment.* Philadelphia, PA, WB Saunders, 1983.

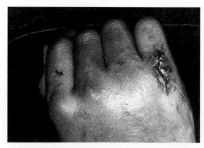

**Figure 2**
Possible tooth injury over the MP joint of the little finger.

# TESTS

## Physical Examination

Measure and record the location of the laceration. A small laceration over the ring or little finger is a sign of a possible clenched fist injury. Be alert for a tooth wound proximal to the metacarpophalangeal (MP) joint when the finger is extended but lies over the knuckle in a clenched fist. Document the location and severity of the swelling, erythema, and any purulent discharge. When the injury is on the dorsum of the hand, significant swelling may occur quickly (within 2 to 3 hours). Assess function of the flexor and extensor tendons and sensory nerves distal to the laceration. Examine the forearm for signs of ascending infection (eg, lymphangitic streaks, enlarged epitrochlear nodes).

## Diagnostic Tests

PA, lateral, and oblique radiographs of the hand should be obtained to rule out an underlying fracture or presence of a foreign body. Aerobic and anaerobic cultures should be obtained when any drainage is present. A white blood cell count can serve as a baseline for following the clinical course, but this test may be within normal limits in the early phases after injury.

# DIFFERENTIAL DIAGNOSIS

Laceration from a sharp object (accurate history)

Septic joint caused by a retained foreign body (possibly evident on radiographs)

# ADVERSE OUTCOMES OF THE DISEASE

Tendon rupture and/or laceration can occur as a result of the bite. An abscess involving the deep palmar space, osteomyelitis, joint sepsis, joint stiffness, and possibly septic tenosynovitis can develop with delay in treatment.

# TREATMENT

Bite wounds can be treated on an outpatient basis if the joint has not been penetrated, if there has been no tendon or bony injury, and when medical treatment is sought within 8 hours of the injury.

Anesthetize the wound with a 1% plain lidocaine solution and carefully examine and débride the skin edges and any underlying necrotic tissue. The extensor mechanism over the MP joints should be examined with the finger flexed to assess for damage to the tendons or penetration of the underlying joint. It is important to explore the wound with the patient's

SECTION 4 ■ HAND AND WRIST

fingers both flexed and extended. If the possibility of joint infection exists, an arthrotomy is necessary to irrigate the joint. Irrigate the wound with a large amount of an antibiotic irrigation solution and apply saline-soaked gauze or a nonadherent dressing. Human bites should never be closed primarily.

Immobilize the hand in a bulky dressing that incorporates a dorsal plaster splint that holds the hand in a safe position (ie, with the MP joint at 60° to 90° of flexion and the interphalangeal joints in a resting, extended position). Appropriate tetanus prophylaxis should be given as outlined in **Table 1**, followed by antibiotics. Penicillin and a first-generation cephalosporin provide adequate coverage in most instances. Tetracycline can be used for patients who are allergic to penicillin. If cultures obtained from specimens taken at the time of initial wound care are positive, antibiotic type and dosage should be adjusted accordingly.

Advise patients who present soon after injury and without an established abscess to return within 24 hours for a recheck to confirm that infection has not developed. After the first 24 hours, daily whirlpool treatment or twice-daily dressing changes can be started. The wound should be allowed to close by secondary intention. For established infections, urgent surgical débridement and intravenous antibiotics are usually necessary. Early referral is necessary in these cases.

## ADVERSE OUTCOMES OF TREATMENT

Inadequate evaluation or treatment can lead to significant complications, including the need for amputation in advanced cases. Infection may develop with primary wound closure. Patients may experience sensitivity to antibiotics.

**Table 1   Guide to Tetanus Prophylaxis in Wound Management**

| History of Tetanus Toxoid (Doses) | Clean, Minor Wound Td | TIG | Contaminated Wound Td | TIG |
|---|---|---|---|---|
| Unknown | Yes | No | Yes | Yes* |
| Fewer than 3 doses | Yes | No | Yes | Yes* |
| 3 or more | Yes, if more than 10 years since last dose | No | Yes, if more than 5 years since last dose | No |

Td = combined tetanus and diphtheria toxoid adsorbed (dose = 0.5 mL IM). TIG = tetanus immune globulin (dose = 250 IU IM).
*Td and TIG should be administered at different sites.
Adapted from the Centers for Disease Control and Prevention.

## Referral Decisions/Red Flags

Wounds that involve the joint, tendon, nerve, or bone require further evaluation. A bite wound that becomes infected despite treatment with antibiotics also needs further evaluation.

Section 4 ■ Hand and Wrist

# KIENBÖCK DISEASE

**ICD-9 Codes**

**715.23**
Osteoarthrosis of the wrist, secondary

**732.3**
Kienböck disease

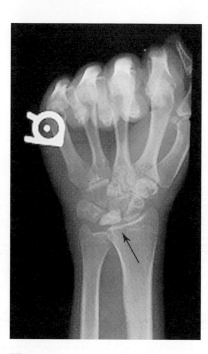

**Figure 1**

PA clenched fist view of left hand of patient with Kienböck disease shows significant sclerosis of the lunate (arrow) and possible early collapse.

## SYNONYMS
Osteonecrosis of the carpal lunate

## DEFINITION
Kienböck disease—osteonecrosis of the carpal lunate—most commonly affects men between the ages of 20 and 40 years (**Figure 1**). Patients may have a history of trauma, but the cause of the disrupted blood supply is frequently difficult to establish. With progression of the disease, the lunate collapses and fragments ultimately lead to end-stage arthritis of the wrist.

## CLINICAL SYMPTOMS
Pain, stiffness, and diffuse swelling over the dorsal aspect of the wrist are common. Patients often report weakness or inability to grasp heavy objects.

## TESTS

### Physical Examination
Examination typically reveals tenderness directly over the lunate bone (mid-dorsal wrist area, just distal to the radius). Grip strength usually is decreased. With progression of the disease, dorsal swelling and limited wrist motion are common.

### Diagnostic Tests
PA and lateral radiographs of the wrist are indicated (**Figure 2**). In the early phase of Kienböck disease, radiographs show increased density (whiteness) of the lunate bone compared with

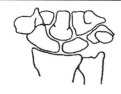

Stage 1:
No visible change
in the lunate

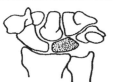

Stage 2:
Sclerosis of the lunate

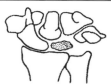

Stage 3A:
Sclerosis and
fragmentation of
the lunate

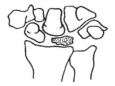

Stage 3B:
Stage 3A with proximal
migration of the
capitate or fixed
rotation of the scaphoid

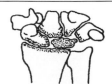

Stage 4:
Stage 3A or 3B
combined with
degenerative changes
at adjacent joints

**Figure 2**

Radiographic classification of Kienböck disease according to the method of Lichtman and associates, modified by Weiss and associates.

Reproduced with permission from the American Society for Surgery of the Hand: *Hand Surgery Update.* Rosemont, IL, American Academy of Orthopaedic Surgeons, 1994, p 86.

the surrounding carpal bones. In later stages, the dead bone will fragment and collapse, resulting in generalized degenerative arthritis of the wrist.

## DIFFERENTIAL DIAGNOSIS

Fracture of the distal radius (evident on radiographs)

Fracture of the scaphoid (evident on radiographs)

Ganglion (discrete mass, normal radiographs)

Scapholunate dissociation (increased distance between the scaphoid and lunate on radiographs)

Tenosynovitis of the extensor tendon (diffuse swelling over extensor tendon extending onto the hand)

Wrist arthritis (narrowing of joint space but normal contour of lunate)

## ADVERSE OUTCOMES OF THE DISEASE

Untreated Kienböck disease can result in progressive arthritis.

## TREATMENT

When radiographs are normal, or when the lunate shows significant sclerosis, splint the wrist in a neutral position for 3 weeks. NSAIDs may make the patient more comfortable. If the pain persists after 3 weeks, further evaluation is indicated.

## ADVERSE OUTCOMES OF TREATMENT

Loss of motion, chronic pain, and decreased grip strength are possible.

## REFERRAL DECISIONS/RED FLAGS

Patients whose plain radiographs show any abnormality of the lunate need further evaluation. Persistent dorsal wrist pain, despite 3 weeks of immobilization, also is an indication for further evaluation.

SECTION 4 ■ HAND AND WRIST

# MALLET FINGER

**ICD-9 Code**

**736.1**
Mallet finger

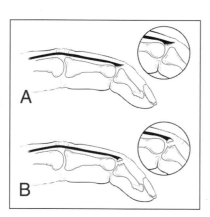

**Figure 1**

Mallet finger caused by rupture of the extensor tendon at its insertion (**A**); mallet finger caused by avulsion of a piece of distal phalanx (**B**).

Adapted with permission from Rockwood CA, Green D P, Bucholz RW, et al (eds): *Rockwood and Green's Fractures in Adults*, ed 4. Philadelphia, PA, Lippincott- Raven, 1996, vol 2, p 617.

## SYNONYMS
Baseball finger
Terminal extensor tendon rupture

## DEFINITION
A mallet finger deformity is caused by rupture, laceration, or avulsion of the insertion of the extensor tendon at the base of the distal phalanx. Sometimes, instead of the tendon tearing, the injury avulses a fragment of the distal phalanx at the tendinous attachment (**Figure 1**).

## CLINICAL SYMPTOMS
Patients report pain and an inability to straighten the fingertip.

## TESTS

### Physical Examination
Examination reveals that the distal interphalangeal (DIP) joint is in flexion and that the patient is unable to actively extend the joint although it can be passively extended. The dorsal area of the DIP joint initially is tender and slightly swollen, but about 2 weeks after the injury occurs, the fingertip usually is not painful.

## DIAGNOSTIC TESTS
A lateral radiograph may reveal a small bony avulsion from the dorsal side of the distal phalanx. With large dorsal avulsion fragments, the distal phalanx may subluxate volarly from the unopposed pull of the flexor tendon.

## DIFFERENTIAL DIAGNOSIS
Fracture of the distal phalanx (evident on radiographs)
Fracture-dislocation of the DIP joint (evident on radiographs)

## ADVERSE OUTCOMES OF THE DISEASE
Permanent flexion of the DIP joint is possible.

# TREATMENT

Continuous splinting of the DIP joint in extension is critical to restoring full function of the extensor tendon. The splint can be applied on either the volar or the dorsal surface of the finger (**Figure 2**). With acute injuries, the splint should be worn for 6 weeks. If the injury is more than 3 months old, a splint should be worn for at least 8 weeks.

Advise patients to maintain the DIP joint in extension when the splint is removed for cleaning. If the fingertip droops at any time after the splint is applied, the healing process is disrupted and the period of splinting must be extended. Four or five days after the splint is applied, check the dorsal skin for maceration or pressure spots. If the joint does not come into full extension by the second visit, the patient should be evaluated for possible surgical pinning.

Visits every 2 to 3 weeks are helpful to monitor progress and usually lead to a better outcome than if the splint is applied and the patient is not seen again until 6 to 8 weeks later. At the end of the splinting period, if no extensor lag is evident, guarded active flexion is started, with splinting continued at night for 2 to 4 weeks.

Certain occupations (eg, cooking, dishwashing, typing) make splint wear difficult, and patients doing these tasks repeatedly should be evaluated for possible surgical pinning.

# ADVERSE OUTCOMES OF TREATMENT

Persistent deformity associated with flexion of the fingertip is possible, despite treatment.

# REFERRAL DECISIONS/RED FLAGS

Patients with volar subluxation of the distal phalanx and/or an avulsed bony fragment that involves more than one third of the joint surface need further evaluation.

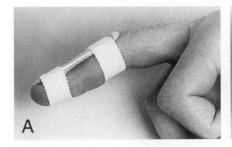
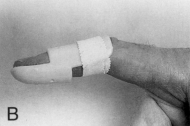

**Figure 2**

Types of splints used in treatment of mallet finger. **A,** Dorsal aluminum splint; **B,** commercial splint.

Reproduced from Culver JE Jr: Office management of athletic injuries of the hand and wrist. *Instr Course Lect* 1989;38:473-482.

SECTION 4 ■ HAND AND WRIST

# Nail Bed Injuries

**ICD-9 Code**

**883.0**
Open wound of finger(s) without
mention of complication

## Synonyms
Smashed finger
Subungual hematoma

## Definition
Many injuries to the fingertip are crushing in nature, resulting
in various degrees of injury to the fingernail, nail bed, and
distal phalanx (**Figure 1**). The types of nail bed injuries include
simple lacerations, stellate lacerations, severe crush injuries, and
avulsions. Approximately 50% are associated with fractures of
the distal phalanx.

## Clinical Symptoms
Patients usually have pain and obvious injury to the fingertip.

## Tests

### Physical Examination
Determine the extent of the injury, noting any subungual
hematoma and its extent, avulsion or laceration of the nail, and
whether an associated fracture of the distal phalanx is displaced
or nondisplaced. When the fingernail is avulsed, note the extent
of injury to the nail bed (both germinal and sterile matrices).
Examine the fingernail for attached remnants of the nail bed.
An avulsion of the fingernail in a child or infant may be
associated with a physeal injury, in which case referral to a
specialist is indicated.

### Diagnostic Tests
PA and lateral radiographs of the finger are necessary when a
fracture of the distal phalanx is suspected.

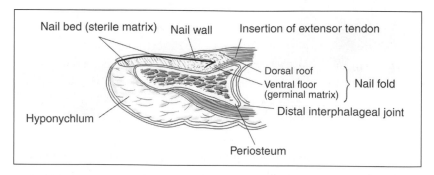

**Figure 1**
Anatomy of the nail bed of the finger: Sagittal view.

# DIFFERENTIAL DIAGNOSIS

Mallet finger (unable to fully extend the distal interphalangeal joint)

# ADVERSE OUTCOMES OF THE DISEASE

If the patient has sustained damage to the nail bed, particularly the germinal matrix, a permanent nail deformity may result.

# TREATMENT

## Subungual Hematomas

Painful subungual hematomas can be treated with decompression. After scrubbing the finger and applying a disinfectant, create a hole in the fingernail over the hematoma, using battery-operated microcautery, if available, or a heated paper clip or 18-gauge needle. The hole must be large enough to allow continued drainage. Penetrate only through the nail and avoid perforating too deeply into the nail bed, as this is extremely painful and may result in scarring of the nail bed.

## Nail Bed Lacerations

For lacerations of the nail bed with injury to the nail plate, the nail plate should be removed and the nail bed repaired. This should be done with adequate anesthesia (see Digital Anesthetic Block [Hand], pp 336-337), with sterile preparation of the finger, and the use of a finger tourniquet. Elevate all or part of the nail plate using a small scissors. The entire nail can be removed or just enough to allow visualization of the laceration and suture placement. Irrigate the wound, remove the hematoma, and meticulously suture the nail bed using No. 6-0 or 7-0 bioabsorbable gut suture. After repair, stent the nail fold open by placing some xeroform gauze or a piece of a red rubber catheter into the nail fold. This gauze can be left in place because it will grow out with the new nail. An associated minimally displaced or nondisplaced fracture usually will be stabilized with the repair.

## Nail Avulsions

The proximal portion of the nail bed (germinal matrix) may be avulsed and lying on top of the nail fold (**Figure 2**). This must be replaced underneath the nail fold and sutured in place. The sutures should be placed through the proximal fold to pull the nail bed into the fold. If the nail avulsion is associated with a fracture, the distal phalanx may need to be stabilized. Any nail bed tissue adherent to the fingernail should be gently removed with a scalpel and sewn in place in the nail bed defect using small bioabsorbable suture. A large fragment of nail or the

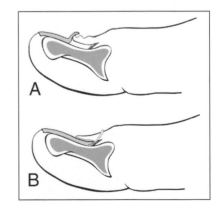

**Figure 2**
Nail avulsion. **A,** The proximal portion of the nail bed (germinal matrix) is avulsed and is lying on top of the nail fold.
**B,** Replacement of the germinal matrix into the nail fold.

SECTION 4 ■ HAND AND WRIST

whole nail itself, when it has a large amount of nail bed still attached to it, should not have the tissue removed; rather, sew the entire fragment anatomically in place. Any injuries to the nail fold should be repaired with No. 5-0 gut, nylon, or monofilament suture. Injuries in children should be repaired with bioabsorbable sutures.

## Wound Care

The finger should be dressed with antibacterial ointment, nonadherent gauze, sterile gauze, and an outer wrap. The finger should be splinted for protection.

# ADVERSE OUTCOMES OF TREATMENT

Abnormal growth and subsequent deformity of the nail can occur.

# REFERRAL DECISIONS/RED FLAGS

Nail bed injuries with complex lacerations or loss of tissue or injury to the germinal matrix may require more involved surgical treatment. Associated open fractures of the distal phalanx require further evaluation.

# PROCEDURE

## FISHHOOK REMOVAL

Retrograde extraction of a fishhook is difficult because of the barb (**Figure 1**). Most fishhook injuries involve the skin and subcutaneous tissues only. Although many techniques of fishhook removal have been described, only two are discussed here (**Figures 2** and **3**). Remember to wear protective gloves at all times during this procedure and use sterile technique.

### TECHNIQUE 1

#### STEP 1
Cleanse the skin with a bactericidal skin preparation solution.

#### STEP 2
Use a 27-gauge needle to infiltrate the skin with 2 to 3 mL of 1% local anesthetic.

#### STEP 3
Grasp the exposed end of the hook (shank) with the thumb and index finger and rotate the hook to force the barb out through the skin.

#### STEP 4
Cut the barbed end of the hook with a wire cutter.

#### STEP 5
Remove the rest of the hook retrograde. It will back out easily once the barb is gone.

#### STEP 6
Apply a topical antibiotic and a sterile bandage to the wound.

**CPT Code**

Appropriate E/M CPT Code (if no incision is used to remove fishhook)

**10120**
Incision and removal of foreign body, subcutaneous tissues; simple (if incision is used to remove fishhook)

*Current Procedural Terminology* © 2004 **American Medical Association. All Rights Reserved.**

### MATERIALS

Sterile gloves

Bactericidal skin preparation solution

24″ length of No. 0 or No. 1 nylon or silk suture

3-mL syringe with a 27-gauge needle

3 mL of a 1% local anesthetic without epinephrine

Wire cutter

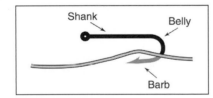

**Figure 1**
Embedded fishhook with parts labeled.

SECTION 4 ■ HAND AND WRIST

# FISHHOOK REMOVAL (CONTINUED)

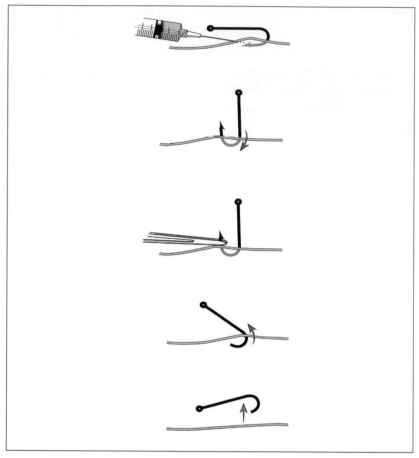

**Figure 2**

Technique 1 for removing a fishhook, in which the barb is removed and the hook is pushed out through the skin.

Adapted with permission from Quadrant HealthCom, Barnett RC: Removal of fish hooks. *Hosp Med* 1980;16:56 57. Copyright © 1980 Quadrant HealthCom, Inc.

## TECHNIQUE 2

### STEP 1
Cleanse the skin with a bactericidal skin preparation solution.

### STEP 2
Inject 2 to 3 mL of 1% local anesthetic about the hook.

### STEP 3
Loop a size No. 0 or No. 1 nylon or silk suture around the belly of the hook at the point where it penetrates the skin.

# FISHHOOK REMOVAL (CONTINUED)

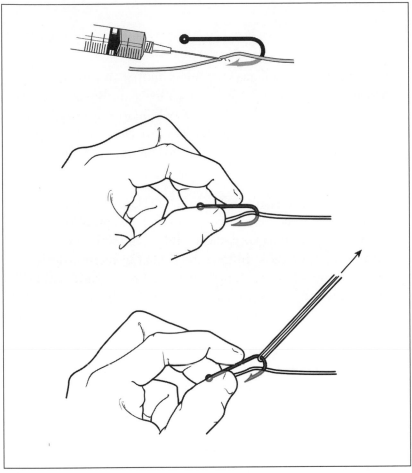

**Figure 3**
Technique 2 for removing a fishhook, in which the barb is pulled out.
**Adapted with permission from Quadrant HealthCom, Barnett RC: Removal of fish hooks.** *Hosp Med*
**1980;16:56-57. Copyright © 1980 Quadrant HealthCom, Inc.**

*STEP 4*
Grasp the shank of the hook with your left thumb and long
finger and press against the skin. At the same time, press
gently downward on the belly of the hook with the left index
finger to disengage the barb from the surrounding tissues.

*STEP 5*
With your right hand, grasp the suture 10″ to 12″ from the
hook and pull sharply to remove the hook. Caution is advised
because the hook often disengages with considerable velocity.

*STEP 6*
Dress the wound with a sterile adhesive bandage.

# FISHHOOK REMOVAL (CONTINUED)

## ADVERSE OUTCOMES

Use of the first technique may inflict further soft-tissue damage by pushing the barb through the skin. Breakage of the hook or infection is possible. Fishhook injuries usually occur in a marine environment and can be associated with unusual infections (vibrio species, atypical mycobacterial organisms).

## AFTERCARE/PATIENT INSTRUCTIONS

Check whether the patient has current tetanus prophylaxis. Advise the patient to keep the wound clean until it is healed, usually in 3 to 4 days. Instruct the patient to return to your office if redness, fever, or proximal swelling occur. Consider the prophylactic administration of an oral cephalosporin.

# SPRAINS AND DISLOCATIONS OF THE HAND

## SYNONYMS

Gamekeeper's thumb
Jammed finger
Skier's thumb
Sprain

**ICD-9 Codes**

**834.00**
Dislocation of finger or thumb, closed, unspecified site

**842.10**
Sprains and strains of hand, unspecified site

## DEFINITION

Sprains of the fingers are common injuries characterized by a partial or complete tear of a collateral ligament and/or volar capsular ligament (**Figure 1**). Most sprains of the fingers are relatively straightforward injuries that can be managed nonsurgically. The exception is rupture of the ulnar collateral ligament of the thumb metacarpophalangeal (MP) joint, which usually requires surgical treatment.

The ulnar collateral ligament of the thumb MP joint is an important stabilizer of the thumb. When this ligament is torn, the thumb deviates outward when the thumb is stressed in a radial direction (**Figure 2**). The name "gamekeeper's thumb" derives from the chronic injury observed in English gamekeepers as a result of their method of killing rabbits. Today, a frequent cause of this injury is forced abduction of the thumb against a ski pole (skier's thumb); however, the injury also occurs during ball-playing sports or from a fall.

Most dislocations in the hand are hyperextension injuries that result from a complete tear of the volar capsule that usually results in dorsal displacement of the distal element. Dislocation is most common at the proximal interphalangeal (PIP) joint. Dorsal dislocations of the MP joint are either simple or complex. The latter is associated with interposition of the volar plate between the metacarpal head and the proximal phalanx (**Figure 3**). Complex dislocations (involving any of the fingers) may require open reduction.

## CLINICAL SYMPTOMS

Patients almost always report a history of trauma and acute onset of pain. With a gamekeeper's thumb, pain and swelling is localized to the inside (ulnar aspect) of the thumb MP joint. With a dislocation, patients describe a deformity that developed immediately after the injury. The patient or a well-meaning friend may have reduced or attempted to reduce a dislocation before the patient seeks medical attention.

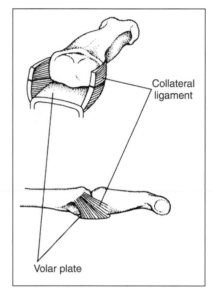

**Figure 1**
Collateral ligaments and volar plates of the PIP joint.

Reproduced with permission from American Society for Surgery of the Hand: *The Hand: Examination and Diagnosis*, ed 3. New York, NY, Churchill Livingstone, p 54.

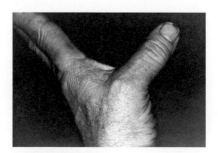

**Figure 2**
Clinical appearance of ulnar collateral ligament tear.

SECTION 4 ■ HAND AND WRIST

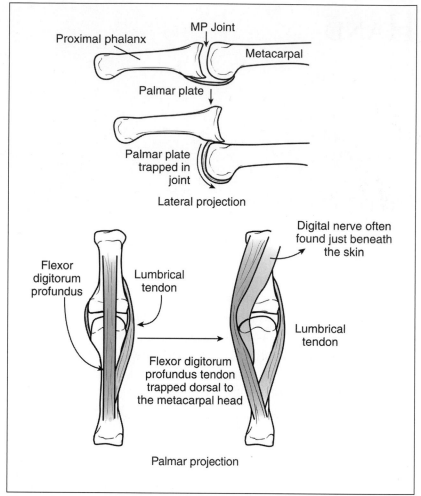

**Figure 3**

Complex dislocation of the MP joint. The lateral projection shows the palmar (volar) plate trapped in the joint. The palmar projection shows the flexor digitorum profundus tendon trapped dorsal to the metacarpal head.

Reproduced with permission from the American Society for Surgery of the Hand: *Hand Surgery Update.* Rosemont, IL, American Academy of Orthopaedic Surgeons, 1994.

# TESTS

### *Physical Examination*

If the joint is swollen but not grossly deformed, palpate both sides of the joint for tenderness over the collateral ligaments (**Figure 4**). Radiographs should be obtained to rule out fractures. If there is no fracture, then joint stability should be tested by applying medial and lateral stresses to the joint (**Figure 5**). If the finger angulates easily under stress, it indicates a complete tear of the collateral ligament; if the patient has pain with stress testing but no instability, assume there has been a sprain.

Dislocations usually are obvious on inspection. Complex dislocations of the MP joint are characterized by fixed

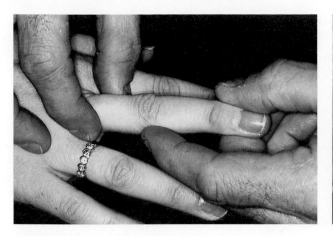

**Figure 4**
Palpation of the collateral ligaments.

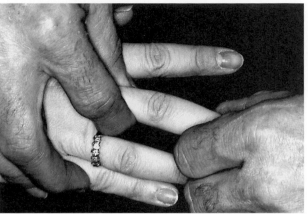

**Figure 5**
Applying medial and lateral stresses to the PIP joint.

displacement of the distal segment. Usually, complex dislocations occur at the MP joint and are characterized by a palmar prominence of the metacarpal head and angulation and dorsal displacement of the proximal phalanx. Patients with complex MP dislocations have limited active flexion.

### Diagnostic Tests

AP and lateral radiographs are necessary to rule out a fracture or a fracture-dislocation (**Figure 6**).

## DIFFERENTIAL DIAGNOSIS

Extensor tendon rupture (boutonnière deformity, inability to extend the PIP joint)

Fracture (evident on radiographs)

## ADVERSE OUTCOMES OF THE DISEASE

Limited motion, stiffness, chronic pain, and swelling may persist. Chronic hyperextension of the PIP joint or flexion contracture can occur.

## TREATMENT

Most sprains of the collateral ligaments can be treated with splinting. The exception is an unstable, complete rupture of the ulnar collateral ligament of the thumb MP joint. These injuries may require surgical stabilization because interposition of the adductor pollicis tendon between the end of the ulnar collateral ligament and the base of the proximal phalanx prevents adequate repair of the avulsed ligament.

Nonsurgical treatment for sprains and dislocations focuses on relocation of the joint and protection of the reduction with splinting. Reduction of a dorsal dislocation of the PIP is usually

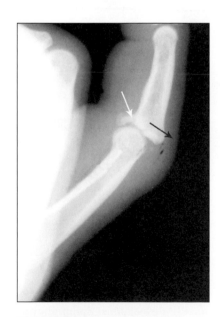

**Figure 6**
Lateral view of finger shows fracture-dislocation of the PIP joint: dorsal translation of the middle phalanx (black arrow) associated with a complex fracture of the base of the middle phalanx (white arrow).

SECTION 4 ■ HAND AND WRIST

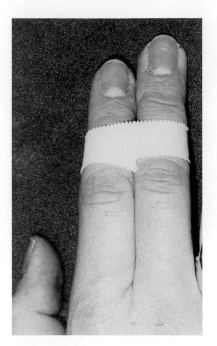

**Figure 7**
Buddy taping.

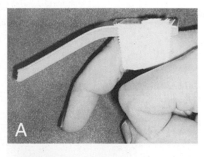

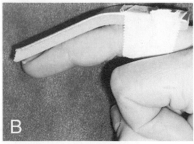

**Figure 8**
**A,** Dorsal extension block splint for PIP dislocations. Splint allows flexion (**A**) but blocks the last 20° to 30° of extension (**B**), preventing excessive motion of the volar plate.

done with axial traction and flexion of the proximal phalanx (see below). Buddy taping to an adjacent finger is effective treatment for collateral ligament injuries in the finger joints (**Figure 7**). Complete rupture of the volar plate, associated with dorsal dislocation, is treated by splinting the joint in 20° to 30° of flexion for 2 to 3 weeks or using buddy taping and early motion. Incomplete tears of the ulnar collateral ligament of the thumb MP joint can be treated in a thumb spica cast with the thumb slightly flexed for 2 to 4 weeks. The duration of treatment is based on subsequent clinical examination and radiographs.

Closed reduction of a PIP or distal interphalangeal (DIP) joint dislocation should be done under a digital block anesthetic (see Digital Anesthetic Block [Hand], pp 336-337). To reduce the dislocation, grasp the distal portion of the finger and apply longitudinal traction while stabilizing the finger or hand proximal to the dislocation. Apply gentle pressure over the dorsum of the deformity to guide the reduction. After reduction, move the finger through a range of motion and then assess collateral ligament stability. If the joint seems stable, the finger can be buddy taped. If the joint has full range of motion after the reduction but tends to dislocate during the last 20° of extension, apply a dorsal extension block splint to allow healing of the volar plate (**Figure 8**). This type of splint blocks the last 20° to 30° of extension. Use the splint for 2 to 3 weeks, then buddy tape the finger to an adjacent finger for an additional 3 weeks.

The relocation of MP joint dislocations may require regional nerve blocks. If the dislocation cannot be reduced with adequate anesthesia, soft tissue could be interposed, and open reduction may be necessary (**Figure 9**).

DIP dislocations are typically dorsal or dorsolateral. With open injuries, suspect an associated tear of the extensor tendon. After adequate digital block anesthesia, apply longitudinal traction to reduce the dislocation. Open dislocations need appropriate débridement and irrigation but tend to be stable after reduction. Next, apply a dorsal aluminum splint over the middle and distal phalanges for 1 to 2 weeks. If the fingertip droops after the reduction and the patient cannot actively extend the distal phalanx, treat the injury as a mallet finger. Carefully examine the flexor digitorum profundus tendon after relocation for discomfort on DIP flexion. Some patients can have a significant partial flexor digitorum profundus injury following dorsal dislocation of the DIP joint.

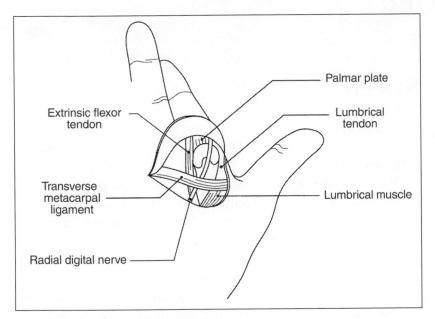

**Figure 9**
Entrapment of the metacarpal head between the lumbrical and extrinsic flexor tendon.

Reproduced with permission from the American Society for Surgery of the Hand: *Hand Surgery Update.* Rosemont, IL, American Academy of Orthopaedic Surgeons, 1994, p 22.

## ADVERSE OUTCOMES OF TREATMENT

Instability, joint stiffness, persistent hyperextension deformity, and/or residual flexion deformity can develop. Arthritis also may develop with an inadequate reduction.

## REFERRAL DECISIONS/RED FLAGS

Patients with an unstable thumb MP joint (suggestive of complete ulnar collateral ligament injury) need further evaluation for possible surgical stabilization. Patients whose dislocations cannot be reduced easily with digital anesthesia are candidates for open reduction. In addition, patients with fracture-dislocations and open dislocations need further evaluation. Open dislocations are best treated surgically to achieve adequate débridement and repair.

# TRIGGER FINGER

## SYNONYMS

Locked finger
Stenosing tenosynovitis of the flexor tendons

## DEFINITION

The flexor tendons of the fingers glide back and forth under four annular and three cruciform pulleys that keep the tendons from bowstringing. The flexor tendon or first annular pulley may become thickened and narrowed from chronic inflammation and irritation. As a result, motion of the tendon is limited and the finger may snap or lock during flexion of the finger or thumb (**Figure 1**). The long and ring fingers are most commonly affected, but any digit may be involved.

Trigger finger may be idiopathic or associated with rheumatoid arthritis or diabetes mellitus. The idiopathic type is more often observed in middle-aged women. A higher prevalence of trigger finger is observed in patients with carpal tunnel syndrome and de Quervain stenosing tenosynovitis.

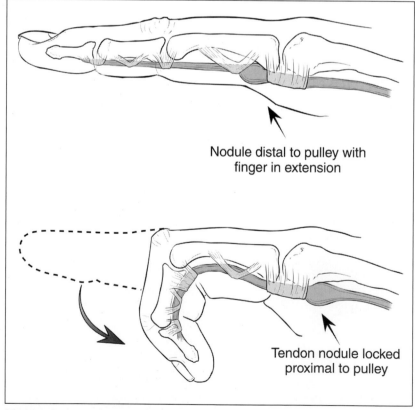

Nodule distal to pulley with finger in extension

Tendon nodule locked proximal to pulley

**Figure 1**
Nodule or thickening in flexor tendon, which strikes the proximal pulley, making finger extension difficult.

## CLINICAL SYMPTOMS

Patients typically report pain and catching when they flex the finger and may describe the finger as going "out of joint." They may awaken with the finger locked in the palm, although the finger gradually unlocks during the day. The proximal interphalangeal (PIP) joint may be identified as the source of the pain, but the stenosis is at the level of the metacarpophalangeal (MP) joint. Some patients have a painful nodule in the distal palm, usually at the level of the distal flexion crease, with no history of triggering. Other patients' only symptoms are swelling and/or stiffness in the fingers, particularly in the morning. In patients with rheumatoid arthritis or diabetes mellitus, several fingers may be involved.

## TESTS

### Physical Examination

Examination reveals tenderness in the palm at the level of the distal palmar crease, usually overlying the MP joint. A nodule also may be palpable at this site. The nodule moves, and the finger may lock when the patient flexes and extends the affected finger. This maneuver is almost always painful for the patient. Full flexion of the finger may not be possible.

### Diagnostic Tests

This is a clinical diagnosis; radiographs are not needed.

## DIFFERENTIAL DIAGNOSIS

Anomalous muscle belly in the palm (swelling more proximal in the palm)

Diabetes mellitus (single and multiple trigger fingers)

Dupuytren disease (palpable cord)

Ganglion of the tendon sheath (tendon mass at the base of the finger that does not move with flexion)

Rheumatoid arthritis (multiple joint involvement)

## ADVERSE OUTCOMES OF THE DISEASE

Flexion contracture of the PIP joint or stiffness in extension may develop.

## TREATMENT

Initial treatment may involve a short course of NSAIDs or injection of corticosteroid into the tendon sheath (see Trigger Finger Injection, pp 391-392). Care must be exercised to avoid injecting the tendon, as corticosteroid injected into a tendon may predispose it to rupture. If symptoms persist, a second injection in 3 to 4 weeks is indicated. However, because patients with rheumatoid disease are already at increased risk for tendon rupture, only one injection is indicated for these patients before surgical release should be considered. If two injections fail to resolve the trigger finger, surgical release should be considered.

## ADVERSE OUTCOMES OF TREATMENT

NSAIDs can cause gastric, renal, or hepatic complications. Repeated corticosteroid injections might lead to rupture of the flexor tendon and also may injure the digital sensory nerve. Infection also is a risk. In patients with diabetes mellitus, steroid injections may increase blood glucose levels.

## REFERRAL DECISIONS/RED FLAGS

Failure of nonsurgical treatment, development of contractures in the PIP joint, and/or a locked finger (in flexion or extension) indicate a need for further evaluation. Patients with rheumatoid arthritis whose problem does not resolve after a single injection also need additional evaluation. Patients with type 1 diabetes mellitus who do not tolerate steroid injection require specialty evaluation.

# Procedure

## Trigger Finger Injection

The flexor tendons pass beneath a pulley situated just distal to the distal palmar crease. Palpating this area as the patient flexes and extends the finger reveals a click or snapping sensation as the enlarged tendon passes beneath the pulley.

**Note:** Opinions differ regarding single- and two-needle injection techniques. Proponents of the single-needle technique believe that one needle is less painful for the patient than two. Because the corticosteroid preparation is thicker than the local anesthetic, however, a slightly larger gauge needle is required at the outset. The DVD uses a two-needle, two-syringe technique.

### Step 1

Wear protective gloves at all times during this procedure and use sterile technique.

### Step 2

Cleanse the palm with a bactericidal skin preparation solution.

### Step 3

Identify the lump on the tendon and infiltrate the skin at the distal palmar crease, which directly overlies the tendon, and inject the anesthetic at that level.

### Step 4

Inject 0.5 mL of a 1% anesthetic solution into the subcutaneous tissue, then advance the needle into the tendon sheath and inject the rest of the anesthetic (**Figure 1**). Continue to insert the needle as the patient moves the affected finger through a small arc of flexion and extension. When the needle touches the moving tendon, the patient will experience a scratchy sensation. If the needle moves, it has penetrated the tendon and should be partially withdrawn until the scratchy sensation occurs. At this point, the needle tip is inside the tendon sheath but external to the tendon.

### Step 5

Leave the needle in place, change syringes, and then inject the corticosteroid preparation.

### Step 6

Check the finger for filling of the tendon sheath with the solution.

### Step 7

Dress the puncture wound with a sterile adhesive bandage.

**CPT Code**

**20550**

Injection(s); single tendon sheath, or ligament, aponeurosis (eg, plantar "fascia")

*Current Procedural Terminology* © 2004 **American Medical Association. All Rights Reserved.**

## MATERIALS

Sterile gloves

Bactericidal skin preparation solution

2 to 3 mL of a 1% local anesthetic without epinephrine

Two 3-mL syringes with a 25-gauge needle

1 mL of a corticosteroid preparation

Adhesive dressing

SECTION 4 ■ HAND AND WRIST

# TRIGGER FINGER INJECTION (CONTINUED)

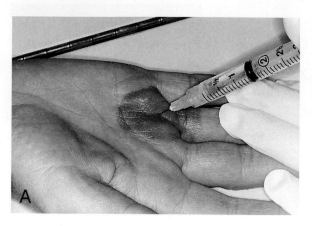
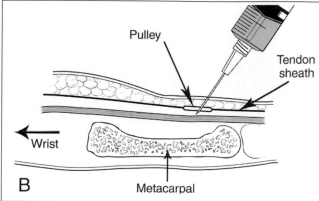

**Figure 1**
**A,** Location for needle insertion for trigger finger injection. **B,** Proper positioning of the needle, through the pulley and into the tendon sheath.

## ADVERSE OUTCOMES

Injection of corticosteroid into the subcutaneous tissues may lead to depigmentation and/or local fat atrophy, resulting in a tender, unsightly depression beneath the skin.

## AFTERCARE/PATIENT INSTRUCTIONS

Advise the patient of possible significant discomfort for 1 to 2 days following any injection of a corticosteroid. Also, the finger may be numb for 1 to 2 hours until the local anesthetic wears off. Instruct the patient to return to your office if swelling, redness, or inordinate pain occurs. The patient should be able to use the finger in a normal fashion after the injection.

# TUMORS OF THE HAND AND WRIST

## DEFINITION

Most tumors in the hand and wrist are benign, with primary malignant tumors and skeletal metastases accounting for less than 1% of these neoplasms. Ganglia are the most common benign soft-tissue tumors, followed by giant cell tumors and epidermal inclusion cysts. Enchondromas are the most common benign neoplasm of the bones of the hand, accounting for 90% of all cases. Squamous cell carcinomas are the most common malignant neoplasm of the hand, and chondrosarcomas are the most common primary malignant bone tumor in the hand. Malignant melanomas are frequently seen in the upper extremity because of the exposure of the arm to sun.

## CLINICAL SYMPTOMS

Many tumors of the hand are painless. The exception is a glomus tumor, which characteristically is extremely painful and sensitive to cold. Enchondromas present with pain after a patient sustains a pathologic fracture through the weakened bone. Lipomas can cause pain and numbness in the fingers if the lesion is compressing an adjacent nerve. Masses located near joints can cause loss of motion.

## TESTS

### Physical Examination

Note the position, size, and characteristics of the mass (**Figures 1** and **2**). These factors help to narrow the diagnostic possibilities.

A ganglion cyst is characterized as a mass located over the dorsal or volar radial aspect of the wrist, the flexion crease of the finger at the level of the web space, or over the top of the distal interphalangeal joint of the finger.

Epidermal inclusion cysts typically occur around the end of the finger (thumb and long) or at the end of an amputation stump. Pressing a small flashlight against an inclusion cyst will not transilluminate the mass, but this same maneuver will transilluminate a ganglion cyst.

A giant cell tumor is characterized by a multinodular, firm, nontender mass located around an interphalangeal joint, usually of the thumb or the index or long finger.

A blue or red area visible under the fingernail could be a glomus tumor, subungual hematoma, or foreign body. However, subungual discoloration in the absence of trauma should raise a

SECTION 4 ■ HAND AND WRIST

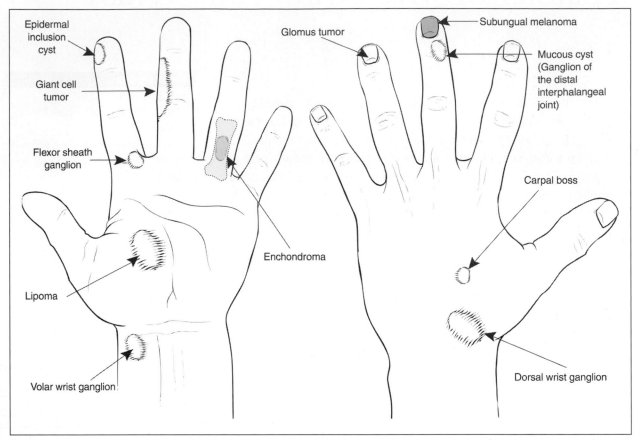

**Figure 1**

Typical locations and types of benign hand tumors.

suspicion of melanoma. Likewise, a mole (nevus) that changes shape or color can indicate a malignant melanoma.

Lipomas typically are superficial, soft, reasonably well defined, and nontender on palpation. A frequent location in the hand is the thenar eminence. When lipomas are located on the palmar surface of the wrist, compression of the median or ulnar nerve may occur.

Recurrent paronychia infections and chronic nail deformities can be caused by underlying squamous cell carcinoma. A diagnosis of Kaposi sarcoma should be suspected in a patient with AIDS who develops skin nodules or red-brown plaques.

A symptomatic enchondroma is characterized by tenderness and swelling over the involved phalanx (usually the proximal). A pathologic fracture may be present.

A carpal boss is a dorsal prominence at the base of the third metacarpal or second metacarpal. These dorsal osteophytes may be confused with a neoplasm. A ganglion is sometimes associated with a carpal boss.

## Diagnostic Tests

PA and lateral radiographs of the involved finger or PA, lateral, and oblique views of the hand should be obtained.

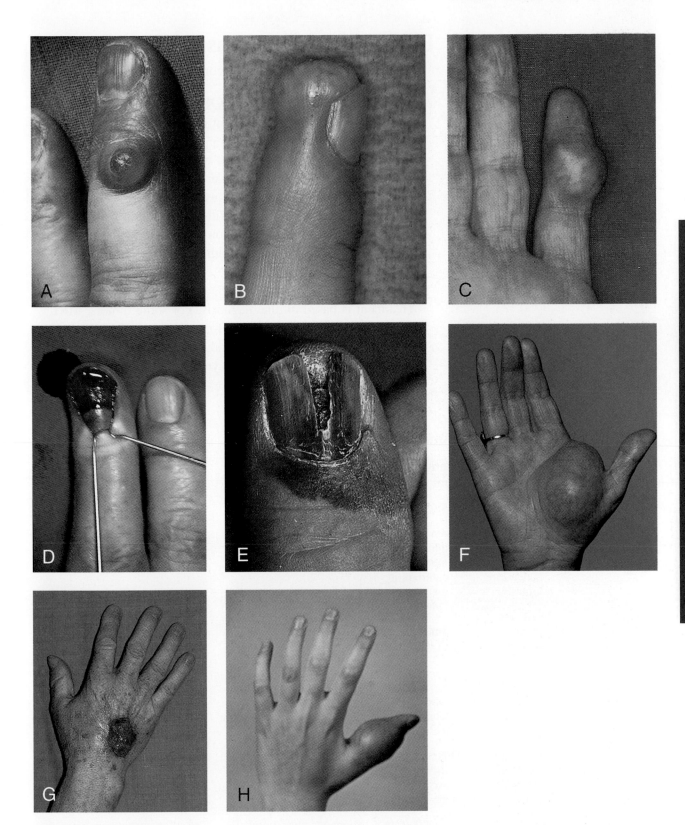

**Figure 2**

Clinical appearance of various hand tumors. **A,** Ganglion (mucous) cyst. **B,** Epidermoid cyst. **C,** Giant cell tumor. **D,** Glomus tumor. **E,** Melanoma. **F,** Lipoma. **G,** Squamous cell carcinoma. **H,** Enchondroma.

(Reproduced from Evers B, Klammer HL: Tumors and tumorlike lesions of the hand. *Arch Am Acad Orthop Surg* 1997;1:37-42.)

SECTION 4 ■ HAND AND WRIST

## DIFFERENTIAL DIAGNOSIS

See **Table 1** and Figure 1 for a complete listing.

## ADVERSE OUTCOMES OF THE DISEASE

Ganglia can result in limited joint motion. Nail changes, skin atrophy, and infection can develop as a result of a mucoid cyst. Drainage is a problem associated with epidermal mucoid cysts. Patients with giant cell tumors can have limited tendon function because of peritendinous adhesions. Nerve compression can develop as a result of lipoma. With an enchondroma, fracture can occur. Squamous cell carcinomas and malignant melanoma can metastasize and result in death.

## TREATMENT

Treatment is based on the diagnosis. For some tumors, MRI will add significant additional information regarding the nature of the mass. Surgical excision and histologic examination are required for most expanding or symptomatic masses.

### Table 1   Common Benign Tumors of the Hand and Wrist

| Type of Tumor* | Common Location(s) | Patient Age and Gender | Signs and Symptoms | Radiographic Findings |
|---|---|---|---|---|
| Ganglion cyst (See Ganglia of the Wrist and Hand, pp 362-366) | | | | |
| Epidermal inclusion cyst | Fingertip or anywhere from penetrating injury | Teens to middle age; more common in men | Painless, slow growing; does not transilluminate | Round soft-tissue mass, also in distal phalanx |
| Giant cell tumor of tendon sheath | Digits on palmar surface | > 30 years; ratio of men to women 2:3 | Slowly enlarging painless mass | 20% show cortical erosion |
| Glomus tumor | 50% occur under fingernail | 30 to 50 years; ratio of women to men 2:1 | Triad of symptoms: marked pain, cold intolerance, very tender, blue discoloration of nail | Some show erosion on lateral view |
| Lipoma | Thenar area in palm and first web space | 30 to 60 years; slight predominance in women | Painless, slow growing; might cause nerve entrapment | No bony involvement, soft-tissue mass |
| Enchondroma | In proximal phalanges or metacarpals | 10 to 60 years; affects men and women equally | Might become painful after trauma because of fracture | Radiolucent expansive lesion, cortex thin, fracture and areas of calcification possibly visible |

*See Figure 1.

## ADVERSE OUTCOMES OF TREATMENT

Ganglia recur at the same site in 5% to 10% of patients. The recurrence rate of giant cell tumors is relatively high after surgical excision. Joint stiffness can develop after treatment of pathologic fractures caused by enchondromas.

## REFERRAL DECISIONS/RED FLAGS

Patients with a painful or expanding mass, one that interferes with function, or one believed to be malignant need further evaluation. Pigmented subungual lesions should be referred for evaluation.

SECTION 4 ■ HAND AND WRIST

# Ulnar Nerve Entrapment at the Wrist

**ICD-9 Code**

**354.2**
Lesion of ulnar nerve

SECTION 4 ■ HAND AND WRIST

## Synonym
Ulnar tunnel syndrome

## Definition
Entrapment of the ulnar nerve at the wrist usually is caused by a space-occupying lesion such as a lipoma, ganglion, ulnar artery aneurysm, or muscle anomaly (**Figure 1**). Repetitive trauma, such as operating a jackhammer or using the base of the hand as a hammer, also may cause ulnar neuropathy at the wrist. Ulnar nerve entrapment at the wrist is less common than ulnar nerve entrapment at the elbow.

## Clinical Symptoms
Patients may or may not have pain, but they often report weakness and numbness.

## Tests

### Physical Examination
Inspect the hypothenar eminence for atrophy. Assess sensory and motor function of the ulnar nerve. In some patients, only the motor branch of the ulnar nerve may be affected, sparing the sensory branches; however, with sensory involvement, tapping over the ulnar nerve in the hypothenar region will produce tingling in the ring and little fingers (Tinel sign).

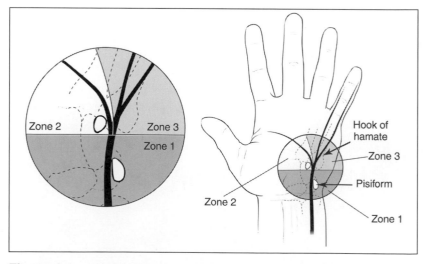

**Figure 1**
Distal ulnar tunnel showing the three zones of entrapment. Lesions in zone 1 cause both motor and sensory symptoms; lesions in zone 2 cause motor deficits; and lesions in zone 3 create sensory deficits.

Sensation over the dorsal and ulnar aspects of the hand is normal. When the ulnar nerve is involved at the elbow, almost all patients will have both sensory and motor involvement, with numbness over the dorsal and ulnar sides of the hand. Motor weakness is detected by atrophy of the hypothenar and intrinsic muscles or weakness of the intrinsic muscles (finger spreaders) (**Figure 2**).

### Diagnostic Tests

Results of electrophysiologic studies may be abnormal and may differentiate ulnar entrapment at the wrist from the more common entrapment at the elbow.

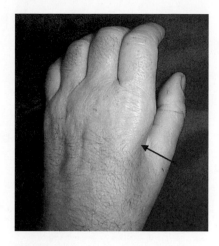

**Figure 2**
Intrinsic muscle wasting indicative of ulnar nerve entrapment at the wrist.

# DIFFERENTIAL DIAGNOSIS

Carpal tunnel syndrome (usually involves the thumb and index, long and ring fingers)

Cervical (C7-C8) radiculopathy (more proximal muscle involvement, numbness on the dorsum of the hand)

Peripheral neuropathy (from diabetes, alcoholism, or hypothyroidism; more generalized numbness)

Thoracic outlet syndrome (symptoms more diffuse)

Ulnar artery thrombosis in the hand (positive Allen test, firm cord on the ulnar side of the hand)

Ulnar neuropathy at the elbow (sensory changes on the dorsum of the hand)

Wrist arthritis (pain, limited motion, evident on radiographs)

# ADVERSE OUTCOMES OF THE DISEASE

Loss of intrinsic muscle function causes decreased grip strength and pinch. Sensory loss, when present, involves the ring and little fingers. In advanced disease, clawing of the ring and little fingers can develop.

# TREATMENT

Because the usual cause of ulnar entrapment at the wrist is extrinsic compression (because of a lipoma, ganglion, or tumor, for example), treatment is usually surgical. When the obvious cause is external pressure, such as resting the hypothenar area on a keyboard or desk, then use of padding or a change in position could help.

# ADVERSE OUTCOMES OF TREATMENT

Postoperative infection, persistent symptoms, or both are possible.

# REFERRAL DECISIONS/RED FLAGS

Patients with ulnar weakness and neuropathy need further evaluation.

# PAIN DIAGRAM—HIP AND THIGH

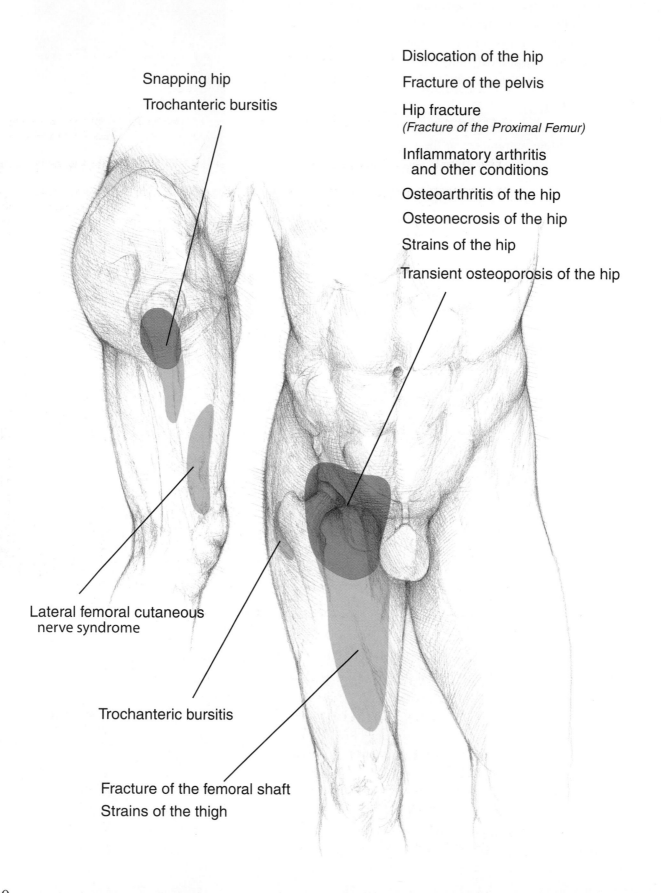

Snapping hip
Trochanteric bursitis

Dislocation of the hip

Fracture of the pelvis

Hip fracture
*(Fracture of the Proximal Femur)*

Inflammatory arthritis
and other conditions

Osteoarthritis of the hip

Osteonecrosis of the hip

Strains of the hip

Transient osteoporosis of the hip

Lateral femoral cutaneous
nerve syndrome

Trochanteric bursitis

Fracture of the femoral shaft
Strains of the thigh

# HIP AND THIGH

**Section Editor**
Joseph D. Zuckerman, MD
Professor and Chairman
Department of Orthopaedic Surgery
NYU Hospital for Joint Diseases
New York, New York

Craig J. Della Valle, MD
Assistant Professor
Department of Orthopaedic Surgery
Rush University Medical Center
Chicago, Illinois

Robert Donatelli, PhD, PT, OCS
National Director of Sports Rehabilitation
Physiotherapy Associates
Las Vegas, Nevada

Gregg R. Klein, MD
Assistant Professor
Department of Orthopaedic Surgery
NYU Hospital for Joint Diseases
New York, New York

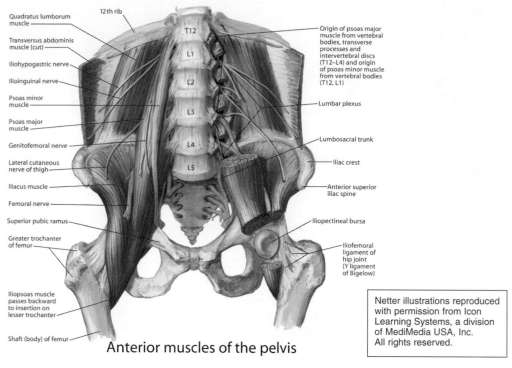

Anterior muscles of the pelvis

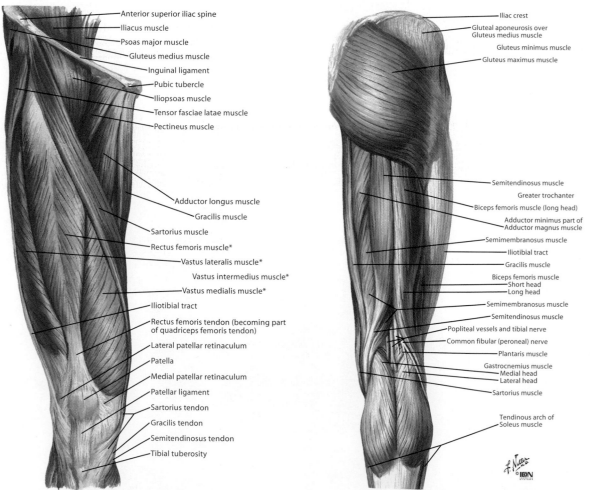

Muscles of the anterior thigh

Muscles of the posterior thigh and gluteus

# HIP AND THIGH—OVERVIEW

In patients with hip or proximal thigh pain, the pain generally comes from one of the following sources: (1) the hip joint itself, (2) the soft tissues around the hip and pelvis, (3) the pelvic bones, or (4) referred pain from the lumbar spine. Diagnosing pathology involving the hip joint and pelvis is often possible with a careful history and physical examination combined with plain radiographs; in some cases, however, advanced imaging studies such as MRI, CT, or nuclear medicine scans may be required.

The hip joint consists of the articulation between the cartilaginous surfaces of the femoral head and the pelvic acetabulum and is a diarthroidal, synovial ball-and-socket joint. The acetabulum is formed by the confluence of the ilium, ischium, and pubis, and the articular surface that is created is horseshoe shaped. The proximal femur consists of the femoral head and neck and the greater and lesser trochanters **(Figure 1)**. The greater trochanter is a large bony prominence found at the lateral base of the femoral neck; it serves as the attachment site for the abductor musculature (the gluteus medius and minimus). The lesser trochanter is a smaller bony prominence located on

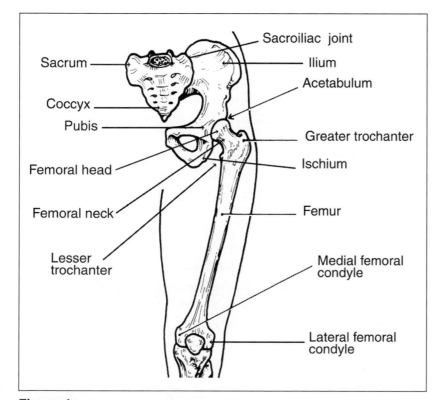

**Figure 1**
Bones of the hip and thigh.

the medial aspect of the proximal femur; it serves as the attachment site for the iliopsoas tendon, a powerful hip flexor.

Radiographic examination of the hip should include an AP radiograph of the pelvis and either a frog-lateral view of the pelvis or an AP and lateral radiograph of the involved hip. Radiographs should be carefully evaluated for displaced or nondisplaced fractures, degenerative changes of the hip joint (including joint space narrowing), and changes in bony architecture, such as lytic or blastic lesions that could suggest a primary or metastatic tumor.

# TYPE OF PAIN

Pain arising from the hip joint may be secondary to osteoarthritis, osteonecrosis, inflammatory conditions (such as rheumatoid arthritis), septic arthritis, fractures of the proximal femur or pelvis, or dislocations of the femoral head. Patients with these conditions usually report pain in the groin or the anterior aspect of the proximal thigh, but pain may be present in the buttock or lateral aspect of the thigh or be referred to the supracondylar region of the knee. Hip joint pathology is often associated with a decrease in range of motion that in degenerative conditions is associated with difficulty in activities such as donning shoes. A limp may also be present, and patients with traumatic injuries (such as proximal femoral or pelvic fractures) may be unable to bear weight on the extremity.

Problems involving the bony pelvis include traumatic high-energy fractures, insufficiency fractures associated with osteoporosis, avulsion fractures from attached tendons, and primary or metastatic tumors. Problems involving both the hip joint and bony pelvis often manifest as pain in the groin, buttock, or lateral thigh.

Conditions that affect the soft tissues around the hip, such as trochanteric bursitis, lateral femoral cutaneous nerve impingement, and snapping hip syndrome, typically cause pain on the lateral or anterolateral aspect of the proximal thigh. Patients with an injury of the adductor muscles will note pain in the groin; hamstring injuries are associated with pain in the buttock or posterior aspect of the thigh.

The sacroiliac joint is relatively immobile and is rarely a focus for pain other than as an associated injury with high-energy pelvic ring disruptions. However, conditions that involve the sacroiliac joint such as seronegative arthritides or traumatic arthritis can cause buttock and posterior thigh pain but are unlikely to restrict function.

Pathology in the lumbar spine can present as referred pain to the buttock and posterior thigh or as pain that radiates down the ipsilateral extremity in a radicular pattern. Patients with degenerative problems of the lumbar spine or strains of the lumbar musculature may have pain limited to the buttock, whereas disorders that cause entrapment of the spinal nerves (such as disk herniations) will cause pain in a radicular pattern. These patients typically do not have symptoms referable to the groin, significant discomfort with rotation of the hip, or limited range of motion of the hip joint, although they often present with what they describe as "pain in the hip."

Nonmusculoskeletal pathology may present as groin or hip pain, and if the source of pain is obviously not the hip joint, these etiologies must be explored. Constitutional symptoms such as fever, chills, and weight loss should be explored to rule out malignancy or infection. Inguinal or abdominal hernias and rectus abdominus strains may present with pain in the groin or anterior thigh and may be difficult for the patient to distinguish from hip pathology. Gastrointestinal disorders such as inflammatory bowel disease, diverticulosis, diverticulitis, or appendicitis may mimic hip pain. Pain from abdominal aortic aneurysms may mimic groin pain. Urinary tract infections or nephrolithiasis may also cause pain referred to the hip region.

Pathology of the male and female reproductive systems may also present as pain in the groin or hip area. Prostatitis, epididymitis, hydroceles, varicoceles, testicular torsions, and testicular neoplasms have all been known to cause groin pain in men. Ectopic pregnancy, dysmenorrhea, endometriosis, and pelvic inflammatory disease may cause pain in this location in women.

# GAIT

A brief examination of the patient's gait can be very helpful in making a diagnosis. Ask the patient to walk up and down the hall several times at a brisk pace. An abductor or gluteus medius lurch is manifested by a lateral shift of the body to the weight-bearing side with ambulation. This type of gait often occurs in patients who have intra-articular hip pathology (osteoarthritis, inflammatory arthritis, or osteonecrosis of the hip). Pain associated with a limp suggests pathology around the pelvis or hip and requires further investigation.

SECTION 5 ■ HIP AND THIGH

# PHYSICAL EXAMINATION
# HIP AND THIGH

## INSPECTION/PALPATION

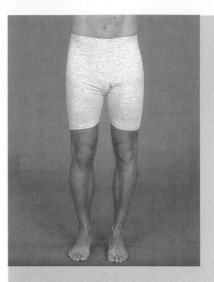

### *Anterior view*

With the patient standing, look for atrophy of the anterior thigh musculature and note the overall alignment of the hip, knee, and ankle.

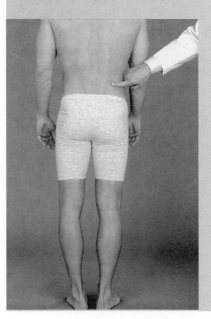

### *Posterior view*

With the patient standing, look for atrophy of the buttock and posterior thigh musculature. Palpate the iliac crests (in the photograph, the examiner is pointing to the right iliac crest), the posterior iliac spine (deep to the dimples of Venus), and the greater trochanter. Note any pelvic obliquity (one iliac crest lower than the opposite side). Limb-length discrepancy will cause one iliac crest to be lower than the other, but this apparent obliquity can be corrected by placing blocks under the shorter limb. Fixed pelvic obliquity from a spinal deformity cannot be corrected by this maneuver. A Trendelenburg test can be conducted at this time. For the Trendelenburg test, the patient is instructed to stand on one leg (the affected leg). With normal hip abductor strength, the pelvis will stay level. With abnormal abductor strength (positive test), the pelvis will drop, with the iliac crest becoming lower on the opposite side (see p 412).

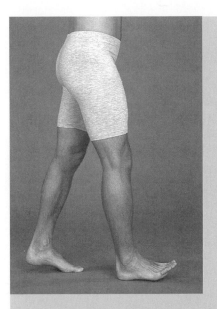

## Gait

Note how the patient walks across the room. Hip deformities often cause a limp that can range in severity from barely detectable to a marked swaying of the trunk and slowing of gait. Patients with a painful hip joint may have an antalgic gait; that is, they shorten the stance phase on the affected side to avoid placing weight across the painful joint. A Trendelenburg gait, characterized by a lateral shift of the body weight, is seen in patients with weakness of the abductor musculature; this is sometimes primary but is more often secondary to a degenerative disorder of the hip. As the hip joint degenerates and friction within the hip joint increases, it becomes more difficult for the abductor musculature to level the pelvis during gait.

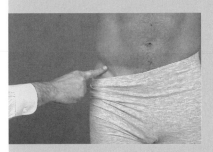

## Anterior view, supine

With the patient supine, palpate to identify any masses, abnormal adenopathy, or tenderness in the region of the anterior superior iliac spine (ASIS) (the examiner is palpating the ASIS in the photograph) or greater trochanter. Patients with avulsion of the sartorius or rectus femoris will report tenderness at or directly inferior to the ASIS. Patients with meralgia paresthetica (entrapment of the lateral femoral cutaneous nerve) will report tenderness immediately medial to the ASIS and hypoesthesia over the distal lateral thigh.

Patients who report a popping sensation in the hip while ambulating most likely have a thickened iliotibial band snapping over the greater trochanter that occurs as the hip moves into flexion and internal rotation. Ask the patient to recreate the snapping and palpate the iliotibial band as it snaps over the greater trochanter.

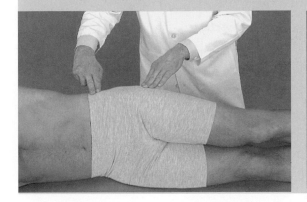

## Lateral view, side-lying

Place the patient in a side-lying position on the unaffected side to facilitate the examination. Structures in the region of the greater trochanter may be palpated in the supine position, but examination of this area is easier with the patient lying on the unaffected side. Tenderness directly over the trochanter reproduces pain with greater trochanteric bursitis. Tenderness at the proximal tip of the trochanter may indicate gluteus medius tendinitis. Tenderness at the posterior margin of the trochanter may indicate external rotator tendinitis.

# RANGE OF MOTION

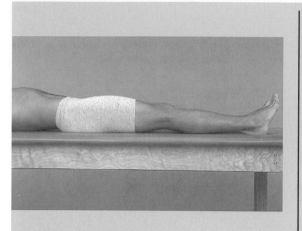

### *Flexion: Zero Starting Position*

Place the patient supine on a firm, flat surface with the opposite hip held in enough flexion to flatten the lumbar spine. Flattening the lumbar spine prevents excessive lordosis, which may camouflage a hip flexion contracture.

Avoid positioning the opposite hip in excessive flexion, as this will rock the pelvis into abnormal posterior inclination, thereby creating a false-positive hip flexion contracture. Instead, flex the opposite hip to a position where the lumbar spine just starts to flatten or, more precisely, to a position where the inclination of the pelvis is similar to that of a normal standing posture (ie, the anterior superior iliac spine is inferior to the posterior iliac spine by only 2° to 3°).

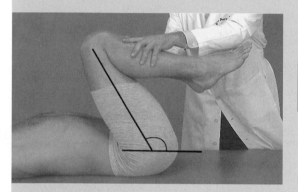

### *Maximum flexion*

Maximum flexion is the point at which the pelvis begins to rotate. Normal hip flexion in adults is 110° to 130°.

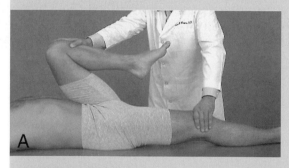

A

B

30°

### *Hip flexion contracture—Thomas test*

With the opposite hip flexed as described in the Zero Starting Position, move the affected hip into flexion and then allow the affected hip to extend until the pelvis starts to rock. The top figure (**A**) demonstrates no hip flexion contracture; (**B**) demonstrates a hip flexion contracture of 30°.

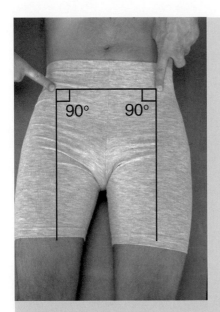

### Abduction and adduction: Zero Starting Position

The Zero Starting Position is with the pelvis level (ie, the limbs are at a 90° angle to a transverse line across the anterior superior iliac spines).

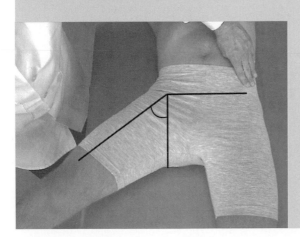

### Abduction

Measure abduction in degrees from the Zero Starting Position. Maximum abduction is reached when the pelvis begins to tilt, a movement that you can detect by keeping your hand on the patient's opposite ASIS when moving the leg. Normal hip abduction in adults is 35° to 50°.

SECTION 5 ■ HIP AND THIGH

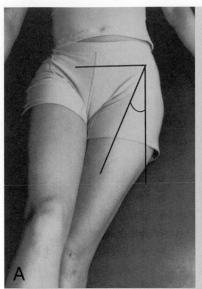

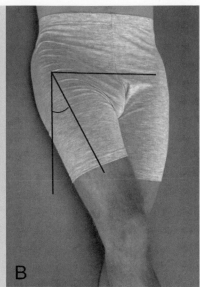

## Adduction

To measure adduction, elevate the opposite extremity to allow adduction of the affected extremity (**A**). Maximum adduction is reached when the pelvis starts to rotate. If elevating the opposite extremity is impractical, measure adduction by moving the affected extremity over the top of the opposite limb (**B**). Normal hip adduction in adults is 25° to 35°.

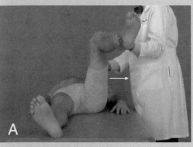

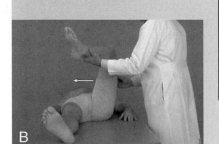

## Internal-external rotation in flexion

For adults, it is more practical to measure rotation with the hips in flexion. However, this approach should not be used in children or when assessment of femoral torsion or a more precise measurement of hip rotation in a "walking" position is required.

Flex the hip and knee to 90°, with the thigh held perpendicular to the transverse line across the anterior superior iliac spines. Measure internal rotation by rotating the tibia away from the midline of the trunk, thus producing inward rotation of the hip (**A**). Measure external rotation by rotating the tibia toward the midline of the trunk, thus producing external rotation at the hip (**B**). (See Intoeing and Outtoeing, pp 889-893.)

# MUSCLE TESTING

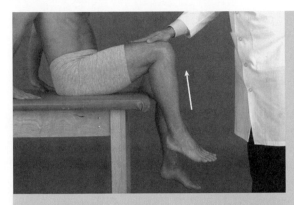

### *Hip flexors*

With the patient seated, ask him or her to flex the hip as you resist the effort.

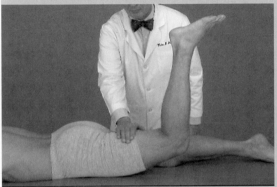

### *Hip extensors*

With the patient prone, place the knee in approximately 90° of flexion and ask the patient to extend the hip as you resist the effort with your hand by pushing against the thigh.

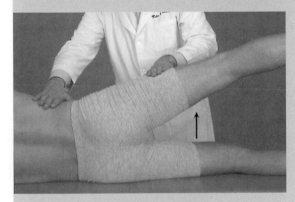

### *Hip abductors*

With the patient lying on the unaffected side, ask him or her to abduct the hip as you resist the effort. Note that hip abductor strength also can be assessed by the Trendelenburg test.

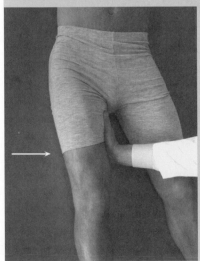

### *Hip adductors*

With the patient supine, place your hand on the medial thigh and ask the patient to adduct the hip as you resist the effort.

SECTION 5 ■ HIP AND THIGH

# SPECIAL TESTS

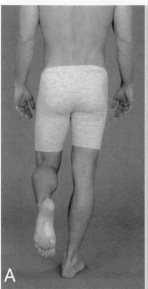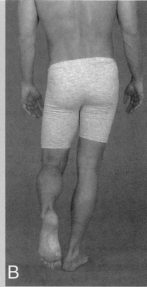

### *Trendelenburg test*

Ask the patient to stand on one leg. With normal hip abductor strength, the pelvis will stay level **(A)**. If hip abductor strength is inadequate on the stance limb side, the pelvis will dip toward the opposite side (positive Trendelenburg test) **(B)**.

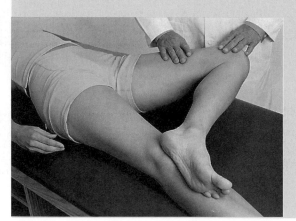

### *FABER test*

The FABER (flexion-abduction-external rotation) test, sometimes called the figure-of-4 test, is a stress maneuver to detect hip and sacroiliac pathology. With the patient supine, place the affected hip in flexion, abduction, and external rotation. Then place the patient's foot on the opposite knee and press down on the thigh of the affected side. If the maneuver is painful, the hip or sacroiliac region may be affected. Increased pain with this test also may be a nonorganic finding.

# DISLOCATION OF THE HIP

**ICD-9 Codes**

**835.01**
Posterior dislocation

**835.02**
Anterior dislocation

## DEFINITION

Dislocation of the hip occurs when the femoral head is displaced from the acetabulum. Because of its strong capsule and deep acetabulum, the hip is rarely dislocated in adults. The causative injury usually is high-energy trauma, such as a motor vehicle accident or fall from a height. Posterior dislocations (femoral head posterior to the acetabulum) are far more common than anterior dislocations, accounting for more than 90% of these injuries.

## CLINICAL SYMPTOMS

Patients have severe pain and are typically unable to move the lower extremity. Patients often have other associated musculoskeletal injuries, and there is a high prevalence of associated head, intra-abdominal, and chest injuries.

## TESTS

### Physical Examination

With a posterior dislocation, the affected limb is short and the hip is fixed in a position of flexion, adduction, and internal rotation (**Figure 1**). Assess the status of distal pulses and function of the sciatic and femoral nerves. Sciatic nerve palsies are common (8% to 20% incidence), with the peroneal division of the sciatic nerve most commonly affected.

With anterior dislocations, the hip assumes a position of mild flexion, abduction, and external rotation. Femoral nerve palsy may be present, but nerve injuries are less frequent with anterior dislocations.

Inspect the extremity for abrasions about the anterior aspect of the knee or for a knee effusion. Significant knee ligament injuries are commonly associated with hip dislocations because most hip dislocations typically occur from a direct blow to the flexed hip and knee. An associated fracture of the ipsilateral femur or acetabulum may be present.

### Diagnostic Tests

An AP radiograph of the pelvis and AP and lateral views of the femur including the knee should be obtained. On the AP radiograph, the size of the femoral heads and joint spaces should appear symmetric. With a posterior hip dislocation (**Figure 2**), the affected femoral head appears smaller than the contralateral femoral head, whereas with an anterior hip

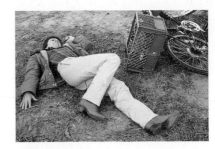

**Figure 1**
The clinical appearance of a posterior dislocation of the right hip.

Reproduced from Heckman JD (ed): *Emergency Care and Transportation of the Sick and Injured*, ed 4. Park Ridge, IL, American Academy of Orthopaedic Surgeons, 1987, p 208.

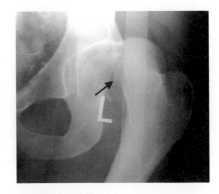

**Figure 2**
Posterior dislocation of the left hip with an associated fracture of the femoral head (arrow).

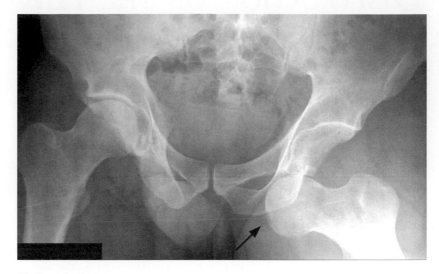

**Figure 3**
AP radiograph of the pelvis demonstrating an anterior dislocation of the left hip (arrow).

dislocation, the femoral head appears larger than the femoral head on the opposite, normal hip (**Figure 3**). Associated fractures of the acetabulum (particularly fractures of the posterior wall) are common, and in these cases, a CT scan should be obtained to fully define the fracture pattern (**Figure 4**). Following reduction of the dislocation, it is imperative to ensure that the reduction is completely concentric without interposition of associated bony fragments or residual subluxation; if there is any question regarding these parameters, a CT scan should be obtained.

## DIFFERENTIAL DIAGNOSIS

Fracture of the acetabulum or pelvis (pain in the groin and/or buttock)

Fracture of the hip or shaft of the femur (pain in the groin, buttock, and thigh)

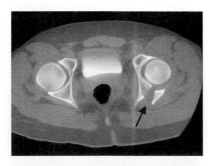

**Figure 4**
CT scan of the pelvis showing a displaced fracture of the posterior wall of the acetabulum.

## ADVERSE OUTCOMES OF THE DISEASE

Osteonecrosis of the femoral head is the most common early complication and occurs in approximately 10% of patients. Dislocation of the hip joint tears the hip capsule and disrupts the blood supply to the femoral head; a delay in reduction increases the risk of osteonecrosis. Osteonecrosis may not be apparent for as long as 2 or 3 years after the injury, and thus these patients require follow-up over several years. Post traumatic arthritis (secondary to the severe impact to the cartilaginous surfaces), sciatic or femoral nerve injury, and chronic pain also may occur.

# TREATMENT

A hip dislocation is an emergency. A reduction should be performed as soon as possible to decrease the risk of osteonecrosis. The reduction should be performed in an atraumatic fashion to avoid damage to the articular cartilage or fracture of the femoral head or acetabulum. Associated fractures of the femoral head or intra-articular loose bodies should be ruled out before the reduction is performed. Repeat radiographs and, frequently, a postreduction CT are necessary to identify unrecognized intra-articular bony fragments and to confirm a perfectly concentric reduction; if retained bony fragments are identified within the joint, they must be surgically removed. Nerve and vascular function should be carefully evaluated both before and after the reduction. Postreduction treatment of an uncomplicated dislocated hip is early crutch-assisted ambulation with weight bearing as tolerated until the patient is free of pain, usually 2 to 4 weeks after the injury. Patients should then begin hip abduction and extension exercises and use a walking aid in the hand opposite the involved hip until they can walk without a limp. Associated fractures of the acetabulum often require surgical treatment to ensure that adequate stability has been restored to the joint.

# ADVERSE OUTCOMES OF TREATMENT

Despite a rapid closed reduction, osteonecrosis may still occur. The impact of the injury itself may cause severe damage to the cartilaginous surfaces of the femoral head or acetabulum, resulting in posttraumatic arthritis.

# REFERRAL DECISIONS/RED FLAGS

All traumatic dislocations of the hip are serious injuries requiring immediate attention.

SECTION 5 ■ HIP AND THIGH

# FRACTURE OF THE FEMORAL SHAFT

**ICD-9 Code**

**821.01**
Fracture of the femoral shaft, closed

## DEFINITION

The shaft, or diaphysis, of the femur is defined as that portion between the regions of the proximal subtrochanteric region and the distal supracondylar area of the knee. In most adults, fractures of the femoral shaft are caused by high-energy trauma such as a motor vehicle accident. As such, this injury is severe and is potentially associated with life-threatening pulmonary, intra-abdominal, and head injuries. Pathologic fractures of the femoral shaft are less common, occur in bone weakened by osteopenia or tumors, result from low-energy injuries such as a simple fall, and have a much lower incidence of associated complications.

## CLINICAL SYMPTOMS

Patients present with severe pain in the thigh along with an obvious deformity and are unable to move, let alone bear weight on the extremity. Patients who have sustained the injury as a result of high-energy trauma are likely to have multisystem injuries and may not be alert or even responsive to questioning.

## TESTS

### Physical Examination

Inspect for deformity, swelling, and open injuries. It is important to recognize that a femoral shaft fracture can act as a distracting injury, causing the examiner to overlook other associated musculoskeletal injuries and thus a thorough examination of the entire extremity is mandatory to rule out associated injuries. Ligamentous injuries of the ipsilateral knee are common; however, often the knee cannot be examined until the patient is anesthetized for surgical treatment. Evaluate the vascular status of the limb distal to the fracture. Assess function of the femoral, peroneal, and posterior tibial nerves. In the presence of deformity and vascular compromise, simple manual longitudinal traction should be applied to determine whether the deformity is the cause of the ischemia. As these are typically high-energy injuries, standard Advanced Trauma Life Support (ATLS) protocols should be applied to evaluate for and potentially treat associated life-threatening injuries.

### Diagnostic Tests

Fracture is confirmed by AP and lateral radiographs of the femur (**Figure 1**). High-energy trauma can disrupt adjacent

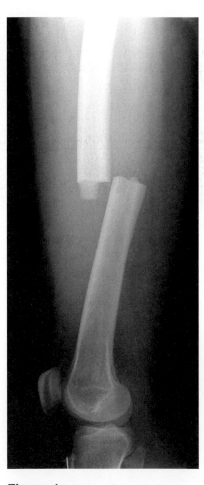

**Figure 1**
Lateral radiograph showing a femoral shaft fracture.

joints, and radiographs of the hip, knee, and pelvis must be obtained. It is particularly important to identify an ipsilateral fracture of the femoral neck because treatment options differ and outcomes can be radically different (**Figure 2**). If vascular compromise is identified, arterial studies are required.

## DIFFERENTIAL DIAGNOSIS

Fracture of the pelvis, acetabulum, or proximal femur (evident on radiographs)

Malignant or metastatic lesion of the femur (pain in the thigh with activity or at rest, evident on radiographs)

Osteomyelitis with bone destruction (pain in the thigh, evident on radiographs)

Soft-tissue injury without fracture (pain, swelling, ecchymosis of the thigh, pain with knee motion)

Stress fracture of the femur (pain in the thigh that increases with weight bearing; may be evident on plain radiographs, but MRI may be needed to confirm the diagnosis)

## ADVERSE OUTCOMES OF THE DISEASE

The most significant adverse outcomes are those associated with violent trauma or long-bone fractures, such as fat embolism, adult respiratory distress syndrome, and multisystem organ failure. Acute arterial injury also is life threatening and requires immediate recognition and treatment. Complications of open fractures, such as infection, may result in chronic osteomyelitis.

## TREATMENT

Immediate, temporary splinting may be applied for comfort during transfers and during immediate patient evaluation, followed by the application of skeletal traction until surgical intervention is undertaken. Skeletal traction pins can be applied to the distal femur or the proximal tibia. These provide patient comfort and prevent shortening of the extremity, which can be difficult to overcome once the fracture is treated surgically. Surgical treatment is indicated for the vast majority of patients to lessen the risk of pulmonary and other systemic complications. Patients with open fractures should receive appropriate tetanus prophylaxis along with immediate systemic antibiotic treatment, followed by emergent surgical débridement of the soft-tissue injury as soon as the patient is medically stabilized.

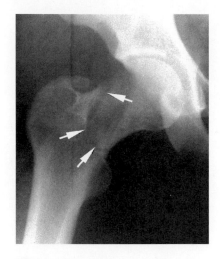

**Figure 2**
AP radiograph showing a femoral neck fracture (arrows) in a patient with a femoral shaft fracture in the same extremity caused by high-energy trauma.

SECTION 5 ■ HIP AND THIGH

## Adverse Outcomes of Treatment

Despite prompt surgical treatment, pulmonary complications and fat embolism syndrome may occur. Nonunion, malunion, and infection are potential problems with any fracture treated surgically. Even if uneventful healing occurs, the high energy associated with these injuries may have effects on the associated soft tissues that are long-lasting. Persistent pain, limp, and difficulty returning to jobs that require manual labor are not uncommon.

## Referral Decisions/Red Flags

Femoral shaft fractures are markers of a high-energy traumatic injury and thus require appropriate evaluation and treatment for associated musculoskeletal, head, thoracic, and intra-abdominal injuries. Open injuries require special attention to ensure that appropriate tetanus boosters and intravenous antibiotics are administered, along with prompt surgical débridement and fracture fixation.

# FRACTURE OF THE PELVIS

## DEFINITION

Pelvic fractures include fractures of the pelvic ring and acetabulum. Pelvic injuries range in severity from stable, low-energy fractures that heal readily when treated nonsurgically with early, assisted ambulation to unstable, high-energy fractures that are associated with massive blood loss and resultant hemodynamic instability that can lead to death if not stabilized emergently. Stable pelvic ring fractures generally involve only one side of the pelvic ring. For example, a unilateral fracture of the superior and inferior pubic ramus is a stable injury. Unstable pelvic ring fractures disrupt the ring at two sites. For example, a fracture of a superior and inferior pubic ramus combined with a fracture of the sacrum or ilium is considered an unstable pelvic fracture. Another unstable pattern is disruption of the symphysis pubis combined with a fracture of the sacrum or disruption of one or both sacroiliac ligaments (**Figure 1**). Acetabular fractures are by definition intra-articular injuries that can lead to posttraumatic arthritis if displaced. Acetabular fractures usually are high-energy injuries.

### ICD-9 Codes

**808.0**
Fracture of the acetabulum

**808.2**
Fracture of the pubis

**808.41**
Fracture of the ilium

**808.42**
Fracture of the ischium

**808.43**
Multiple pelvic fractures with disruption of pelvic circle

SECTION 5 ■ HIP AND THIGH

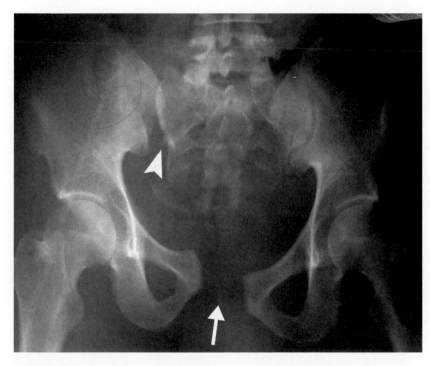

**Figure 1**

AP view of the pelvis revealing an unstable pelvic fracture with disruption of the symphysis pubis (white arrow) and sacroiliac joint (white arrowhead).

# CLINICAL SYMPTOMS

Low-energy pelvic fractures are often seen in elderly patients. Presenting symptoms are similar to those in patients with a fracture of the hip, including pain in the groin with attempts at weight bearing or an inability to bear weight on the extremity. Most pelvic and acetabular fractures are high-energy injuries that cause pain in the groin, lateral hip, or buttock and are associated with other musculoskeletal injuries as well as traumatic injuries of the head, chest, and abdomen.

# TESTS

## Physical Examination

Low-energy pelvic fractures are associated with pain on attempted range of motion of the hip and on attempted straight leg raising. Patients who are able to ambulate have an antalgic gait pattern. Patients should be screened for a loss of consciousness, chest pain, or shortness of breath that either caused the fall or has occurred since the fall. The cervical spine should be examined to ensure that there is no pain with attempted range of motion.

Patients with high-energy pelvic fractures require treatment in a trauma center with the application of standard trauma protocols including an initial evaluation of the airway, breathing, and circulatory status of the patient. Inspect the pelvic area for swelling, ecchymosis, and obvious deformity as well as for lacerations, which may represent an open fracture of the pelvis. Palpation and gentle compression of the pelvis often will localize the area of injury. The neurovascular status of the lower extremities should be evaluated carefully because peripheral nerve injuries are not uncommon and pelvic fractures that involve the sacrum can directly damage the spinal nerve roots. Unstable fractures may also be associated with genitourinary injuries of the prostate and bladder. If blood is present in the perineal area, a urologic consultation should be obtained prior to placing a Foley catheter.

## Diagnostic Tests

Standard trauma protocols include an AP radiograph of the chest, a lateral radiograph of the cervical spine, and an AP radiograph of the pelvis; this view of the pelvis will identify most pelvic fractures. If a pelvic fracture is seen on this view, pelvic inlet and outlet views (**Figure 2**) should be obtained to assist with identification of the injury pattern. If an acetabular fracture is demonstrated, oblique views of the pelvis are required to fully define the extent of the fracture. CT scans are

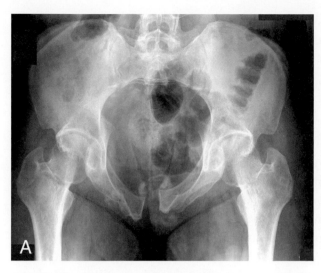
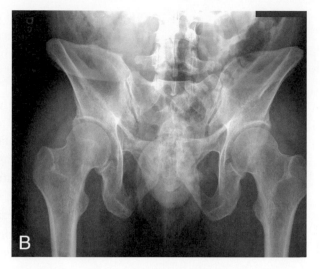

**Figure 2**
Pelvic inlet (**A**) and outlet (**B**) views are useful for determining rotational and vertical displacement of the pelvis. Note the displacement and rotation of the left pubic ramus.

often needed to define these complex injuries and plan for appropriate surgical intervention (**Figure 3**).

## DIFFERENTIAL DIAGNOSIS

Hip arthritis (pain in the groin or buttock, limited hip motion, evident on radiographs)

Hip fracture (pain in the groin or buttock, shortened and externally rotated leg)

Hip strain (pain in the groin or buttock)

Tumors involving the bony pelvis or sacrum (pain in the low back, groin, rectum, and/or buttock; evident on radiographs)

## ADVERSE OUTCOMES OF THE DISEASE

High-energy injuries are associated with a significant prevalence of musculoskeletal injuries as well as head, chest, and abdominal injuries that can have serious sequelae, including death. Associated genitourinary injuries are common and can lead to pain and/or sexual dysfunction. Neurologic injuries may be permanent, leading to abnormal motor and/or sensory dysfunction of the ipsilateral lower extremity. Although nonunion of these fractures is uncommon, malunion of the pelvis sometimes occurs and may lead to deformity of the pelvis and/or limb-length discrepancy with persistent pain. With acetabular fractures, which are intra-articular injuries, if the cartilage itself has been damaged by the impact, posttraumatic arthritis can result even if the fracture is fixed anatomically with rigid internal fixation. Patients with pelvic ring and acetabular fractures are at substantial risk for thromboembolic complications. Even if these injuries go on to uneventful bony

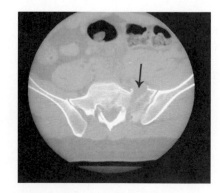

**Figure 3**
CT scan of the pelvis shows an unstable fracture of the left side of the sacrum (arrow).

union, the psychosocial implications of these injuries are substantial because many patients have persistent pain that requires changes in occupation.

## TREATMENT

Treatment of pelvic fractures is determined by the degree of pelvic instability and the presence of associated injuries. Pelvic fractures associated with minor injuries, such as falls in the elderly patient, are common and typically have a stable pattern. Treatment consists of analgesics, gait training for protected weight bearing with a walker, and protection against complications related to immobility, such as venous thromboembolism and skin breakdown. Most patients require protected weight bearing for about 6 weeks, until the pain has subsided and the fracture demonstrates early healing. These patients should also undergo evaluation and treatment for osteoporosis to prevent the occurrence of similar fragility fractures.

Pelvic fractures sustained in high-energy injuries often are life threatening. Initial treatment focuses on hemodynamic resuscitation along with identification and treatment of associated injuries. As a temporizing measure, a sheet can be tautly but carefully applied around the patient's pelvis to decrease pelvic volume, affect a temporary reduction, and thereby potentially reduce pelvic bleeding. Definitive treatment of unstable pelvic and acetabular fractures usually requires surgical intervention.

## ADVERSE OUTCOMES OF TREATMENT

Degenerative arthritis of the sacroiliac or hip joint, heterotopic ossification, malunion, nonunion, or neurovascular injury may occur.

## REFERRAL DECISIONS/RED FLAGS

High-energy displaced pelvic fractures and open pelvic fractures are best managed at a level I trauma center, where a multidisciplinary approach can be applied to optimize patient survival. Fractures involving the acetabulum or sacroiliac joint require evaluation for possible surgical reduction and fixation.

# FRACTURE OF THE PROXIMAL FEMUR

## SYNONYM
Hip fracture

## DEFINITION

Hip fractures are a common problem in elderly individuals with osteoporosis. These fractures generally involve either the femoral neck, which is susceptible to a twisting injury, or the intertrochanteric region, which is susceptible to a fall on the greater trochanter. Both types occur with approximately the same frequency and affect a similar patient population; however, surgical treatment of the two injuries differs. Femoral neck fractures are also known as intracapsular hip fractures and thus by definition occur in the region of the proximal femur that is within the hip capsule itself (**Figure 1**). Intracapsular hip fractures often lead to a disruption of the blood supply to the femoral head, and thus nonunion and osteonecrosis are frequent complications of this injury. Intertrochanteric hip fractures are extracapsular, occurring in the region of the proximal femur between the base of the femoral neck and the distal aspect of the lesser trochanter (**Figure 2**), and require more robust fixation than do femoral neck fractures. They are associated with lower rates of osteonecrosis or nonunion, as the blood supply to the femoral head is not typically disrupted; however, implant failure is a much more common problem with these injuries.

Advanced age is the most important risk factor for a proximal femoral fracture. The frequency of hip fractures generally doubles with each decade beyond age 50 years. There are several reasons for this. Decreased proprioceptive function and loss of protective responses increase the likelihood that elderly individuals will fall. Also, because they have a decreased ambulatory speed, when they fall they tend to fall to the side as opposed to forward, so the lateral thigh and hip region often strikes the ground first. Dizziness, stroke, syncope, peripheral neuropathies, and medications are other factors that can compromise balance and predispose elderly patients to hip fractures.

White women are two to three times more likely to be affected than African-American or Hispanic women. Other risk factors include sedentary lifestyle, smoking, alcoholism, use of psychotropic medication, dementia, and living in an urban area.

**ICD-9 Codes**

**820.00**
Femoral neck (transcervical) fracture

**820.21**
Intertrochanteric femur fracture

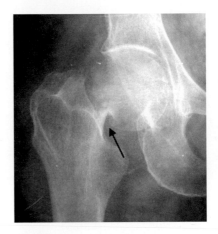

**Figure 1**
AP view showing a displaced femoral neck fracture (arrow).

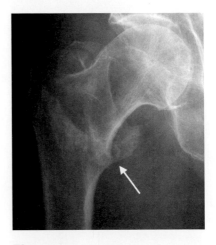

**Figure 2**
AP view showing an intertrochanteric fracture of the hip (arrow).

SECTION 5 ■ HIP AND THIGH

## CLINICAL SYMPTOMS

Most patients report a fall followed by the inability to bear weight on the extremity or ambulate and pain in the groin. A few can walk with assistance (crutches, cane, or walker) but have groin or buttock pain on weight bearing that seems to get worse with ambulation. Occasionally, patients report pain referred to the supracondylar region of the knee. Elderly patients with hip pain after a fall should be treated as if they have a hip fracture until proved otherwise.

## TESTS

### Physical Examination

Patients with a displaced femoral neck or intertrochanteric fracture lie with the limb externally rotated, abducted, and shortened. Patients with stress fractures or nondisplaced fractures of the femoral neck may have no obvious deformity. Attempts to gently rotate the limb while the hip is extended are painful, and patients are unable to straight-leg raise (lift the heel on the affected side off of the bed while keeping the knee straight).

### Diagnostic Tests

An AP radiograph of the pelvis and a cross-table lateral radiograph of the involved hip reveal most fractures of the proximal femur. It is important to avoid a frog-lateral radiograph in patients suspected of a proximal femoral fracture as this will cause severe pain and may cause displacement of a nondisplaced fracture. An MRI scan should be obtained if the history and physical examination are suggestive of a fracture but plain radiographs are negative (**Figure 3**).

## DIFFERENTIAL DIAGNOSIS

Pathologic fracture (underlying or associated tumor, benign or malignant)

Pelvic fracture (normal hip joint motion, pain on external rotation)

## ADVERSE OUTCOMES OF THE DISEASE

Proximal femoral fractures are, in general, markers of poor health, and medical complications frequently accompany these injuries, including thromboembolic events, pneumonia, decubitus ulcers, and urinary tract infections. One-year mortality following proximal femoral fractures in elderly patients has been reported at 10% to 30%, and patients often lose both ambulatory capacity and functional independence. Complications directly related to the fracture include nonunion and osteonecrosis.

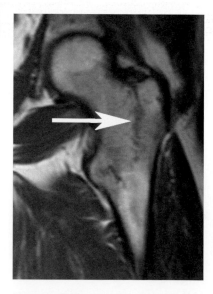

**Figure 3**
T1-weighted MRI scan showing a nondisplaced intertrochanteric hip fracture (arrow).

# Treatment

Most proximal femoral fractures are treated surgically because the risks of nonsurgical treatment (primarily related to the extended period of bed rest required, with the associated risk of thromboembolic events, pneumonia, decubitus ulcers, and general deconditioning) generally outweigh the risks of surgical treatment for all except the most medically unstable patients and nonambulatory and/or demented patients who have minimal pain associated with transfers. Patients diagnosed with a proximal femoral fracture should be evaluated by an orthopaedic surgeon, an internist, and an anesthesiologist in a timely manner to expedite surgical treatment. Patients should undergo a thorough evaluation to determine if medical comorbidities are present that can be optimized preoperatively to decrease the risk of perioperative morbidity and mortality. Thromboembolic prophylaxis of some form should be instituted immediately (mechanical, pharmacologic, or both in combination) because these patients are at extraordinarily high risk for thromboembolic events. Numerous studies have suggested that a delay of more than 48 hours from the time of injury to surgical intervention is associated with increased mortality. Therefore, surgical intervention should not be delayed longer than 48 hours unless some other intervention will substantially decrease the patient's perioperative risk from surgical treatment. Although skin traction has been commonly used in the past to relieve preoperative discomfort, recent prospective randomized studies have shown that it is less effective than a pillow placed beneath the patient's knee.

The form of surgical treatment selected is determined primarily by fracture location (femoral neck versus intertrochanteric), displacement, and patient activity level. Intertrochanteric fractures are treated with either a screw and side plate (**Figure 4, A**) or an intramedullary nail (**Figure 4, B**). Nondisplaced or valgus impacted femoral neck fractures are treated by percutaneous fixation with multiple (typically three) screws (**Figure 4, C**). Displaced fractures in elderly patients are typically treated with prosthetic replacement (**Figure 4, D**) (either hemiarthroplasty or total hip arthroplasty) because the risks of nonunion and osteonecrosis approach 50% if surgical fixation is performed, with a substantial rate of secondary surgical interventions to treat these complications. Femoral neck fractures in patients younger than 60 years are typically associated with high-energy trauma and constitute a surgical emergency, as anatomic surgical fixation in a timely manner is required for optimal outcomes. As part of their evaluation, patients who present with fractures of the femoral neck or intertrochanteric area of the femur should have their bone

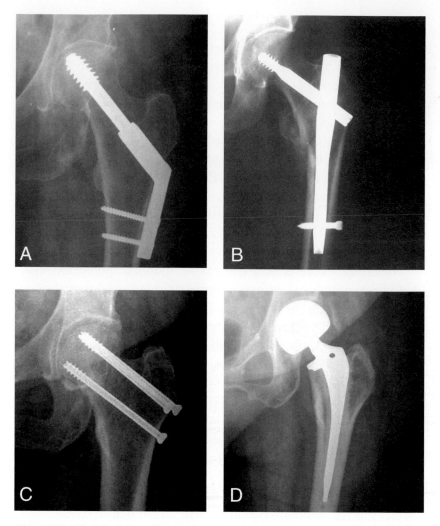

**Figure 4**

Postoperative AP radiographs. **A,** Intertrochanteric hip fracture treated with a screw and side plate. **B,** Intertrochanteric hip fracture treated with an intramedullary nail. **C,** Nondisplaced femoral neck fracture treated with three cannulated screws. **D,** Displaced femoral neck fracture treated with a cemented arthroplasty of the hip.

density measured. If low bone mineral density is found, the physician should advise the patient of the advantages of adequate calcium intake.

## ADVERSE OUTCOMES OF TREATMENT

With femoral neck fractures, osteonecrosis of the femoral head and fracture nonunion are common complications of internal fixation, and prosthetic dislocation can occur if the proximal femur has been replaced. With intertrochanteric fractures, the most common complication of surgical treatment is failure of fixation and secondary arthritis (**Figure 5**). All patients with proximal femoral fractures should undergo evaluation and treatment for osteoporosis because they are at substantial risk for fracture of the contralateral hip and other fragility fractures such as distal radius and lumbar compression fractures.

## REFERRAL DECISIONS/RED FLAGS

A femoral neck fracture in a patient younger than age 60 years constitutes a surgical emergency because the risk of osteonecrosis and fracture nonunion are significant, and prompt surgical fixation decreases the risk of these complications. In a patient with a history and physical examination suggestive of a fracture but with negative plain radiographs, an MRI scan should be obtained to definitively diagnose or rule out a proximal femoral fracture. All proximal femoral fractures should be considered for surgical treatment given the high risk of complications when nonsurgical treatment is undertaken.

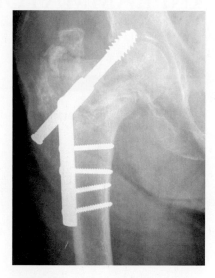

**Figure 5**
AP radiograph showing a failed fixation following intertrochanteric hip fracture.

SECTION 5 ■ HIP AND THIGH

# INFLAMMATORY ARTHRITIS

## SYNONYM

Synovitis of the hip

## DEFINITION

Most inflammatory conditions that involve the hip are local manifestations of systemic disorders; however, these conditions may first present with symptoms referable to the hip. Although any of the inflammatory arthritides listed in the differential diagnosis may involve the hip, the prevalence of hip involvement is highest in rheumatoid arthritis and ankylosing spondylitis. End-stage arthritis of the hip also is commonly observed in patients with systemic lupus erythematosus, but this is often secondary to osteonecrosis.

With few exceptions, the pathophysiology of inflammatory arthropathies results from an immunologic host response to antigenic challenge. The exact cause remains unclear, but epidemiologic and genetic evidence supports a genetic component to many inflammatory arthritides.

## CLINICAL SYMPTOMS

Inflammatory arthritis of the hip is characterized by a dull, aching pain in the groin, lateral thigh, or buttocks region. The pain is often episodic, with patients experiencing morning stiffness, improvement with moderate activity, and increased pain and stiffness following more vigorous activity. Patients often will note a progressive limp as well as limited range of motion, which may manifest as difficulty with dressing or with donning shoes. With increasing time and disease progression, symptoms are indistinguishable from osteoarthritis of the hip.

## TESTS

### Physical Examination

Gait abnormalities such as an antalgic gait (short stance phase on the affected side) are common in the earlier phases of the disease, whereas a Trendelenburg gait develops with progressive loss of articular cartilage. Hip range of motion is often restricted, with a loss of internal rotation the most sensitive finding in adults with hip joint disease. Synovial inflammation can be detected by placing the patient in a prone position with the knee flexed and applying gentle rotation to the extremity (as if rolling a rolling pin), moving only the hip. If synovial inflammation is present, this maneuver will cause pain.

## Diagnostic Tests

An AP view of the pelvis as well as AP and frog-lateral radiographs of the involved hip are obtained. In the early stages of inflammatory conditions these may show subtle osteopenia and/or a joint effusion. In later stages of inflammatory arthritis, symmetric joint space loss and periarticular bone erosions are typical (**Figure 1**).

For a patient with a history and physical examination consistent with an acute synovitis of the hip, laboratory studies should include complete blood count, acute phase reactants (erythrocyte sedimentation rate or C-reactive protein), rheumatoid factor, and antinuclear antibody tests. When an effusion is present, aspiration performed with radiographic assistance can be considered. The aspirate should be sent for culture, cell count with differential analysis, and inspection for crystalline deposits.

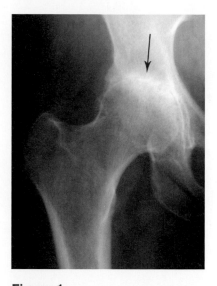

**Figure 1**
AP view of the hip showing inflammatory arthritis of the hip with concentric joint space narrowing (arrow), minimal osteophytes, and generalized osteopenia.

# DIFFERENTIAL DIAGNOSIS

Ankylosing spondylitis (stiffness of the spine and hips, low back pain, evident on radiographs)

Calcium pyrophosphate deposition disease (uncommon in the hip)

Gout (rare in hip, previous diagnosis of gout most probable, pain in groin or buttock)

Hemophilic arthropathy (previous diagnosis of hemophilia, pain with motion, evident on radiographs)

Infection (acute onset, pain in the groin, fever, marked restriction of motion)

Inflammatory bowel disease (previous diagnosis of bowel disease most probable, groin and buttock discomfort)

Osteoarthritis of the hip (pain in the groin or buttock, limited range of motion)

Osteonecrosis (dull ache in groin or buttock, evident on radiographs and/or MRI)

Reiter syndrome (arthritis, conjunctivitis, pain in the hip, urethritis)

Rheumatoid arthritis (pain in the groin or buttock, decreased range of motion, evident on radiographs)

Stress fracture (pain in the groin or buttock with activity, evident on MRI)

Systemic lupus erythematosus (pain in the groin or buttock, limited range of motion)

Trochanteric bursitis (pain in the lateral aspect of the thigh)

# ADVERSE OUTCOMES OF THE DISEASE

Adverse outcomes of the disease include persistent pain and progressive gait abnormalities, which may lead to decreased ambulatory capacity and loss of functional independence.

# TREATMENT

For noninfectious inflammatory arthritis, a nonsurgical treatment plan administered in conjunction with a rheumatologist can include anti-inflammatory medications, disease-modifying agents, acetaminophen or other analgesics, the use of an assistive device held in the hand contralateral to the affected hip, and activity modification. Intra-articular corticosteroid injections can be considered, but they generally require fluoroscopic guidance for accurate placement. A physical therapy program emphasizing range-of-motion exercises and judicious strengthening can be helpful but may exacerbate the patient's symptoms. Total hip arthroplasty is the treatment of choice for patients with advanced symptoms that have failed to respond to nonsurgical treatment. Septic arthritis of the hip is a surgical emergency and requires immediate surgical drainage followed by long-term (typically 6 weeks) intravenous antibiotic therapy.

# ADVERSE OUTCOMES OF TREATMENT

Adverse outcomes of nonsurgical treatment include complications related to the chronic use of NSAIDs, such as gastric, renal, or hepatic problems. Extended treatment with acetaminophen in large doses can lead to hepatic toxicity. Corticosteroids are often used as part of the treatment algorithm and can lead to osteonecrosis of the femoral head. The most common short-term complications related to total hip arthroplasty include neurovascular injury, thromboembolic events, infection, leg-length inequality, and prosthetic dislocation. Wear-related complications are unusual because this patient population is typically inactive; however, prosthetic loosening requiring revision surgery may still occur.

# REFERRAL DECISIONS/RED FLAGS

Septic arthritis of the hip is a surgical emergency that requires immediate surgical drainage. For noninfectious arthritis, symptoms recalcitrant to nonsurgical treatment that lead to persistent pain and function disability indicate the need for further evaluation.

# LATERAL FEMORAL CUTANEOUS NERVE SYNDROME

## SYNONYM
Meralgia paresthetica

**ICD-9 Code**

**355.1**
Meralgia paresthetica

## DEFINITION
Compression or entrapment of the lateral femoral cutaneous nerve is characterized by pain, burning (dysesthesia), or hypoesthesia over the lateral thigh. Motor nerve dysfunction does not occur because the lateral femoral cutaneous nerve is a sensory nerve. The nerve is most susceptible to compression where it exits the pelvis just medial to the anterosuperior iliac spine. This syndrome can be caused by a number of factors, including obesity, compression from tight clothing or straps around the waist (eg, tool belt or backpack), scar tissue from previous operations, significant trauma (especially involving hip extension), or mild repetitive trauma over the course of the nerve. The nerve can also be injured during anterior surgical approaches to the hip, pelvis, or acetabulum. Rarely, pathologic intrapelvic or abdominal processes (cecal tumors) cause compression of the lateral femoral cutaneous nerve.

## CLINICAL SYMPTOMS
Symptoms associated with this condition include pain and dysesthesia in the anterolateral or lateral thigh that sometimes extends to the lateral knee. Uncommonly, patients report aching in the groin area and, if the condition is acute, pain radiating to the sacroiliac joint area. Joggers describe the pain as an "electric jab" each time the affected hip extends, usually after running a short distance.

## TESTS

### Physical Examination
Hypoesthesia or dysesthesia in the distribution of the lateral femoral cutaneous nerve is typical, with the most reproducible spot of hypoesthesia above and lateral to the knee (**Figure 1**). Burning is most consistent in this area. Pressure over the nerve where it exits the pelvis just medial to or directly over the anterosuperior iliac spine can produce tenderness or reproduce paresthesias along the distribution of the nerve. Muscle weakness and reflex changes are absent. Abdominal and pelvic examinations are needed to exclude intra-abdominal pathology.

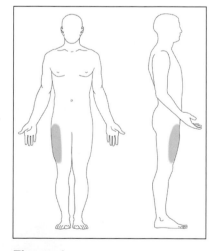

**Figure 1**
Location of hypoesthesia or dysesthesia associated with lateral femoral cutaneous nerve entrapment.

### Diagnostic Tests

An AP radiograph of the pelvis will rule out any bony abnormality, and AP and lateral radiographs of the hip may be appropriate when the patient has restricted internal rotation of the hip and groin pain. CT or MRI is appropriate to investigate a suspected intrapelvic mass.

## DIFFERENTIAL DIAGNOSIS

Diabetes mellitus or other causes of peripheral neuropathy (numbness in the feet)

Hip arthritis (limited internal rotation, limp)

Intra-abdominal tumor (pelvic or abdominal mass, hematochezia, weight loss)

Lumbar disk herniation (L1 through L4 motor and sensory changes, positive prone rectus femoris stretch test)

Trochanteric bursitis (tenderness over trochanter, stiffness when rising)

## ADVERSE OUTCOMES OF THE DISEASE

Pain and dysesthesia will continue if the patient is not treated.

## TREATMENT

Numbness is often well tolerated, but burning dysesthesia can become intolerable. Removing the source of compression, such as a tight waistband or mild repetitive trauma to the nerve, can relieve the symptoms of burning. In obese patients, significant weight loss often relieves symptoms. Infiltration of the area around the nerve where it exits the pelvis near the anterosuperior iliac spine with a corticosteroid preparation may reduce symptoms. Surgical release of the nerve is rarely required, but its most common indication is in patients with persistent burning dysesthesia.

## ADVERSE OUTCOMES OF TREATMENT

In some instances, symptoms persist despite treatment.

## REFERRAL DECISIONS/RED FLAGS

A suspected pelvic or abdominal mass signals the need for immediate further evaluation. The presence of intolerable symptoms that have failed to respond to nonsurgical treatment also indicates the need for further evaluation.

# OSTEOARTHRITIS OF THE HIP

## SYNONYMS

Degenerative arthritis of the hip

Osteoarthrosis of the hip

## DEFINITION

Osteoarthritis of the hip is characterized by loss of articular cartilage of the hip joint. The osteoarthrosis may be primary (idiopathic) or secondary to hip diseases during childhood, trauma, osteonecrosis, previous joint infection, or other conditions.

## CLINICAL SYMPTOMS

The classic presentation is a gradual onset of anterior thigh or groin pain. Some patients have pain in the buttock or the lateral aspect of the thigh. The pain may be referred to the distal thigh (knee) and may be perceived only in the knee. Initially, pain occurs only with activity, but gradually the frequency and intensity of the pain increase to the point that pain at rest and at night occurs. As osteoarthritis progresses, patients develop decreased range of motion, which may manifest as a limp and as difficulty putting on trousers or donning shoes. Ambulatory capacity gradually decreases as pain increases. Occasionally, patients will have a severe limp and stiffness but little pain.

Careful questioning may reveal a history of hip problems as an infant or toddler (indicative of developmental dysplasia of the hip), as a small child (indicative of Legg-Calvé-Perthes disease), or as an adolescent (suggestive of slipped capital femoral epiphysis). Patients with osteoarthritis of the hip may have other coexisting conditions, as listed in the differential diagnosis.

## TESTS

### Physical Examination

The earliest sign of osteoarthritis of the hip is a loss of internal rotation as determined by range-of-motion testing. Gradually, global decreases in range of motion occur and many patients develop a fixed external rotation and flexion contracture. Flexion contractures are particularly problematic because they greatly affect gait patterns, as the patient must compensate by increasing lumbar spine extension to afford hip extension. In addition, an antalgic gait (short stance on the painful leg) and

SECTION 5 ■ HIP AND THIGH

an abductor lurch (swaying the trunk far over the affected hip) develop as the body tries to compensate for the pain and secondary weakness in the hip abductor muscles.

## Diagnostic Tests

AP and lateral radiographs of the hip are indicated for patients with pain and limited internal rotation of the hip. The classic radiographic features of osteoarthritis of the hips are joint space narrowing, osteophyte formation, subchondral cyst formation, and subchondral sclerosis (**Figure 1**).

# DIFFERENTIAL DIAGNOSIS

Degenerative lumbar disk disease (normal hip motion)

Femoral cutaneous nerve entrapment (sensory changes, burning, normal motion)

Herniated lumbar disk (diminished knee reflex, sensory changes)

Inflammatory arthritis of the hip (rheumatoid arthritis, systemic lupus erythematosus, ankylosing spondylitis)

Osteonecrosis of the femoral head (evident on radiographs)

Trochanteric bursitis (local tenderness, normal motion)

Tumor of the pelvis or spine (back pain, night pain, normal motion)

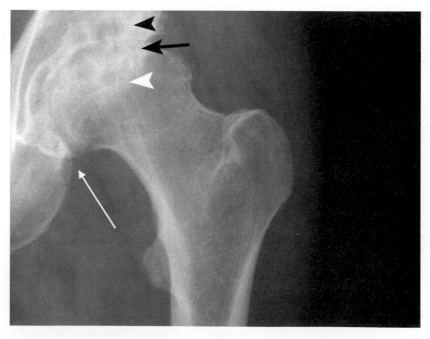

**Figure 1**

AP radiograph showing degenerative joint disease of the hip with joint space narrowing (black arrow), osteophyte formation (white arrow), subchondral cyst formation (black arrowhead), and subchondral sclerosis (white arrowhead).

## ADVERSE OUTCOMES OF THE DISEASE

Osteoarthritis of the hip is a progressive condition with a natural history of increasing pain and a subsequent decrease in function associated with progressive gait abnormality. In the end stages of the disease, pain is severe, occurring at night and at rest and severely limiting ambulation, and large fixed contractures of the hip develop secondarily. Progressive bone loss of the femoral head or acetabulum may occur but is uncommon.

## TREATMENT

Initial treatment for all patients is nonsurgical and consists of a combination of acetaminophen, NSAIDs, activity modification, and the use of an assistive device held in the hand contralateral to the affected hip. Non–weight-bearing exercise (such as the use of a stationary bicycle or swimming) is occasionally helpful but often exacerbates patient symptoms. Intra-articular injections with corticosteroids are used occasionally; they generally require fluoroscopic guidance for accurate placement.

Vigorous, young patients in whom nonsurgical treatment fails and who have a biomechanical derangement of the hip may be candidates for a realignment osteotomy of the proximal femur or acetabulum. Hip fusion is another alternative for young, vigorous patients who either must return to work as a manual laborer or who lead a vigorous lifestyle. The vast majority of patients in whom nonsurgical treatment fails, however, are most appropriately treated with total hip replacement surgery (**Figure 2**). Total hip replacement is associated with dramatic decreases in pain as well as increases in function and is among the most cost-effective medical interventions available when quality-adjusted years of life are considered.

## ADVERSE OUTCOMES OF TREATMENT

Adverse outcomes of nonsurgical treatment include complications related to the chronic use of NSAIDs such as gastric, renal, or hepatic problems. Extended treatment with acetaminophen in large doses can lead to hepatic toxicity. The most common short-term complications related to total hip arthroplasty include neurovascular injury, thromboembolic events, infection, leg-length inequality, and prosthetic dislocation. Long-term complications of total hip arthroplasty are more common in younger, active patients and relate primarily to wear of the bearing surface and loosening of the components that may require revision surgery. Patients who are treated with osteotomy or hip fusion may require further

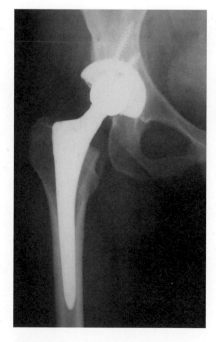

**Figure 2**
AP radiograph of the hip of a patient with osteoarthritis following total hip arthroplasty.

surgical intervention in the form of total hip replacement if the surgery is unsuccessful, if subsequent arthritis develops later, or if pain relief is incomplete.

## Referral Decisions/Red Flags

Patients who have persistent pain despite nonsurgical treatment including acetaminophen, multiple different NSAIDs, activity modification, and/or the use of an assistive device require appropriate referral for further evaluation of potential surgical intervention. Younger patients may be referred earlier to determine if alternatives to total hip replacement (such as a redirectional osteotomy) are appropriate.

# OSTEONECROSIS OF THE HIP

## SYNONYMS
Aseptic necrosis of the hip
Avascular necrosis of the hip

**ICD-9 Code**

**733.42**
Aseptic necrosis of femoral head and neck

## DEFINITION

Osteonecrosis of the hip results from the death of varying amounts of bone in the femoral head. The causative event may be traumatic disruption of the vascular supply to the femoral head or deficient circulation from other causes (eg, microvascular thrombosis in patients with sickle cell anemia). Initially, only the osteocytes and other cells are affected, but with time the bone structure fragments and collapses. As a result, the overlying articular surface collapses as well and progressive arthritis develops.

Osteonecrosis affects 10,000 to 20,000 new patients per year in the United States, occurs with greater frequency in the third through fifth decades of life, and often is bilateral. Risk factors include trauma (hip dislocation or femoral neck fracture), history of corticosteroid use, alcohol abuse, sickle cell disease, rheumatoid arthritis, and systemic lupus erythematosus. A list of clinical entities commonly associated with osteonecrosis appears in **Table 1**. Of note, the association with corticosteroids generally is associated with the amount and duration of medication; however, osteonecrosis sometimes develops after only one or two doses of intravenous corticosteroids.

## CLINICAL SYMPTOMS

Patients usually report the indolent onset of a dull ache or a throbbing pain in the groin, lateral hip, or buttock area. Patients may report severe pain during the initial phases of the disease when bone death occurs. Secondary arthritis develops with progressive collapse of the femoral head, and symptoms may be indistinguishable from osteoarthritis. Limited range of motion may occur, and patients often report a progressive limp. The history should focus on risk factors for the disease as outlined in Table 1.

## TESTS

### Physical Examination

Patients have pain with attempted straight-leg raising (lifting the heel off of the examination table with the knee held straight) as well as with range of motion of the hip. Range of motion may be decreased (particularly internal rotation) in addition to being

**Table 1    Risk Factors for Osteonecrosis**

Alcohol abuse

Caisson disease (scuba diving)

Chronic pancreatitis

Corticosteroid use

Crohn's disease

Gaucher disease

HIV Infection

Myeloproliferative disorders

Radiation treatment

Rheumatoid arthritis

Trauma

Sickle cell disease

Smoking

Systemic lupus erythematosus

SECTION 5 ■ HIP AND THIGH

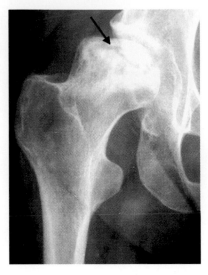

**Figure 1**
AP view of the hip showing osteonecrosis of the femoral head with collapse (arrow).

painful. Patients often have an antalgic gait (short stance phase) but may develop a Trendelenburg gait once secondary arthritis develops.

## Diagnostic Tests

An AP view of the pelvis and AP and frog-lateral radiographs of the hip should be obtained. In the earliest stages of the disease, plain radiographs may be normal. With time, patchy areas of sclerosis and lucency may be present. With disease progression, a "crescent sign" appears, which is a well-defined sclerotic area just beneath the articular surface that represents a subchondral fracture. The femoral head typically becomes progressively more aspherical with time, leading to secondary degenerative changes of the acetabulum, which may appear indistinguishable from degenerative arthritis (**Figure 1**).

In patients in whom osteonecrosis is suspected but radiographic findings are normal or equivocal, MRI is indicated (**Figure 2**). Patients with unilateral atraumatic osteonecrosis may benefit from MRI of the contralateral hip to diagnose asymptomatic disease on that side that may benefit from surgical treatment to prevent disease progression.

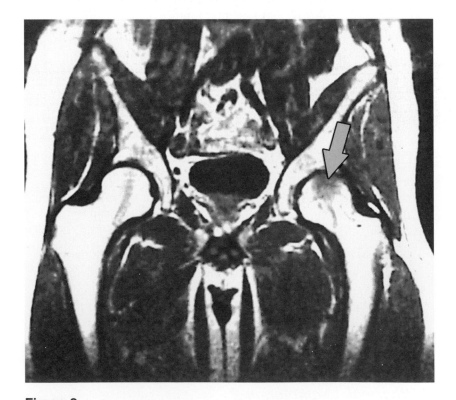

**Figure 2**
MRI scan reveals significant involvement of the weight-bearing surface of the left hip consistent with osteonecrosis (arrow). The opposite hip is normal.

Reproduced from Poss R (ed): *Orthopaedic Knowledge Update 3*. Park Ridge, IL, American Academy of Orthopaedic Surgeons, 1990, p 540.

## DIFFERENTIAL DIAGNOSIS

Fracture of the femoral neck (evident on radiographs, MRI)

Lumbar disk disease (back pain, reflex changes, radiation below knee)

Muscle strain or groin pull (normal radiographs, intermittent limp)

Osteoarthritis of the hip (no risk factors, absence of sclerosis within the femoral heads on radiographs)

Septic arthritis of the hip (fever, constitutional symptoms)

Transient osteoporosis of the hip (disabling pain without previous trauma, osteopenia, patient a women in third trimester of pregnancy or a middle-aged man)

## ADVERSE OUTCOMES OF THE DISEASE

The natural history of osteonecrosis is not well understood. In general, in patients with smaller lesions in non–weight-bearing areas and limited exposure to vascular insult, symptoms tend to resolve without femoral head collapse and arthritis developing. In patients with larger lesions and/or sustained insult to the vascular supply of the femoral head, however, femoral head collapse and secondary degenerative arthritis develop. End-stage degenerative changes also develop in these patients, including progressive pain, decreased range of motion, decreased ambulatory capacity, and limp.

## TREATMENT

Treatment options prior to collapse are controversial. A myriad of different treatment options have been attempted, including protected weight bearing, pulsed magnetic electrical fields, and surgical interventions, but few studies have adequate randomization or statistical power to provide guidance with regard to selecting among these options. Surgical choices for the patient without collapse aimed at maintaining the native femoral head include core decompression (removing a core of bone from the femoral head and neck to decrease bone marrow pressure and encourage blood flow) with or without bone grafting, vascularized fibular grafting (harvesting a portion of the ipsilateral fibula with a vascular pedicle and transplanting it to the femoral head and neck to stimulate revascularization), and fresh osteochondral allografting of the femoral head. The former two options aim to relieve pressure in the femoral head that may be causing pain and stimulate healing of the lesion. Once femoral head collapse has occurred, most recommend replacement arthroplasty, although some have advocated core decompression for short-term pain relief.

SECTION 5 ■ HIP AND THIGH

## ADVERSE OUTCOMES OF TREATMENT

If attempts to preserve the femoral head fail, degenerative arthritis may develop subsequently, requiring further surgical intervention in the form of total hip arthroplasty. A unique complication of core decompression is a fracture of the femoral shaft if the core biopsy tract is placed below the level of the greater trochanter. The results of total hip arthroplasty in this patient population are often inferior because patients may be young and vigorous and bone metabolism may be altered, placing higher demands on the prosthesis and increasing the risk of prosthetic loosening.

## REFERRAL DECISIONS/RED FLAGS

Plain radiographic evidence of or clinical suspicion for osteonecrosis requires further evaluation to determine if surgical intervention to preserve the femoral head is indicated.

# SNAPPING HIP

## DEFINITION

Snapping hip is characterized by a snapping or popping sensation that occurs as tendons around the hip move over bony prominences. The most common site is the iliotibial band snapping over the greater trochanter. Snapping also can occur when the iliopsoas tendon slides over the pectineal eminence of the pelvis or from intra-articular tears of the acetabular labrum (fibrocartilage rim at the periphery of the acetabulum).

## CLINICAL SYMPTOMS

Iliotibial band subluxation usually occurs with walking or rotation of the hip. Patients will point to the trochanteric area (**Figure 1**). Some patients notice the snapping when they lie with the affected side up and rotate the leg. If a trochanteric bursitis subsequently develops, patients will report increased pain when first rising in the morning, pain at night, and difficulty lying on the affected side.

Snapping caused by subluxation of the iliopsoas tendon usually is felt in the groin as the hip extends from a flexed position, as when rising from a chair. Many patients feel the snapping but have no disability. In a few patients, the snapping is either annoying or painful.

Snapping from intra-articular causes is more disabling and more likely to cause patients to grab for support.

## TESTS

### Physical Examination

Iliotibial band subluxation can be recreated by having the patient stand and then rotate the hip while holding it in an adducted position. A snap can be palpated as the iliotibial band slides over the greater trochanter. Snapping of the iliopsoas tendon may be palpated as the hip extends from a flexed position and the tendon moves over the pectineal eminence of the pelvis. Restricted internal rotation of the involved hip, a limp, or shortening of the limb suggests problems within the hip joint.

### Diagnostic Tests

AP radiographs of the pelvis and lateral hip can exclude bony pathology or intra-articular hip disease. Radiographs typically are normal for patients with a snapping hip. A CT arthrogram may be necessary to rule out intra-articular loose bodies. MRI with gadolinium may be necessary to rule out a tear of the acetabular labrum.

**ICD-9 Code**

**719.65**
Snapping hip

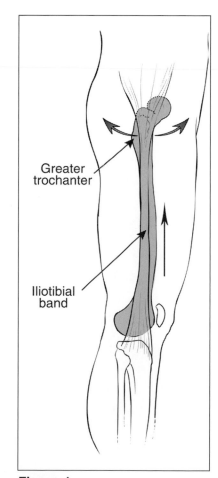

**Figure 1**
The iliotibial band slips anteriorly and posteriorly over the prominent greater trochanter.

# DIFFERENTIAL DIAGNOSIS

Osteoarthritis of the hip (limited internal rotation)

Osteochondral loose body (fragment of bone and cartilage within the joint, pain with hip motion)

Osteonecrosis of the femoral head (compromised blood supply to the femoral head, groin pain)

Tear of the acetabular labrum (pain or instability with hip motion)

# ADVERSE OUTCOMES OF THE DISEASE

Pain and annoyance are commonly reported.

# TREATMENT

Snapping hip is often painless, and once the diagnosis is made with certainty, patients often require only an explanation of the source of the symptoms for reassurance. Patients who are significantly bothered by the symptoms should be advised to avoid provocative maneuvers and activities so that the symptoms can subside. Treatment consisting of stretching and strengthening exercises (iliotibial band, hip abductors, hip adductors, and hip flexors) and a short course of NSAIDs may reduce the discomfort associated with tendon snapping and secondary bursitis. Corticosteroid injection into the greater trochanteric bursa (for snapping iliotibial band) or into the psoas tendon sheath (for snapping iliopsoas tendon) may reduce pain.

Surgery is reserved for the uncommon cases that are disabling and fail to resolve with nonsurgical management.

# PHYSICAL THERAPY PRESCRIPTION

The functional goal of rehabilitation for a patient with a snapping hip is to reduce the pain and increase the ability of the patient to return to functional activities such as walking and running. Stretching exercises for tight muscles around the hip should be performed in conjunction with strengthening exercises. Weakness of the hip abductors is very commonly associated with tightness of the iliotibial band.

The home exercise program (see p 444) should include stretching and strengthening exercises. If the pain does not diminish within 2 or 3 weeks on a home program, physical therapy may be ordered. The prescription should include a complete evaluation of the hip strength and the flexibility of the soft-tissue structures such as the iliotibial band, hamstrings, and hip flexors. Increasing the endurance of the trunk muscles should be part of the physical therapy prescription.

# ADVERSE OUTCOMES OF TREATMENT

NSAIDs can cause gastric, renal, or hepatic complications. Postoperative infection or persistent pain is possible if surgical intervention is undertaken.

# REFERRAL DECISIONS/RED FLAGS

Unclear diagnosis, intra-articular pathology, and/or failure of nonsurgical measures indicate the need for further evaluation.

SECTION 5 ■ HIP AND THIGH

# HOME EXERCISE PROGRAM FOR SNAPPING HIP

Perform the exercises in the order listed. Apply dry or moist heat to the hip for 5 to 10 minutes before the exercises to prepare the tissues. Alternatively, riding a stationary bicycle for 10 minutes will also prepare the tissues for stretching. Apply a bag of crushed ice or frozen peas to the hip for 20 minutes after the exercises to help reduce inflammation. If you experience pain in the hip during or after the exercises, discontinue the exercises and call your doctor.

| Exercise Type | Muscle Group | Number of Repetitions/Sets | Number of Days per Week | Number of Weeks |
|---|---|---|---|---|
| Iliotibial band stretch | Tensor fascia | 4 repetitions/2 to 3 sets | 5 to 7 | 2 to 3 |
| Hip abduction | Gluteus medius | 8 repetitions/2 sets, progressing to 15 repetitions/3 sets | 3 | 2 to 3 |

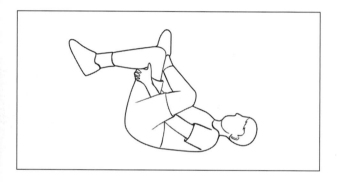

## *Iliotibial Band Stretch*

Lie on your back and bend both knees so that your feet are flat on the floor. Place the ankle of the affected leg on the opposite knee and clasp your hands behind the thigh as shown. Pull the thigh toward you until you feel a stretch in the hip. Hold the stretch for 30 seconds, then relax for 30 seconds. Perform 2 to 3 sets of 4 repetitions 5 to 7 days a week, continuing for 2 to 3 weeks.

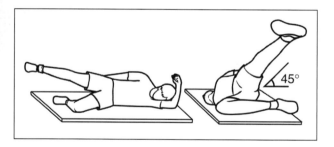

## *Hip Abduction*

Lie on your side with the affected hip on top, cradling your head in your arm, and with the bottom leg bent to provide support. Slowly move the top leg up and back to 45°, keeping the knee straight. Hold this position for 5 seconds. Slowly lower the leg and relax it for 2 seconds. Ankle weights should be used, starting with light enough weight to allow 2 sets of 8 repetitions. Progress to 3 sets of 15 repetitions. Then return to 2 sets of 8 repetitions and add weight. Perform the exercise 3 times per week, continuing for 2 to 3 weeks.

# STRAINS OF THE HIP

## DEFINITION

Hip strain is a general term applied to injuries of the muscle-tendon units around the hip. Vigorous muscular contraction while the muscle is on stretch frequently causes the injury. For example, forceful hip flexion can strain the iliopsoas muscle, as when a soccer player forcibly flexes the hip to kick a ball and the leg is blocked or forcefully extended by an opponent. Overuse injuries are a second cause of hip strains. Several muscles, including the abdominals, hip flexors (iliopsoas, sartorius, or rectus femoris), and adductors, should be considered when a patient has pain around the hip after an acute or overuse injury (**Figure 1**).

## CLINICAL SYMPTOMS

The most common presenting symptom is pain over the injured muscle that is exacerbated when that area continues to be used during strenuous activities.

## TESTS

### Physical Examination

The deep location of the hip muscles compromises the examination, and precise localization of the injured muscle is not always possible. A strain of the hip adductors is identified

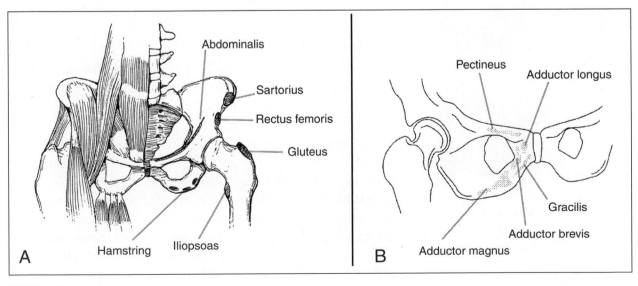

**Figure 1**

**A,** Anterior view of pelvis: muscle origins and insertions. **B,** Anterior view of pelvis: adductor muscle insertions.

(A, Reproduced with permission from Delee JC, Drez D Jr (eds): *Orthopaedic Sports Medicine: Principles and Practice.* Philadelphia, PA, WB Saunders, 1994, vol 2, pp 1063-1085.)

SECTION 5 ■ HIP AND THIGH

by tenderness in the groin and increased pain with passive abduction. Injury to the abdominal muscles is identified by increased pain when the patient flexes the trunk. When a hip flexor is injured, the pain is worse with flexion of the hip against resistance or with passive extension of the hip. Strain of the rectus femoris is delineated by increased pain when putting the rectus femoris on stretch. Injury to the iliopsoas typically causes pain in the deep groin or inner thigh, whereas pain from a proximal sartorius strain is more superficial and lateral.

### Diagnostic tests

AP radiographs of the pelvis and a frog-lateral view of the involved hip can rule out a fracture or other bony lesion. A bone scan or MRI (**Figure 2**) can contribute useful information to help the physician arrive at the correct diagnosis, but these studies are rarely necessary except in the elite athlete.

## DIFFERENTIAL DIAGNOSIS

Hip avulsion fractures (may be seen with strains of the sartorius [avulsion fracture of the anterior superior iliac spine] or rectus femoris [avulsion fracture of the anterior inferior iliac spine])

Osteonecrosis of the hip (chronic dull ache in groin, inner thigh, or buttock; evident on radiographs, MRI)

Pelvic or proximal femoral tumors (pain at rest or at night, increased pain with weight bearing)

## ADVERSE OUTCOMES OF THE DISEASE

Chronic injury can be debilitating and threaten athletic performance. If pain persists, the patient's gait may be altered, resulting in secondary injuries.

## TREATMENT

Rehabilitation enhances full recovery and should be initiated after confirmation of the injury. For most patients, modification of activities, followed by a home exercise program, is sufficient. Elite athletes usually are treated with a more aggressive and costly regimen (**Table 1**). Rehabilitation can be divided into five phases that generally are completed within approximately 6 weeks. Phase I includes rest, ice, compression, and protected weight bearing with the use of crutches if needed (48 to 72 hours). Phase II includes passive range-of-motion exercises, accompanied by heat, electrical stimulation, or ultrasound (72 hours up to 1 week). The final three phases include different isometric exercises and sport-specific training. The purpose of the final phases is to increase strength and flexibility and focus on returning the patient to the preinjury level of

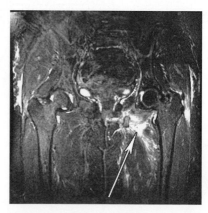

**Figure 2**
Coronal STIR MRI scan of the pelvis demonstrates high signal intensity, indicating edema, at the origin and proximal muscle belly of several of the adductor muscles. This is consistent with a muscle strain.

## Table 1　Rehabilitation Guidelines for Muscle Injuries in Elite Athletes

|  | Goals | Treatment | Time Frame |
|---|---|---|---|
| Phase I | Reduce pain, inflammation, and bleeding | Rest, ice, and compression; crutches if needed | 48 to 72 hours |
| Phase II | Regain range of motion | Passive range of motion, heat, ultrasound, electrical muscle stimulation | 72 hours to 1 week |
| Phase III | Increase strength, flexibility, and endurance | Isometrics, well-leg cycling | Weeks 1 to 3 |
| Phase IV | Increase strength and coordination | Isotonic and isokinetic exercises | Weeks 3 to 4 |
| Phase V | Return to competition | Sport-specific training | Weeks 4 to 6 |

Reproduced with permission from Delee JC, Drez D Jr (eds): *Orthopaedic Sports Medicine: Principles and Practice.* Philadelphia, PA, WB Saunders, 1994, vol 2, pp 1063-1085.

activity. If pain is exacerbated during the rehabilitation process, the patient should return to the phase of treatment before symptoms recurred. Anti-inflammatory medications can be a useful adjunct to a physical therapy program to reduce pain and inflammation.

## PHYSICAL THERAPY PRESCRIPTION

Strains of the hip are usually secondary to overuse and/or muscle imbalances. For example, running long distances can result in muscle fatigue. The hip abductors, extensors, and internal and external rotators are among the weakest muscle groups in the hip, so a home exercise program that attempts to strengthen these muscles is appropriate provided that there is no pain with the exercise (see pp 449-450).

If pain persists after the patient has been on a home program for 3 to 4 weeks, formal physical therapy may be ordered. The prescription should include an evaluation of the trunk and hip muscles, including testing of the quadratus lumborum, abdominals, and back extensors. Once the deficits are determined, an extensive strengthening program should be initiated.

## ADVERSE OUTCOMES OF TREATMENT

Recalcitrant pain may indicate a more serious injury or tendinous disruption that requires further evaluation. Recurrent injuries also are possible and are more likely to occur in competitive or weekend athletes who fail to maintain flexibility of the affected muscle.

## REFERRAL DECISION/RED FLAGS

Symptoms that do not respond to treatment require further evaluation to ensure that a more serious injury has not occurred and that a malignancy or osteonecrosis of the hip is not mimicking symptoms of hip strain.

# HOME EXERCISE PROGRAM FOR STRAINS OF THE HIP

Perform the exercises in the order listed. After each set of exercises, apply ice, such as a bag of ice cubes or crushed ice or a bag of frozen peas, to the hip for 20 minutes. If the pain in the hip is aggravated by the exercises or does not go away within 3 to 4 weeks, call your doctor.

| Exercise Type | Muscle Group | Number of Repetitions/Sets | Number of Days per Week | Number of Weeks |
|---|---|---|---|---|
| Hip abduction | Gluteus medius | 8 repetitions/2 sets, progressing to 12 repetitions/3 sets | 3 | 3 to 4 |
| Hip extension | Gluteus maximus | 8 to 12 repetitions/2 to 3 sets | 3 | 3 to 4 |
| Hip rotations | *External*: Piriformis *Internal*: Medial hamstring | 8 to 12 repetitions/2 to 3 sets | 3 | 3 to 4 |

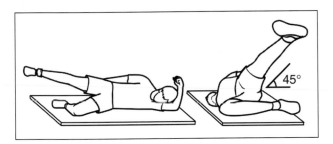

## Hip Abduction

Lie on your side with the affected hip on top, cradling your head in your arm, and the bottom leg bent to provide support. Slowly move the top leg up and back to 45°, keeping the knee straight. Hold this position for 5 seconds. Slowly lower the leg and relax it for 2 seconds. Ankle weights should be used, starting with light enough weight to allow 2 sets of 8 repetitions, progressing to 3 sets of 12 repetitions. Then return to 2 sets of 8 repetitions and add weight. Perform the exercise 3 days a week, continuing for 3 to 4 weeks.

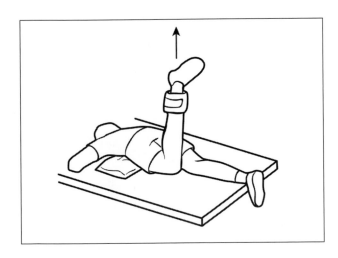

## Hip Extension

Lie face down with a pillow under your hips and the knee on the affected side bent 90°. Elevate the leg off the floor to a count of 5, lifting the leg straight up with the knee bent. Ankle weights should be used, starting with light enough weight to allow 2 sets of 8 repetitions, progressing to 3 sets of 12 repetitions. Then return to 2 sets of 8 repetitions and add weight. Perform the exercise 3 days a week, continuing for 3 to 4 weeks.

SECTION 5 ■ HIP AND THIGH

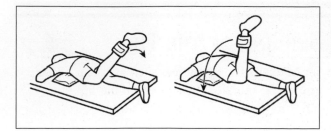

## Hip Rotations

Lie face down with a pillow under your hips and the knee on the affected side bent 90°. Rotating from the hip, move the ankle slowly from side to side, attempting to touch the floor. Ankle weights should be used, starting with light enough weight to allow 2 sets of 8 repetitions, progressing to 3 sets of 12 repetitions. Then return to 2 sets of 8 repetitions and add weight. Perform the exercise 3 days a week, continuing for 3 to 4 weeks.

# STRAINS OF THE THIGH

## DEFINITION

Injury to the thigh muscles can be temporarily painful and devastating to the avid elite or weekend athlete. The posterior thigh muscles (hamstring muscles) are injured more often than the anterior thigh muscles (quadriceps). Most hamstring strains occur when one of these muscles (biceps femoris, semimembranosus, or semitendinosus) is put on stretch during an active contraction. The strain or tear usually occurs at the musculotendinous junction. The quadriceps may sustain a similar injury; however, the quadriceps is more often injured by a direct blow.

## CLINICAL SYMPTOMS

A patient with a hamstring strain typically reports a sudden onset of posterior thigh pain that occurred while running, water skiing, or some other rapid movement. A "pop" may have been perceived at the onset of pain. Quadriceps contusions are associated with a direct blow during contact sports.

## TESTS

### Physical Examination

Physical examination reveals local tenderness at the site of the injured muscle. With time, the inflammation spreads and the tenderness can become less localized. Muscle injury and associated hemorrhage may be evident by ecchymosis located in the posterior thigh. The hamstrings span two joints, originating above the hip on the ischial tuberosity and inserting below the knee on the tibia and fibula. Therefore, placing the hamstring on stretch to confirm the diagnosis requires flexion of the hip followed by extension of the knee. Three components of the quadriceps muscle (vastus medialis, vastus intermedius, and vastus lateralis) only span one joint. Therefore, pain associated with strain or contusion of this part of the quadriceps muscle is exacerbated by flexion of the knee and is not related to the position of the hip. However, the rectus femoris component of the quadriceps muscle spans the hip and knee. To put this muscle on stretch, perform the prone rectus femoris test by flexing the knee with the hip in extension.

**ICD-9 Code**

**843.9**
Sprains and strains of hip and thigh, unspecified site

SECTION 5 ■ HIP AND THIGH

## *Diagnostic Tests*

Radiographs or other specialized imaging studies usually are not needed in patients with a typical history and physical examination. If there is a suspicion of a fracture or bony avulsion injury, plain radiographs can be obtained. MRI can confirm the thigh strain (**Figure 1**) but is rarely indicated because the history and physical examination can adequately provide a correct diagnosis.

# DIFFERENTIAL DIAGNOSIS

Adductor injuries (pain in the groin and inner thigh, ecchymosis, occasional sharp, stabbing pain)

Iliopsoas strains (pain in the groin with hip flexion)

Muscle strain of other pelvic/hip muscles (pain with ambulation)

Pelvic avulsion fractures (pain and ecchymosis over the anterosuperior iliac spine, evident on radiographs)

Proximal femoral tumor (pain in the groin or thigh at rest or at night, pain with weight bearing, evident on radiographs)

# ADVERSE OUTCOMES OF THE DISEASE

Chronic hamstring injuries are debilitating and can end an elite athlete's career. Contusion (hemorrhage) in the quadriceps muscle may progress to myositis ossificans with a resulting restriction of knee flexion and a possible diagnostic dilemma because the clinical appearance may simulate a malignant tumor.

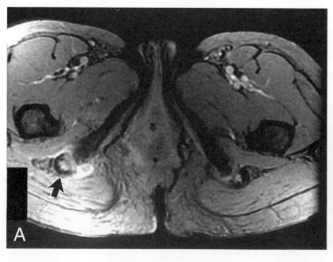
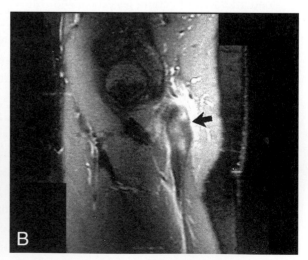

**Figure 1**

**A,** Axial MRI scan of the pelvis of a 39-year-old woman who sustained an acute injury while water skiing. Area of signal change (arrow) indicates an acute hamstring injury. **B,** Sagittal MRI scan of the hip and thigh of the same patient also demonstrates the hamstring injury (arrow).

# TREATMENT

Initial treatment includes prevention of further swelling and hemorrhage by having the patient rest and elevate the limb while applying ice and compressive wraps as needed. As time passes, the patient should begin a program of rehabilitation with stretching and strengthening of the injured muscle. The degree of rehabilitation necessary depends on the patient's general activity level and the severity of the injury. Most patients can be treated with a home exercise program. Elite athletes usually are treated with a more aggressive and costly regimen. The long-term results are generally similar. If myositis ossificans develops in the quadriceps muscle, the rehabilitation process is typically longer. However, surgical excision of the ossific mass is rarely needed. NSAIDs may be used as an adjunct to a physical therapy program to reduce pain and inflammation.

# PHYSICAL THERAPY PRESCRIPTION

The hamstrings, adductors, and quadriceps muscle groups of the thigh are commonly injured. Sometimes a muscle imbalance of the hip and trunk is responsible for strains of these muscle groups. Early treatment consists of rest, ice, compression, and elevation (RICE) of the affected limb. Depending on the severity of the injury, 1 to 3 weeks of rest may be required. Following the period of rest, early mobilization of the muscle is important to the healing process. Gentle stretching of the involved muscle group is important to regain flexibility, and strengthening is important to prevent a recurrence of the injury. An early home exercise program might include gentle stretching of the hamstrings and strengthening of the hip muscles, especially the abductors (see pp 454-455).

If pain and stiffness persist, formal physical therapy may be ordered. The prescription should include a detailed assessment of the trunk and hip muscle strength, a flexibility assessment of the involved muscle, and pain-relieving modalities to promote healing of the muscle.

# ADVERSE OUTCOME OF TREATMENT

NSAIDs can cause gastric, renal, or hepatic complications. Failure to rehabilitate the injury adequately can result in chronic problems.

# REFERRAL DECISIONS/RED FLAGS

Patients with symptoms that fail to respond to appropriate rehabilitation require further evaluation.

SECTION 5 ■ HIP AND THIGH

# HOME EXERCISE PROGRAM FOR STRAINS OF THE THIGH

Perform the exercises in the order listed. Apply dry or moist heat to the thigh for 5 to 10 minutes before exercising to prepare the tissues, and apply a bag of crushed ice or frozen peas for 20 minutes after exercising to prevent inflammation. If the exercises increase pain or the pain does not go away after adhering to the program for 3 to 4 weeks, call your doctor.

| Exercise Type | Muscle Group | Number of Repetitions/Sets | Number of Days per Week | Number of Weeks |
|---|---|---|---|---|
| 2-person hamstring stretch *or* 1-person hamstring stretch | Hamstrings | 4 repetitions/2 to 3 sets | Daily | 3 to 4 |
| Hip abduction | Gluteus medius | 8 to 12 repetitions/2 to 3 sets | 3 | 3 to 4 |

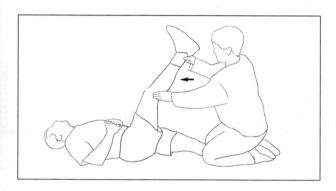

## *2-Person Hamstring Stretch*

Lie on the floor with your legs straight or with one leg bent slightly at the knee if that is more comfortable. Your partner raises one leg just to the point of tightness and applies resistance for 30 seconds while you try to lower the leg. Do the same with the other leg. Repeat the cycle 4 times. Perform 2 to 3 sets of 4 repetitions daily, continuing for 3 to 4 weeks.

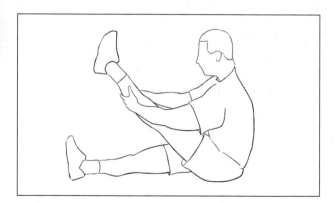

## *1-Person Hamstring Stretch*

Sit on the floor with your legs straight. Grasp the calf of one leg and slowly pull the leg toward your ear, keeping your back straight. Hold for 5 seconds. Do the same with the other leg. Repeat the cycle 4 times. Perform 2 to 3 sets of 4 repetitions daily, continuing for 3 to 4 weeks.

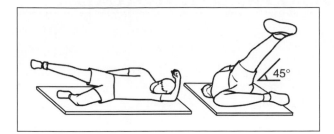

## Hip Abduction

Lie on your side with the affected hip on top, cradling your head in your arm, and with the bottom leg bent to provide support. Slowly raise the top leg up and back to 45°, keeping the knee straight. Slowly lower the leg to a count of 5 and relax it for 2 seconds. Ankle weights should be used, starting with a weight that allows 2 sets of 8 repetitions and progressing to 3 sets of 12 repetitions. Then return to 2 sets of 8 repetitions and add weight in 2- to 3-pound increments, progressing each time to 3 sets of 12 repetitions. Perform the exercise 3 days a week for 3 to 4 weeks.

SECTION 5 ■ HIP AND THIGH

# STRESS FRACTURE OF THE FEMORAL NECK

## ICD-9 Codes

**733.95**
Stress fracture of other bone; stress reaction of bone

**820.00**
Femoral neck fracture (transcervical) fracture

## SYNONYM

Stress fracture of the hip

## DEFINITION

Femoral neck stress fractures are often misdiagnosed or missed, and failure to identify this injury may be catastrophic. Stress fractures are usually the result of a dynamic continuing process rather than a single acute traumatic event. Stress fractures of the femoral neck occur most commonly in military recruits and athletes, especially runners. These fractures may be classified based on the anatomic location of the fracture. Tension stress fractures, which tend to occur in older patients, are usually transverse and occur on the superior aspect of the proximal femoral neck. These injuries have a high tendency to displace. Fractures on the inferior medial side of the femur, which are usually designated compression injuries, occur more commonly in younger athletes and do not usually displace.

## CLINICAL SYMPTOMS

Patients usually present with vague pain in the groin, anterior thigh, or knee that is associated with activity or weight bearing and usually subsides after cessation of activity. Athletes usually report that an increased activity level occurred in the few weeks preceding the symptoms.

## TESTS

### Physical Examination

Examination of the hip may reveal pain at extreme range of motion or a limited range of motion, most significantly in internal rotation. Occasionally, the patient will walk with an antalgic gait. Tenderness at the proximal thigh or groin may be present, related to soft-tissue irritation in the area. A resisted straight-leg raising maneuver (lifting the heel of the affected side off the examination table with the knee held straight) may reproduce the groin or thigh pain.

### Diagnostic Tests

Although plain radiographs are the first diagnostic test ordered, they are not diagnostic in most patients. Classic radiographic signs of stress fracture including radiolucent lines, sclerosis, or periosteal new bone formation are usually not apparent until

2 to 4 weeks after the onset of symptoms. Bone scans may detect stress fractures as soon as 24 to 48 hours after the injury (**Figure 1**). MRI is extremely sensitive for stress fractures of the femoral neck and should be considered in all patients with clinical evidence of a stress fracture but negative radiographs.

# DIFFERENTIAL DIAGNOSIS

Acute fracture of the femoral neck (evident on radiographs and MRI, history of trauma)

Muscle strain or groin pull (normal radiographs, intermittent limp)

Osteoarthritis of the hip (no risk factors, absence of sclerosis within the femoral heads on radiographs)

Osteonecrosis (dull ache in groin or buttock, evident on radiographs and/or MRI)

Pathologic fracture (underlying or associated benign or malignant tumor) (evident on bone scan, MRI, or radiographs)

Pelvic fracture (normal hip joint motion, pain on external rotation)

Tear of the acetabular labrum (pain or instability with hip motion)

# ADVERSE OUTCOMES OF THE DISEASE

Unlike patients with acute femoral neck fractures, patients with stress fractures are usually healthy and active. Adverse outcomes are associated with fracture displacement and include nonunion, osteonecrosis, and progressive varus deformity.

# TREATMENT

Treatment of stress fractures is usually guided by the type and the presence of fracture displacement. Displaced fractures in the young patient are treated as a surgical emergency, and

SECTION 5 ■ HIP AND THIGH

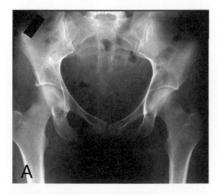
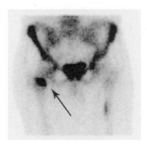

**Figure 1**

Stress fracture of the femoral neck. **A,** Initial AP radiograph demonstrates no apparent sign of fracture. **B,** Bone scan showing markedly increased uptake at site of femoral neck fracture (arrow). **C,** AP radiograph following a period of rest from impact activities shows increased osseous density at site of fracture healing (arrow).

immediate anatomic reduction and internal fixation is mandatory.

Nondisplaced compression or medial-side stress fractures are treated with cessation of activity and non–weight bearing with crutches until the fracture is healed. Healing usually takes 6 to 8 weeks. During this time period, serial radiographs are essential to monitor for fracture displacement or widening. Internal fixation may be necessary if the fracture progresses or the symptoms persist despite appropriate nonsurgical treatment.

All tension-side stress fractures are treated surgically whether the fracture is displaced or nondisplaced. These injuries have a high tendency to displace, and an aggressive approach is necessary. Internal fixation is the treatment of choice in these patients.

## ADVERSE OUTCOMES OF TREATMENT

Osteonecrosis of the femoral head and fracture nonunion are potential complications of internal fixation of femoral neck stress fractures.

## REFERRAL DECISIONS/RED FLAGS

A displaced femoral neck fracture in a patient younger than 60 years constitutes a surgical emergency because the risks of osteonecrosis and fracture nonunion are significant, and prompt surgical fixation decreases the risk of these complications. All stress fractures require consideration for surgical treatment given the high risk of displacement of tension-side fractures.

# TRANSIENT OSTEOPOROSIS OF THE HIP

## SYNONYM
Bone marrow edema syndrome

**ICD-9 Code**
**733.09**
Osteoporosis not elsewhere
classified or drug-induced

## DEFINITION
Transient osteoporosis of the hip is an uncommon idiopathic condition characterized by spontaneous onset of hip pain associated with radiographic osteoporosis of the femoral head and neck. The condition is most common in middle-aged men and in women during the third trimester of pregnancy. Resolution is spontaneous, usually within 6 to 12 months.

## CLINICAL SYMPTOMS
Patients typically have spontaneous onset of pain in the anterior thigh (groin), lateral hip, or buttock. Pain is usually worse with weight bearing and better at rest. Symptoms typically worsen for the first several months and then gradually abate.

## TESTS

### Physical Examination
Patients usually have an antalgic gait and pain at the limits of hip motion.

### Diagnostic Tests
Plain radiographs of the hip typically demonstrate diffuse osteoporosis of the femoral head and neck, although signs may not be evident in the early phase of the disease. MRI is helpful to rule out other diagnoses and help confirm the diagnosis of transient osteoporosis. The typical MRI findings are of bone marrow edema of the femoral neck with diffuse decreased signal intensity on T1-weighted images and diffuse increased signal intensity on T2-weighted images. The signal change usually extends into the intertrochanteric region (**Figure 1**).

## DIFFERENTIAL DIAGNOSIS
Infections involving the proximal femur or hip joint (pain, constitutional symptoms)

Osteonecrosis of the femoral head (pain in the groin or buttock, sclerosis on radiographs)

Pigmented villonodular synovitis of the hip (pain in the groin or buttock, evident on MRI and biopsy)

Stress fracture of the femoral neck (pain in the groin or buttock, evident on radiographs or MRI)

Tumors involving the proximal femur (pain in the groin, buttock, or thigh; evident on radiographs or MRI)

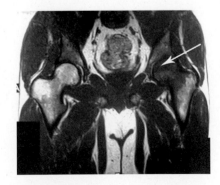

**Figure 1**
Coronal T1-weighted MRI scan of the pelvis showing diffuse decreased signal intensity (arrow) indicating transient osteoporosis of the hip.

## ADVERSE OUTCOMES OF THE DISEASE

Fracture of the femoral neck can occur during the time the bone is weakened by osteoporosis. Pregnant women with the disease appear to be at higher risk for femoral neck fracture.

## TREATMENT

The disease is a self-limited process that typically resolves spontaneously within 6 to 12 months after the onset of symptoms. After other diseases have been excluded and a firm diagnosis is established (usually by the characteristic MRI appearance), supportive treatment is begun. Patients are provided with mild analgesics and placed on crutches to limit weight bearing until symptoms resolve and radiographs demonstrate reconstitution of normal bone density.

## REFERRAL DECISIONS/RED FLAGS

The diagnosis may be difficult to make with certainty. In pregnant women, decisions regarding imaging studies and choice of analgesics should be made in consultation with the patient's obstetrician. Pregnant women with the disease appear to be at greater risk for femoral neck fracture.

# TROCHANTERIC BURSITIS

## SYNONYM
Greater trochanteric bursitis

**ICD-9 Code**
**726.5**
Enthesopathy of hip region

## DEFINITION
Inflammation and hypertrophy of the greater trochanteric bursa may develop without apparent cause or in association with lumbar spine disease, intra-articular hip pathology, significant limb-length inequalities, inflammatory arthritis, or previous surgery around the hip (particularly when internal fixation devices are placed in or near the greater trochanter) (**Figure 1**).

## CLINICAL SYMPTOMS
Patients usually have pain and tenderness over the greater trochanter. The pain may radiate distally to the knee or ankle (but not to the foot) or proximally into the buttock. The pain is worse when first rising from a seated or recumbent position,

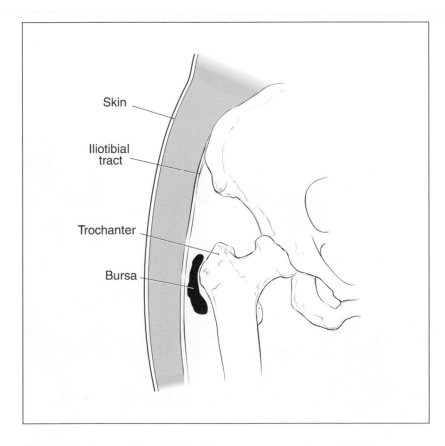

**Figure 1**
Location of trochanteric bursa, between the iliotibial band and the greater trochanter.

SECTION 5 ■ HIP AND THIGH

feels somewhat better after a few steps, and recurs after walking for half an hour or more. Patients report night pain and are unable to lie on the affected side. Inflammation (tendinitis) of the gluteal tendons may cause a similar pain pattern.

# Tests

## Physical Examination

With the patient in the lateral decubitus position, palpate the greater trochanter (**Figure 2**). Point tenderness over the lateral greater trochanter is the essential finding. Pain is often exacerbated with active hip abduction. Tenderness above the trochanter suggests tendinitis of the gluteus medius tendon. Patients report increased discomfort with adduction of the hip or adduction combined with internal rotation.

## Diagnostic Tests

AP radiographs of the pelvis and lateral radiographs of the hip are necessary to rule out bony abnormalities and intra-articular hip pathology. Occasionally, rounded or irregular calcific deposits may be seen above the trochanter at the attachment of the gluteus medius. Bone scans and MRI rarely are needed to make the diagnosis but occasionally may be helpful to rule out uncommon conditions such as occult fractures, tumors, or osteonecrosis of the femoral head.

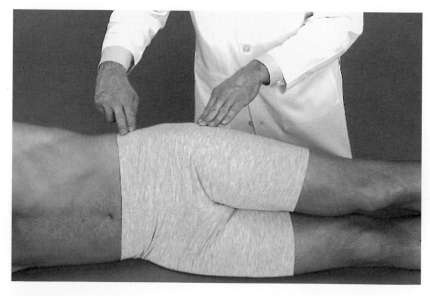

**Figure 2**
Palpation with the patient in the lateral decubitus position. With trochanteric bursitis, there is point tenderness over the lateral greater trochanter.

## DIFFERENTIAL DIAGNOSIS

Metastatic tumor (evident on radiographs, weight loss, constitutional symptoms)

Osteoarthritis of the hip (painful internal rotation, evident on radiographs)

Sciatica (pain posteriorly, pain radiating to the foot, motor and sensory changes, reflex changes)

Septic arthritis of the hip (fever, severe pain with motion)

Snapping hip (obvious snap of the iliotibial band)

Trochanteric fracture (evident on radiographs, persistent limp when walking, positive Trendelenburg sign)

## ADVERSE OUTCOMES OF THE DISEASE

Chronic pain, a limp, and/or sleep disturbances are possible.

## TREATMENT

NSAIDs, activity modifications, and short-term use of a cane are sufficient for most patients. Injection of a local anesthetic and corticosteroid preparation into the greater trochanteric bursa (see Trochanteric Bursitis Injection, pp 464-466) can be helpful in relieving symptoms. Occasionally, repeat injections are required for symptomatic relief. Surgery is indicated only rarely, for intransigent cases.

## ADVERSE OUTCOMES OF TREATMENT

NSAIDs can cause gastric, renal, or hepatic complications. In some patients, pain may persist. Although rare, infection from the injection can develop. Infection largely can be avoided by the careful use of sterile technique.

## REFERRAL DECISIONS/RED FLAGS

Failure of treatment, diagnostic uncertainty, and/or suspected fracture are indications for further evaluation.

SECTION 5 ■ HIP AND THIGH

# PROCEDURE

**CPT Code**

**20610**

Arthrocentesis, aspiration and/or injection; major joint or bursa (eg, shoulder, hip, knee joint, subacromial bursa)

*Current Procedural Terminology* © 2004 American Medical Association. All Rights Reserved.

## MATERIALS

Sterile gloves

Bactericidal skin preparation solution

10-mL syringe

20-gauge or 22-gauge 1½″ needle (use a spinal needle in larger patients)

3 to 5 mL of 1% lidocaine

40 to 80 mg of a corticosteroid preparation

Sterile adhesive sponge

Adhesive dressing

**Note:** Opinions differ regarding single- versus two-needle injection techniques. Proponents of the single-needle technique believe that one needle is less painful for the patient than two. Because the corticosteroid preparation is thicker than the local anesthetic, however, a slightly larger gauge needle is required at the outset. Physicians who prefer the two-needle technique point out that the smaller gauge needle is easier for patients to tolerate and that the pain of the second injection is dulled by the anesthetic. A two-syringe, two-needle technique is described on the DVD.

## STEP 1

Wear protective gloves at all times during the procedure and use sterile technique.

## STEP 2

Ask the patient to lie in the lateral decubitus position with the affected hip turned upward. Place a pillow between the patient's knees to relax the iliotibial band and reduce the pressure required to inject the solution.

## STEP 3

Cleanse the skin with a bactericidal skin preparation.

## STEP 4

Draw lidocaine into a 10-mL syringe.

## STEP 5

Draw the chosen dose of corticosteroid preparation into the same syringe and mix the two solutions.

## STEP 6

Palpate the greater trochanter and identify the point of maximum tenderness.

## STEP 7

Insert the needle until it contacts bone, then withdraw it 1 or 2 mm so that the tip is in the bursa and not in the bone (**Figure 1**). Usually, a 1½″ needle is sufficient, but for larger patients a spinal needle might be needed to reach the trochanteric bursa. Do not withdraw the needle too far or it will be outside the trochanteric bursa.

## STEP 8

Aspirate to ensure that the needle is not in an intravascular position, then inject one 1- to 2-mL aliquot of the corticosteroid preparation/local anesthetic mixture.

# TROCHANTERIC BURSITIS INJECTION (CONTINUED)

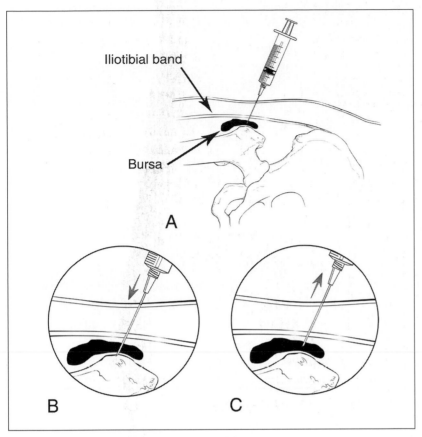

Iliotibial band

Bursa

A

B

C

**Figure 1**

Trochanteric bursitis injection. **A,** Location for needle insertion
showing anatomic landmarks. **B,** The needle is first inserted until it
contacts bone. **C,** The needle is then withdrawn 1 or 2 mm so that the
tip is in the bursa.

**Adapted with permission from the Mayo Foundation, Rochester, MN.**

## STEP 9
Partially withdraw the needle, then reinsert it and inject
another 1- to 2-mL aliquot. Continue this to infiltrate the
entire bursa, an area of several square centimeters around the
point of maximum tenderness.

## STEP 10
Withdraw the needle completely and apply gentle pressure
over the injection site with a sterile dressing sponge.

## STEP 11
Dress the puncture wound with a sterile adhesive bandage.

SECTION 5 ■ HIP AND THIGH

## Adverse Outcomes

Although rare, infection or allergic reactions to the local anesthetic or corticosteroid preparation are possible. Always query the patient about medication allergies before the procedure. In some patients with diabetes mellitus, poor control of blood glucose levels may occur, but this is usually temporary. Deposition of the steroid subcutaneously may cause fat atrophy or depigmentation. A minority of patients will require a series of injections to achieve lasting pain relief; however, repeated injections with corticosteroids should be avoided.

## Aftercare/Patient Instructions

Advise the patient that as the local anesthetic wears off, pain often persists or becomes worse for a few days until the corticosteroid takes effect. Instruct the patient to attempt weight bearing as tolerated and to contact you if symptoms recur or if redness, fever, immobilizing pain, or any other evidence of a local problem related to the injection occurs.

# PAIN DIAGRAM—KNEE AND LOWER LEG

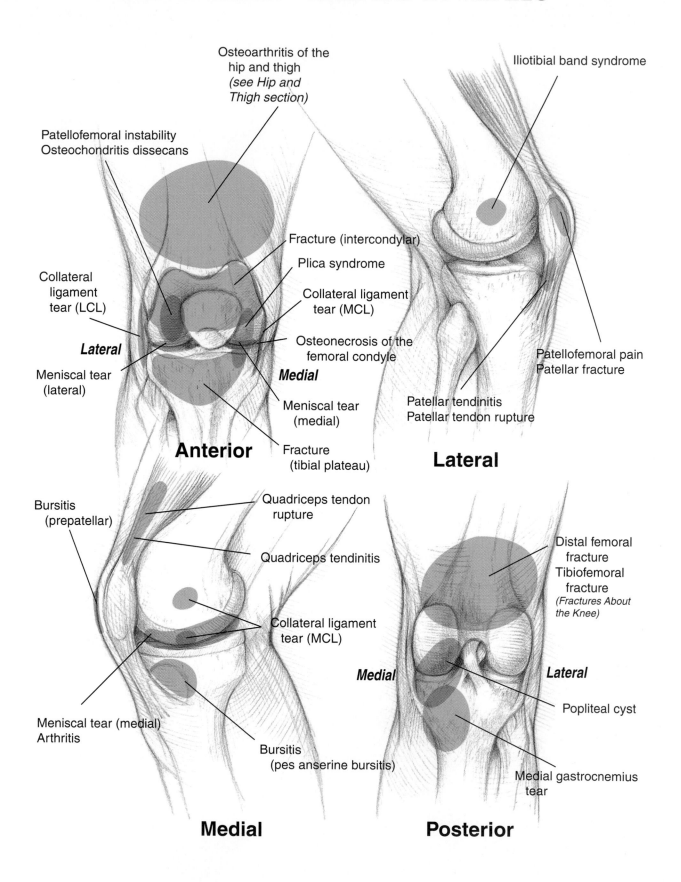

Osteoarthritis of the hip and thigh *(see Hip and Thigh section)*

Iliotibial band syndrome

Patellofemoral instability
Osteochondritis dissecans

Fracture (intercondylar)

Plica syndrome

Collateral ligament tear (MCL)

Collateral ligament tear (LCL)

Osteonecrosis of the femoral condyle

*Medial*

*Lateral*

Meniscal tear (lateral)

Meniscal tear (medial)

Fracture (tibial plateau)

**Anterior**

Patellofemoral pain
Patellar fracture

Patellar tendinitis
Patellar tendon rupture

**Lateral**

Bursitis (prepatellar)

Quadriceps tendon rupture

Quadriceps tendinitis

Collateral ligament tear (MCL)

Distal femoral fracture
Tibiofemoral fracture
*(Fractures About the Knee)*

*Medial*

*Lateral*

Popliteal cyst

Meniscal tear (medial)
Arthritis

Bursitis (pes anserine bursitis)

Medial gastrocnemius tear

**Medial**

**Posterior**

# KNEE AND LOWER LEG

**Section Editor**
Christopher D. Harner, MD
Professor of Orthopaedic Surgery
Chief, Division of Sports Medicine
Department of Orthopaedic Surgery
University of Pittsburgh
Pittsburgh, Pennsylvania

Robert Donatelli, PhD, PT, OCS
National Director of Sports Rehabilitation
Physiotherapy Associates
Las Vegas, Nevada

Craig S. Mauro, MD
Department of Orthopaedic Surgery
University of Pittsburgh
Pittsburgh, Pennsylvania

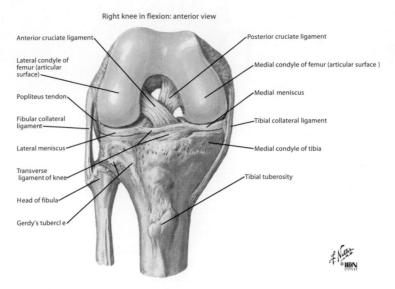

Right knee in flexion: anterior view

Anterior cruciate ligament

Lateral condyle of femur (articular surface)

Popliteus tendon

Fibular collateral ligament

Lateral meniscus

Transverse ligament of knee

Head of fibula

Gerdy's tubercle

Posterior cruciate ligament

Medial condyle of femur (articular surface )

Medial meniscus

Tibial collateral ligament

Medial condyle of tibia

Tibial tuberosity

## Knee: Cruciate and Collateral Ligaments

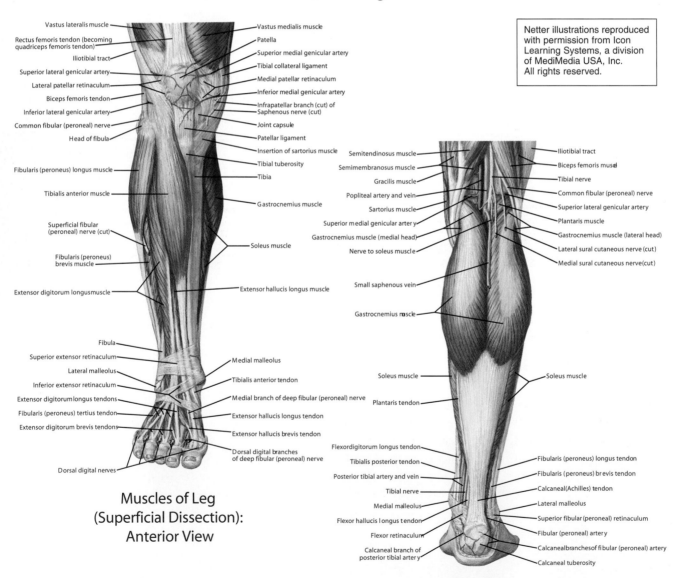

Vastus lateralis muscle

Rectus femoris tendon (becoming quadriceps femoris tendon)

Iliotibial tract

Superior lateral genicular artery

Lateral patellar retinaculum

Biceps femoris tendon

Inferior lateral genicular artery

Common fibular (peroneal) nerve

Head of fibula

Fibularis (peroneus) longus muscle

Tibialis anterior muscle

Superficial fibular (peroneal) nerve (cut)

Fibularis (peroneus) brevis muscle

Extensor digitorum longus muscle

Fibula

Superior extensor retinaculum

Lateral malleolus

Inferior extensor retinaculum

Extensor digitorum longus tendons

Fibularis (peroneus) tertius tendon

Extensor digitorum brevis tendons

Dorsal digital nerves

Vastus medialis muscle

Patella

Superior medial genicular artery

Tibial collateral ligament

Medial patellar retinaculum

Inferior medial genicular artery

Infrapatellar branch (cut) of Saphenous nerve (cut)

Joint capsule

Patellar ligament

Insertion of sartorius muscle

Tibial tuberosity

Tibia

Gastrocnemius muscle

Soleus muscle

Extensor hallucis longus muscle

Medial malleolus

Tibialis anterior tendon

Medial branch of deep fibular (peroneal) nerve

Extensor hallucis longus tendon

Extensor hallucis brevis tendon

Dorsal digital branches of deep fibular (peroneal) nerve

## Muscles of Leg (Superficial Dissection): Anterior View

Semitendinosus muscle

Semimembranosus muscle

Gracilis muscle

Popliteal artery and vein

Sartorius muscle

Superior medial genicular artery

Gastrocnemius muscle (medial head)

Nerve to soleus muscle

Small saphenous vein

Gastrocnemius muscle

Soleus muscle

Plantaris tendon

Flexor digitorum longus tendon

Tibialis posterior tendon

Posterior tibial artery and vein

Tibial nerve

Medial malleolus

Flexor hallucis longus tendon

Flexor retinaculum

Calcaneal branch of posterior tibial artery

Iliotibial tract

Biceps femoris muscle

Tibial nerve

Common fibular (peroneal) nerve

Superior lateral genicular artery

Plantaris muscle

Gastrocnemius muscle (lateral head)

Lateral sural cutaneous nerve (cut)

Medial sural cutaneous nerve (cut)

Soleus muscle

Fibularis (peroneus) longus tendon

Fibularis (peroneus) brevis tendon

Calcaneal (Achilles) tendon

Lateral malleolus

Superior fibular (peroneal) retinaculum

Fibular (peroneal) artery

Calcaneal branches of fibular (peroneal) artery

Calcaneal tuberosity

## Muscles of Leg (Superficial Dissection): Posterior View

# KNEE AND LOWER LEG—OVERVIEW

Most knee and lower leg problems can be diagnosed by obtaining an appropriate medical history, performing a thorough examination of the knee, and taking appropriate radiographs. Patients with knee problems often report pain, instability, stiffness, swelling, locking, or weakness. These findings may occur in or around any aspect of the knee. Careful localization of the pain and tenderness will significantly narrow the differential diagnosis. Examination of patients with knee problems also includes a screening evaluation of hip joint rotation because some patients with problems intrinsic to the hip present with distal thigh pain and other symptoms that mimic knee disorders.

Radiographic examination of the knee should include AP and lateral radiographs. If the patient is able to stand, obtain weight-bearing AP radiographs of both knees to allow comparison of the injured knee with the opposite, uninjured knee. When symptoms are localized to the patellofemoral joint, an axial patellofemoral view, such as a Merchant or Laurin view, is helpful. All radiographs should be evaluated for changes in bony architecture, including lytic and blastic lesions.

AP radiographs are best used to evaluate medial and lateral compartment arthritis, fractures of the distal femur and proximal tibia, and alignment of the femur with the tibia. Lateral radiographs are helpful in assessing the patella for fractures and malposition (patella alta and patella baja) and in analyzing the bony architecture of the distal femur and proximal tibia. Axial patellofemoral views are best used to assess subluxation of the patella and arthritis of the patellofemoral joint.

MRI rarely is needed in the initial diagnostic workup but sometimes plays an important role in surgical planning.

## ACUTE PAIN

Acute leg and knee pain usually occurs secondary to an injury. With the exception of a compartment syndrome, the different conditions that cause acute leg pain are temporarily painful but, with proper treatment, resolve without sequelae. Possible diagnoses fall into six basic categories, any of which can be painful: (1) fractures, (2) meniscal injuries, (3) ligamentous injuries, (4) musculotendinous strains, (5) extensor mechanism injuries, and (6) contusions.

Fractures may involve the distal femur, the patella, the proximal tibia, and the fibula. Inspect for swelling and deformity, palpate for tenderness in the bone itself, and obtain appropriate radiographs. Patellar fractures may result from indirect forces, such as falls, but fractures of the tibia and femur at the knee usually result from major trauma. Patellar dislocations are often reduced at the scene when a helper extends the knee for transportation.

Obtaining a history of the mechanism of injury is key in diagnosing meniscal tears. A history of a twisting injury sustained with the foot planted on the ground and locking (inability to extend the knee completely) with localized pain and tenderness along the joint line are indicative of meniscal pathology. Some patients report that manipulating or pushing on the knee enabled them to "unlock" it.

Patients with ligamentous injuries have acute pain, swelling, and instability. Strains of various musculotendinous structures around the knee also cause acute pain and swelling, but most do not result in instability. Patients with injuries to the extensor mechanism report a fall followed by sudden weakness or collapse of the knee. Contusions result from direct blows and cause localized pain and tenderness.

# CHRONIC PAIN

Conditions that cause chronic knee pain include arthritis, tumors, sepsis, and overuse syndromes (including bursitis/tendinitis and anterior knee pain). Arthritis is relatively easy to diagnose because symptoms localize to the joint line and are associated with loss of motion and radiographic changes. Chronic leg pain is defined as pain that has been present for more than 2 or 3 weeks. The etiology includes a spectrum of disorders. In addition to the unique conditions discussed in this chapter, chronic pain in the calf region also may be secondary to infection (osteomyelitis or pyomyositis), tumors (soft-tissue or bone), and other general disorders.

Tumors are characterized by night pain (relentless pain in which the patient is unable to sleep) and often can be palpated or identified on radiographs. The most common malignant tumors are osteosarcoma (in adolescents) and chondrosarcoma (in adults). The most common benign tumor is giant cell tumor, which typically occurs in adults aged 20 to 30 years. Metastatic disease in the knee region is uncommon.

Sepsis in the knee joint is rare in adults; it is more commonly located in the prepatellar bursa. Inspection and palpation of the involved area easily determine the location of the infection. Swelling, erythema, and loss of knee motion are characteristic of sepsis in either location, but infection in the prepatellar bursa causes swelling over the patella. With sepsis in the knee joint, swelling occurs around (medial, lateral, and suprapatellar regions) but not over the patella.

Bursitis/tendinitis and anterior knee pain have similar characteristics: both usually are chronic, often secondary to overuse, and often bilateral. The pain typically is worse with rising or walking after sitting, at night, and with prolonged exercise or use.

# LOCATION OF PAIN

## Anterior Knee Pain

Tenderness at the upper pole of the patella indicates tendinitis or a partial tear of the quadriceps insertion on the patella. Tendinitis or overuse injury of the patellar tendon (also called the patellar ligament) produces pain at the inferior pole of the patella or at the tibial tubercle.

## Medial Knee Pain

Pain at the medial joint line, midway between the front and back of the knee, is common with a torn meniscus, especially with degenerative tears that occur as the result of minor trauma such as twisting or rising from a squat. When the meniscal tear is sufficiently large or loose, patients also might report catching or locking. Tenderness in this area also is common with arthritis that affects the medial compartment of the knee. Pain proximal to and/or at the medial joint line, with localized swelling and a history of recent injury, usually indicates a sprain or tear of the medial collateral ligament either at its origin on the medial femoral epicondyle or in the midsubstance of the ligament.

Distal to the medial joint line lies the pes anserinus (composed of the insertion of the sartorius, gracilis, and semitendinosus tendons; so named because it resembles the foot of a goose) and the superficial portion of the medial collateral ligament. Pain in this area in the absence of trauma suggests a bursitis under the pes anserine tendons. This condition often is associated with osteoarthritis of the medial knee joint.

## Lateral Knee Pain

Pain over the lateral femoral condyle suggests iliotibial band syndrome, usually associated with overuse or erratic exercise habits. Pain over the lateral joint line usually indicates a disorder of the lateral meniscus or osteoarthritis of the lateral joint (more common in women or obese patients).

## Posterior Knee Pain

Pain at the posteromedial corner of the knee may indicate a tear of the medial meniscus (at the joint line), a popliteal cyst, or both. Popliteal aneurysms also may be painful in the popliteal area. Patients with knee effusions may perceive popliteal pain from the distention of the joint capsule.

SECTION 6 ■ KNEE AND LOWER LEG

# INSTABILITY

The knee joint comprises articulations between the tibia and the femur (tibiofemoral joint), between the patella and the femur (patellofemoral joint), and between the tibia and fibula, although this latter articulation is rarely the source of knee symptoms. True instability means that one bony component moves on another in an abnormal fashion, such as the patella sliding laterally on the femur in recurrent subluxation of the patella, or the tibia moving anteriorly on the femur in the anterior cruciate ligament–deficient knee. Patients typically use the terms "giving way," "slippage," or "buckling," which can refer to true instability or to collapse of the knee (often secondary to pain or muscle weakness in the axis of the quadriceps mechanism).

## Tibiofemoral Instability

Identifying the specific ligament injury that is responsible for instability can be difficult in a painful, traumatized knee because of muscle guarding. During examination, four ligament complexes should be gently assessed with the patient as relaxed as possible: (1) anterior cruciate ligament, (2) posterior cruciate ligament, (3) medial collateral ligament, and (4) lateral collateral ligament.

Chronic instability of the knee also occurs with severe arthritis because, with the loss of articular cartilage and bone height from the arthritis (relative laxity), the ligaments are not at full tension. In these instances, the knee may have "increased play" when the ligament is tested but there will be a defined end point when the intact ligament finally tightens.

## Patellofemoral Instability

Instability in the extensor mechanism is usually caused by a lateral dislocation or subluxation of the patella. The diagnosis is made by palpation. When the patella remains dislocated, the patient's knee often will be locked in approximately 45° of flexion with an obvious deformity present. Following an acute subluxation or dislocation that has reduced spontaneously, the patient usually exhibits dramatic apprehension when an attempt is made to displace the patella laterally.

# STIFFNESS

Stiffness of the knee is the most common symptom that accompanies an effusion. The distention of the knee cavity prevents full flexion, and the patient feels that the knee is "stiff" but might not notice that it is also swollen.

Arthritis is the other common cause of stiffness. Patients with arthritis often report that the knee sticks or locks momentarily as they walk. This occurs because the articular surfaces are rough and incongruous and act like two pieces of sandpaper rubbing together.

Stiffness also may result from any inflammatory condition at the knee, including arthritis, overuse syndromes, and traumatic effusion.

## SWELLING

With an intra-articular effusion, distention occurs around and above the patella in the knee cavity. Patients often notice this as stiffness; they cannot fully flex the knee because the knee cavity is filled with synovial fluid or blood and therefore cannot be compressed.

Patients may also report knee swelling when they see soft-tissue puffiness in the infrapatellar bursa. This bursa is located behind and to either side of the patellar tendon (infrapatellar tendon). Think of this structure as the knee's thermometer: it swells with a variety of knee disorders and is obvious to patients because it feels tense when they kneel, is prominent when they rub their knees, and is obvious when they look at their knees in the mirror.

## LOCKING

True locking occurs when a torn meniscus prevents the knee from extending fully. The knee can flex from the stuck position (although the range of flexion also is typically limited). Patients also note that the knee is stiff after prolonged sitting, with the stiffness gradually loosening when they start moving. Often patients are able to "unlock" their knee by forcefully flexing or extending or by some other maneuver they have learned works for them.

Pseudolocking occurs with arthritis of the patellofemoral joint or between the femur and tibia, when the adjacent rough surfaces stick momentarily as they glide onto one another. It also can occur with minor knee conditions such as a medial synovial plica, when the synovial tissue becomes momentarily stuck under the patella as the knee extends.

## WEAKNESS

Weakness of the muscles around the knee may occur acutely or gradually. Acute catastrophic weakness usually occurs as a result of one of three types of disruption of the extensor mechanism: (1) a tear of the patellar tendon below the patella, (2) a tear of the quadriceps tendon above the patella, or (3) a fracture through the patella. With partial ruptures, the extensor mechanism might continue to function, but without proper protection, the tear may become complete.

SECTION 6 ■ KNEE AND LOWER LEG

# PHYSICAL EXAMINATION
# KNEE AND LOWER LEG

## INSPECTION/PALPATION

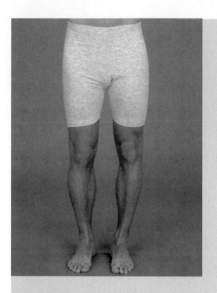

### *Anterior view*

With the patient standing and facing you, look for valgus (knock-knee) or varus (bowleg) deformities, asymmetry of alignment, and quadriceps atrophy. Internal femoral torsion will rotate the knees so that the patellae point inward when the feet are pointing straight ahead.

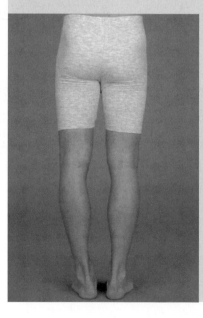

### *Posterior view*

With the patient standing, look for atrophy of the hamstrings or calf muscles.

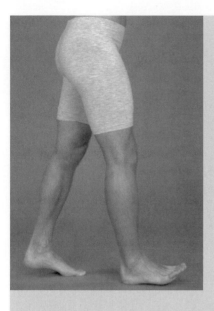

### Gait

Watch the patient walk. With arthritic knee conditions, the patient will limit motion and shorten the duration of the stance phase on the affected side.

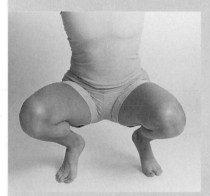

### Squat

Ask the patient to squat. The patient should be able to flex both knees symmetrically.

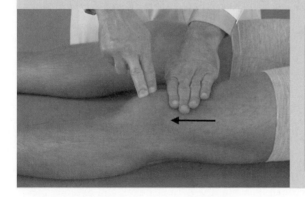

### Knee effusion

Inspect the suprapatellar region. If a large knee effusion is present, it will be readily visible in this region. Subtle knee effusions can be demonstrated by "milking down" joint fluid from the suprapatellar pouch. Hold the fluid wave in place with one hand and push straight down on the patella (patellar ballottement) with the other hand. Excessive fluid will create a spongy feeling as the patella is pushed down.

SECTION 6 ■ KNEE AND LOWER LEG

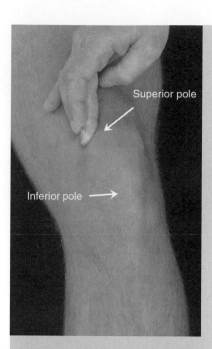

### Patella

Palpate the superior and inferior poles of the patella. Quadriceps tendinitis or rupture causes tenderness at the superior pole, whereas patellar tendinitis (jumper's knee) or rupture creates tenderness at the inferior pole. Displace the patella laterally to palpate the lateral facet on the undersurface of the patella and then displace it medially to assess the medial facet.

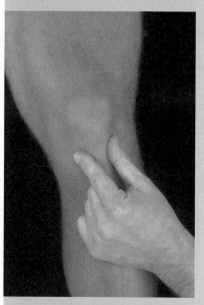

### Infrapatellar bursa

Palpate below the patella, on either side of the patellar tendon, for swelling. Often this condition is visible as a dumbbell-like swelling on either side of the tendon. The asymmetry is easily seen with the patient seated or standing.

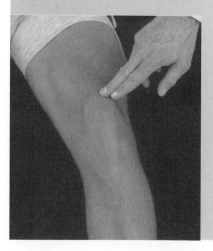

### Patellar tracking

Palpate the patella as the patient flexes and extends the knee. Crepitus is noted with patellofemoral arthritis; however, the degree of crepitus does not correlate with the severity of the arthritis.

Watch movement of the patella while the patient flexes and extends the knee. As the knee moves from extension to flexion, the patella normally moves in a gentle arc from a relatively lateral position when the knee is extended, to a more medial position during early flexion, and then back to a relatively lateral position as flexion continues. With patellar instability, this arc of movement is increased and may make an inverted-J–shaped motion (the "J sign"), a sudden lateral movement of the patella as the knee nears full extension.

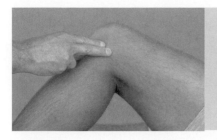

### Joint line tenderness

Flex the patient's knee and identify the joint line (soft spot between the femur and tibia). Feel along the joint margin on both the medial and lateral sides of the knee. An area of increased tenderness supports the diagnosis of a torn meniscus.

# RANGE OF MOTION

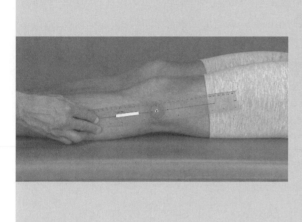

### Active

Knee motion consists primarily of flexion and extension. In adults, knee flexion normally ranges from 135° to 145°, and extension is to at least 0°. Knee hyperextension (past 0°) is more often seen in young children or individuals with "loose joints." Active flexion measurements may be taken while the patient squats, using the knee straight as the starting position. Extension or hyperextension is motion opposite to flexion, which is measured relative to full extension and compared with the contralateral knee.

### Passive

Measurements of passive flexion and extension may be taken with the patient supine or prone, with the examiner's hands placed on the ankle and knee to flex and extend the patient's knee. Passive extension may also be measured with the patient supine and the heel resting on a support that elevates the leg 5 cm above the examination table.

# MUSCLE TESTING

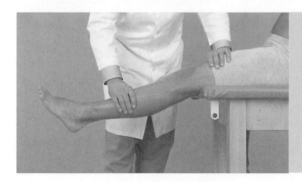
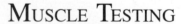

### Quadriceps

With the patient seated, ask him or her to extend the knee. Resist the effort by pushing down on the tibia after the knee is in full extension.

SECTION 6 ■ KNEE AND LOWER LEG

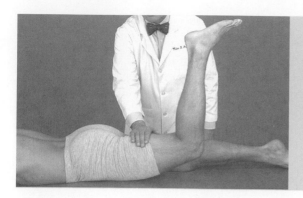

### Hamstrings

With the patient prone, place the knee in approximately 90° of flexion. Ask the patient to extend the hip as you resist the effort by pushing down on the thigh.

## SPECIAL TESTS

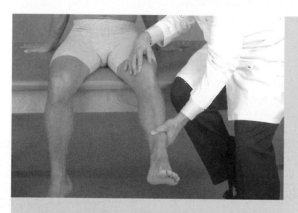

### Patellar apprehension sign

With the patient seated and the quadriceps relaxed, place the knee in extension. Displace the patella laterally and then flex the knee to 30°. With patellar instability, this maneuver displaces the patella to an abnormal position on the lateral femoral condyle. The patient often anticipates or perceives pain and becomes apprehensive, not allowing the examiner to displace the patella or flex the knee.

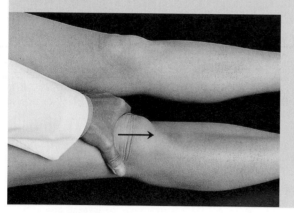

### Patellar grind test

With the patient supine and the knee extended, place one hand superior to the patella and gently push the patella inferiorly. Ask the patient to tighten the quadriceps against this patellar resistance. A grinding sound and/or pain is indicative of patellofemoral chondromalacia. Pain may accompany the maneuver.

SECTION 6 ■ KNEE AND LOWER LEG

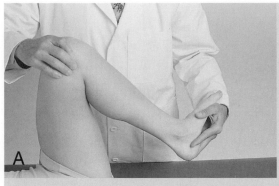

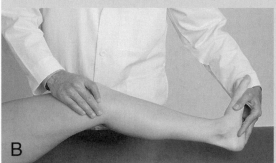

### McMurray test

Flex the knee to the maximum pain-free position. Hold the leg in that position while externally rotating the foot (**A**), and then gradually extend the knee while maintaining the tibia in external rotation (**B**). This maneuver stresses the medial meniscus and often elicits a localized medial compartment click and/or pain in patients with a tear of the posterior horn of the medial meniscus. The same maneuver performed while rotating the foot internally will stress the lateral meniscus. Pain-free flexion beyond 90° is necessary for this test to be useful.

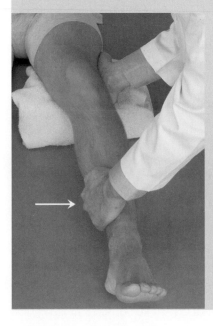

### Valgus stress test

Assess medial collateral ligament (MCL) stability by applying the valgus stress test to both knees, once with the knee extended, and once with the knee flexed to 25°. With the thigh supported to relax the quadriceps, place one hand on the lateral side of the knee, grasp the medial distal tibia with the other hand, and abduct the knee. At 25° of flexion, if the affected knee opens up in a valgus direction more than the opposite knee, the patient has either a complete or partial tear of the MCL. If the knee opens up in full extension, the patient has a severe injury involving more than the MCL.

SECTION 6 ■ KNEE AND LOWER LEG

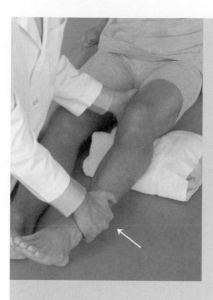

### Varus stress test

Assess lateral collateral ligament (LCL) stability by applying the varus stress test to both knees, once with the knee in extension and once with the knee in 25° of flexion. Place one hand on the medial side of the knee, grasp the lateral distal tibia with the other hand, and adduct the knee. At 25° of flexion, if the knee opens up more than the opposite knee in a varus direction, the patient has either a complete or partial tear of the LCL. If the knee opens up in full extension, the patient has a severe injury involving more than the LCL.

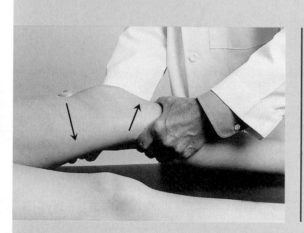

### Lachman test

This test assesses the anterior cruciate ligament (ACL). With the thigh supported and the thigh muscles relaxed, flex the knee to 25° and grasp the distal femur from the lateral side with one hand and the proximal tibia from the medial side with the other hand. Maintain the knee in neutral rotation, then initiate a "shucking" motion by pulling anteriorly on the tibia while stabilizing the femur, focusing on the amount of bony translation of the tibia relative to the femur. Increased anterior tibial translation indicates a partial or complete tear of the ACL.

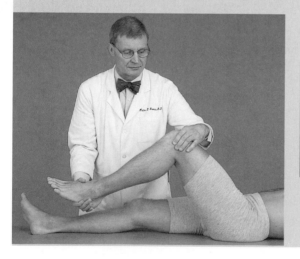

### Pivot shift test

The pivot shift test is used to assess dysfunction in the knee with ACL and secondary restraint deficiency. To perform the test, the knee is placed in full extension and then slowly flexed while the examiner applies a valgus stress and an internal rotation stress. With a positive test, a subluxation will occur at 20° to 40° of knee flexion.

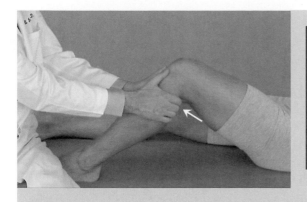

### Anterior drawer test

The anterior drawer test assesses ACL stability. It is easier to perform than the Lachman test but is not as sensitive. With the patient supine and the knee flexed to 90°, stabilize the leg by sitting on the patient's foot. Palpate the hamstring tendons to ensure that they are relaxed. Grasp the proximal tibia with both hands and slide the tibia anteriorly. Compare the results with the uninjured knee, which should always be examined first.

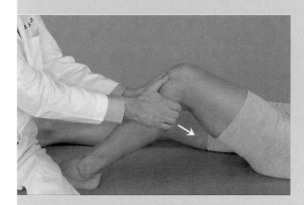

### Posterior drawer test

The posterior drawer test assesses posterior cruciate ligament (PCL) stability. With the patient supine, flex the knee to 90° with the foot supported on the table. Grasp the proximal tibia with both hands and place your thumbs on top of the medial and lateral tibial plateaus. Normally, the anterior tibial plateaus sit 10 mm anterior to the femoral condyles. Slide the tibia posteriorly. If the PCL is injured, the proximal tibia falls back. When the tibial plateaus are flush with the femoral condyles, there is 10 mm or more of posterior laxity, consistent with a complete tear of the PCL. Compare results with the uninjured knee, which should always be examined first.

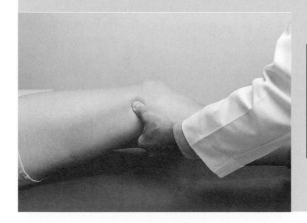

### Noble's test

Noble's test assesses for the presence of iliotibial band (ITB) syndrome. With the patient supine and the knee flexed to 90°, apply pressure to the ITB over the lateral femoral condyle and then extend the knee. Tenderness elicited between 30° and 40° of knee flexion is a positive sign.

SECTION 6 ■ KNEE AND LOWER LEG

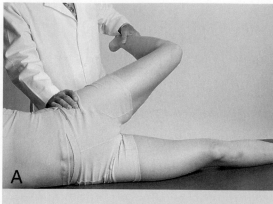

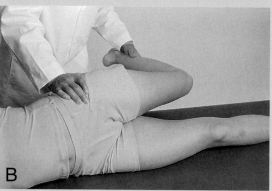

### Ober's test

Ober's test assesses ITB tightness. The patient lies on the unaffected side with the unaffected knee and hip flexed. With the affected knee flexed to 90°, the examiner abducts and hyperextends the ipsilateral hip while stabilizing the pelvis (**A**). The leg is then slowly lowered as far as possible (**B**). Inability of the extremity to drop below horizontal to the level of the table indicates a tight ITB.

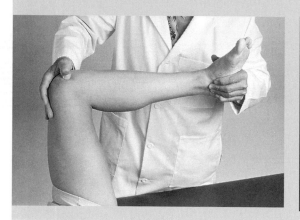

### Wilson test

The Wilson test is used to assess the presence of osteochondritis dissecans (OCD). The test is performed with the patient supine. The examiner flexes the hip and knee 90° and internally rotates the tibia. The knee is then slowly extended. The Wilson test is positive when the patient reports pain as the knee reaches approximately 20° to 30° of flexion and when pain is relieved with external rotation of the tibia while maintaining the same flexion angle. This maneuver causes the tibial spine to abut and then rotate away from the OCD lesion on the medial femoral condyle.

SECTION 6 ■ KNEE AND LOWER LEG

# ANTERIOR CRUCIATE LIGAMENT TEAR

## SYNONYMS
ACL tear
Anterior cruciate insufficiency
Crucial ligament tear
Torn cruciate

**ICD-9 Codes**
**717.83**
Chronic disruption of anterior
cruciate ligament
**844.2**
Acute anterior cruciate ligament tear

## DEFINITION
The anterior cruciate ligament (ACL) is a primary stabilizer of the knee (**Figure 1**). A tear of the ACL results from a rotational (twisting) or hyperextension force applied to the knee joint that overcomes the strength of the ligament. Although partial tears can occur, injuries involving the ACL more often result in complete tears. About half the time, an ACL tear is accompanied by a significant meniscal tear. An ACL tear also can occur in association with a tear of the medial collateral ligament or, more rarely, with tears of the lateral ligaments or the posterior cruciate ligament. Uncommonly, knee injuries that disrupt multiple ligaments and result in knee instability also may injure the popliteal artery, a limb-threatening emergency.

## CLINICAL SYMPTOMS
Patients with ACL tears usually report sudden pain and giving way of the knee from a twisting or hyperextension-type injury. One third of patients report an audible pop as the ligament tears. A patient who sustains an ACL tear during athletic activity usually is unable to continue participating because of pain and/or instability. The pain increases because an effusion caused by bleeding into the joint (hemarthrosis) develops over the ensuing 24 hours.

As the swelling resolves, the patient temporarily may have no trouble moving the knee; however, if the tear is left untreated, recurrent instability develops, particularly with attempts to return to agility sports. Chronic knee instability from an untreated ACL tear can lead to further meniscal and articular cartilage damage, with resulting degenerative arthritis.

## TESTS

### Physical Examination
The most sensitive test for ACL insufficiency is the Lachman test, in which the knee is flexed to 25° and the tibia is gently pulled forward while the femur is stabilized (**Figure 2**). Because of the subcutaneous location of the medial tibia, it is easier to grasp the tibia on the medial side (right hand for right

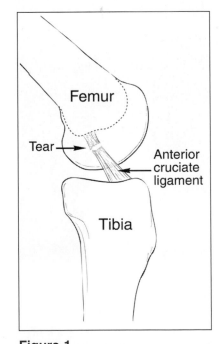

**Figure 1**
Lateral view of the knee showing a complete ACL tear.

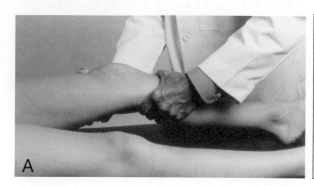
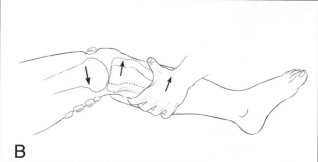

**Figure 2**

Lachman test. **A,** The knee is flexed approximately 25°. The examiner gently pulls the tibia forward with the medial hand while stabilizing the distal femur with the lateral hand. In a relaxed patient, increased anterior translation of the tibia with a soft end point constitutes a positive test. **B,** Diagram showing movement of the tibia relative to the femur.

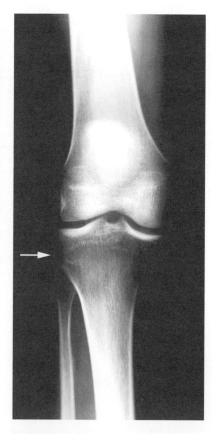

**Figure 3**

AP view of the knee showing a Segond fracture, indicative of an ACL injury. Note the fleck of bone (arrow) next to the lateral tibial plateau.

knee, left hand for left knee) while stabilizing the femur from the lateral side with the opposite hand. If the thigh is large, the examiner may find it difficult to support the thigh in one hand. In this situation, the patient's thigh may be placed on the examiner's thigh. The examiner uses one hand to support the thigh in this position. The examiner's other hand distracts the tibia from the supported femur. Increased motion of the tibia with no solid end point indicates a tear of the ACL. The anterior drawer test, performed with the knee flexed 90°, is negative in 50% of acute ACL tears and so is less helpful.

*Diagnostic Tests*

AP, lateral, and tunnel views of the knee are optimal for every patient with a suspected ACL tear. Usually these radiographs are positive only for an effusion and possibly an avulsion fracture of the lateral capsular margin of the tibia (lateral capsular sign or Segond fracture) (**Figure 3**); however, radiographs are helpful in ruling out other pathology.

MRI, although quite sensitive at detecting ACL tears, is expensive and rarely necessary. Usually the diagnosis can be made on physical examination by an experienced examiner.

# DIFFERENTIAL DIAGNOSIS

Fracture (tenderness over the bone, evident on radiographs)

Meniscal tear (continued tenderness along the joint line, pain or trapping with circumduction)

Patellar dislocation/subluxation (positive apprehension sign when displacing the patella laterally)

Patellar tendon or quadriceps rupture (inability to perform straight-leg raise)

Posterior cruciate ligament tear (positive posterior drawer test, firm end point on Lachman test)

## ADVERSE OUTCOMES OF THE DISEASE

Untreated, the recurring instability resulting from an ACL tear may cause subsequent meniscal tears and degenerative disease. The instability also makes successful return to participation in agility sports such as soccer, football, or basketball unlikely.

## TREATMENT

Initial treatment of an acute ACL injury includes rest, ice, and use of crutches until the patient is able to ambulate without a limp. If the knee effusion (hemarthrosis) is tense, aspiration may be indicated to relieve symptoms (see Knee Joint Aspiration/Injection, pp 571-573). A knee immobilizer or range-of-motion brace may be used for comfort when necessary until acute pain subsides.

Early range-of-motion exercises are important. With the patient sitting, the injured knee should be actively extended and flexed as comfort allows. Exercises should be performed repeatedly for several minutes four or five times daily. Full extension and flexion should be regained as soon as pain and swelling permit.

Definitive treatment of an ACL injury depends on the patient's age, desired activity level, and any associated injuries. For young, active patients, ACL reconstruction offers the best chance for a successful return to agility sports. Older or less active individuals may be treated with physical therapy aimed at controlling the instability. ACL functional bracing, although controversial, also may be helpful with older or less active patients.

## PHYSICAL THERAPY PRESCRIPTION

Initial treatment of a torn ACL is to control the inflammation and pain with the use of rest, ice, compression, and elevation (RICE) of the leg. In addition, maintaining the range of motion and regaining muscle strength are important to the rehabilitation. Strengthening of the quadriceps and the hamstring muscle group is critical for knee stability following an ACL injury, as is balance training. Excessive anterior shearing forces during knee extension from 60° to 0°, and especially from 30° to 10°, can cause damage, as can varus and valgus stress in full knee extension. Therefore, exercises that protect the ACL injury by avoiding these ranges of motion and positions, such as hamstring curls to strengthen the hamstring muscle group and isometric quadriceps contraction and straight-leg raises to strengthen the quadriceps, are used initially (see p 489).

SECTION 6 ■ KNEE AND LOWER LEG

If instability, pain, and inflammation continue after 2 to 3 weeks and surgery is not a patient option, formal physical therapy may be ordered. The prescription should include an assessment of the strength of the hip and trunk muscles, especially the hip external rotators and abductors. Outpatient physical therapy for rehabilitation of an ACL-deficient knee should emphasize strengthening of these muscle groups as well as neuromuscular training such as plyometrics and perturbation training. In addition, the physical therapist's evaluation might include structural deviations that sometimes contribute to ACL injury, such as a large Q angle, excessive foot pronation, hip anteversion, and genu recurvatum and valgum, to help determine the appropriate treatment.

## Adverse Outcomes of Treatment

Nonsurgical treatment carries the risk of recurrent instability, meniscal tears, and degenerative joint disease. Scarring of the knee joint (arthrofibrosis) with loss of motion can occur after ACL injury or postoperatively after ACL reconstruction. Surgical reconstruction carries several risks: the usual risks of surgery (infection, phlebitis, pulmonary emboli, neurovascular insult, scarring, etc); the possibility that the ACL can tear again; or failure of the ACL graft to incorporate or successfully remodel, resulting in recurrence of laxity. Fracture of the tibial or patellar graft site also may occur after ACL reconstruction when a portion of the patellar tendon is used for the ACL graft.

## Referral Decisions/Red Flags

Patients with suspected ACL tears and/or posttraumatic knee effusions require further evaluation and treatment. Even patients who are not candidates for ACL reconstruction can benefit from regular monitoring of the ACL tear.

# HOME EXERCISE PROGRAM FOR ACL TEAR

Perform all five exercises, in the order listed. After each exercise session, apply ice (such as a bag of crushed ice or a bag of frozen peas) to the knee for 20 minutes, keep the leg elevated, and apply a compression bandage to the knee. If pain or swelling increases at any time or if it does not improve after you have adhered to the program for 3 to 4 weeks, call your doctor.

| Exercise Type | Muscle Group | Number of Repetitions/Sets | Number of Days per Week | Number of Weeks |
|---|---|---|---|---|
| Hamstring curls (standing) | Hamstrings | 20 repetitions/3 sets | 4 to 5 | 3 to 4 |
| Straight-leg raises | Quadriceps | 20 repetitions/3 sets | 4 to 5 | 3 to 4 |
| Hip abduction | Gluteus medius | 20 repetitions/3 sets | 4 to 5 | 3 to 4 |
| Straight-leg raises (prone) | Gluteus maximus | 20 repetitions/3 sets | 4 to 5 | 3 to 4 |
| Wall slides | Quadriceps Hamstrings | 20 repetitions/3 sets | 4 to 5 | 3 to 4 |

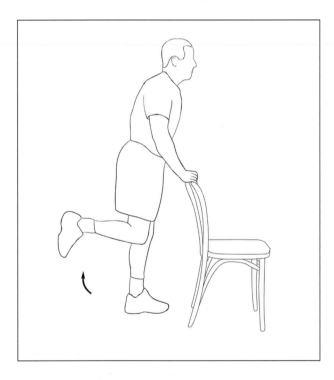

## *Hamstring Curls*

Stand on a flat surface with your weight evenly distributed on both feet. Hold onto the back of a chair or the wall for balance. Bend the injured knee, raising the heel of the affected leg toward the ceiling as far as you can without pain. Hold this position for 5 seconds and then relax. Perform 3 sets of 20 repetitions, 4 to 5 days a week, continuing for 3 to 4 weeks.

SECTION 6 ■ KNEE AND LOWER LEG

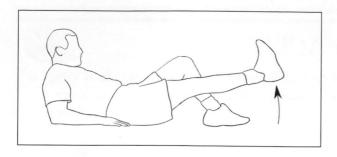

### Straight-Leg Raises

Lie on the floor, supporting your torso with your elbows as shown. Keep the injured leg straight and bend the other leg at the knee so that the foot is flat on the floor. Tighten the thigh muscle of the injured leg and slowly raise it 6 to 10 inches off the floor. Hold this position for 5 seconds and then relax. Perform 3 sets of 20 repetitions, 4 to 5 days a week, continuing for 3 to 4 weeks.

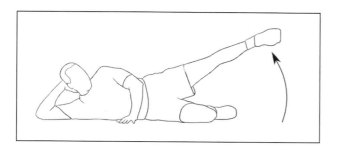

### Hip Abduction

Lie on your side with the injured side on top and with the bottom leg bent to provide support. Slowly raise the top leg to 45°, keeping the knee straight. Hold the position for 5 seconds. Slowly lower the leg and relax it for 2 seconds. Perform 3 sets of 20 repetitions, 4 to 5 days a week, continuing for 3 to 4 weeks.

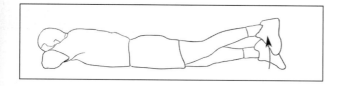

### Straight-Leg Raises (Prone)

Lie on the floor on your stomach with your legs straight. Tighten the hamstrings of the injured leg and raise the leg toward the ceiling as far as you can. Hold the position for 5 seconds. Lower the leg and rest it for 2 seconds. Perform 3 sets of 20 repetitions, 4 to 5 days a week, continuing for 3 to 4 weeks.

### Wall Slides

Lie on your back with the uninjured leg extending through a doorway and the injured leg extended against the wall. Let the foot gently slide down the wall. Hold the position of maximum flexion for 5 seconds and then slowly straighten the leg. Perform 3 sets of 20 repetitions, 4 to 5 days a week, continuing for 3 to 4 weeks.

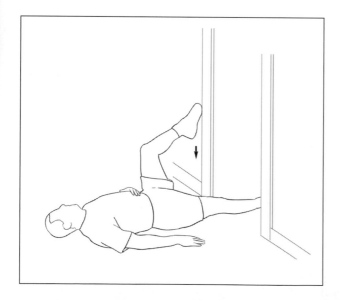

# ARTHRITIS OF THE KNEE

## SYNONYMS
Degenerative joint disease
Osteoarthritis
Rheumatoid arthritis
"Wear and tear" arthritis

## DEFINITION
Osteoarthritis (OA) is the most common form of knee arthritis and can involve each of the three compartments of the knee individually or in combination. The knee can be divided into the medial compartment, including the medial tibial plateau and the medial femoral condyle; the lateral compartment, including the lateral tibial plateau and lateral femoral condyle; and the patellofemoral joint, including the patella and the femoral trochlear groove. The medial compartment of the knee is the area most frequently involved in OA, resulting in a bowleg or genu varum deformity. Knock-knees or genu valgum occurs when the destructive arthritic process primarily involves the lateral compartment. Isolated patellofemoral OA can exist, especially in patients with subluxation or patella alta or baja; however, it is most frequently associated with concomitant tibiofemoral OA.

Secondary knee arthropathy usually occurs in individuals with a strong history of trauma, including fractures, meniscal tears, and/or meniscectomy, or with chronic ligament insufficiencies, such as anterior cruciate ligament–deficient knees. OA of the knee also may occur secondary to intra-articular fractures (posttraumatic) and inflammatory arthritides such as rheumatoid arthritis.

## CLINICAL SYMPTOMS
OA most commonly affects patients older than 55 years, particularly those who are obese and genetically predisposed. Insidious onset of pain is common. As the OA progresses, the patient will have pain on weight bearing, regardless of the initial cause. Common symptoms include buckling or giving way, which is caused by bony areas impinging upon each other. The patient usually reports a history of difficulty climbing and descending stairs. Stiffness and intermittent joint swelling can limit motion at the extremes of flexion and extension. Symptoms of locking or catching, often mimicking a meniscal tear, can result from the impingement or sticking of rough joint

SECTION 6 ■ KNEE AND LOWER LEG

surfaces and reflexive dysfunction of the quadriceps muscle or the impingement of inflamed synovial tissue between the joint surfaces. With severe OA, pain can occur when the patient is resting or even sleeping.

# TESTS

## Physical Examination

Examination commonly reveals an angular (varus or valgus) deformity through the knee, which can be confirmed by a weight-bearing examination. Sometimes the opposite knee can be used for comparison; however, it is not uncommon for a patient to have windswept deformities (one knee valgus, one knee varus). The osteoarthritic knee often will have a mild effusion, with diffuse tenderness along the joint lines at times extending into the medial hamstring tendon insertion on the anteromedial tibia. Careful palpation may reveal thickening and osteophytes along the articular margin of the femur. Crepitus around the patellofemoral joint is often present. Loss of range of motion often parallels progression of the arthritis.

## Diagnostic Tests

Weight-bearing AP radiographs of both knees in full extension will show narrowing of the joint space (**Figure 1**).

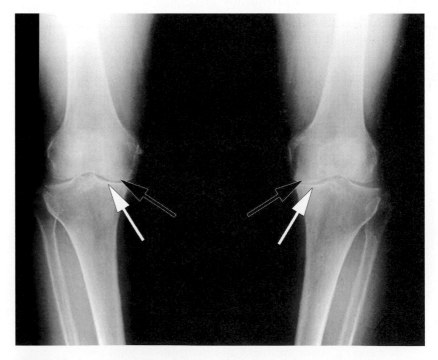

**Figure 1**
Weight-bearing AP radiograph of both knees showing substantial collapse of the medial joint space (black arrows) and subchondral sclerosis (white arrows).

Radiographic findings of degenerative arthritis include asymmetric joint narrowing, bone sclerosis, periarticular cysts, and osteophytes. Radiographic findings of inflammatory arthritis include symmetric joint narrowing, disuse osteopenia, and bony erosions at the articular margins. The overall condition of the patellofemoral and tibiofemoral joints may be further assessed with lateral and axial patellofemoral views. In addition, weight-bearing AP radiographs with the knee in approximately 40° of flexion can help identify narrowing of the articular surface because they profile different weight-bearing areas of the tibia and femur. The tunnel view (also called intercondylar notch view) often will reveal osteophytes, as well as demonstrate osteochondral loose bodies.

## DIFFERENTIAL DIAGNOSIS

Herniated L3 or L4 disk with radiculopathy (diminished knee reflex, numbness)

Meniscal tear (history of trauma and/or locking and catching)

Osteonecrosis of the femur or tibia (over age 50 years, female, history of steroid use, blood dyscrasia)

Pigmented villonodular synovitis (unexplained recurring hemarthrosis)

Primary hip pathology (dermatomal referred pain to the knee, limited range of hip motion)

Septic arthritis (fever, malaise, abnormal joint fluid)

Tendinitis/bursitis (tenderness directly over a tendon or bursa)

## ADVERSE OUTCOMES OF THE DISEASE

Chronic pain may ensue, with substantial loss of knee function. Weight-bearing activity and walking may produce significant discomfort. The overall physical condition of the patient declines because a high level of activity cannot be maintained. Weight gain also often occurs.

## TREATMENT

Nonsurgical management includes NSAIDs and perhaps the use of intra-articular injections (corticosteroids or viscosupplementation). Concomitant use of acetaminophen is often helpful. Modality treatments including ice, heat, and liniments also may temporarily relieve stiffness and aching. Mechanical aids such as neoprene sleeves and elastic bandages can help control swelling that occurs with activity. Shock-absorbing shoe insoles or heels decrease impact on the knee with heel strike. Nonimpact exercises such as water aerobics and recumbent cycling help maintain muscle tone. Progressive resistance exercises (weight training) in pain-free arcs of motion

SECTION 6 ■ KNEE AND LOWER LEG

help diminish muscle atrophy and improve muscle endurance. Use of a cane or single crutch in the hand opposite the painful limb (so that the limb can be protected when it is in heel-strike phase) may help decrease pain while ambulating. A patient with poor balance or a history of falling should use an ambulatory assistive device, such as a walker. Severe functional limitations and pain at rest or at night indicate the failure of nonsurgical management and the need for surgical treatment. Surgical management of advanced cases often entails total knee replacement.

## ADVERSE OUTCOMES OF TREATMENT

Gastrointestinal or hepatic complications may result from chronic use of NSAIDs, as well as concomitant fluid retention and diminished renal function, which can lead to edema and hypertension. Repeated intra-articular injections of corticosteroids typically provide only temporary relief and may result in iatrogenic sepsis and/or accelerated destruction of cartilage.

## REFERRAL DECISIONS/RED FLAGS

Any patient with pain at rest, decreased range of motion, or significant functional limitations requires further evaluation.

# BURSITIS OF THE KNEE

## SYNONYMS

Pes anserine bursitis

Prepatellar bursitis

## DEFINITION

Bursae are sacs that lie between the skin and bony prominences or between tendons, ligaments, and bone. They are lined by synovial tissue, which produces a small amount of fluid to decrease friction between adjacent structures. Chronic pressure or friction (overuse) causes thickening of this synovial lining and subsequent excessive fluid formation, thereby leading to localized swelling and pain.

The prepatellar bursa on the anterior aspect of the knee is superficial and lies between the skin and the bony patella. This bursa can become inflamed (bursitis) or infected (septic bursitis) as a result of trauma to the anterior knee, such as a direct blow, or from chronic irritation from activities that require extensive kneeling, such as wrestling or carpet installation (housemaid's knee). Bacterial infections typically result from direct penetration, which may be an unrecognized event in patients who kneel extensively. *Staphylococcus aureus* and *Streptococcus* species are the most common infecting organisms.

The pes anserinus bursa lies under the insertion site of the sartorius, gracilis, and semitendinosus muscles on the medial flare of the tibia just below the tibial plateau. Although pes anserine bursitis may result from overuse, it occurs more commonly in patients with early osteoarthritis in the medial compartment of the knee.

## CLINICAL SYMPTOMS

At first, pain will be present only with activity or direct pressure. The pain often is more severe after the patient has been sedentary for some time, and patients may notice a limp when first arising from a chair. Patients also note localized swelling over the involved structure. This swelling is most marked with prepatellar bursitis, as this bursa forms a dome-shaped swelling over the anterior aspect of the knee when it becomes inflamed and filled with fluid. Pes anserine bursitis also can be confused with medial meniscal pathology because the bursitis pain is located along the anteromedial aspect of the proximal tibia (**Figure 1**).

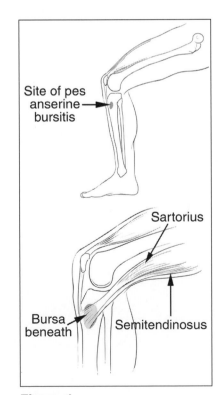

**Figure 1**

Medial view of region of pes anserine tenderness.

SECTION 6 ■ KNEE AND LOWER LEG

These symptoms must be differentiated from those of arthritis. The patient with septic knee arthritis usually reports intense joint pain, swelling, erythema, guarding of the limb, and a low-grade fever.

## TESTS

### Physical Examination

Inspect the knee for areas of swelling and palpate structures for localized tenderness. Compression of the saphenous nerve and its infrapatellar branch by swelling of the pes anserinus bursa may cause numbness below the patella. Measure range of knee motion and then watch the patient walk. Patients with acute prepatellar bursitis typically have swelling superficial to the patella such that the patella may not be palpable in its subcutaneous position.

A patient with septic bursitis may have increased pain, warmth, and erythematous changes over the patella. With noninfectious traumatic bursitis, the area may be warm but is typically not painful or erythematous. Systemic signs (fever, elevated white blood cell count, etc) usually are not as dramatic with an infected prepatellar bursa as they are with septic arthritis of the knee. However, the clinical appearance of infectious and noninfectious bursitis may be the same. Therefore, aspiration of the bursa should be performed in all patients.

### Diagnostic Tests

AP and lateral radiographs should be obtained in patients with chronic pain to rule out bony conditions. Radiographs will be normal with the exception of anterior soft-tissue swelling. With prepatellar bursitis, aspiration should be performed to rule out infection. Septic bursitis may demonstrate purulent or seropurulent material. This aspiration should be done in a manner that does not seed the knee joint. The fluid should be sent for Gram stain and culture, crystal analysis, and synovial fluid analysis.

## DIFFERENTIAL DIAGNOSIS

Inflammatory arthritis (multiple joint involvement, abnormal laboratory studies)

Medial meniscal tear (catching, locking, effusions)

Osteoarthritis of the knee (intra-articular effusion, osteophytes)

Patellar fracture (intra-articular hemarthrosis, history of trauma)

Patellar tendinitis (jumper's knee) (tenderness at the inferior pole of the patella)

Saphenous nerve entrapment (numbness over the medial shin, dysesthesia)

Septic knee (flexion contracture, pain with knee motion, intra-articular swelling)

Tumor (pain, mass)

Septic arthritis of the knee (effusion of the joint but the patella can be palpated in its subcutaneous position, knee held in more flexion)

# ADVERSE OUTCOMES OF THE DISEASE

Chronic bursitis may lead to continued pain and thickening of the bursal wall. Pressure from continued swelling may cause weakening of overlying ligaments and/or tendons. Progression of a septic bursitis may result in chronic drainage or spread to the knee joint.

# TREATMENT

Most patients with noninfected bursitis respond to nonsurgical treatment, including a short-term course of NSAIDs, ice, and activity modifications. Therapeutic modalities such as ultrasound and phonophoresis may help. Patients with identifiable tightness should perform quadriceps, hamstring, or iliotibial band stretching/flexibility exercises to prevent atrophy and maintain strength. Injection of a corticosteroid preparation is appropriate in recalcitrant cases. Surgical treatment for bursitis of the knee is the exception rather than the rule. Early-onset, mild septic bursitis can be treated with oral antibiotics. More severe infections require initial treatment with intravenous antibiotics. Repeat aspiration may help in decompressing the bursa. Surgical drainage may be necessary but is not often required.

# ADVERSE OUTCOMES OF TREATMENT

NSAIDs may lead to concomitant gastric, renal, or hepatic complications. Infection from corticosteroid injection is possible. Tendon or ligament weakening as a result of corticosteroid injection theoretically may lead to spontaneous rupture. Chronic or recurrent infection, septic arthritis, or emergence of resistant organisms may occur.

# REFERRAL DECISIONS/RED FLAGS

Any patient whose symptoms do not respond to nonsurgical treatment or who has signs of ligament or tendon insufficiency requires further evaluation. The associated osteoarthritis in recurrent pes anserine bursitis requires evaluation. Prepatellar bursa infections may require surgical treatment when they cannot be aspirated, do not respond to antibiotics, or become recurrent.

SECTION 6 ■ KNEE AND LOWER LEG

# CLAUDICATION

## DEFINITION

Claudication is activity-associated discomfort in the legs with a neurogenic or vascular etiology. Neurogenic claudication is associated with spinal stenosis. Ischemia to the cauda equina is the underlying pathology, induced by postures that mechanically compress the nerve roots with resultant paresthesias and dysesthesias. Vascular claudication is secondary to peripheral vascular disease and compromised blood flow with walking activities. It can result in a similar type of leg pain.

## CLINICAL SYMPTOMS

Patients with neurogenic claudication experience vague pain that begins in the buttocks and spreads to the legs while walking. Walking down inclines significantly increases symptoms secondary to the associated increased lordotic posture. Symptoms typically resolve when the patient sits or lies down. In general, the pain of neurogenic claudication tends to progress from proximal to distal in the lower extremity, whereas the pain of vascular claudication tends to start distally and radiate proximally. Claudication may lead to paresthesias and dysesthesias. Pain and paresthesias do not resolve immediately on cessation of walking in patients with neurogenic claudication. This differs from the pain associated with vascular claudication, which typically subsides when walking stops.

## TESTS

### Physical Examination

Patients with neurogenic claudication may have no abnormal physical findings at rest, but weakness and reflex changes may develop after activities that provoke leg pain. Patients with vascular claudication have diminished or absent pulses below the waist, along with redness and pallor changes with elevation.

### Diagnostic Tests

AP and lateral radiographs of the spine in patients with neurogenic claudication show degenerative changes. MRI and CT can define the pathology, although neither imaging study is necessary as a primary screening tool. Doppler studies and arteriography will demonstrate vascular disease in patients with vascular claudication.

SECTION 6 ■ KNEE AND LOWER LEG

## DIFFERENTIAL DIAGNOSIS

Chronic compartment syndrome (athlete, pain following or during exercise)

Herniated L3 or L4 disk with radiculopathy (diminished knee reflex, numbness)

Meniscal tear (history of trauma and/or locking and catching)

Osteonecrosis of the femur or tibia (patient age over 50 years, women more often than men, history of steroid use, blood dyscrasia)

## ADVERSE OUTCOMES OF THE DISEASE

Patients with either vascular or neurogenic claudication may experience significant compromise in quality of life because of their inability to walk.

## TREATMENT

Patients with neurogenic claudication can be treated with over-the-counter analgesic medications, intermittent NSAIDs, epidural corticosteroid injections, flexion exercises for the lumbar spine, and surgical decompression. Therapeutic options for vascular claudication include supportive measures, pharmacologic treatment, nonsurgical interventions, and surgery. Supportive measures include meticulous foot care, well-fitting and protective shoes, and avoidance of elastic support hose.

## ADVERSE OUTCOMES OF TREATMENT

NSAIDs may lead to concomitant gastric, renal, or hepatic complications.

## REFERRAL DECISIONS/RED FLAGS

Any patient with neurogenic claudication whose symptoms do not respond to nonsurgical treatment requires further evaluation. Patients with vascular claudication require evaluation by a vascular surgeon.

# COLLATERAL LIGAMENT TEAR

## DEFINITION

The shape of the knee provides limited inherent stability. Stability of the knee joint is largely dependent on its ligaments and periarticular muscles. Therefore, injuries to knee ligaments are common. Four ligaments provide primary stabilization of the knee. The medial and lateral collateral ligaments are outside the joint and stabilize the knee against valgus and varus stresses (**Figure 1**). The anterior and posterior cruciate ligaments are inside the joint and stabilize the knee against anterior and posterior stresses.

The mechanism of injury in a medial collateral ligament (MCL) tear (or sprain) is commonly a valgus (abduction) force without rotation, such as in a football clipping injury. The less common lateral collateral ligament (LCL) tear is the result of a pure varus (adduction) force to the knee. Variable external rotation stress frequently occurs with MCL sprains. Injuries to the collateral ligaments can occur alone or in association with a meniscal tear or an anterior or posterior cruciate ligament tear.

## CLINICAL SYMPTOMS

Most patients are able to ambulate after an acute collateral ligament injury and may be able to return to play for the remainder of the game. Patients report localized swelling or stiffness and medial or lateral pain and tenderness, but instability and mechanical symptoms, such as locking or popping, are infrequent after an isolated collateral ligament injury. Within 24 to 48 hours, localized ecchymosis and a small effusion develop. Pain may increase and motion may become limited over the first 6 to 8 hours following injury.

## TESTS

### Physical Examination

The uninjured knee should be examined first to understand what is normal for the patient. This also reduces the patient's fears about examining the painful limb. Swelling in and around the injured ligament is common, but the presence of a significant knee effusion might indicate an associated intra-articular injury.

The MCL may be tender along its entire course, from the medial femoral condyle to its tibial insertion. Isolated tenderness at the most proximal or distal extent of the MCL may signify an avulsion-type injury. The LCL may be tender anywhere along its course, from the lateral femoral epicondyle

SECTION 6 ■ KNEE AND LOWER LEG

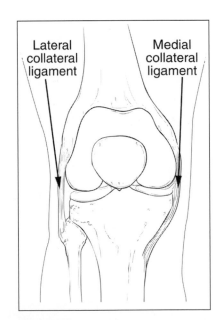

**Figure 1**
Medial and lateral knee structures.

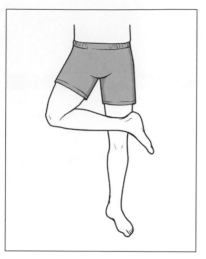

**Figure 2**
The "figure-of-4" position.

to its insertion on the fibular head. The MCL is best palpated with the knee in slight flexion, but the LCL is best examined with the leg in the "figure-of-4" position (**Figure 2**).

Apply a varus and then a valgus stress with the knee first in full extension and then at 25° of flexion (to relax the cruciate ligaments and posterior capsule). Laxity in full extension indicates a more extensive injury that includes the anterior and posterior cruciate ligaments plus posterior capsule rather than just the MCL or LCL. These injuries are knee dislocations with spontaneous reduction in which there may be a major neurovascular injury.

Increased joint space opening of less than 5 mm compared with the normal knee is considered a grade I (interstitial) tear, whereas increased opening of more than 10 mm is considered a grade III (complete) tear. A grade II (partial) tear falls between these extremes. The degree of instability may be masked in a patient with significant pain and involuntary muscle contraction. Be aware of the possibility of a false-negative examination for laxity because of muscle guarding.

### Diagnostic Tests
AP and lateral radiographs, although usually negative, may reveal an avulsion from the femoral origin of the MCL or the fibular insertion of the LCL.

## DIFFERENTIAL DIAGNOSIS

Anterior cruciate ligament tear (moderate to marked knee effusion, positive Lachman test)

Epiphyseal fracture of the distal femur (tenderness at epiphyseal plate, evident on radiographs)

Meniscal tear (mild to moderate knee effusion, joint line tenderness)

Osteochondral fracture (radiographic evidence of loose osteochondral fragment)

Patellar subluxation or dislocation with spontaneous reduction (positive apprehension sign)

Posterior cruciate ligament tear (positive posterior drawer test)

Tibial plateau fracture (bony tenderness and radiographic evidence of fracture)

## ADVERSE OUTCOMES OF THE DISEASE
Although instability of the knee is rare, it may occur in association with disruption of the anterior and/or posterior cruciate ligament. Lateral instability may occur after isolated LCL tears, especially in patients with varus alignment.

# TREATMENT

Treatment of isolated MCL tears, even complete tears, usually is nonsurgical. Grade I sprains with no effusion usually resolve within a couple of weeks. Rest, ice, compression, and elevation (RICE), coupled with a short-term course of crutches and NSAIDs, usually are adequate. With grade II sprains, use of a hinged brace and weight bearing as tolerated are appropriate. For grade III injuries, use of a hinged brace with gradual return to full weight bearing over the course of 4 to 6 weeks is indicated. Rehabilitation includes early range-of-motion exercises (including bicycling) and quadriceps and hamstring progressive resistance exercises. Grade III injuries frequently require 3 to 4 months of protective bracing before the patient can return to unrestricted activity.

Although grade I and II LCL tears also should be treated nonsurgically, grade III LCL tears invariably involve a tear of the posterolateral capsular complex and are best treated surgically to avoid late instability, especially in varus knees.

# PHYSICAL THERAPY PRESCRIPTION

Initial treatment for a torn collateral ligament is rest, ice, compression, and elevation (RICE) to control the inflammation and pain. Early movement (7 days postinjury) is very important in reestablishing tensile strength and mobility of the ligament. Healing of the collateral ligament is enhanced with movement and delayed with immobilization. A home exercise program should consist of active flexion and passive extension range-of-motion exercises for the knee and isometric exercises for the quadriceps muscle (see pp 505-506).

If pain and inflammation continue after 3 to 4 weeks, formal physical therapy may be ordered. The prescription should include an evaluation of hip and knee muscle strength, followed by exercises targeting the weak muscles. If the range of motion of the knee joint is limited, mobilization is indicated.

# ADVERSE OUTCOMES OF TREATMENT

Frank instability is very uncommon after an isolated collateral ligament injury, but chronic pain and recurrence are possible. Patients are vulnerable to recurrence for 6 months; therefore, bracing for high-risk activities (contact sports) is recommended. Missed associated diagnoses, such as of meniscal and anterior cruciate ligament tears, which can cause persistent pain or swelling or a persistent sense of instability, can complicate the course of nonsurgical treatment, and patients may ultimately require surgical intervention.

SECTION 6 ■ KNEE AND LOWER LEG

## REFERRAL DECISIONS/RED FLAGS

Patients with hemarthrosis, significant joint effusion, or instability need further evaluation. Failure to respond to nonsurgical treatment might mean a missed diagnosis, such as an associated cruciate or posterior capsule rupture or meniscal tear.

SECTION 6 ■ KNEE AND LOWER LEG

# HOME EXERCISE PROGRAM FOR COLLATERAL LIGAMENT TEAR

Perform the exercises in the order listed. Dry or moist heat may be applied to the back of the knee during the passive knee extension. Apply a bag of crushed ice or frozen peas to the injured side of the knee for 20 minutes after completing the exercises to prevent additional inflammation. If pain increases at any time or does not improve after performing these exercises for 3 to 4 weeks, call your doctor.

| Exercise Type | Muscle Group | Number of Repetitions/Sets | Number of Days per Week | Number of Weeks |
|---|---|---|---|---|
| Hamstring curls | Hamstrings | 25 to 45 repetitions/3 sets | 5 to 6 | 3 to 4 |
| Passive knee extension (prone) | Hamstrings | 1 repetition/2 to 3 sets | 5 to 6 | 3 to 4 |
| Passive knee extension (seated) | Quadriceps | 25 to 50 repetitions/3 sets | 5 to 6 | 3 to 4 |

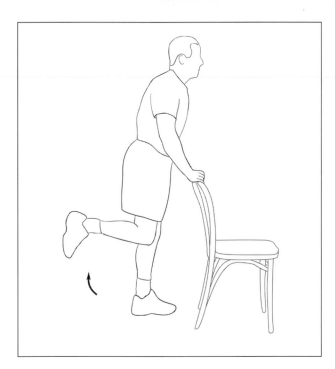

## Hamstring Curls

Stand on a flat surface with your weight evenly distributed on both feet. Hold onto the back of a chair or the wall for balance. Bend the injured knee, lifting the heel toward the ceiling as far as possible without pain. Hold this position for 5 seconds and then relax. Perform 3 sets of 25 to 45 repetitions, 5 to 6 days a week, continuing for 3 to 4 weeks. Seated version: Sit on a chair with your feet flat on the floor. Raise the injured knee off the chair and hold the position for 5 seconds.

SECTION 6 ■ KNEE AND LOWER LEG

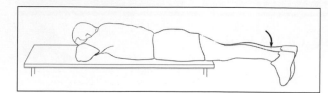

## Passive Knee Extension (Prone)

Lie face down on a table or bed with your thighs supported just above the knee. Relax your legs and let gravity pull the knees down (into extension). Stay in this position for 5 to 10 minutes. Repeat this 2 to 3 times per day, 5 to 6 days a week, continuing for 3 to 4 weeks.

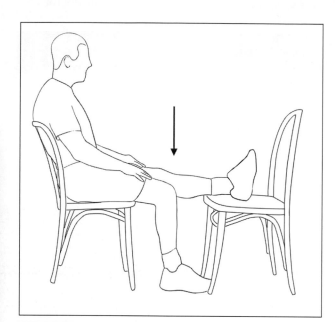

## Passive Knee Extension (Seated)

Sit in a chair with your injured leg propped up on another chair of equal height, as shown. Relax your leg and let gravity pull the knee down (into extension). Hold the position for 10 seconds. Perform 3 sets of 25 to 50 repetitions, 5 to 6 days a week, continuing for 3 to 4 weeks.

SECTION 6 ■ KNEE AND LOWER LEG

# COMPARTMENT SYNDROME

## DEFINITION

The muscles of the leg are divided by fibrous septae into four compartments: anterior, lateral, superficial posterior, and deep posterior (**Figure 1**). Compartment syndromes are characterized by an elevation of intracompartmental pressure to a degree that compromises blood flow to the involved muscles and nerves. Although acute compartment syndromes most often develop after fractures of the tibia, any condition that has the potential to cause significant swelling, such as contusions, muscle strains, or crush injuries, also can result in this limb-threatening condition. Compartment syndrome of the leg may affect one or more of the four compartments. The anterior compartment is the most frequently involved.

Exertional compartment syndrome of the leg, sometimes called chronic compartment syndrome, is an exercise-induced pathologic increase in tissue pressure (typically greater than 40 mm Hg) in one or more of the four muscle compartments. The result is leg pain and occasionally paresthesias radiating into the foot.

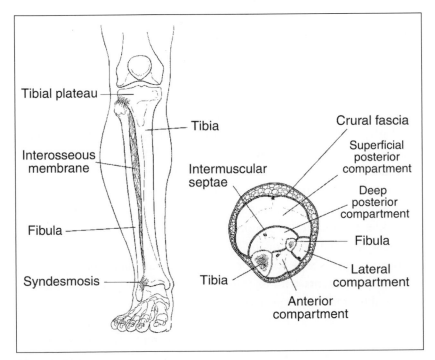

**Figure 1**

Frontal and cross-sectional views of leg showing compartmental anatomy.

Reproduced from Sullivan JA, Anderson SJ (eds): *Care of the Young Athlete*. Rosemont, IL, American Academy of Orthopaedic Surgeons, 1999, p 406.

SECTION 6 ■ KNEE AND LOWER LEG

# CLINICAL SYMPTOMS

The hallmark of an acute compartment syndrome is severe leg pain that is out of proportion to what would otherwise be expected. As the condition progresses, patients also may experience paresthesias or numbness on the dorsum of the foot (with anterior or lateral compartment involvement) or on the plantar aspect of the foot (with involvement of the deep posterior compartment).

Exertional compartment syndrome is associated with prolonged walking or running. Symptoms develop gradually with exercise, but with cessation of the activity, the compartment tissue pressure returns to normal (less than 10 mm Hg), and symptoms gradually resolve within 30 minutes. Patients with an exertional compartment syndrome do not experience pain at rest. The anterior compartment is most commonly involved, and patients may note weakness of the foot dorsiflexors and paresthesias in the dorsum of the first web space. Deep posterior compartment syndromes may result in paresthesias on the plantar aspect of the foot secondary to tibial nerve involvement.

# TESTS

## Physical Examination

Acute compartment syndromes cause marked swelling, tenseness, and tenderness of the involved compartment. Increased pain with passive stretching of the muscles of the involved compartment is characteristic. For example, with an anterior compartment syndrome, passive stretch of the extensor hallucis longus (eg, flexing the great toe) causes marked pain. With involvement of the lateral compartment, inversion of the foot will passively stretch the peroneus longus and brevis. With a deep posterior compartment syndrome, extension of the great toe will place the flexor hallucis longus on stretch. Superficial compartment muscles are put on stretch by dorsiflexing the ankle. Decreased sensation of the involved nerves is often present at the onset of the syndrome, but paralysis and loss of dorsalis pedis and posterior tibial pulses are late findings.

Most patients with exertional compartment syndrome have no abnormal physical findings when they are not exercising, although some will have defects of the anterior compartment fascia. If the leg is examined during exercise, the involved compartment musculature may appear swollen and tense and may be tender to palpation.

*Diagnostic Tests*

The best way to confirm the diagnosis is to measure compartment pressures (anterior, lateral, superficial, and deep posterior) using an indwelling catheter. A clinically significant acute compartment syndrome is present when the diastolic pressure minus the compartment pressure is less than 30 mm Hg. Patients with exertional compartment syndromes develop pressures that exceed 40 mm Hg with exercise and remain elevated for a prolonged period after activity, taking 30 minutes or longer to return to normal.

# DIFFERENTIAL DIAGNOSIS

*Chronic compartment syndrome*

Shin-splints (tenderness along tibia)

Stress fracture (pain at rest, radiographic findings)

*Acute compartment syndrome*

Contusion (clinical differentiation, low compartment pressure)

# ADVERSE OUTCOMES OF THE DISEASE

Tissue necrosis from compromised blood flow to muscles and nerves with acute compartment syndrome may be limb threatening. Patients with exertional compartment syndrome may experience significant compromise in quality of life because of their inability to exercise.

# TREATMENT

Treatment of an acute compartment syndrome is immediate four-compartment fasciotomy, or "opening" the compartment by incising longitudinally the fascial tissues that form the compartment. Nonsurgical treatment of exertional compartment syndrome requires discontinuing an activity or decreasing its intensity to an asymptomatic level. Because exertional compartment syndrome typically involves only one or two rather than all four compartments, surgical treatment is fasciotomy of the involved compartment(s).

# ADVERSE OUTCOMES OF TREATMENT

Incomplete fasciotomy and continued tissue necrosis is possible following treatment of acute compartment syndrome.

# REFERRAL DECISIONS/RED FLAGS

Acute compartment syndromes are surgical emergencies. Failure to diagnose and immediately treat a compartment syndrome may result in tissue necrosis and permanent muscle contracture,

SECTION 6 ■ KNEE AND LOWER LEG

pain, weakness, and neurologic injury. Do not be misled by the presence of intact pulses or intact sensation. In rare situations, a patient with a chronic exertional compartment syndrome will develop an acute compartment syndrome. Presumably, this occurs when the swelling and pressure increase to such an extent that they do not return to normal after cessation of exercise. This condition requires emergent treatment.

SECTION 6 ■ KNEE AND LOWER LEG

# CONTUSIONS

## SYNONYM
Bruise

**ICD-9 Code**
**924.10**
Contusion of lower limb

## DEFINITION
Contusions are injuries to the leg sustained from a direct, blunt blow. Although the resulting disability usually is minor, some contusions are quite painful, with significant swelling and tenderness. Excessive swelling may result in a compartment syndrome, which therefore should be considered in the clinical evaluation.

## CLINICAL SYMPTOMS
Contusions cause swelling, tenderness, and ecchymosis of the involved muscle. Active muscle contraction and passive stretch may be painful.

## TESTS

### Physical Examination
Physical examination usually reveals a tense, swollen, tender extremity, which is larger in circumference than the contralateral leg.

### Diagnostic Tests
AP and lateral radiographs should be obtained in patients involved in high-energy trauma or with severe pain to rule out a fracture about the knee.

## DIFFERENTIAL DIAGNOSIS
Compartment syndrome (disproportionate pain with passive movement, elevated compartment pressures)

Fracture about the knee (evident on radiographs)

Knee dislocation (evident on radiographs)

## ADVERSE OUTCOMES OF THE DISEASE
Heterotopic ossification is the formation of mature lamellar bone in soft tissues. Myositis ossificans traumatica, a type of heterotopic ossification, occurs from direct injury to the muscles. Fibrous, cartilaginous, and osseous tissues near bone are affected. Myositis ossificans traumatica may follow any contusion, but it is most common following contusions of the

thigh. With myositis ossificans, a firm mass develops at the site of injury 3 to 4 weeks after the injury. Radiographic changes begin at 3 to 4 weeks and mature as a bony mass by 3 to 6 months.

## TREATMENT

Contusions are treated with minor analgesics, rest, ice, elevation, range-of-motion exercises, calf stretching, and strengthening exercises (bilateral heel raises, heel raises with weights, single-leg heel raises). Treatment is the same with myositis ossificans. In rare patients with myositis ossificans and persistent loss of motion, a painful bony mass, or significant limitation, the heterotopic bone should be surgically excised.

## ADVERSE OUTCOMES OF TREATMENT

NSAIDs may lead to concomitant gastric, renal, or hepatic complications.

## REFERRAL DECISIONS/RED FLAGS

Contusions must not be confused with fractures about the knee or knee dislocations, as the latter require immediate referral and treatment. An acute compartment syndrome resulting from a contusion must be identified and treated immediately.

# FRACTURES ABOUT THE KNEE

## DEFINITION

Distal femur fractures may be classified as supracondylar, condylar involving the medial or lateral femoral condyle, or combinations of these injuries (**Figure 1**). They account for 4% to 7% of all femur fractures. Fractures of the proximal tibial metaphysis are called tibial plateau fractures (**Figure 2**).

In young patients, these fractures usually occur as a result of high-energy trauma and are often associated with other injuries. In elderly patients with osteoporosis, these fractures occur as a result of a low-energy force. Tibial plateau fractures often result from a valgus force (lateral plateau fracture) or varus force (medial plateau fracture). Many of these fractures are intra-articular. These fractures may be associated with collateral ligament injuries.

## CLINICAL SYMPTOMS

Patients report an injury with immediate onset of pain and swelling.

**ICD-9 Codes**
**821.2**
Fracture of other and unspecified parts of femur, lower end, closed
**823.0**
Fracture of tibia and fibula, upper end, closed

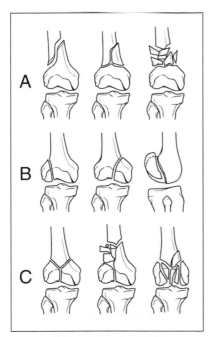

**Figure 1**
Supra- and intercondylar fracture patterns of the distal femur.
**A,** Distal shaft fractures (extra-articular). **B,** Unicondylar fractures. **C,** Intercondylar/bicondylar fractures.
Adapted with permission from Canale TS (ed): *Campbell's Operative Orthopaedics,* ed 10. Philadelphia, PA, Elsevier, 2002, p 2806.

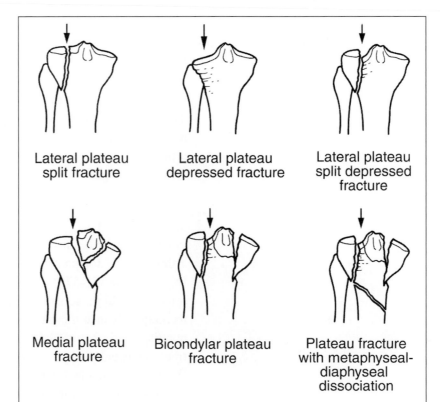

Lateral plateau split fracture

Lateral plateau depressed fracture

Lateral plateau split depressed fracture

Medial plateau fracture

Bicondylar plateau fracture

Plateau fracture with metaphyseal-diaphyseal dissociation

**Figure 2**
Tibial plateau fracture patterns.
Adapted from Perry CR: Fractures of the tibial plateau. *Instr Course Lect* 1994;43:119-126.

# TESTS

## Physical Examination

Swelling of the knee is often marked because bleeding from intra-articular fractures extends into the joint. Inspect the extremity for skin integrity. Assess function of deep peroneal, superficial peroneal, and posterior tibial nerves, as well as distal pulses. Inspect for other injuries, particularly in the patient who has sustained high-energy trauma.

## Diagnostic Tests

Initial radiographic examination should include AP and lateral views of the knee. Oblique radiographs and CT scans may be necessary for preoperative planning. When distal pulses are absent, Doppler examination is useful.

# DIFFERENTIAL DIAGNOSIS

Cruciate ligament disruption (no fracture on radiographs)

Knee dislocation (evident on radiographs)

Quadriceps rupture (no fracture on radiographs, inability to extend the knee against gravity)

Thigh contusion and/or compartment syndrome (negative radiographs, compartment pressure measurements if in question)

# ADVERSE OUTCOMES OF THE DISEASE

Nonunion or malunion of the fracture is possible, with resultant loss of function and the need for surgical salvage procedures. The instability of an unrecognized fracture also may cause neurovascular injury or skin breakdown. Uncorrected intra-articular step-off (articular surface displacement) may lead to arthritic changes.

# TREATMENT

For patients with tense, painful knee effusions, consider arthrocentesis for pain relief (see Knee Joint Aspiration/Injection, pp 571-573). Because a fracture is present, the risk of infection is high, so extreme care should be taken to use sterile technique. Nonsurgical treatment is often indicated for nondisplaced or minimally displaced fractures. Displaced fractures usually require open reduction and internal fixation. With intra-articular fractures, the goal of surgical treatment is restoration of joint alignment and congruity. Emergent treatment is required for open fractures, vascular injuries requiring repair, and compartment syndrome.

## ADVERSE OUTCOMES OF TREATMENT

Complications of treatment include stiffness of the knee, nonunion, failure of fixation, malunion, infection, and injury to neurovascular structures.

## REFERRAL DECISIONS/RED FLAGS

These injuries require further evaluation. Even nondisplaced fractures in this region are at increased risk for displacement.

SECTION 6 ■ KNEE AND LOWER LEG

# ILIOTIBIAL BAND SYNDROME

## SYNONYMS

Iliotibial band tendinitis
Runner's knee

## DEFINITION

The iliotibial band (ITB) is a dense, fibrous band of tissue that originates from the anterior superior iliac spine region, extends down the lateral portion of the thigh, and inserts on the lateral tibia at Gerdy's tubercle. When the knee is extended, the ITB sits anterior to the lateral femoral condyle. When the knee is flexed past 30°, the ITB moves posterior to the lateral femoral condyle (**Figure 1**). ITB syndrome develops when the distal portion of the ITB rubs against the lateral femoral condyle, causing irritation and subsequent inflammation of the ITB. Occurring with repetitive flexion and extension of the knee, ITB syndrome is seen most commonly in long distance runners and cyclists, but any athlete, especially those with predisposing factors for ITB tightness, such as genu varum, internal tibial rotation, and excessive foot pronation, may develop this syndrome.

## CLINICAL SYMPTOMS

Patients with ITB syndrome usually describe pain at the anterolateral aspect of the knee that worsens with running, especially downhill, or cycling. This pain is usually most intense at heel strike. Also, patients may report an audible popping in the knee with walking or running. The patient is usually asymptomatic at rest both before and after activity.

## TESTS

### Physical Examination

Tenderness to direct palpation is most evident directly over the lateral femoral epicondyle, 2 to 3 cm proximal to the lateral joint line. Noble's and Ober's tests (see Physical Examination—Knee and Lower Leg: Special Tests, pp 483 and 484) may help to confirm the diagnosis of ITB syndrome. Functional testing, such as eliciting lateral knee pain when the patient hops with a flexed knee, is also confirmatory.

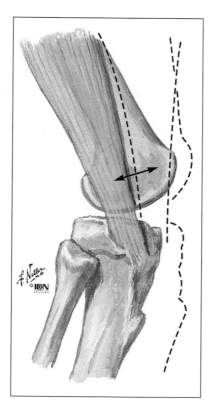

**Figure 1**

Movement of the ITB over the lateral femoral condyle with flexion and extension of the knee.

(Reproduced with permission from Icon Learning Systems.)

SECTION 6 ■ KNEE AND LOWER LEG

*Diagnostic Tests*

AP and lateral radiographs are usually negative with ITB syndrome but should be ordered to exclude other pathology presenting as lateral knee pain.

## DIFFERENTIAL DIAGNOSIS

Hamstring strain

Lateral collateral ligament sprain (opening with varus stress)

Meniscal injury (joint line tenderness, mechanical symptoms, positive McMurray test)

## ADVERSE OUTCOMES OF THE DISEASE

Continued lateral knee pain may lead to decreased activity and associated lowered fitness level.

## TREATMENT

Most patients respond to nonsurgical treatment, including physical therapy, a short-term course of NSAIDs, ice, and activity modifications. Physical therapy interventions must address the entire lower limb. A program to improve hamstring flexibility and hip abductor weakness should be initiated. Iliotibial band, tensor fasciae latae, and hip external rotator flexibility also must be addressed. Acute management may include modalities to decrease inflammation, such as phonophoresis or iontophoresis and cryotherapy. NSAIDs are also effective to help control the acute inflammatory process.

Following the initial period of inflammation control, alterations in training may be helpful for long-term prevention. Runners may alter their duration or pace of training, adjust their stride length, or reverse direction if they run on a circular track. Cyclists may adjust their seat height or foot position on the pedals. Runners with excessive pronation or excessive lateral wear may need special orthoses.

Local injection with corticosteroids or even surgery may be warranted only when the symptoms do not respond to stretching, physical therapy, and exercise modification.

## ADVERSE OUTCOMES OF TREATMENT

NSAIDs may lead to concomitant gastric, renal, or hepatic complications. Infection and ITB weakening from corticosteroid injection are possible.

# REFERRAL DECISIONS/RED FLAGS

Symptoms that do not respond to nonsurgical treatment require further evaluation. Further evaluation is also indicated if signs of ligament or tendon insufficiency are present.

# MEDIAL GASTROCNEMIUS TEAR

## SYNONYM
Tennis leg

**ICD-9 Code**

**844.9**
Medial gastrocnemius tear

## DEFINITION
Acute strains or ruptures of the medial head of the gastrocnemius muscle usually occur at the muscle-tendon junction. The injury often occurs while playing tennis, running on a hill, or jumping. These injuries are most common in athletes over 30 years of age.

## CLINICAL SYMPTOMS
The patient typically feels a pulling or tearing sensation in the calf. Most of the pain is located proximally and medially. This injury can result in diffuse calf pain, swelling, and tenderness.

## TESTS

### Physical Examination
The patient typically has tenderness and swelling over the medial gastrocnemius. The patient holds the ankle in plantar flexion to avoid placing tension on the injured muscle and typically ambulates with the ankle in a plantar flexed position. The patient is unable to perform a single-leg toe raise. Ecchymosis can develop in the calf over 24 hours. The patient has a negative Thompson test (see p 590), which would be positive with an Achilles tendon rupture.

### Diagnostic Tests
No specific diagnostic tests are necessary to evaluate a medial gastrocnemius tear.

## DIFFERENTIAL DIAGNOSIS
Achilles tendinitis (more distal localization)

Achilles tendon rupture (positive Thompson test)

Popliteal cyst rupture (no trauma, no plantar flexion)

## ADVERSE OUTCOMES OF THE DISEASE
Scar tissue may form, resulting in chronic pain, dysfunction, or reinjury due to shortening of the muscle-tendon unit. Another potential complication of a medial gastrocnemius tear is deep venous thrombosis (DVT) formation, due to inactivity and trauma.

SECTION 6 ■ KNEE AND LOWER LEG

## TREATMENT

Medial gastrocnemius tears are treated nonsurgically initially with such measures as minor analgesics, rest, ice, elevation, a ½-inch heel lift, a calf sleeve or compression hose, and crutches. These are followed by isometric calf contractions in plantar flexion and gentle range-of-motion, stretching, and strengthening exercises (bilateral heel raises, heel raises with weights, single-leg heel raises).

## PHYSICAL THERAPY PRESCRIPTION

The initial treatment goal is to control the pain and inflammation with the use of rest, ice, compression, and elevation (RICE). A home exercise program (see pp 521-522) should include early movement: within 7 to 21 days postinjury, gentle active and passive range-of-motion exercises should be initiated. The active exercises should include calf raises, and the passive exercises should include gentle stretching of the gastrocnemius muscle group.

If pain and limited function continue for more than 3 to 4 weeks, formal physical therapy may be ordered. The prescription should include an evaluation of the extent of gastrocnemius and soleus muscle tightness and weakness of the gastrocnemius, and the physical therapist should design a program to increase the range of motion and improve muscle strength.

## ADVERSE OUTCOMES OF TREATMENT

NSAIDs can lead to concomitant gastric, renal, or hepatic complications. Loss of dorsiflexion may occur if range-of-motion exercises are not encouraged.

## REFERRAL DECISIONS/RED FLAGS

Persistent symptoms indicate the need for further evaluation.

# HOME EXERCISE PROGRAM FOR MEDIAL GASTROCNEMIUS TEAR

Perform the exercises in the order listed. After performing the calf raises, apply a bag of crushed ice or frozen peas to the injured area for 20 minutes to prevent further inflammation. Apply moist or dry heat to the injured area before and during the heel cord stretch. If the exercises increase the pain or if the pain does not improve after you have performed the exercises for 3 to 4 weeks, call your doctor.

| Exercise Type | Muscle Group | Number of Repetitions/Sets | Number of Days per Week | Number of Weeks |
|---|---|---|---|---|
| Calf raises | Gastrocnemius/ soleus | 10 repetitions/3 sets | 3 to 4 | 3 to 4 |
| Heel cord stretch | Gastrocnemius/ soleus | 4 repetitions/2 to 3 sets | Daily | 3 to 4 |

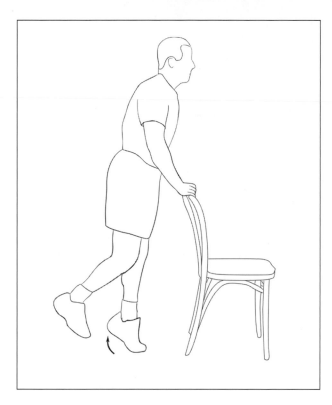

## Calf Raises

Stand on a flat surface with your weight evenly distributed on both feet. Hold onto the back of a chair or the wall for balance and lift the foot on the uninjured side. Keeping the knee of the injured leg straight, raise the heel off the floor as high as you can, using your body weight as resistance. Work up to 3 sets of 10 repetitions, 3 to 4 days a week, continuing for 3 to 4 weeks.

SECTION 6 ■ KNEE AND LOWER LEG

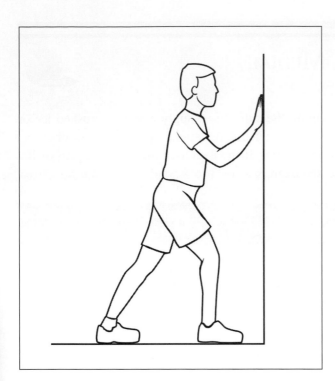

## Heel Cord Stretch

Stand facing the wall with the affected leg straight and the knee of the unaffected leg bent, as shown. The toe of the affected leg should be pointed in, and the heel should not come off the ground. Hold the stretch for 30 seconds with the knee straight and then relax for 30 seconds. Perform 2 to 3 sets of 4 repetitions daily, continuing for 3 to 4 weeks.

# Meniscal Tear

## Synonyms

Locked knee

Torn cartilage

## Definition

The medial and lateral menisci are fibrocartilaginous pads that function as shock absorbers between the femoral condyles and tibial plateaus. Meniscal tears occur alone or in association with ligament injuries such as anterior cruciate ligament tears. Meniscal tears disrupt the mechanics of the knee, leading to varying degrees of symptoms and predisposing the knee to degenerative arthritis.

## Clinical Symptoms

Patients with traumatic tears typically report a significant twisting injury to the knee. Older patients with degenerative tears may have a history of minimal or no trauma, with the injury occurring during an activity such as simply rising from a squatting position. Patients usually can ambulate after an acute injury and frequently are able to continue to participate in athletics.

Traumatic tears are typically followed by the insidious onset of knee swelling and stiffness over 2 to 3 days. Mechanical symptoms such as locking, catching, and popping may then develop. Patients usually experience pain on the medial or lateral side of the knee, particularly with twisting or squatting activities. In some cases, large unstable fragments of meniscal tissue become incarcerated in the knee joint, leading to a "locked knee." More frequently, motion is limited by a feeling of tightness in the knee secondary to the effusion. The mechanical symptoms and degree of pain tend to wax and wane.

## Tests

### Physical Examination

The most common finding on physical examination is tenderness over the medial or lateral joint line. Young patients who have traumatic tears that disrupt the peripheral blood supply typically present with a large effusion or hemarthrosis. In degenerative tears or tears that involve the avascular central body of the meniscus, effusions are typically small or absent.

SECTION 6 ■ KNEE AND LOWER LEG

Knee motion may be limited secondary to pain or an effusion. During provocative testing, forced flexion and circumduction (internal and external rotation of the foot) frequently elicit pain on the side of the knee with the meniscal tear. The McMurray test is positive when the flexion-circumduction maneuver is associated with a painful click.

### Diagnostic Tests

AP, lateral, and axial patellofemoral views are indicated for patients with a history of trauma or an effusion. For patients with chronic conditions, the AP and lateral views should be weight bearing. A weight-bearing AP view with the knees flexed 45° is sensitive for early osteoarthritis and is recommended in older patients. MRI is highly specific and sensitive for meniscal pathology. Knee aspiration is indicated when a diagnosis of infection or crystal arthropathy is considered.

## DIFFERENTIAL DIAGNOSIS

Anterior cruciate ligament tear (hemarthrosis, positive Lachman test)

Crystal disease (crystals in aspirate)

Loose body (fragment may be evident on radiographs, but purely cartilaginous loose body may not)

Medial collateral ligament tear (pain and instability with valgus stress)

Osteoarthritis (joint space narrowing may be evident on weight-bearing radiographs)

Osteochondritis dissecans (evident on radiographs, especially medial femoral condyle)

Osteonecrosis of the femoral condyle (patient age over 50 years, pain, evident on radiographs or MRI)

Patellar subluxation or dislocation (tender medial patella, apprehension sign)

Pes anserine bursitis (tender distal to medial joint line)

Saphenous neuritis (tender to palpation along the course of the saphenous nerve)

Tibial plateau fracture (bony tenderness, evident on radiographs)

## ADVERSE OUTCOMES OF THE DISEASE

Recurrent episodes of locking and damage to the adjacent articular cartilage with subsequent osteoarthritis are possible, particularly with a delay in definitive treatment. With the exception of the outer rim, the blood supply to the meniscus is poor. Although small peripheral tears can heal, most tears are more central and cannot heal. Patients with recurrent stiffness, locking, or pain have a mechanically significant tear, which suggests ongoing internal damage. Failure to recognize and treat a traumatic tear may lead to progressive damage and a lost opportunity for surgical repair.

# TREATMENT

In the absence of mechanical symptoms and particularly when a degenerative tear is present, initial treatment should consist of rest, ice, compression, and elevation (RICE). A short course of oral analgesics, such as acetaminophen or ibuprofen, may facilitate return to normal activity. Traumatic tears in younger patients should be evaluated and treated aggressively. Sports activity should be restricted until MRI evaluation is made or symptoms resolve. Surgical débridement or repair is indicated in younger patients with significant tears and in older patients whose symptoms do not respond to nonsurgical treatment.

# PHYSICAL THERAPY PRESCRIPTION

Initial treatment should consist of RICE to control soft-tissue edema, joint effusion, and pain. Early controlled movement is generally effective in improving mobility and reducing pain. The type of meniscal injury called a bucket handle tear, however, is beyond the scope of rehabilitation.

A home exercise program should include early pain-free movement such as knee bends and straight-leg raises (see p 527). In addition, use of a stationary bicycle may be helpful in reducing pain and increasing range of motion. If the pain continues for more than 3 to 4 weeks, formal physical therapy is an option. The prescription should include a thorough evaluation of quadriceps and hamstring strength and of the trunk and hip to determine core muscle deficits. In addition, exercises to promote healing should be initiated.

# ADVERSE OUTCOMES OF TREATMENT

NSAIDs may cause gastric, renal, or hepatic complications. Meniscal repair has a 10% to 30% failure rate, sometimes necessitating subsequent re-repair or partial meniscectomy. Persistent pain after a partial meniscectomy may occur secondary to concomitant pathology, such as osteoarthritis or saphenous neuritis. Traumatic osteoarthritis may be a late complication in the involved compartment following partial meniscectomy. Postoperative infection is rare.

SECTION 6 ■ KNEE AND LOWER LEG

# REFERRAL DECISIONS/RED FLAGS

A patient with a traumatic effusion, mechanical symptoms, or ligamentous instability requires further evaluation. Patients who do not respond to nonsurgical treatment and have persistent joint line tenderness or effusions also may require further evaluation.

# HOME EXERCISE PROGRAM FOR MENISCAL TEAR

Perform the exercises in the order listed. To prevent inflammation, apply a bag of crushed ice or frozen peas to the injured side of the knee for 20 minutes after completing the exercises. If the exercises increase the pain in your knee or if the pain does not improve after performing the exercises for 3 to 4 weeks, call your doctor.

| Exercise Type | Muscle Group | Number of Repetitions/Sets | Number of Days per Week | Number of Weeks |
|---|---|---|---|---|
| Hamstring curls | Hamstrings | 25 repetitions/3 sets | 4 to 5 | 3 to 4 |
| Straight-leg raises | Quadriceps | 10 repetitions/3 sets | 4 to 5 | 3 to 4 |

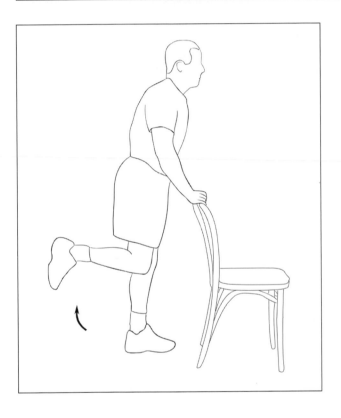

## Hamstring Curls

Stand on a flat surface with your weight evenly distributed on both feet. Hold onto the back of a chair or the wall for balance. Bend the injured knee, raising the heel toward the ceiling as far as possible without pain. Hold this position for 5 seconds and then relax. Perform 3 sets of 25 repetitions 4 to 5 days a week, continuing for 3 to 4 weeks. Scated version: Sit on a chair with your feet flat on the floor. Raise the injured knee off the chair and hold the position for 5 seconds.

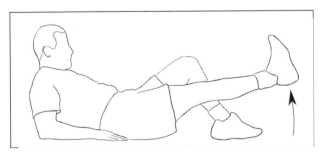

## Straight-Leg Raises

Lie on the floor, supporting your torso with your elbows as shown. Keep the injured leg straight and bend the other leg at the knee so that the foot is flat on the floor. Tighten the thigh muscle of the injured leg and slowly raise it 6 to 10 inches off the floor. Hold this position for 5 seconds and then relax. Perform 3 sets of 10 repetitions 4 to 5 days a week, continuing for 3 to 4 weeks.

SECTION 6 ■ KNEE AND LOWER LEG

# OSTEOCHONDRITIS DISSECANS

**ICD-9 Code**

**732.7**
Osteochondritis dissecans

## DEFINITION

Osteochondritis dissecans (OCD) is osteonecrosis of subchondral bone. This disorder most commonly occurs in the knee but also may develop in other locations such as the talus and distal humerus. The most common location in the knee is the posterolateral side of the medial femoral condyle (**Figure 1**), but it also occurs in other areas of the distal femur and, uncommonly, in the patella.

The lesion is thought to result from repetitive small stresses to the subchondral bone that disrupt the blood supply to an area of bone. The osteonecrotic bone becomes separated from surrounding viable bone by fibrous tissue. Over time, the resultant osteonecrosis weakens the involved area, and shear forces gradually fracture (dissect) the articular cartilage surface. Ultimately the osteonecrotic fragment may completely fragment and become loose bodies in the joint.

## CLINICAL SYMPTOMS

Patients usually report the gradual onset of knee pain. They also may report knee effusions and catching or locking symptoms,

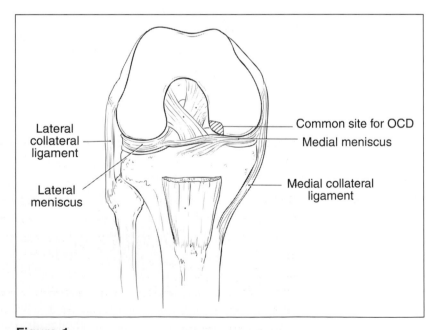

**Figure 1**
Diagram of the knee. Note the most common location for OCD of the knee, on the posterolateral aspect of the medial femoral condyle.

Adapted with permission from Mercier LR: *Practical Orthopedics*, ed 4. St. Louis, MO, Mosby Year Book, 1995, p 208.

particularly when the overlying articular cartilage has been disrupted. Walking with the foot rotated outward may relieve the pain.

## TESTS

### Physical Examination

Examination will reveal tenderness with palpation of the involved area. The most common site for OCD, on the medial femoral condyle, can be palpated with the knee flexed 90°. Pressure is directed over the medial femoral condyle, just medial to the inferior pole of the patella. The Wilson test (see Physical Examination—Knee and Lower Leg: Special Tests, p 484) may be positive.

### Diagnostic Tests

The lesion is best seen on tunnel and lateral views, although it can also usually be seen on an AP radiograph. MRI can help in visualizing the integrity of the overlying articular cartilage and in staging the lesion.

## DIFFERENTIAL DIAGNOSIS

Cruciate ligament injury (positive diagnostic tests, negative radiographs)

Meniscal tear (joint line tenderness, negative radiographs)

## ADVERSE OUTCOMES OF THE DISEASE

Untreated or unsuccessfully treated OCD lesions may fragment, forming loose bodies and leaving defects in the articular cartilage that may lead to degenerative joint disease.

## TREATMENT

The goal of treatment is to obtain healing of the lesion. If shear forces are minimized, new bone formation can replace the osteonecrotic bone. This process requires creeping substitution of new bone formation. Whether treated nonsurgically or surgically, OCD lesions take months to heal.

Nonsurgical treatment is appropriate when the overlying articular cartilage is intact; however, nonsurgical treatment is not likely to succeed after skeletal maturity. Nonsurgical treatment includes activity modifications to the point that symptoms are relieved, specifically, avoiding running and jumping activities, and possibly a period of crutch ambulation. Immobilization is reserved for refractory symptoms or noncompliant patients.

SECTION 6 ■ KNEE AND LOWER LEG

Surgical treatment is necessary after skeletal maturity and in children in whom the lesion has progressed to the stage that the articular cartilage has partially or totally separated. If the lesion is intact (still in place), it is drilled to promote vascular ingrowth and creeping substitution. Unstable lesions require temporary internal fixation to promote healing. When the fragment is loose, treatment consists of removing the free fragment and débriding the articular surface defect.

## ADVERSE OUTCOMES OF TREATMENT

Unsuccessful treatment of OCD may lead to a defect in the joint surface, with progressive osteoarthritis. This may require a cartilage replacement procedure. Possible complications of surgical treatment are infection or further damage to the joint caused by the hardware or failure of the hardware.

## REFERRAL DECISIONS/RED FLAGS

Children with lesions < 1 cm in width usually do well with nonsurgical treatment; however, those with lesions > 2 cm usually have progressive problems. Children with lesions between 1 and 2 cm should be treated based on symptoms and radiographic findings. After the physis has closed, the prognosis for healing is significantly poorer, and these patients require further evaluation.

# OSTEONECROSIS OF THE FEMORAL CONDYLE

## SYNONYM
Avascular necrosis

**ICD-9 Code**

**733.43**
Aseptic necrosis of bone, medial
femoral condyle

## DEFINITION
Osteonecrosis literally means "bone death." It occurs in the femoral condyle when a segment of bone loses its blood supply. The etiology is unknown, but it may begin as a stress fracture and probably involves some combination of trauma and altered blood flow. A portion of the weight-bearing surface of the medial femoral condyle is most often involved. The typical patient is a woman (female:male ratio is 3:1) who is over 60 years of age.

Osteonecrosis of the femoral condyle may be idiopathic or may be associated with chronic steroid therapy, renal transplantation, systemic lupus erythematosus, sickle cell anemia, and Gaucher disease. Microfracture of the subchondral bone occurs along with segmental collapse. Ultimately, progression to osteoarthritis is likely.

## CLINICAL SYMPTOMS
Patients typically describe a sudden, sharp pain localized to the medial compartment. This pain probably develops when a shear force causes a subchondral fracture or disruption of the articular surface. An effusion may be present, and the patient may limit motion secondary to pain. Bilateral symptoms occur in less than 20% of patients.

## TESTS

### Physical Examination
Physical examination will reveal an effusion, some loss of motion, and often a flexion contracture when the condition has gone unrecognized. Pain to palpation over the medial femoral condyle also is common.

### Diagnostic Tests
Radiographically, osteonecrosis of the medial femoral condyle has been divided into stages to better define the extent of the pathology and outline appropriate care. These signs begin with flattening of the convexity of the condyle and progress through joint space narrowing, sclerosis, and osteophyte formation. The two determinants for accurate diagnosis are the area of the

lesion and the percentage of involvement of the condyle. MRI or a bone scan can be helpful in making the diagnosis and determining the extent of involvement.

## DIFFERENTIAL DIAGNOSIS

Meniscal tears (evident on MRI)
Osteoarthritis (tricompartmental involvement)
Osteochondritis dissecans (sex and age predilection, location)
Pes anserine bursitis (location)

## ADVERSE OUTCOME OF THE DISEASE

Unrecognized or untreated symptomatic osteonecrosis will progress to osteoarthritis. Current treatment seeks to slow this progression.

## TREATMENT

Nonsurgical management includes an unloading brace, NSAIDs, pain medication, and a conditioning program to restore quadriceps strength and endurance with modifications as necessary to avoid knee pain when exercising. Water exercise is an excellent option. Surgical intervention, which is indicated when symptoms persist despite a course of nonsurgical treatment, can include débridement and drilling, procedures to alter the weight-bearing axis and unload the medial compartment, and, for advanced cases, total knee replacement.

## ADVERSE OUTCOMES OF TREATMENT

Surgical complications may occur. The results of procedures that alter the weight-bearing axis are mixed: risk to neurovascular structures and overcorrection are the two main concerns. Total knee replacement provides excellent pain relief and improved function but carries the possible need for future revision.

## REFERRAL DECISIONS/RED FLAGS

Failure to improve with nonsurgical treatment warrants consideration of surgical intervention. Disproportionate pain, which can indicate complex regional pain syndrome, also indicates the need for further evaluation.

# PATELLAR/QUADRICEPS TENDINITIS

## SYNONYMS

Extensor mechanism tendinitis

Jumper's knee

## DEFINITION

Extensor mechanism tendinitis is an overuse or overload syndrome involving either the quadriceps tendon at its insertion on the superior pole of the patella, or the patellar tendon at the inferior pole of the patella or at its insertion at the tibial tubercle. Younger adults (under age 40 years) with this condition often engage in jumping or kicking sports (jumper's knee) or have erratic exercise habits. Patellar or quadriceps tendinitis also sometimes develops in older patients after a lifting strain or a significant change in exercise level. Weight gain is sometimes a factor.

## CLINICAL SYMPTOMS

Anterior knee pain is the hallmark. Patients often point to a tender spot where symptoms concentrate. The pain is often noted immediately at the end of exercise or following sitting that has been preceded by exercise. Pain also may be reported with prolonged sitting, squatting, or kneeling. Climbing or descending stairs, running, jumping, or squatting often increases the pain.

## TESTS

### Physical Examination

Palpate for tenderness at the bony attachment of the quadriceps tendon or the infrapatellar tendon. Increased heat, mild swelling, and soft-tissue crepitus also may be evident in the tender region. Examination in the area of the infrapatellar bursa (below the patella and behind the infrapatellar tendon) often reveals puffiness (**Figure 1**). Knee motion is normal but frequently is painful with resisted full extension. Pain is most exacerbated by hyperflexion of the knee, which increases the stresses on the extensor mechanism. When the condition is long-standing, quadriceps atrophy may be evident. Other general knee tests are negative in isolated cases.

**ICD-9 Codes**

**726.60**
Enthesopathy of knee, unspecified

**726.64**
Patellar tendinitis

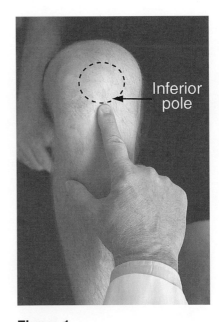

Inferior pole

**Figure 1**
Palpation of the infrapatellar bursa.

SECTION 6 ■ KNEE AND LOWER LEG

*Diagnostic Tests*

AP and lateral radiographs of the knee typically are negative, but lateral views may show small osteophytes or heterotopic ossification at the upper or lower pole of the patella. MRI is reserved for recalcitrant cases for which surgical treatment is being considered or for cases in which partial rupture is possible (significant weakness in extension but no palpable defect).

# DIFFERENTIAL DIAGNOSIS

Anterior or posterior cruciate ligament injury (positive Lachman or posterior drawer test)

Inflammatory conditions (multisystem findings, elevated erythrocyte sedimentation rate)

Partial rupture of the extensor mechanism (weakness, palpable defect, difficulty with straight-leg raising test)

Patellofemoral pain syndrome (anterior knee pain, other abnormal patellofemoral signs but not superior or inferior pole tenderness)

Septic arthritis of the knee (fever, warmth, painful motion, elevated erythrocyte sedimentation rate)

# ADVERSE OUTCOMES OF THE DISEASE

Pain and, rarely, spontaneous rupture of the quadriceps or infrapatellar tendon may occur.

# TREATMENT

Treatment is primarily symptomatic but involves three critical aspects. First is a period of relative rest from aggravating activities. Depending on the severity of the condition, this period can vary from 3 to 5 days to as long as 3 to 6 weeks or more. In some instances, patients may need to use a knee immobilizer intermittently. NSAIDs may help control symptoms, but local injections of corticosteroids should be avoided because these injections significantly increase the risk of rupture of the extensor mechanism. Analgesic creams, ice after activity, and heat before activity may be helpful.

The second phase of treatment focuses on regaining a pain-free range of motion, flexibility of the quadriceps and hamstrings, and strength. Exercises focusing on pain-free quadriceps strengthening and flexibility should be initiated, often in conjunction with ultrasound and phonophoresis or other physical therapy modalities. Use of a knee sleeve with a patellar cutout or a compression strap at the level of the patellar tendon (infrapatellar strap) is sometimes helpful.

The third phase of treatment is gradual resumption of the activities that caused the symptoms while continuing the exercises that have restored strength and flexibility. Use of heat before activity and ice after also is often helpful.

## PHYSICAL THERAPY PRESCRIPTION

The early rehabilitation of patellar tendinitis includes rest from eccentric loading activities, ice, and compression of the patellar tendon area. The home exercise program (see p 536-537) should include pain-free activities that promote range of motion, provide gentle stretching, return normal muscle strength to the quadriceps, and reduce any muscle weakness in the hip. Straight-leg raises, knee flexion, and stretching the quadriceps are important to early rehabilitation. If pain persists after 3 to 4 weeks, formal physical therapy may be ordered. The prescription should include assessment of the hip and trunk muscles and of patellar mobility, as well as further strengthening of the quadriceps and hamstring muscle groups.

## ADVERSE OUTCOMES OF TREATMENT

NSAIDs may cause gastric, renal, or hepatic complications. Pain is possible, and occasionally spontaneous rupture of the tendon occurs. Persistent functional impairment is the most common disability.

## REFERRAL DECISIONS/RED FLAGS

Patients with a possible rupture of the extensor mechanism need further evaluation as soon as possible. Cases recalcitrant to nonsurgical management also require further evaluation.

SECTION 6 ■ KNEE AND LOWER LEG

# HOME EXERCISE PROGRAM FOR PATELLAR/QUADRICEPS TENDINITIS

Perform the exercises in the order listed. To prevent inflammation, apply a bag of crushed ice or frozen peas just below the kneecap after completing all the exercises. If the pain continues or gets worse, call your doctor.

| Exercise Type | Muscle Group | Number of Repetitions/Sets | Number of Days per Week | Number of Weeks |
|---|---|---|---|---|
| Straight-leg raises | Quadriceps | 10 repetitions/3 sets | Daily | 3 to 4 |
| Knee flexion | Hamstrings | 25 repetitions/3 sets, progressing to 45 repetitions/3 sets | 4 to 5 | 3 to 4 |
| Prone quadriceps stretch | Quadriceps | 4 repetitions/2 to 3 sets | 5 to 6 | 3 to 4 |

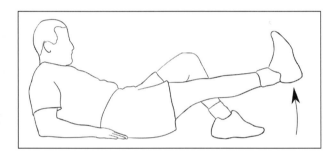

## Straight-Leg Raises

Lie on the floor, supporting your torso with your elbows as shown. Keep the affected leg straight and bend the other leg at the knee so that the foot is flat on the floor. Tighten the thigh muscle of the affected leg and slowly raise it 6 to 10 inches off the floor. Hold this position for 5 seconds and then relax. Perform 3 sets of 10 repetitions daily, continuing for 3 to 4 weeks.

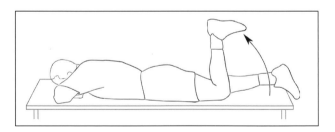

## Knee Flexion

Lie face down on a flat surface with your legs together. Slowly flex the affected knee (bend it up toward your buttocks) as far as possible without pain and then lower it. To add resistance, use rubber tubing while doing the exercise. Perform 3 sets of 25 repetitions, progressing to 3 sets of 45 repetitions. Perform the exercise 4 to 5 days a week, continuing for 3 to 4 weeks.

SECTION 6 ■ KNEE AND LOWER LEG

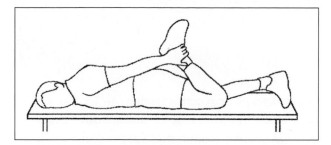

## Prone Quadriceps Stretch

Lie face down on a flat surface with your arms at your sides and your legs straight. Bend the affected knee and grasp the ankle with your hand (or use a towel or rubber tubing). Keeping your thigh flat on the surface, pull gently and hold for 30 seconds; then relax for 30 seconds. Perform 2 to 3 sets of 4 repetitions 5 to 6 days a week, continuing for 3 to 4 weeks.

SECTION 6 ■ KNEE AND LOWER LEG

# PATELLAR/QUADRICEPS TENDON RUPTURES

**ICD-9 Codes**

**822.0**
Fracture of patella

**844.8**
Sprains and strains of knee and leg, other specified sites

**959.7**
Injury, other and unspecified, knee, leg, ankle, and foot

## DEFINITION

A rupture of the quadriceps or patellar tendon, as well as a patellar fracture, will disrupt the extensor mechanism of the knee. Quadriceps and patellar tendon disruptions typically occur with a fall on a knee that is partially flexed. When the quadriceps muscle forcibly contracts to break the impact of the fall, the quadriceps or patellar tendon may be overwhelmed. Fractures of the patella more often result from a direct blow from a motor vehicle accident but also may occur by the indirect mechanism of a fall.

Most patients with ruptures of the quadriceps or patellar tendon are between 30 and 60 years old. A history of previous quadriceps or patellar tendinitis is surprisingly uncommon.

## CLINICAL SYMPTOMS

Patients report significant pain and swelling after an acute injury. Walking may be possible, especially in subtotal ruptures, but patients note a sense of instability or "giving way" with ambulation.

## TESTS

### Physical Examination

A large effusion is usually present. Palpate the knee for defects indicating the area of rupture (**Figure 1**). Fractures of the patella are usually obvious, but ruptures of the quadriceps or patellar tendon may be missed. The key to diagnosis is the patient's inability to extend the knee against gravity or perform a straight-leg raising test.

### Diagnostic Tests

Plain radiographs are appropriate to rule out a patellar fracture. The lateral view may show that, with rupture of the patellar tendon, the patella is in a higher than usual location or that, with rupture of the quadriceps tendon, the patella is in a slightly lower than usual location. MRI will confirm rupture of a tendon but is rarely necessary in the presence of the strong clinical findings.

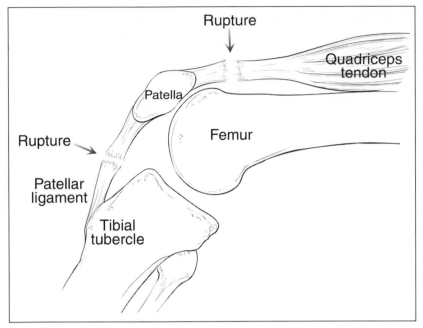

**Figure 1**
Common areas of rupture. These should be palpated during the physical examination.

## DIFFERENTIAL DIAGNOSIS

Collateral ligament tear (varus or valgus injury, medial or lateral tenderness and instability)

Cruciate ligament disruption (effusion may be similar, but the patient is able to extend the knee)

Meniscal tear (effusion relatively small, joint line tenderness, circumduction pain)

## ADVERSE OUTCOMES OF THE DISEASE

Unless the rupture is surgically repaired, marked disability will develop secondary to the deficient extensor mechanism. Delay in treatment significantly increases the difficulty of surgery and may compromise the outcome.

## TREATMENT

Surgical repair is the treatment of choice for a complete rupture of the quadriceps or patellar tendon and for a displaced fracture of the patella. Partial tears of the tendons and nondisplaced fractures, which are uncommon, can be treated by immobilization.

## ADVERSE OUTCOMES OF TREATMENT

Postoperative infection, pain, and weakness of the extensor mechanism are possible.

## REFERRAL DECISIONS/RED FLAGS

All patients with a history and physical examination that suggest extensor mechanism rupture require further evaluation for surgery.

# PATELLOFEMORAL INSTABILITY AND MALALIGNMENT

## SYNONYMS

Miserable malalignment syndrome
Patellar dislocation
Patellar subluxation

### ICD-9 Codes

**718.36**
Recurrent dislocation of joint, lower leg

**836.3**
Dislocation of patella, closed

## DEFINITION

Patellofemoral instability and malalignment encompass a spectrum of pathologic conditions that range from abnormal motion of the patella as it glides over the distal femur, to recurrent subluxation of the patella, to recurrent dislocation of the patella. Patellofemoral instability usually occurs in a lateral direction (**Figure 1**). Medial patellar instability is quite rare. The term "patellofemoral malalignment" indicates that the patella is tilted laterally or predisposed to lateral subluxation, usually because of one or more anatomic factors. Patellar subluxation and dislocation may occur with minimal trauma (eg, a minor twist with a foot planted) in individuals with one or more anatomic predisposing factors such as patella alta, a shallow trochlear groove, a relatively flat patellar undersurface, a laterally tipped patella, "loose ligaments," and hypermobility of the patella. In individuals with normal patellofemoral mechanics, subluxation or dislocation may be caused by direct trauma or, more frequently, by an indirect

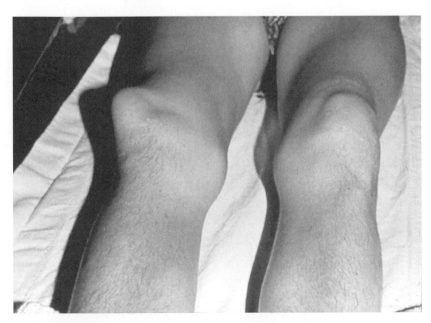

**Figure 1**
Acute lateral patellar dislocation.

Reproduced from Crosby LA, Lewallen DG (eds): *Emergency Care and Transportation of the Sick and Injured*, ed 6. Rosemont, IL, American Academy of Orthopaedic Surgeons, 1995, p 555.

SECTION 6  ■  KNEE AND LOWER LEG

mechanism of injury. A common history is that of a right-handed softball player who dislocates the right patella while swinging the baseball bat. When the right foot is planted firmly on the ground as the torso rotates to the left, the patella lags behind, resulting in a lateral dislocation.

# CLINICAL SYMPTOMS

Patients usually describe severe pain, sometimes report hearing a pop, and occasionally see a deformity of the knee. Patients frequently think that the kneecap has dislocated medially because of the unusual prominence of the medial femoral condyle, which is no longer covered by the patella. The knee is usually maintained in a flexed position. The patella often reduces spontaneously, although sometimes a manual reduction is required.

Subluxation or dislocation of the patella causes tearing of the restraining medial retinacular tissue and the medial patellofemoral ligament, leading to pain, hemarthrosis, and loss of knee motion. Patients who have sustained one episode of instability are likely to sustain additional episodes, particularly when the medial soft tissues have healed in a "stretched-out" position and anatomic predisposing factors are present. Recurrent episodes of instability tend to be less traumatic than the initial episode, with patients experiencing milder symptoms.

In contrast to patients with patellar instability, the primary symptom in patients with symptomatic malalignment is retropatellar pain. This type of anterior knee pain usually is exacerbated when the patient uses stairs, especially when descending. Patients also may report pain with prolonged sitting (movie theater sign) or during squatting. With long-standing maltracking, progressive degenerative changes may occur, leading to patellofemoral arthrosis.

# TESTS

## Physical Examination

Patients with acute patellar instability show apprehension at attempts to manipulate the patella, demonstrating fear and anxiety (apprehension sign) when the patella is translated laterally. Range of motion may be limited in extension and flexion because of pain or fluid in the joint. If the retinaculum is torn, there will be tenderness along the medial edge of the patella. If the medial patellofemoral ligament is torn at its origin, there will be tenderness just proximal to the medial femoral epicondyle. Patients with chronic instability exhibit the apprehension sign but may not have tenderness.

The signs of malalignment are more subtle. During gait, the patellae may tend to point inward (femoral anteversion, tibial torsion), or assume a knock-knee alignment (genu valgum). Genu valgum may be increased, and the distal portion of the vastus medialis may be dysplastic or atrophied. Increased patellar mobility also is common (lateral translation greater than one half the width of the patella), along with tightness of the lateral retinaculum (inability to elevate the lateral edge of the patella to a horizontal position). A high-riding patella (patella alta) and abnormal tracking (positive J sign) also may be observed.

## Diagnostic Tests

AP, lateral, and axial patellofemoral views are necessary. The axial patellofemoral view, such as the Merchant or Laurin view, shows the relationship of the patella to the femoral trochlea. Normally, the patella is centered in the trochlea. In patients with malalignment or previous episodes of instability, radiographs may demonstrate lateral tilt or subluxation of the patella (**Figure 2**). A shallow trochlear groove with a relatively flat patellar undersurface or a patella with an acutely slanted lateral facet may be evident. In patients with excessive lateral pressure syndrome that has progressed to frank patellofemoral arthrosis, radiographs reveal joint space narrowing and other degenerative changes, especially in the lateral articulation. Axial CT may be useful in better delineating the exact nature of the patellar and trochlear relationship, particularly when surgical treatment is considered.

# DIFFERENTIAL DIAGNOSIS

Anterior cruciate ligament tear (increased anterior laxity with Lachman test)

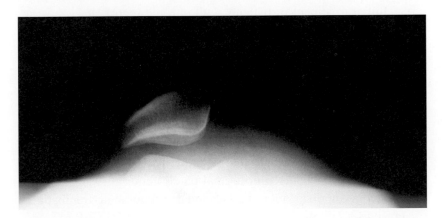

**Figure 2**
Axial patellofemoral view (Laurin view) of the knee showing patellar tilt and subluxation.

SECTION 6 ■ KNEE AND LOWER LEG

Medial collateral ligament tear (pain and laxity with valgus testing)

Medial meniscal tear (medial joint line tenderness)

Patellofemoral pain syndrome (pain without malalignment or instability)

## ADVERSE OUTCOMES OF THE DISEASE

Anterior knee pain secondary to patellar instability or maltracking may lead to secondary quadriceps weakness, further compromising stability and exacerbating the underlying problem. Recurrent episodes of patellar instability and prolonged maltracking may limit activities of daily living and sports activities and also lead to patellofemoral arthrosis.

## TREATMENT

The initial treatment of an acute patellar subluxation or dislocation includes application of a compressive dressing and protective splint with the knee in extension. These measures approximate the torn medial supporting structures. Aspiration of the knee should be considered in patients who have a significant effusion. Adjunctive measures include the use of oral analgesics, frequent application of ice in the first 24 to 48 hours, and modified weight bearing. The patient is instructed in isometric exercises of the quadriceps that are done initially with the splint on. The patient is reevaluated every 2 weeks. When tenderness has resolved over the medial structures, range-of-motion and more vigorous strengthening exercises are started. The total duration of immobilization varies, depending on symptoms, but should not exceed 6 weeks, and quadriceps exercises may be begun even during this early stage of immobilization. Loose bodies seen on radiographs after patellar reduction may need to be removed.

Initial treatment of patients with chronic recurrent maltracking or instability should include exercises emphasizing quadriceps strengthening and flexibility. An elastic brace with a lateral buttress can facilitate the return to occupational or recreational activities. Occasionally, physical therapy modalities such as electrical stimulation or taping can be useful.

When nonsurgical measures fail, proximal or distal realignment of the extensor mechanism may be indicated, with attention toward repair of the medial patellofemoral ligament, especially in patients with normal patellofemoral mechanics and in whom the dislocation was secondary to an acute traumatic episode.

## ADVERSE OUTCOMES OF TREATMENT

The most common adverse outcome after treatment is residual patellofemoral pain. Patellar instability may recur after lateral retinacular release or proximal realignment, but instability is unlikely after distal bony realignment. Even when successful stabilization of the patella is achieved, patellofemoral pain may persist, particularly with concomitant degenerative articular cartilage.

## REFERRAL DECISIONS/RED FLAGS

Patients with a significant effusion after a traumatic knee injury require further evaluation, as do patients with an osteochondral fracture from an acute patellar dislocation. Patients with patellofemoral malalignment or pain that fails to respond to nonsurgical measures also require further evaluation.

SECTION 6 ■ KNEE AND LOWER LEG

# PATELLOFEMORAL PAIN

**ICD-9 Codes**

**717.7**
Chondromalacia of patella

**719.46**
Pain in joint, knee

## SYNONYMS

Anterior knee pain
Chondromalacia
Patellofemoral pain syndrome

## DEFINITION

Patellofemoral pain syndrome refers to a constellation of problems characterized by a diffuse, aching anterior knee pain that increases with activities that place additional loads across the patellofemoral joint, such as running, climbing up or down stairs, kneeling, and squatting. Forces on the articular surface of the patella in a typical 200-lb man can vary from 600 to 3,000 lb per square inch in activities ranging from walking to running. The etiology of this syndrome is multifactorial and in many situations is related to overuse and overloading of the patellofemoral joint. Although patellar malalignment sometimes causes anterior knee pain, it is not a necessary component.

The term chondromalacia should not be used to describe this condition because chondromalacia indicates that pathologic changes are present in the articular surface of the patella, which may not necessarily be true. In addition, many patients who undergo arthroscopy are found to have degenerative changes on the undersurface of the patella consistent with chondromalacia, yet they have no symptoms referable to the patellofemoral joint. For this reason, the terms patellofemoral pain syndrome or anterior knee pain are preferable.

## CLINICAL SYMPTOMS

Patients most commonly report a diffuse, aching anterior knee pain that is worse after prolonged sitting (movie theater sign), climbing stairs, jumping, or squatting. Some patients report a sense of instability or a retropatellar catching sensation. Usually no history of swelling is reported. Often the pain develops after an increase in activity level or in weight training. In most instances, patients will report no preexisting trauma, but on occasion there may be a history of a direct blow to the patella.

## TESTS

### Physical Examination

When the patellofemoral joint is thought to contribute to the patient's pain, its evaluation should be deferred until the end of the examination; otherwise, the patient likely will resist the entire examination.

The patient should first be examined in weight-bearing stance. Watch the patient walk to see whether the patellae point toward each other (a sign of increased femoral anteversion). Look for genu valgum (knock-knees), for inadequate development of the vastus medialis obliquus muscle at the distal and medial thigh, and for foot pronation, which may result in a functional increase in genu valgum.

The Q angle, which is the angle formed by a line drawn from the anterosuperior iliac spine through the center of the patella and a line drawn from the center of the patella to the center of the tibial tubercle, should be measured next (**Figure 1**). In women, the Q angle should be less than 22° with the knee in extension and less than 9° with the knee in 90° of flexion. In men, the Q angle should be less than 18° with the knee in extension and less than 8° with the knee in 90° of flexion.

Excessive femoral anteversion (where the internal rotation of the hip exceeds external rotation by more than 30°) should be checked. Tracking of the patella as the knee moves through flexion and extension also should be observed. As the knee nears full extension, the patella may move laterally more than 1 cm (the J sign) or might even subluxate (a sign of instability). Soft-tissue restraints to medial and lateral patellar translation also should be evaluated. With the knee fully extended, the examiner should be able to elevate the lateral patellar facet to at least a neutral position. At 30° of flexion, the examiner should be able to translate the patella at least one quadrant medially but not more than two quadrants laterally.

The patellar apprehension sign (see Physical Examination—Knee and Lower Leg: Special Tests, p 480) may be performed to evaluate the possibility of patellar instability. Palpate the patella as the patient places the knee through a range of motion to determine whether crepitus occurs and, if so, at what position. Hamstring and quadriceps muscle tightness also should be evaluated.

## Diagnostic Tests

AP, lateral, and bilateral axial patellofemoral views are necessary. The axial patellofemoral view helps to rule out malalignment and arthritis (**Figure 2**).

# DIFFERENTIAL DIAGNOSIS

Meniscal tear (joint line tenderness, possible locking)
Patellar malalignment (malalignment seen clinically and on radiographs)

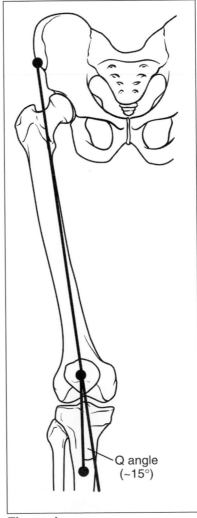

**Figure 1**
Diagram of the Q angle.

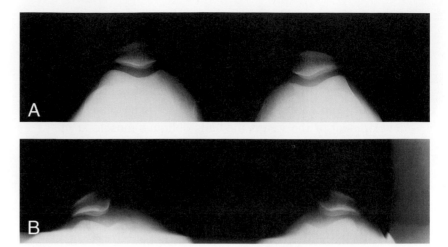

**Figure 2**
Bilateral axial patellofemoral radiographs. **A,** Patellae well aligned in the femoral groove. **B,** Bilateral patellar subluxation.

> Patellar osteoarthritis (in older patients; effusion, crepitus, and evidence on axial radiograph)
>
> Patellar tendinitis (jumper's knee) (inferior pole tenderness, local tenderness at patellar tendon)
>
> Pathologic plica (medial parapatellar pain and tenderness, palpable cord in the medial parapatellar region)
>
> Quadriceps tendinitis (local tenderness at insertion)

## ADVERSE OUTCOMES OF THE DISEASE

Pain and dysfunction are the principal problems.

## TREATMENT

Activity should be adjusted to a pain-free level. A program of quadriceps strengthening and quadriceps and hamstring flexibility should be initiated. Quadriceps exercises need to be individually modified as necessary to avoid causing knee pain (short-arc open or closed chain, or isometric). Using a patellar pad or simple knee sleeve with a patellar cutout, taping the patella to decrease lateral pressure (McConnell taping), or using an infrapatellar strap may help. Some patients benefit from intermittent, short-term use of acetaminophen or NSAIDs. Weight loss is recommended for obese patients. Patients with persistent pain despite nonsurgical treatment may be candidates for surgery.

## PHYSICAL THERAPY PRESCRIPTION

A home exercise program (see pp 550-551) should include exercises to strengthen the quadriceps and gain full flexion range of motion to strengthen the hamstrings. Such exercises include straight-leg raises, knee bends, and prone straight-leg raises.

If pain persists after 3 to 4 weeks, formal physical therapy may be ordered. The prescription should include an assessment of the hip and trunk muscles, patella mobility, and quadriceps/hamstring muscle group strength. In addition to exercises, mobilization is an important component in the treatment of patellofemoral pain.

# ADVERSE OUTCOMES OF TREATMENT

NSAIDs may cause gastric, renal, or hepatic complications. Aggressive full-arc quadriceps exercises typically aggravate the symptoms.

# REFERRAL DECISIONS/RED FLAGS

Persistent symptoms, including pain or recurrent effusions, or findings suggestive of patellar instability indicate the need for further evaluation.

SECTION 6 ■ KNEE AND LOWER LEG

# HOME EXERCISE PROGRAM FOR PATELLOFEMORAL PAIN

Perform the exercises in the order listed. To prevent inflammation, apply a bag of crushed ice or frozen peas along the sides of the kneecap for 20 minutes after completing the exercises. If the pain worsens or does not improve, call your doctor.

| Exercise Type | Muscle Group | Number of Repetitions/Sets | Number of Days per Week | Number of Weeks |
|---|---|---|---|---|
| Hamstring curls | Hamstrings | 25 repetitions/3 sets, progressing to 45 repetitions/3 sets | 4 to 5 | 3 to 4 |
| Straight-leg raises | Quadriceps | 10 repetitions/3 sets | 4 to 5 | 3 to 4 |
| Straight-leg raises (prone) | Quadriceps | 10 repetitions/3 sets | 4 to 5 | 3 to 4 |

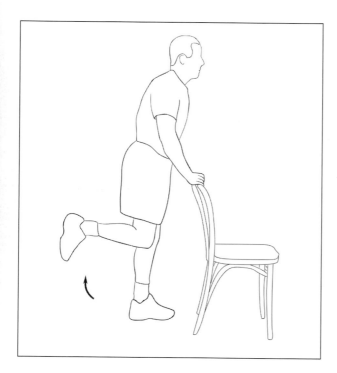

## Hamstring Curls

Stand on a flat surface with your weight evenly distributed on both feet. Hold onto the back of a chair or the wall for balance. Bend the affected knee, raising the heel toward the ceiling as far as possible without pain. Hold this position for 5 seconds and then relax. Perform 3 sets of 25 repetitions, progressing to 3 sets of 45 repetitions. Perform the exercise 4 to 5 days a week, continuing for 3 to 4 weeks. Seated version: Sit on a chair with your feet flat on the floor. Raise the affected knee off the chair and hold the position for 5 seconds.

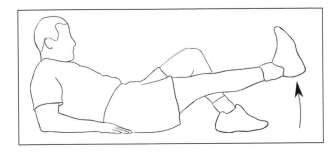

## Straight-Leg Raises

Lie on the floor, supporting your torso with your elbows as shown. Keep the affected leg straight and bend the other leg at the knee so that the foot is flat on the floor. Tighten the thigh muscle of the affected leg and slowly raise it 6 to 10 inches off the floor. Hold this position for 5 seconds and then relax. Perform 3 sets of 10 repetitions 4 to 5 days a week, continuing for 3 to 4 weeks.

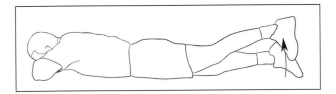

## Straight-Leg Raises (Prone)

Lie on the floor on your stomach with your legs straight. Tighten the hamstrings of the affected leg and raise the leg toward the ceiling as far as you can. Hold the position for 5 seconds. Lower the leg and rest it for 2 seconds. Perform 3 sets of 10 repetitions 4 to 5 days a week, continuing for 3 to 4 weeks.

SECTION 6 ■ KNEE AND LOWER LEG

# PLICA SYNDROME

**ICD-9 Codes**

**717.9**
Unspecified internal derangement of knee

**727.00**
Synovitis and tenosynovitis, unspecified

## DEFINITION

A plica is a normal fold in the synovium. The synovium of the knee joint has five basic plicae. Three of them (suprapatellar, medial, and infrapatellar) are considered distinct structures, and two are considered minor folds. The suprapatellar plica extends from the undersurface of the quadriceps tendon to the medial or lateral capsule of the knee. The medial plica extends from the medial joint capsule to the medial anterior fat pad. The infrapatellar plica (ligamentum mucosa) extends anterior to, and may sometimes cover, the anterior cruciate ligament.

A plica that becomes inflamed and thickened from trauma or overuse may interfere with normal joint motion because the pathologic structure "bowstrings" over the femoral condyle or other structures. Plica syndromes usually result from a combination of trauma and mechanical malalignment and may occur at any age. The medial plica is the plica that most often becomes pathologic.

## CLINICAL SYMPTOMS

The onset of pain is often insidious but may be related to a fall or injury. Patients most often describe activity-related aching in the anterior or anteromedial aspect of the knee. Some patients note a painful snapping or popping in the knee. Buckling or a sense of instability may occur, but true giving way, locking, or obvious effusion is uncommon.

## TESTS

### Physical Examination

Inspect the knee for tenderness. With a pathologic medial plica, tenderness is localized to the medial aspect of the patella. With the knee flexed, a pathologic plica may be palpated as a thickened band. Place the knee in 90° of flexion and then extend the knee. With a pathologic plica, a pop may occur at about 60° of flexion.

Other conditions such as patellofemoral disorders may present with similar symptoms and should be excluded.

### Diagnostic Tests

AP, lateral, and axial patellofemoral views will be normal with plica syndrome but should be obtained to rule out other conditions.

SECTION 6 ■ KNEE AND LOWER LEG

# Differential Diagnosis

Meniscal tear (giving way, joint line tenderness, pain with circumduction)

Osteochondritis dissecans (spontaneous onset, evident on radiographs)

Patellofemoral instability (positive apprehension sign)

Prepatellar bursitis (location)

Quadriceps or patellar tendinitis (tenderness at tendon insertion sites)

Septic arthritis (severe pain, fever, effusion, diagnostic joint aspiration)

# Adverse Outcomes of the Disease

Continued discomfort and interference with running activities can occur, as well as erosive changes in the femoral condyle cartilage, because of the snapping of the thickened plica over the condyle.

# Treatment

Initial management is aimed at decreasing the inflammation and thickening of the plica. Activity modifications and NSAIDs should be considered. An injection of local anesthetic and corticosteroid preparation into the plica can be both diagnostic and therapeutic. Based on the physical examination, an appropriate flexibility and strengthening program should be initiated. With persistent symptoms, and no other evidence of other intra-articular disorders, arthroscopic resection of the plica should be considered.

# Physical Therapy Prescription

Early rehabilitation should include rest, ice, compression, and elevation (RICE) of the affected knee. The home exercise program (see pp 555-556) should include range-of-motion exercises such as knee flexion and hamstring curls to reduce pain and prevent joint stiffness. In addition, atrophy of the quadriceps muscle can be prevented with early isometric exercises such as straight-leg raises.

If symptoms do not respond to the home program after 3 to 4 weeks, a more complex problem involving abnormal patellofemoral mechanics is usually present, and formal physical therapy should be ordered. The prescription should include an evaluation of foot mechanics, patellofemoral mobility, and strength of the hip and trunk muscles. After determining the extent of the muscle imbalances and mechanics, the physical therapist can develop a treatment plan.

Section 6 ■ Knee and Lower Leg

## ADVERSE OUTCOMES OF TREATMENT

NSAIDs may cause gastric, renal, or hepatic complications. Repeated intra-articular injections of corticosteroid may lead to accelerated destruction of articular cartilage and/or iatrogenic sepsis. Surgical resection may be ineffective or complicated by infection and stiffness.

## REFERRAL DECISIONS/RED FLAGS

Continued discomfort and symptoms of instability indicate the need for further evaluation.

# HOME EXERCISE PROGRAM FOR PLICA SYNDROME

Perform the exercises in the order listed. To prevent inflammation, apply a bag of crushed ice or frozen peas to the injured side of the knee for 20 minutes after completing the exercises. You should experience improved range of motion and less pain in your knee. If the pain does not change or becomes worse, call your doctor.

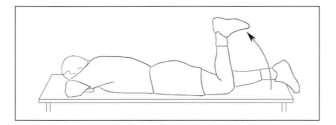

| Exercise Type | Muscle Group | Number of Repetitions/Sets | Number of Days per Week | Number of Weeks |
|---|---|---|---|---|
| Knee flexion | Hamstrings | 25 repetitions/3 sets, progressing to 45 repetitions/3 sets | 4 to 5 | 3 to 4 |
| Hamstring curls | Hamstrings | 25 to 45 repetitions/3 sets | 4 to 5 | 3 to 4 |
| Straight-leg raises | Quadriceps | Work up to 10 repetitions/3 sets | Daily | 3 to 4 |

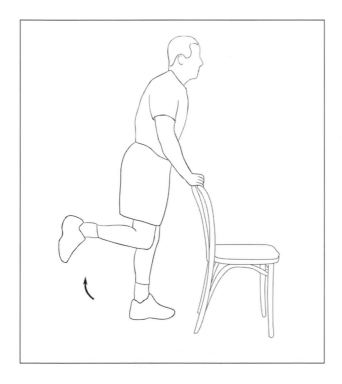

## Knee Flexion

Lie face down on a flat surface with your legs together. Slowly flex the affected knee (bend it up toward your buttocks) as far as possible without pain and then lower it. To add resistance, use rubber tubing while you do the exercise. Perform 3 sets of 25 repetitions, progressing gradually to 3 sets of 45 repetitions. Perform the exercise 4 to 5 days a week, continuing for 3 to 4 weeks.

## Hamstring Curls

Stand on a flat surface with your weight evenly distributed on both feet. Hold onto the back of a chair or the wall for balance. Bend the affected knee, raising the heel toward the ceiling as far as possible without pain. Hold this position for 5 seconds and then relax. Perform 3 sets of 25 repetitions, progressing gradually to 3 sets of 45 repetitions. Perform the exercise 4 to 5 days a week, continuing for 3 to 4 weeks. Seated version: Sit on a chair with your feet flat on the floor. Raise the affected knee off the chair and hold the position for 5 seconds.

SECTION 6 ■ KNEE AND LOWER LEG

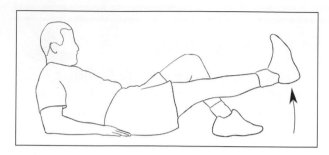

## Straight-Leg Raises

Lie on the floor, supporting your torso with your elbows as shown. Keep the affected leg straight and bend the other leg at the knee so that the foot is flat on the floor. Tighten the thigh muscle of the affected leg and slowly raise it 6 to 10 inches off the floor. Hold this position for 5 seconds and then relax. Work up to 3 sets of 10 repetitions daily, continuing for 3 to 4 weeks.

# POPLITEAL CYST

## SYNONYMS
Baker cyst
Synovial cyst

ICD-9 Code
**727.51**
Popliteal cyst

## DEFINITION
A popliteal cyst, commonly known as a Baker cyst, is the most common synovial cyst in the knee. It develops in the popliteal bursa located at the posteromedial aspect of the knee joint. This normally thin bursa communicates with the knee joint and becomes more prominent (cystic) when synovitis or trauma creates excessive joint fluid that then tracks into the popliteal bursa. Popliteal cysts are associated with degenerative meniscal tears and systemic inflammatory conditions such as rheumatoid arthritis.

## CLINICAL SYMPTOMS
Patients present with swelling or fullness in the popliteal fossa with accompanying pain or tenderness and no history of trauma. Mechanical complaints referable to the knee are common. Smaller cysts may be asymptomatic, but change in size is common. Larger cysts may dissect down the posterior calf and/or rupture, resulting in severe calf pain and decreased motion at the ankle. When they rupture, these cysts may cause severe calf pain and swelling and may be mistaken for a deep venous thrombosis. Ruptures of popliteal cysts usually occur in older patients with degenerative arthritis or rheumatoid arthritis.

## TESTS

### Physical Examination
Inspect the popliteal fossa and compare it with that of the opposite leg. Palpate the area to determine the size, consistency, and amount of tenderness. Cyst locations vary, but most are found to course between the semimembranosus muscle and the medial head of the gastrocnemius muscle. Examine the knee for signs of meniscal or other pathology. Effusion and accompanying mechanical signs indicate an intra-articular irritant causing the generation of excessive joint fluid. Examine the leg to determine whether the cyst has extravasated, causing swelling and tenderness in the calf.

Popliteal cysts are sometimes identified as an incidental finding on a symptomatic knee examination.

**SECTION 6 ■ KNEE AND LOWER LEG**

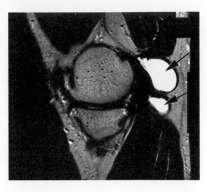

**Figure 1**

MRI scan showing a popliteal cyst. Areas of high signal intensity (arrows) on T2-weighted image indicate fluid, indicative of a cyst.

*Diagnostic Tests*

Radiographs of the knee are usually negative but may show the outline of the cyst or show calcification present in the cyst or within the knee. MRI usually is not necessary but can demonstrate the location and character of the cystic fluid, as well as determine the presence of intra-articular pathology (**Figure 1**).

Cyst aspiration should be approached with caution because of the proximity of neurovascular structures in the popliteal fossa. Furthermore, the cyst fluid may be gelatinous and not easily retrievable with a standard-bore needle.

# DIFFERENTIAL DIAGNOSIS

Deep venous thrombosis (evident on ultrasound or venogram)

Exertional compartment syndrome (evident on physical examination)

Inflammatory arthritis (positive serologic studies)

Medial gastrocnemius strain (evident on physical examination)

Soft-tissue tumor (evident on MRI)

Superficial phlebitis (superficial tenderness, negative ultrasound or venogram)

# ADVERSE OUTCOMES OF THE DISEASE

A cyst rupture may cause severe pain in the posterior calf that, with the swelling, may mimic a deep venous thrombosis. The mass of a cyst may cause compression of surrounding neurovascular structures with sensory or motor changes or venous occlusion.

# TREATMENT

Aspiration has been suggested, but this provides only transient relief because the cyst lining remains intact and the fluid often reaccumulates. Treatment should be directed at the cause of increased synovial fluid. When intra-articular lesions resulting in increased production of synovial fluid can be successfully treated (usually by arthroscopic excision of a torn medial meniscus), the cyst usually resolves spontaneously and excision is unnecessary. Cysts associated with severe arthritis typically resolve after knee replacement. Cyst excision may be required in some patients. Ruptured popliteal cysts are treated symptomatically with minor analgesics, rest, and elevation.

## ADVERSE OUTCOMES OF TREATMENT

Open excision carries the risk of injury to neighboring nerves and blood vessels; dissection should be performed with caution. Recurrence rate when excision is combined with resolution of any internal derangement is low (around 5%).

## REFERRAL DECISIONS/RED FLAGS

Night pain, weight loss, fever and/or chills, or other constitutional symptoms indicate the possibility of a neoplastic process and therefore the need for further evaluation.

SECTION 6 ■ KNEE AND LOWER LEG

# POSTERIOR CRUCIATE LIGAMENT TEAR

## SYNONYM
PCL sprain

## DEFINITION
The posterior cruciate ligament (PCL) is considered the strongest ligament in the knee and serves as the primary restraint to posterior translation of the tibia relative to the femur. Anatomically, it originates on the medial intercondylar wall of the femur and inserts on the posterior aspect of the tibia, running in an oblique direction. Injury to the PCL may be either a stretch injury or a complete rupture, is less common than injuries to the anterior cruciate ligament (ACL), and is often overlooked. Isolated PCL injuries occur less frequently than combined ligament injuries (PCL with ACL and/or collateral ligament injury).

## CLINICAL SYMPTOMS
Four injury patterns suggest the possibility of a PCL injury:

- a dashboard injury (that is, a posteriorly directed force to the anterior knee with the knee in flexion, as in a motor vehicle accident)
- a fall onto a flexed knee with the foot in plantar flexion, resulting in impact to the tibial tubercle; in comparison, the foot in dorsiflexion results in patellofemoral impact
- a pure hyperflexion injury to the knee
- a hyperextension injury to the knee. Typically, the ACL ruptures first; then, with sufficient force, injury to the PCL follows. This combination most commonly occurs in contact sports, secondary to a direct load on the anteromedial proximal tibia with the knee in extension. This mechanism of injury frequently results in a knee dislocation with or without spontaneous reduction.

An effusion commonly develops within the first 24 hours after injury, and range of motion usually is limited. Patients also may report pain and feelings of instability with weight bearing, especially with combined ligamentous injuries.

## TESTS

### Physical Examination
Examination typically reveals a significant effusion and decreased range of motion. Tenderness to palpation may not be exhibited. A thorough examination for knee stability is needed

because PCL injuries are often a component of a combined ligamentous injury. In the acute setting, the physical examination may be difficult because of loss of motion and muscle guarding, which may mask increases in translation. Therefore, reexamining the patient once swelling has decreased is often helpful.

The most sensitive test is the posterior drawer test (see Physical Examination—Knee and Lower Leg: Special Tests, p 483). Be aware, though, that if increased posterior translation of the tibia relative to the femur is present, it can be easily misinterpreted as a positive anterior drawer sign when the tibia is pulled back to the anterior position. This misinterpretation is further complicated by the frequent coexistence of an ACL tear. Observing the resting position of the tibial plateau relative to the femoral condyles helps to remove this uncertainty. With a PCL injury, the tibia will be in a posterior position relative to the femur because of gravity, and there will be no place to sit your thumbs on the anterior tibial plateaus (**Figure 1**).

In acute multiple ligament disruption, with or without spontaneous reduction, distal neurovascular status should be assessed because deficits can be seen.

## Diagnostic Tests

AP and lateral radiographs of the knee obtained in the acute setting can identify bony pathology, aid in diagnosis, and help in planning surgical management. MRI can be useful in confirming PCL tears, as well as any concomitant injuries to ligaments, menisci, and articular cartilage.

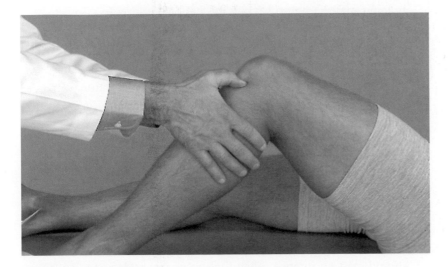

**Figure 1**
The examiner's thumb palpates the position of the tibial plateau relative to the femoral condyles. With a normal PCL, the tibial plateau will lie 1 cm anterior to the femoral condyles.

## DIFFERENTIAL DIAGNOSIS

ACL tear (positive Lachman test, positive pivot shift test)

Articular cartilage injury (pain on palpation, evident on radiographs or MRI)

Combined ligament injury (laxity in multiple directions, evident on MRI)

Medial or lateral collateral ligament tear (pain on palpation and varus/valgus laxity)

Meniscal tear (joint line tenderness)

Patellar or quadriceps tendon rupture (inability to achieve straight-leg raise)

Patellofemoral dislocation (apprehension with lateral patellar displacement)

Tibial plateau fracture (evident on radiographs)

## ADVERSE OUTCOMES OF THE DISEASE

Limb-threatening vascular injury may be present if a dislocated knee with spontaneous reduction has not been recognized and fully evaluated. Recurrent instability, subsequent meniscal tears, and osteoarthritis of the knee are all possible.

## TREATMENT

Isolated PCL injuries typically are treated with a structured program that initially concentrates on resolving swelling and restoring range of motion. Once these goals have been achieved, progression to strengthening exercises may be initiated, with an emphasis on the quadriceps (short-arc terminal extension exercises from 30° of flexion to 0°). Functional bracing may be helpful when the patient returns to contact sports.

Failure of nonsurgical treatment typically manifests as recurrent instability and/or subsequent meniscal tears. These patients require PCL reconstruction to restore functional stability. After reconstructive procedures, instability is improved but increased translation relative to the normal side may remain.

Patients with injuries to the PCL and other ligaments, with or without knee dislocation, usually require surgical reconstruction.

## PHYSICAL THERAPY PRESCRIPTION

A patient with a PCL injury who is not a candidate for surgery should start an intense rehabilitation program designed to improve range of motion and muscle strength of the quadriceps and hamstrings, including neuromuscular training and hip and trunk strengthening. Early rehabilitation should include rest, ice, compression, and elevation (RICE). After the initial healing stage of 1 to 5 days, range-of-motion exercises and quadriceps muscle strengthening should be begun (see pp 564-565). The patient should avoid activities that involve a high knee flexion angle until the hamstrings and quadriceps muscles become stronger. Wall slides are a safe exercise to promote an increase in mobility. Straight-leg raises, both prone and supine, are helpful in the prevention of quadriceps atrophy. The physical therapy prescription should include an evaluation of quadriceps, hip, and trunk muscle strength.

## ADVERSE OUTCOMES OF TREATMENT

Osteoarthritic changes involving the medial and patellofemoral compartments are well-documented sequelae to both nonsurgical and surgical management. Surgical reconstruction may be complicated by infection, graft failure, and recurrent instability.

## REFERRAL DECISIONS/RED FLAGS

Neurovascular compromise or deficits indicate the possibility of a knee dislocation. Any patient with a PCL injury and the possibility of damage to other ligamentous structures requires specialty evaluation.

SECTION 6 ■ KNEE AND LOWER LEG

# HOME EXERCISE PROGRAM FOR PCL INJURY

Perform the exercises in the order listed. Apply a bag of crushed ice or frozen peas to the back of the knee for 20 minutes after completing all the exercises to prevent inflammation. If pain does not improve or worsens or if the knee joint becomes inflamed, call your doctor.

| Exercise Type | Muscle Group | Number of Repetitions/Sets | Number of Days per Week | Number of Weeks |
|---|---|---|---|---|
| Wall slides | Hamstrings/ quadriceps | 25 repetitions/3 sets, progressing to 45 repetitions/3 sets | 6 to 7 | 3 to 4 |
| Straight-leg raises | Quadriceps | 10 repetitions/3 sets | 6 to 7 | 3 to 4 |
| Straight-leg raises (prone) | Quadriceps | 10 repetitions/3 sets | 6 to 7 | 3 to 4 |

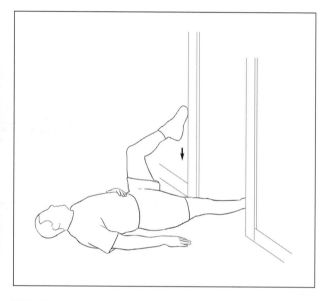

## Wall Slides

Lie on your back with the uninjured leg extending through a doorway and the injured leg resting against the wall. Let the leg gently slide down the wall to a position of maximum flexion. Hold this position for 5 seconds and then slowly straighten the leg. Begin with 3 sets of 25 repetitions, progressing to 3 sets of 45 repetitions. Perform the exercise 6 to 7 days a week, continuing for 3 to 4 weeks.

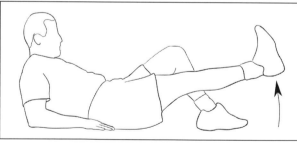

## Straight-Leg Raises

Lie on the floor, supporting your torso with your elbows as shown. Keep the injured leg straight and bend the other leg at the knee so that the foot is flat on the floor. Tighten the thigh muscle of the injured leg and slowly raise it 6 to 10 inches off the floor. Hold this position for 5 seconds and then relax. Perform 3 sets of 10 repetitions 6 to 7 days a week, continuing for 3 to 4 weeks.

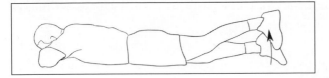

## Straight-Leg Raises (Prone)

Lie on the floor on your stomach with your legs straight. Tighten the hamstrings of the injured leg and raise the leg toward the ceiling as far as you can. Hold the position for 5 seconds. Lower the leg and rest it for 2 seconds. Perform 3 sets of 10 repetitions 6 to 7 days a week, continuing for 3 to 4 weeks.

**SECTION 6 ■ KNEE AND LOWER LEG**

# SHIN-SPLINTS

## DEFINITION

Shin-splints are a poorly understood condition characterized by the gradual onset of pain in the posteromedial aspect of the distal third of the leg. This condition commonly develops in response to exercise and probably represents inflammation of the tibial periosteum secondary to repetitive muscle contraction.

## CLINICAL SYMPTOMS

Shin-splints are generally associated with prolonged walking or running activity. Symptoms develop gradually with exercise, such as running on hard surfaces, early-season hill training, or with increased training intensity, pace, or distance. Pain is localized to the distal third of the medial tibia, the site of the origin of the posterior tibial muscle, and the patient may demonstrate pes planus associated with overpronation.

## TESTS

### Physical Examination
Examination reveals tenderness along the posterior medial crest of the tibia in the middle or distal third of the leg.

### Diagnostic Tests
AP and lateral radiographs should be obtained to identify any stress fractures present.

## DIFFERENTIAL DIAGNOSIS

Exertional compartment syndrome (no symptoms at rest)
Stress fracture (radiographic findings)

## ADVERSE OUTCOMES OF THE DISEASE

No adverse outcomes of shin-splints are known, except continued pain and inability to walk or run.

## TREATMENT

Mild shin-splints may be relieved by limiting activity to soft surfaces, decreasing training, and avoiding hills. NSAIDs, ice massage, and analgesic creams may also be helpful. Further measures include cushioned antipronation inserts, local ultrasound with phonophoresis, foot and ankle range-of-motion and strengthening exercises, and a calf sleeve. Moderate shin-splints may require replacing running with nonprovocative exercise, and severe shin-splints may respond only to restricting all but non–weight-bearing sports.

## ADVERSE OUTCOMES OF TREATMENT

NSAIDs may lead to concomitant gastric, renal, or hepatic complications.

## REFERRAL DECISIONS/RED FLAGS

Conditions such as stress fractures and exertional compartment syndromes must be ruled out before a diagnosis of shin-splints is made.

SECTION 6 ■ KNEE AND LOWER LEG

# STRESS FRACTURE

## SYNONYM
Dreaded black line

## DEFINITION
A stress fracture is a hairline or microscopic break in a bone caused by nontraumatic, cumulative overload on bone. Several factors, including overtraining, incorrect biomechanics, fatigue, hormonal imbalance, poor nutrition, and osteoporosis, have been implicated as contributing causes.

## CLINICAL SYMPTOMS
Stress fractures of the tibia and fibula typically follow a relatively rapid increase in exercise intensity. The pain initially occurs only in association with exercise, but with continued activity, the pain also is noted with normal walking or even at rest or at night. Patients usually describe an extremely painful focal area of the tibia.

## TESTS

### Physical Examination
Tenderness is localized to the affected area of bone. Impact as well as varus, valgus, anterior, and posterior stress on the bone may cause pain. In bones that lie deep within muscle and cannot be easily palpated (eg, femoral neck), eliciting pain with stress placed across the area of injured bone is a critical part of the examination. Six or more weeks after the onset of symptoms, swelling secondary to the bony callus may be palpable.

### Diagnostic Tests
AP and lateral radiographs of the tibia should be obtained; however, stress fractures may not be visible on plain radiographs for 3 weeks or longer after injury. When the pain is not severe, the patient is not involved in an occupation or athletic activity that puts him or her at risk for further injury, and the patient can keep his or her activity level below the pain threshhold, radiographs may be repeated 3 to 4 weeks after initial examination. When immediate confirmation of the suspected diagnosis is necessary, however, a bone scan will show increased uptake at the location of the stress fracture

(**Figure 1**). Alternatively, MRI can confirm the diagnosis. Correlating these findings with the area of pain and tenderness is important because bone scans of athletes who place repetitive stresses on the legs often show areas of increased uptake in asymptomatic locations.

## DIFFERENTIAL DIAGNOSIS

Exertional compartment syndrome (no radiographic findings)

Shin-splints (no radiographic findings)

## ADVERSE OUTCOMES OF THE DISEASE

In most situations, the pain of a stress fracture limits participation in competitive or recreational activities and thus prevents further injury. Some patients continue activity, however, causing a displaced fracture. Prolonged healing time is a more likely outcome of delaying diagnosis of a painful stress fracture.

## TREATMENT

When diagnosed early, most stress fractures of the tibia and fibula respond well to a period of rest. Mild pain may respond to activity modifications. Long leg pneumatic splints or other removable fracture braces may be useful early in the healing process for patients with moderate pain. When significant pain occurs with walking, initial treatment is cast immobilization and limited weight bearing. Low-impact exercise, such as bicycling

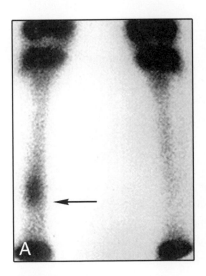 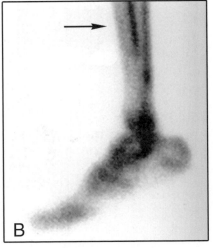

**Figure 1**

Bone scans. **A,** Stress fracture with focal uptake. **B,** Medial tibial stress syndrome with more diffuse uptake along the posteromedial shaft of the tibia.

Reproduced from Sullivan JA, Anderson SJ (eds): *Care of the Young Athlete*. Rosemont, IL, American Academy of Orthopaedic Surgeons, 1999, p 408.

and swimming, may be substituted to maintain cardiovascular conditioning. Return to activity depends on the severity and duration of symptoms before diagnosis, but averages about 2 months.

## ADVERSE OUTCOMES OF TREATMENT

NSAIDs may lead to concomitant gastric, renal, or hepatic complications.

## REFERRAL DECISIONS/RED FLAGS

Patients whose symptoms do not significantly improve after 2 to 3 weeks of rest require further evaluation. Menstrual cycle frequency and calcium intake should be discussed with women. An unusual and difficult stress injury to diagnose is a fatigue fracture of the anterior cortex of the midshaft of the tibia, referred to as the "dreaded black line" because of its radiographic appearance. Treatment of this injury is controversial and ranges from cast immobilization with no weight bearing to intramedullary rod insertion.

SECTION 6 ■ KNEE AND LOWER LEG

# PROCEDURE

## KNEE JOINT ASPIRATION/INJECTION

Aspiration of the knee joint can serve both diagnostic and therapeutic purposes. Traumatic injuries such as single- or multiple-ligament injuries, chondral or osteochondral injuries, or other fractures may produce large effusions around the knee. Pain can be relieved by draining a tense hemarthrosis. Aspiration also can help identify the etiology of an effusion. Gram stain, culture, and crystal analysis help differentiate infectious from inflammatory processes. With an injury, fat droplets from the bone marrow will accumulate on the surface of bloody aspirate placed in a small cup if an intra-articular fracture (distal femur, patella, or tibial plateau) is present.

Injection into the knee joint is the method commonly used to administer corticosteroids or other medications to an inflamed joint. Patients with an arthritic condition of the knee may obtain improvement of symptoms for significant periods with the appropriate administration of a corticosteroid or viscosupplement preparation (hyaluronic acid).

### STEP 1

Wear protective gloves at all times during this procedure and use sterile technique.

### STEP 2

Have the patient lie supine on the examining table with the abdominal and lower extremity muscles as relaxed as possible and the knee extended.

### STEP 3

Mentally, or with a marking pen, outline the landmarks for entry into the joint. Understand that the knee joint will extend almost one hand-width above the superior aspect of the patella, especially when a joint effusion is present. Typical entry will occur from the lateral aspect of the knee 1 cm superior and 1 cm lateral to the superolateral aspect of the patella (**Figure 1**).

### STEP 4

Prepare the skin with a bactericidal solution.

### STEP 5

Use the 25-gauge needle to infiltrate the skin with 3 to 5 mL of local anesthetic at the point of entry.

### CPT code

**20610**
Arthrocentesis, aspiration and/or injection; major joint or bursa (eg, shoulder, hip, knee joint, subacromial bursa)

*Current Procedural Terminology* © 2004 American Medical Association. All Rights Reserved.

### MATERIALS

Sterile gloves

Bactericidal skin preparation solution

25-gauge needle

30-mL or 60-mL syringe with an 18-gauge, 1½″ needle

5 mL of a local anesthetic

Corticosteroid or viscosupplement preparation (optional)

Adhesive dressing

SECTION 6 ■ KNEE AND LOWER LEG

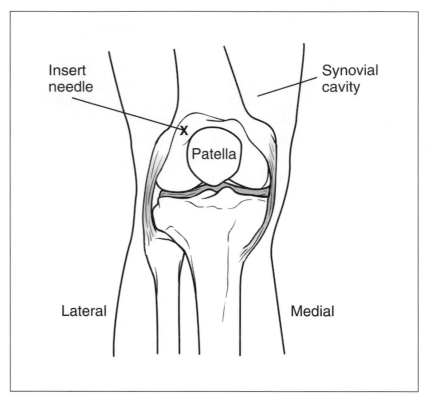

**Figure 1**
Location for needle insertion for knee joint aspiration.

## STEP 6

Using an 18-gauge, 1½″ needle attached to a 30-mL or 60-mL syringe, enter the knee joint at the anesthetized site. Penetration of the joint capsule will be felt as a give or "pop." Withdraw the plunger of the syringe to aspirate the fluid; in a large effusion, the flow should be easy. If establishing flow is difficult, try changing the path of the needle slightly; the needle might be within a fat pad or thick synovium. Manual pressure can be applied to the suprapatellar region to milk more fluid out of the knee. As fluid is withdrawn, the needle may become blocked with synovium; again, a slight change in direction, with the application of forward pressure to the plunger, will usually free the needle tip and allow flow to continue.

## STEP 7

Once the aspiration is complete, inject medication or local anesthetic into the joint if indicated. The aspirating syringe may be removed from the needle while maintaining the needle within the knee, and a syringe with the solution to be injected can be attached.

## STEP 8

When the aspiration and/or injection is complete, apply a sterile dressing.

## ADVERSE OUTCOMES

As with any invasive procedure, extreme care should be taken to use sterile technique. Infection, although not common, may be introduced into the knee. Be sure that the needle's path to the knee joint does not pass through any area of the skin that appears to be compromised or potentially colonized.

## AFTERCARE/PATIENT INSTRUCTIONS

After removal of a large effusion, apply a compressive wrap to minimize reaccumulation of fluid. In addition, rest and elevation of the lower extremity are recommended. Instruct the patient to notify you immediately at any sign of infection, rapid reaccumulation of fluid, or severe pain.

SECTION 6 ■ KNEE AND LOWER LEG

# PAIN DIAGRAM—FOOT AND ANKLE

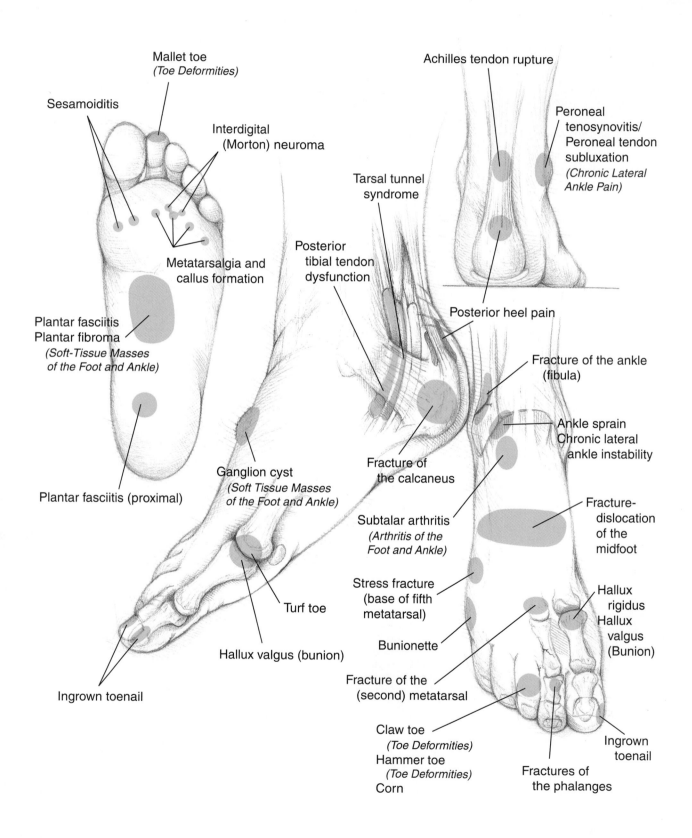

Mallet toe
*(Toe Deformities)*

Sesamoiditis

Interdigital
(Morton) neuroma

Metatarsalgia and
callus formation

Plantar fasciitis
Plantar fibroma
*(Soft-Tissue Masses
of the Foot and Ankle)*

Plantar fasciitis (proximal)

Ganglion cyst
*(Soft Tissue Masses
of the Foot and Ankle)*

Ingrown toenail

Turf toe

Hallux valgus (bunion)

Achilles tendon rupture

Peroneal
tenosynovitis/
Peroneal tendon
subluxation
*(Chronic Lateral
Ankle Pain)*

Tarsal tunnel
syndrome

Posterior
tibial tendon
dysfunction

Posterior heel pain

Fracture of the ankle
(fibula)

Ankle sprain
Chronic lateral
ankle instability

Fracture-
dislocation
of the
midfoot

Hallux
rigidus
Hallux
valgus
(Bunion)

Ingrown
toenail

Fracture of
the calcaneus

Subtalar arthritis
*(Arthritis of the
Foot and Ankle)*

Stress fracture
(base of fifth
metatarsal)

Bunionette

Fracture of the
(second) metatarsal

Claw toe
*(Toe Deformities)*
Hammer toe
*(Toe Deformities)*
Corn

Fractures of
the phalanges

# FOOT AND ANKLE

**Section Editor**
Carol Frey, MD
Clinical Assistant Professor of Orthopaedic Surgery
University of California, Los Angeles
Fellowship Director, West Coast Sports Medicine Fellowship
Manhattan Beach, California

Robert Donatelli, PhD, PT, OCS
National Director of Sports Rehabilitation
Physiotherapy Associates
Las Vegas, Nevada

# Bones of the ankle and foot

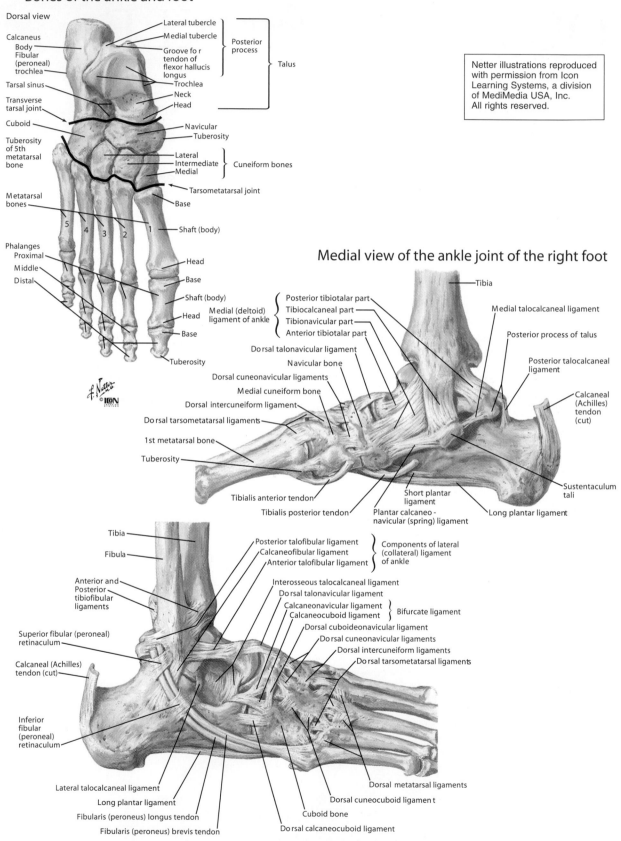

Dorsal view

Lateral tubercle
Medial tubercle
Posterior process

Calcaneus
Body
Fibular (peroneal) trochlea
Groove for tendon of flexor hallucis longus
Trochlea
Neck
Head
Talus

Tarsal sinus
Transverse tarsal joint
Cuboid
Navicular
Tuberosity

Tuberosity of 5th metatarsal bone
Lateral
Intermediate
Medial
Cuneiform bones

Tarsometatarsal joint
Base

Metatarsal bones
5 4 3 2 1
Shaft (body)

Phalanges
Proximal
Middle
Distal

Head
Base
Shaft (body)
Head
Base
Tuberosity

## Medial view of the ankle joint of the right foot

Tibia
Medial talocalcaneal ligament
Posterior process of talus
Posterior talocalcaneal ligament
Calcaneal (Achilles) tendon (cut)

Posterior tibiotalar part
Tibiocalcaneal part
Tibionavicular part
Anterior tibiotalar part
Medial (deltoid) ligament of ankle

Dorsal talonavicular ligament
Navicular bone
Dorsal cuneonavicular ligaments
Medial cuneiform bone
Dorsal intercuneiform ligament
Dorsal tarsometatarsal ligaments
1st metatarsal bone
Tuberosity

Tibialis anterior tendon
Tibialis posterior tendon
Short plantar ligament
Plantar calcaneo-navicular (spring) ligament
Long plantar ligament
Sustentaculum tali

## Lateral view of the ankle joint of the right foot

Tibia
Fibula

Anterior and Posterior tibiofibular ligaments

Superior fibular (peroneal) retinaculum
Calcaneal (Achilles) tendon (cut)
Inferior fibular (peroneal) retinaculum

Posterior talofibular ligament
Calcaneofibular ligament
Anterior talofibular ligament
Components of lateral (collateral) ligament of ankle

Interosseous talocalcaneal ligament
Dorsal talonavicular ligament
Calcaneonavicular ligament
Calcaneocuboid ligament
Bifurcate ligament
Dorsal cuboideonavicular ligament
Dorsal cuneonavicular ligaments
Dorsal intercuneiform ligaments
Dorsal tarsometatarsal ligaments

Lateral talocalcaneal ligament
Long plantar ligament
Fibularis (peroneus) longus tendon
Fibularis (peroneus) brevis tendon
Cuboid bone
Dorsal calcaneocuboid ligament
Dorsal cuneocuboid ligament
Dorsal metatarsal ligaments

# FOOT AND ANKLE—OVERVIEW

During standing and gait, the foot provides support, shock absorption, adaptation to uneven surfaces, balance, power, and direction. During more complex motions such as running and jumping, the functions provided by the foot and ankle increase. Therefore, it is not surprising that more than 20% of musculoskeletal problems affect the foot and ankle. Most of these disorders can be treated in the office setting.

The key to the successful diagnosis of foot and ankle pathology is to find the exact location of the problem. This requires an understanding of the anatomy of the foot and ankle. Furthermore, certain systemic illnesses such as diabetes mellitus, peripheral vascular disease, neuropathy, and inflammatory arthritis may affect the foot and therefore should be evaluated in the medical history. A history of bilateral foot pain should prompt a search for a possible systemic or spinal etiology.

Most patients with foot problems report pain. Chronic pain (more than 2 weeks' duration) is more common than acute pain. A fracture, sprain, or infection should be suspected if the patient presents with acute pain. Always consider a stress fracture when a patient reports recent onset of pain over the metatarsals, especially in the distal aspects of the second or third metatarsals.

Foot problems may result from trauma, congenital abnormalities, overuse, systemic illness, or ill-fitting shoes. The standard radiographic views of the foot for all these problems are the AP, lateral, and 45° oblique views.

## FOREFOOT PROBLEMS

Forefoot problems occur nine times more often in women than in men, a fact that is directly attributable to women's wearing high-heeled and ill-fitting shoes. Shoe modification (lower heels, wider shoes) is always the first line of treatment. Bunions, hammer toes, claw toes, ingrown toenails, metatarsalgia, and interdigital neuromas account for most instances of forefoot pain. These problems are detailed in subsequent chapters.

Other common problems in the forefoot are hallux rigidus (arthritis of the metatarsophalangeal [MTP] joint of the great toe) and stress fractures. Limited extension (dorsiflexion) of the great toe is consistent with hallux rigidus. Pain and tenderness directly over the second or third metatarsals suggest a stress fracture. Synovitis of the lesser MTP joints is common in patients with hallux valgus (caused by pressure from the great toe against the second MTP joint) and inflammatory disorders. Synovitis of the MTP joint causes pain over the affected joint and is often confused with the pain of an interdigital neuroma (pain in the web space).

# MIDFOOT PROBLEMS

Chronic dorsal pain at the midfoot most commonly occurs secondary to degenerative arthritis involving one or more of the midfoot joints. Patients are often able to pinpoint the exact location of the pain. A bony prominence, or osteophyte, referred to as dorsal bossing, can be palpated and corresponds to the underlying arthritic joint. Pain on the plantar aspect of the midfoot is unusual and occurs with plantar fasciitis or plantar fibromas.

# HINDFOOT PROBLEMS

Plantar heel pain secondary to plantar fasciitis is the most common problem in the hindfoot. The pain associated with this condition is often severe with the first few steps taken in the morning; patients normally are pain free during rest. Patients have focal tenderness directly over the plantar medial heel (the origin of the plantar fascia); often, on examination, considerable pressure must be applied in this area to duplicate the patient's symptoms.

Posterior heel pain may be related to irritation from shoes and associated with a prominent superior process of the calcaneus (Haglund deformity) and/or pathology in the Achilles tendon at its insertion. Often an associated superficial bursitis of the posterior heel is present. When evaluating a patient with posterior heel pain, make sure that the problem is not more proximal within the Achilles tendon; otherwise, a partial or even complete rupture of the tendon might be missed.

A commonly overlooked problem in the hindfoot is posterior tibial tendon dysfunction. This condition is characterized by pain and tenderness posterior and distal to the medial malleolus in the region of the posterior tibial tendon. Progressive dysfunction results in an acquired unilateral flatfoot that may be associated with pain on the lateral side of the ankle as the tip of the fibula abuts the collapsing foot.

# ANKLE PROBLEMS

More than 25,000 ankle sprains occur each day in the United States. Acute anterolateral ankle pain, swelling, and, frequently, ecchymosis are the hallmarks of this condition.

A history of the ankle "giving way" suggests a diagnosis of ankle instability. Patients with this history often report pain only when the ankle gives way and not at other times. On the other hand, patients with chronic ankle pain, which commonly occurs at the anterolateral aspect of the ankle, may have constant low-grade pain. Chronic pain and swelling on the posterolateral aspect of the ankle are consistent with injury to the peroneal tendons. An occult fracture (osteochondral lesion) of the ankle joint may present with diffuse ankle pain and an intra-articular effusion. Subtalar synovitis or arthritis also may present in a similar fashion.

Arthritis of the ankle is most often secondary to previous trauma. Rheumatoid arthritis may also affect the ankle. Tarsal tunnel syndrome may cause chronic medial ankle pain but almost always is associated with neurologic symptoms and pain that radiates into the plantar aspect of the foot.

# PHYSICAL EXAMINATION FOOT AND ANKLE

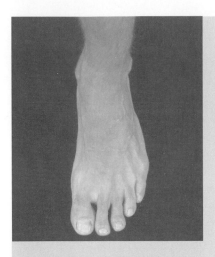

### Anterior view, standing

Inspect the foot and ankle from the front and look at the alignment of the great and lesser toes, the position of the foot in relation to the limb, and the medial curvature of the forefoot (metatarsus adductus).

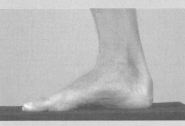

### Medial view

Inspect for a high arch (cavus foot), flatfoot posture (pes planus), or undue prominence of the medial midfoot (accessory navicular). The arches of both feet should be symmetric.

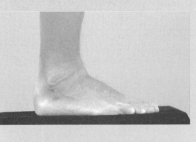

### Lateral view

Inspect for callosities, ankle swelling, or prominence of the posterior calcaneus.

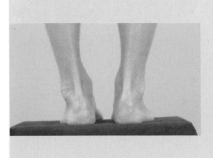

### Posterior view

Assess heel alignment. Normal alignment is neutral or slight valgus (turned-out heel), with no more than one or two lateral toes visible from behind. A patient with an acquired flatfoot from posterior tibial tendon dysfunction will have increased valgus of the calcaneus and more than two visible toes ("too many toes" sign). A varus calcaneus (turned-in heel) occurs with a cavus foot. An inflamed prominence of the posterior heel is called a "pump bump." The patient in the photograph has mild varus of the heel.

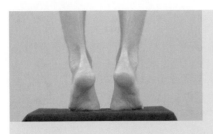

### Standing on toes

With the patient standing on the toes, look to see that the heels move into a normal varus position. A patient with an acquired flatfoot secondary to posterior tibial tendon dysfunction will not be able to rise up on the toes of the affected foot.

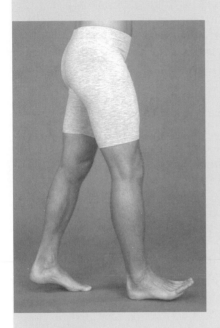

### Gait

Gait is best observed with the patient barefoot. Look for deviations from normal while the patient walks. Normal gait demonstrates equal stride length, foot position, and weight distribution. At heel strike the heel everts and the ankle plantar flexes. The weight transfers along the lateral side of the foot. Pronation occurs in the foot with dorsiflexion of the ankle and internal rotation at the leg, knee, and hip. As the body and leg move forward, supination begins with plantar flexion of the ankle.

Analyze alignment of the foot during the different phases of gait: heel strike, midstance, toe-off, swing phase. Look for obvious limp, lurch, dragging of the feet, intoeing, outtoeing, and drop-foot gait.

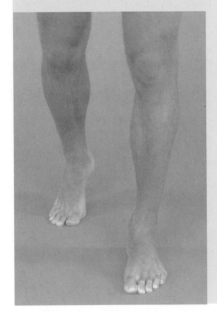

### Angle of gait

Assess the angle of gait, which is the angle of the foot in relation to the axis of the limb when the patient is walking, to identify problems of intoeing and outtoeing. When walking, the foot is normally positioned in 0° to 20° of external rotation. Because tibial torsion is typically asymmetric, one foot is normally positioned in more external rotation.

SECTION 7 ■ FOOT AND ANKLE

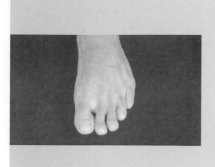

## Anterior view, supine

Inspect the top of the foot for a bunion and associated hallux valgus at the great toe metatarsophalangeal (MTP) joint or a bunionette at the fifth MTP joint. Inspect the lesser toes for abnormalities in alignment (eg, hammer toe, mallet toe, claw toe). Claw toe, in which the MTP joint is extended and the proximal interphalangeal (PIP) and distal interphalangeal (DIP) joints are flexed, commonly occurs in patients with diabetes mellitus, rheumatoid arthritis, Charcot-Marie-Tooth disease, or cavus foot deformities. Multiple toes tend to be involved, and often a corn (hard callus) is apparent over the PIP joint. A corn or callus develops where a deformity rubs against a shoe. Inspect the nails for poor techniques in trimming and signs of infection from an ingrown toenail.

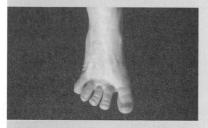

## Spread toes

Ask the patient to spread or fan the toes as widely as possible. Look for corns or ulcerations between the toes. Inability to actively spread the toes may indicate loss of intrinsic muscle function.

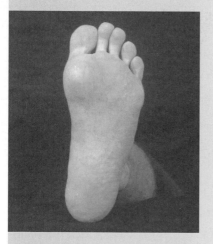

## Plantar surface

With the patient supine, inspect the bottom of the foot for plantar warts (which usually do not occur beneath the metatarsal head), a plantar callus (which occurs beneath the metatarsal head), prominence of the metatarsal heads, ulceration (especially in diabetic feet), or a thin fat pad.

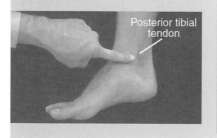

Posterior tibial tendon

## Medial malleolus

Palpate the area posterior and inferior to the medial malleolus in the region of the tibial nerve. In patients with tarsal tunnel syndrome, percussion over the nerve should reproduce symptoms, often described as "shooting" pains (paresthesias) in the heel and plantar aspect of the foot. Patients with posterior tibial tendon dysfunction will have swelling and tenderness along the course of the tendon in this region.

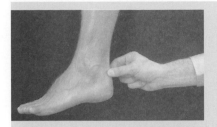

### *Posterior heel*

Palpate both sides of the Achilles tendon insertion to identify swelling or tenderness, which are signs of retrocalcaneal bursitis, a condition that is often associated with a prominence of the posterior superior calcaneus (pump bump or Haglund deformity). Swelling and tenderness of the Achilles tendon at its insertion is associated with tendinitis or calcific tendinosis.

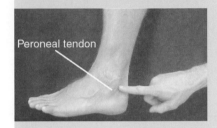

Peroneal tendon

### *Peroneal tendons*

Palpate behind and below the fibular malleolus for tenderness or swelling associated with peroneal tenosynovitis or for subluxation of the tendons during active dorsiflexion and plantar flexion of the ankle.

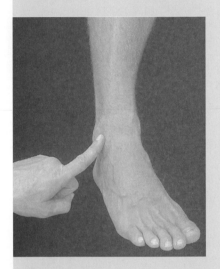

### *Anterior ankle*

Palpate over the anterior talofibular ligament and/or calcaneofibular ligament for tenderness associated with a sprain, often the result of an acute inversion injury. In patients with chronic ankle pain, palpate at the anterolateral corner of the ankle joint (soft junction of the tibia, fibula, and talus) for synovitis. Take care to differentiate pain in the anterolateral corner of the ankle from pain in the sinus tarsi, which may indicate inflammation or pathology of the subtalar joint.

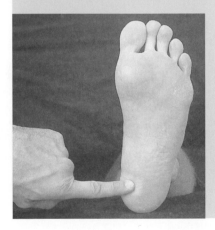

### *Plantar fascia*

Palpate the plantar fascia for tenderness or swelling. With plantar fasciitis, tenderness is noted with considerable pressure over the medial proximal aspect of the plantar fascia. Rupture of the plantar fascia is associated with tenderness and swelling in the middle third of the plantar fascia. Plantar fibromatosis causes swelling and thickening of the plantar fascia, typically beginning in the middle portion.

SECTION 7 ■ FOOT AND ANKLE

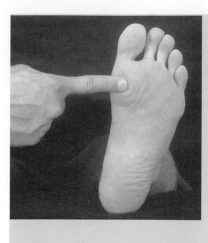

### Sesamoid

Palpate the area beneath the first metatarsal head for tenderness. If the sesamoids are the source of the pain, the tender spot will move as the toe is flexed and extended. The medial sesamoid is more commonly injured or inflamed than is the lateral sesamoid.

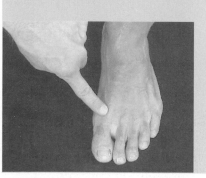

### MTP joint

Palpate the top of the foot for tenderness and swelling of the MTP joints, which may be present with rheumatoid arthritis, idiopathic synovitis, Freiberg infraction, or metatarsalgia. With hallux rigidus, dorsal osteophytes are present at the great toe MTP joint.

# RANGE OF MOTION

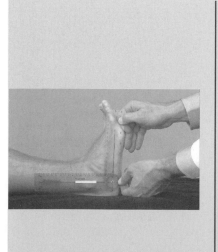

### Ankle motion: Zero Starting Position

Ankle dorsiflexion (ankle extension) is movement of the foot toward the anterior surface of the tibia, and ankle plantar flexion is movement of the foot in the opposite direction. Active ankle motion typically is greater than passive motion. Normal ankle dorsiflexion is 10° to 20°, and normal plantar flexion is 35° to 50°.

As the foot moves from dorsiflexion to plantar flexion, much of the motion occurs at the ankle joint, but other joints in the foot also contribute to this movement. Distinguishing the dorsiflexion/plantar flexion motion that occurs at the ankle joint from that at other joints is difficult; fortunately, it is not critical. From a functional standpoint, the total arc of motion is more important. Therefore, it is understood that clinical measurements of ankle motion also record motion of other joints of the foot.

The Zero Starting Position is with the foot perpendicular to the tibia. Align the goniometer with the axis of the leg and the lateral side of the plantar surface of the foot. To relax the gastrocnemius, measure ankle motion with the knee flexed. To assess heel cord tightness, measure ankle motion with the knee extended.

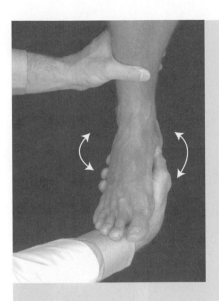

## Inversion and eversion

Inversion (turning the heel inward) and eversion (turning the heel outward) primarily reflect motion at the talocalcaneal (subtalar) joint. Precise measurements are difficult with standard techniques; therefore, in the clinical setting, these motions usually are estimated visually. The Zero Starting Position is with the ankle in slight dorsiflexion. This position limits lateral motion at the ankle joint and, therefore, provides better assessment of talocalcaneal mobility.

Restricted motion may be seen in patients following an acute ankle sprain and with subtalar arthritis, end-stage posterior tibial tendon dysfunction, or tarsal coalition (bony connection between talus and calcaneus).

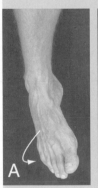
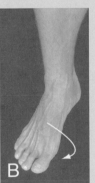

## Supination and pronation

Supination and pronation refer to rotation of the foot about an anterior/posterior axis.

Supination (**A**) includes inversion of the heel, as well as adduction and plantar flexion of the midfoot.

Pronation (**B**) is the opposite motion and includes eversion of the heel and abduction and dorsiflexion of the midfoot.

Supination and pronation of the foot are difficult to quantify. Compare motion of the affected foot with that on the unaffected side for the most useful information.

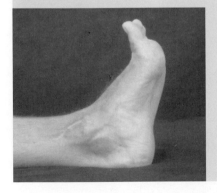

## Great toe: Zero Starting Position

Motion at the MTP and interphalangeal (IP) joints occurs in the dorsiflexion/plantar flexion plane. Dorsiflexion (extension) is the primary motion of the MTP joint, but this plane of motion is virtually nonexistent at the IP joint.

The Zero Starting Position for measuring motion at the MTP joint is the functional neutral position. This position aligns the great toe with the plantar surface of the foot. Reduced motion at the MTP joint may indicate hallux rigidus.

SECTION 7 ■ FOOT AND ANKLE

# MUSCLE TESTING

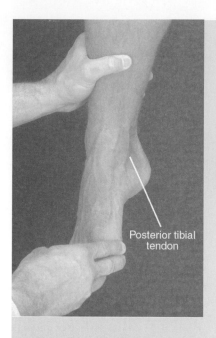

Posterior tibial
tendon

## Posterior tibialis

To test the strength of the posterior tibialis muscle or integrity of the posterior tibial tendon, stabilize the tibia and, with the foot in plantar flexion (to eliminate activity of the tibialis anterior), resist the patient's attempt to invert the foot. Weakness indicates injury or dysfunction of the posterior tibialis or a lesion involving the posterior tibial nerve or L5 nerve root.

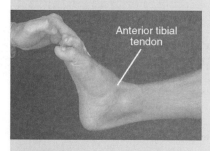

Anterior tibial
tendon

## Anterior tibialis

To test the strength of the anterior tibialis muscle, ask the patient to flex the toes (to eliminate activity of the toe extensors) and then invert and dorsiflex the foot against resistance. Weakness indicates a lesion involving the L4 nerve root or deep peroneal nerve.

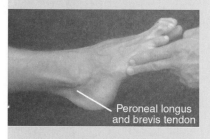

Peroneal longus
and brevis tendon

## Peroneus longus and brevis

To test the strength of the peroneus longus and brevis muscles, stabilize the tibia and position the foot in plantar flexion (to eliminate activity of the lateral toe extensors). Resist the patient's attempt to evert the foot. Weakness indicates injury or dysfunction of the peroneal tendons or a lesion involving the superficial peroneal nerve.

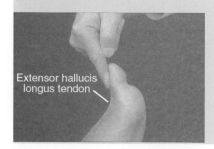

Extensor hallucis
longus tendon

## Extensor hallucis longus

With the ankle in neutral, ask the patient to extend the great toe against resistance. Weakness indicates deep peroneal nerve dysfunction with weakness of the extensor hallucis longus muscle. Note that the extensor hallucis muscle is the easiest and most specific muscle to assess for L5 nerve root dysfunction.

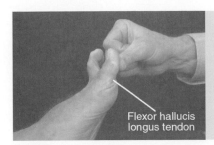

Flexor hallucis
longus tendon

### Flexor hallucis longus

With the ankle in neutral, ask the patient to flex the great toe against resistance. Weakness indicates tibial nerve dysfunction. The flexor hallucis muscle is the easiest and most specific muscle to assess for S1 nerve root dysfunction.

# SPECIAL TESTS

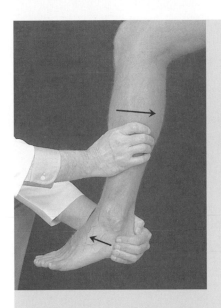

### Anterior drawer test

To test stability of the anterior talofibular ligament, place the ankle in approximately 20° of plantar flexion. Stabilize the tibia, grasp the hindfoot, and pull forward. Asymmetric or excessive motion will occur with chronic ankle laxity and severe acute ankle sprains. When performing this test, always compare the affected ankle with the opposite (normal) side. If this test elicits pain, the results may be unreliable.

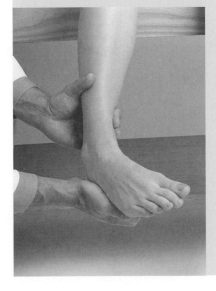

### Varus stress test

With the tibia stabilized and the ankle in neutral, grasp the calcaneus and invert the hindfoot. Excessive or asymmetric motion will occur with chronic laxity of the calcaneofibular ligament. When performing this test, always compare the affected ankle with the opposite (normal) side. If the patient has pain during this test, the results may be unreliable.

SECTION 7 ■ FOOT AND ANKLE

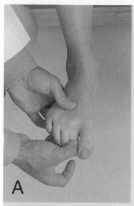
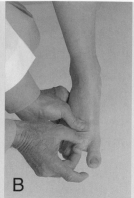

### MTP instability

With the patient sitting, stabilize the foot, then grasp the proximal phalanx of each toe and move the joint in a plantar (down) (**A**) and dorsal (up) (**B**) direction. Instability is often present after chronic synovitis or a long-standing claw toe deformity. In a patient with active synovitis, this test may be painful. The second toe is most often affected.

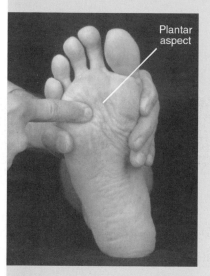

Plantar aspect

### Interdigital (Morton) neuroma test

Apply upward pressure between adjacent metatarsal heads, and then compress the metatarsals from side to side with the free hand. The upward pressure places the neuroma between the metatarsal heads, allowing it to be compressed during side-to-side compression. Interdigital neuromas are almost always located between either the second and third or the third and fourth metatarsal heads. The most common location is between the third and fourth metatarsal heads.

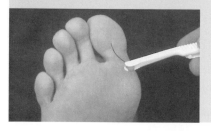

### Sensitivity test

Use a 0.10-g (5.07-mm) filament to identify protective sensation in a patient with diabetes mellitus.

SECTION 7  ■  FOOT AND ANKLE

# ACHILLES TENDON RUPTURE

## SYNONYMS
Heel cord rupture
Tendoachilles rupture

### ICD-9 Code
**845.09**
Sprains and strains of ankle and
foot; Achilles tendon

## DEFINITION
Disruption of the Achilles tendon (heel cord) usually occurs
5 to 7 cm proximal to the insertion of the tendon on the
calcaneus. This condition commonly affects middle-aged men
who play quick, stop-and-go sports such as tennis and
basketball.

## CLINICAL SYMPTOMS
The sudden, severe calf pain typically is described as a
"gunshot wound" or as a "direct hit from a racquet." The severe
acute pain may resolve quickly, and the injury may be
misdiagnosed as an ankle sprain. When the rupture is missed,
significant weakness develops, impairing ambulation.

## TESTS

### Physical Examination
Swelling in the lower calf is common. The patient often has
difficulty bearing weight and often has a palpable defect in the
tendon. With the patient lying prone and the foot hanging off
the edge of the table, the foot with a ruptured Achilles tendon
will rest at a 90° angle to the tibia, whereas a foot with an
intact Achilles tendon will rest in slight plantar flexion because
of the resting tension in the tendon. Perform the Thompson test
by placing the patient prone with the knee and ankle at 90°.
The test also can be done with the patient kneeling on a chair.
Squeezing the calf normally results in passive plantar flexion of
the ankle (**Figure 1**); a positive test is the absence of plantar
flexion. The Thompson test is most reliable within 48 hours of
the rupture.

### Diagnostic Tests
None usually are needed.

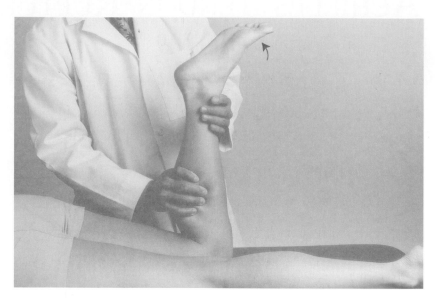

**Figure 1**

The Thompson test. With the patient kneeling on a chair or lying prone on the examining table, squeeze the calf. If the Achilles tendon is normal, this maneuver will result in passive plantar flexion of the ankle (arrow). If the Achilles tendon is torn, passive plantar flexion will be absent (positive Thompson test).

## DIFFERENTIAL DIAGNOSIS

Achilles tendinitis or tendinosis (thick, tender Achilles tendon or crepitus may be noted on palpation)

Deep vein thrombosis (no history of injury, negative Thompson test)

Medial gastrocnemius tear (pain on palpation over the medial head of the gastrocnmeius-soleus complex)

Plantaris rupture (pain but little loss of function)

Stress fracture of the tibia (constant pain over a localized area of the tibia)

## ADVERSE OUTCOMES OF THE DISEASE

Weakness during the stance phase of gait and decreased athletic function are possible. Patients note that when they are walking, they feel as if they are on soft sand.

## TREATMENT

Nonsurgical treatment consists of a graduated program of casting or bracing with the foot in plantar flexion. Surgical repair also requires cast immobilization, typically for 8 weeks, followed by 8 to 12 weeks with a tapered heel lift, for the Achilles tendon to heal. Physical therapy may be necessary if full range of motion and balance are not obtained by 6 months after surgery, but almost all patients obtain full range of motion, especially dorsiflexion, by this time. The decision whether to treat the patient surgically or nonsurgically is based on the degree of tendon retraction as well as the patient's level of activity, age, medical condition, and surgical risk. When either treatment is delayed beyond a few days, Achilles tendon rupture becomes more complicated to treat because retraction of the proximal muscle widens the gap. Whatever treatment modality is selected, a progressive strength and conditioning program is recommended during the rehabilitation phase, followed by a gradual return to sports.

## PHYSICAL THERAPY PRESCRIPTION

An Achilles tendon rupture can be very painful and debilitating. The type of rehabilitation depends on the extent of the tendon tear. For both severe and minor tears, pain-free immobilization, rest, ice, compression, and elevation (RICE) are indicated for the first 5 or 6 days postinjury. Use of crutches is also helpful to prevent further injury. The home exercise program (see p 592) may be begun on day 7. Minor tears usually do well with gentle active mobilization, such as obtained by using a stationary bicycle. The amount of dorsiflexion and stretch to the Achilles tendon can be controlled by adjusting the seat higher (farther from the pedals) or lower (closer to the pedals). The closer the seat is to the pedals, the greater amount of dorsiflexion and stretch to the Achilles tendon. Heel cord stretching may be initiated on day 14. The stretch should be pain free. If the patient has difficulty achieving pain-free ankle range of motion, formal physical therapy may be ordered. The prescription should include an evaluation of the mobility of the tendon, the ankle, and the subtalar and midtarsal joints. The therapist should be careful to respect the stage of soft-tissue healing.

## ADVERSE OUTCOMES OF TREATMENT

Surgical risks include infection and wound problems such as delayed healing. A second rupture may occur with either type of treatment but is more common after nonsurgical treatment.

## REFERRAL DECISIONS/RED FLAGS

A history of a sudden pop with pain and swelling in the calf indicates probable rupture of the Achilles tendon and the need for further evaluation within 24 hours.

SECTION 7 ■ FOOT AND ANKLE

# HOME EXERCISE PROGRAM FOR ACHILLES TENDON RUPTURE

Begin gentle movement of the ankle, such as by using a stationary bicycle, on day 7 after the injury. Add the heel cord stretch on day 14 after the injury. Before stretching, warm up the tissues by applying moist heat or riding a stationary bicycle for 10 minutes. To prevent inflammation, apply a bag of crushed ice or frozen peas to the heel for 20 minutes after exercising. You should not experience pain with the exercises. If you are unable to perform the exercise because of pain or stiffness or if your symptoms do not improve in 3 to 4 weeks, call your doctor.

| Exercise | Muscle Group | Number of Repetitions/Sets | Number of Days per Week | Number of Weeks |
| --- | --- | --- | --- | --- |
| Heel cord stretch | Gastrocnemius-soleus complex | 4 repetitions/2 or 3 sets | Daily | 3 to 4 |

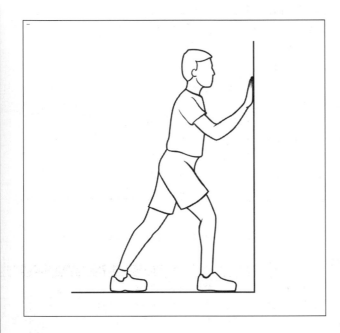

## Heel Cord Stretch

Stand facing a wall with the knee of the unaffected limb bent for support, the affected limb straight, and the toes pointed in slightly. Keeping the heels of both feet flat on the floor, lower your hips toward the wall. Hold the stretch for 30 seconds and then relax for 30 seconds. Repeat 4 times. Perform this exercise 2 or 3 times a day, 6 or 7 days a week.

# ANKLE SPRAIN

## SYNONYMS
Inversion injury
Lateral collateral ligament tear

**ICD-9 Code**
**845.00**
Sprains and strains of the ankle and foot

## DEFINITION
More than 25,000 ankle sprains occur every day. Ankle sprains are not always simple injuries. Residual symptoms occur in up to 40% of patients.

The lateral ligaments (anterior talofibular and calcaneofibular) are the only structures injured in most ankle sprains, but other ligament tears may occur with an inversion injury (**Figure 1**). Additional injury to the anterior tibiofibular syndesmosis, the thick ligaments connecting the distal tibia and fibula, also may occur. This combined injury, referred to as a "high" ankle sprain, increases recovery time. Injury to the subtalar joint is commonly associated with a severe ankle sprain. The most common injury to the subtalar joint after an inversion injury is a tear of one of the interosseous ligaments. Associated injuries to the medial deltoid ligament also occur but are less common.

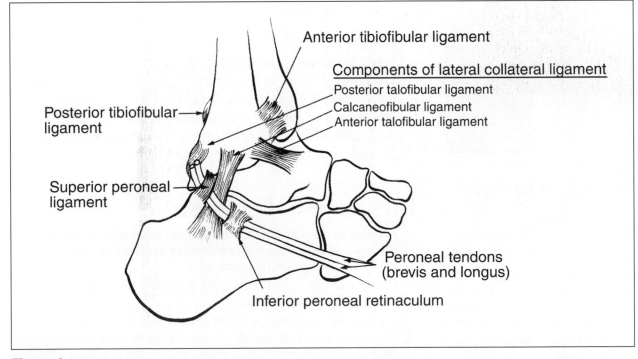

**Figure 1**
Ligaments of the ankle.

SECTION 7 ■ FOOT AND ANKLE

## CLINICAL SYMPTOMS

Pain over the injured ligaments, swelling, and loss of function are common. A severe sprain is more common in patients who report feeling a pop, followed by immediate swelling and the inability to walk. Determine whether the patient has a history of ankle sprains and giving way to identify whether an acute injury is superimposed on chronic ankle instability.

## TESTS

### Physical Examination

Examination often reveals ecchymosis and swelling around the entire ankle joint, not just the lateral side. Tenderness on palpation over the anterior talofibular and calcaneofibular ligaments can help identify which ligaments are injured. Palpate the lateral and medial malleoli and the base of the fifth metatarsal; crepitus or tenderness suggests a fracture.

Injury to the tibiofibular syndesmosis is suggested by two tests: the squeeze test (**Figure 2**) and the external rotation test. The squeeze test is performed by compressing the tibia and fibula at midcalf. The external rotation test is performed by placing the ankle in dorsiflexion and then externally rotating the foot. A positive result is the presence of pain over the distal tibiofibular syndesmosis.

After an injury to the subtalar joint there is tenderness over the sinus tarsi and there may be ecchymosis on the medial aspect of the heel.

### Diagnostic Tests

When tenderness is present over the distal fibula, ankle joint, tibiofibular syndesmosis, or other bony structure, radiographs of the ankle and/or foot are needed to rule out a fracture or syndesmosis disruption. Radiographs also are indicated when the patient has marked swelling and cannot bear weight on the affected extremity.

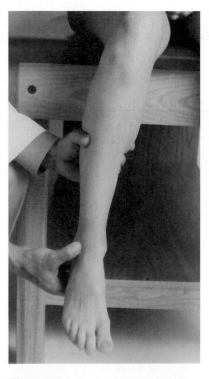

**Figure 2**

The squeeze test for injury to the tibiofibular syndesmosis. Pain over the distal tibiofibular syndesmosis when the examiner squeezes the tibia and fibula at midcalf is a positive result.

## DIFFERENTIAL DIAGNOSIS

Fracture of the calcaneus, talus, lateral malleolus, or base of the fifth metatarsal (focal tenderness over the fractured anatomic structure, evident on radiographs)

Fracture of the lateral process of the talus (focal tenderness, swelling below the fibula)

Fracture of the proximal fibula (Maisonneuve fracture associated with tear of deltoid and disruption of syndesmotic ligament) (focal tenderness, crepitus over the proximal fibula)

Osteochondral fracture of the talar dome (evident on ankle radiographs, bone scan, or MRI)

Peroneal tendon tear or subluxation (retrofibular tenderness and swelling)

## ADVERSE OUTCOMES OF THE DISEASE

An untreated severe sprain may result in chronic pain, instability, and the possibility of ankle arthritis. Chronic pain may result from subtalar stiffness. Chronic instability is most common after incomplete rehabilitation.

## TREATMENT

The goal of treatment is to prevent chronic pain and instability. Phase 1 consists of NSAIDs, ice, compression, and elevation. The use of a brace or air stirrup is indicated for protection and to promote soft-tissue healing (**Figure 3**). Encourage weight bearing as tolerated, with the use of crutches as needed. For severe sprains or sprains in children, the use of a cast or cast boot for 2 to 3 weeks may facilitate walking and healing.

Phase 2 begins when the patient can bear weight without increased pain or swelling, usually 2 to 4 weeks after the injury. Continue use of the air stirrup or brace. Begin exercises to increase peroneal and dorsiflexor strength; also, the Achilles tendon should be stretched. Continue this phase until the patient has full range of motion and 80% of normal ankle strength. Plantar flexion exercises are not included in the exercise program because they place the ankle in a position of minimal stability.

Phase 3 usually begins 4 to 6 weeks after injury. This phase of functional conditioning includes proprioception, agility, and endurance training. Exercises that are helpful for proprioception include standing on the sprained ankle with the opposite foot elevated and the eyes closed. Balance boards are very useful during this phase of treatment. Running in progressively smaller figures-of-8 is excellent for agility and peroneal strength. During this time, the patient should be weaned from the air stirrup or ankle brace.

This three-phase treatment program may take only 2 weeks to complete for minor sprains or up to 6 to 8 weeks for severe injuries. For athletes with moderate to severe sprains who are returning to sports, the use of a functional brace or air stirrup, or taping on a long-term basis, will help prevent recurrent injury. The use of a brace is particularly indicated for athletes in sports associated with a high risk for ankle sprains, such as basketball, volleyball, and soccer. Long-term exercises should include peroneal strengthening in both dorsiflexion and plantar flexion, as well as continued Achilles tendon stretching.

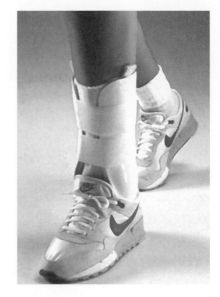

**Figure 3**
An air stirrup–type ankle brace.

SECTION 7 ■ FOOT AND ANKLE

## PHYSICAL THERAPY PRESCRIPTION

The most important part of early rehabilitation is to control the inflammation with rest, ice, compression, and elevation (RICE) for the first 5 or 6 days postinjury. Use of crutches during this same period can be helpful to control further damage to the healing ligament. Early mobilization of the ankle can begin as part of a home program of active pain-free exercises beginning on day 7 (see p 597). If the patient continues to have pain and limited mobility of the ankle after 2 to 3 weeks on a home exercise program, formal physical therapy may be ordered. The prescription should include an evaluation by the therapist to determine the mobility of the ankle and subtalar joints. Strengthening exercises combined with balance training may be initiated at the therapist's discretion.

## ADVERSE OUTCOMES OF TREATMENT

Casting and ankle immobilization for more than 3 weeks may cause stiffness and a slower return to normal activity. Incomplete rehabilitation is the most common cause of chronic instability after an ankle sprain. Subtalar stiffness may result in persistent anterolateral pain.

## REFERRAL DECISIONS/RED FLAGS

Fractures of the foot and ankle, tears or subluxation of the peroneal tendons, nerve injury, a history of repeated giving way (chronic instability), and failure to improve in 6 weeks with appropriate treatment all indicate serious injury and the need for further evaluation.

# HOME EXERCISE PROGRAM FOR ANKLE SPRAIN

To prevent inflammation, apply a bag of crushed ice or frozen peas to the ankle for 20 minutes after performing the exercises. You should not experience pain with the exercise. If you continue to experience pain or limited mobility of the ankle after performing the exercises for 2 to 3 weeks, call your doctor.

| Exercise | Muscle Group | Number of Repetitions/Sets | Number of Days per Week | Number of Weeks |
|---|---|---|---|---|
| Ankle curls | Anterior tibialis Gastrocnemius-soleus complex | 25 repetitions/3 sets, progressing to 45 repetitions/3 sets | Daily | 2 to 3 |
| Ankle eversion/inversion | Posterior tibialis Peroneus longus and peroneus brevis | 25 repetitions/3 sets, progressing to 45 repetitions/3 sets | Daily | 2 to 3 |

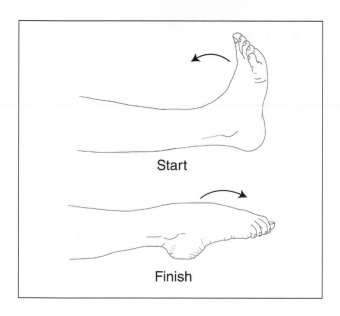

## Ankle Curls

Find a position where your weight is off your feet, such as lying on a bed or on the floor or seated on a chair. Pull your toes toward you and then extend them as far as possible. Begin with 3 sets of 25 repetitions and increase gradually to 3 sets of 45 repetitions. Perform the exercise daily, continuing for 2 to 3 weeks.

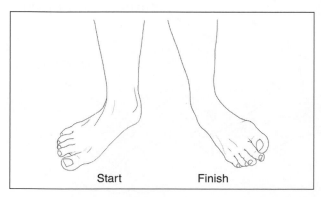

## Ankle Eversion/Inversion

Find a position where your weight is off your feet, such as lying on a bed or on the floor or seated on a chair. Slowly move your foot from side to side, keeping the lower leg motionless and moving only at the ankle. Begin with 3 sets of 25 repetitions and increase gradually to 3 sets of 45 repetitions. Perform the exercise daily, continuing for 2 to 3 weeks.

SECTION 7 ■ FOOT AND ANKLE

# ARTHRITIS OF THE FOOT AND ANKLE

## SYNONYMS
Osteoarthritis
Posttraumatic arthritis

## DEFINITION
The most common types of arthritis of the foot and ankle are osteoarthritis (degenerative arthritis) and posttraumatic arthritis. Frequent locations of arthritis in the foot and ankle are the first metatarsophalangeal (MTP) joint (MTP joint of the great toe), the midfoot (tarsometatarsal joint), the talonavicular joint, the subtalar (talocalcaneal) joint, and the ankle (talonavicular) joint (**Figure 1**).

## CLINICAL SYMPTOMS
Patients with arthritis of the first MTP joint report pain, loss of dorsiflexion, and swelling of the great toe joint (see Hallux Rigidus, pp 645-647).

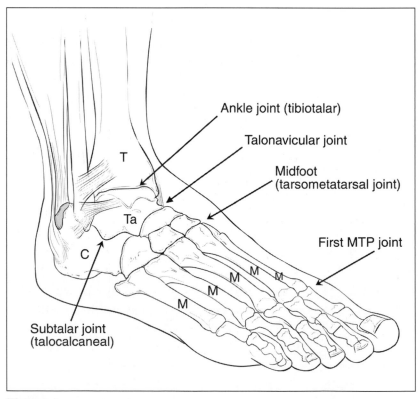

**Figure 1**
Common sites of foot and ankle arthritis. C = calcaneus, T = tibia, Ta = talus, M = metatarsal.

Midfoot osteoarthritis commonly occurs in older patients and also after a Lisfranc (tarsometatarsal) dislocation. The patient usually reports diffuse aching in the midfoot that worsens with prolonged walking or standing as well as difficulty pushing off with the foot.

Talonavicular arthritis causes focal pain over the joint (medial aspect of the hindfoot). This is a common site for rheumatoid arthritis.

Subtalar arthritis produces pain over the subtalar joint and frequently follows calcaneal fractures. Difficulty walking on uneven surfaces (such as sand or rocky terrain) results because the motion of this joint primarily involves inversion and eversion of the foot.

Most patients with ankle arthritis have a history of trauma. Pain, swelling, and stiffness in the anterior ankle are common symptoms. Patients with ankle arthritis have difficulty flexing and extending the ankle and therefore tend to walk with the leg externally rotated.

## TESTS

### Physical Examination

With hallux rigidus, loss of motion in the first MTP joint and difficulty pushing off with the great toe are common. In patients with midfoot arthritis, palpation reveals tenderness and often a dorsal bump on the midfoot. Patients with talonavicular or subtalar arthritis may show a loss of inversion and eversion of the hindfoot compared with the opposite foot; however, ankle joint motion is relatively normal. Patients with ankle joint arthritis have swelling and loss of ankle motion, and often walk with the leg externally rotated.

### Diagnostic Tests

Weight-bearing radiographs reveal the typical signs of degenerative or posttraumatic arthritis, including osteophytes (spurs) and joint space narrowing. The first MTP joint usually shows dorsal osteophytes protruding from the metatarsal head. In midfoot arthritis, joint space narrowing is especially evident at the second tarsometatarsal joint (**Figure 2**). Talonavicular arthritis is best viewed on an AP radiograph of the foot. With subtalar arthritis, the lateral view of the foot reveals loss of the normal talocalcaneal joint space. Ankle joint arthritis usually causes loss of joint space, which can be seen on both AP (**Figure 3**) and lateral ankle views, as well as spur formation anteriorly and posteriorly.

When the extent of arthritis is uncertain, CT can be helpful in the midfoot where the bony anatomy is sometimes difficult to view on plain radiographs.

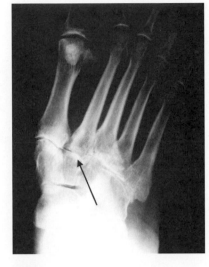

**Figure 2**
AP view shows primary degenerative arthritis of the midfoot. Note the joint space narrowing at the second tarsometatarsal joint (arrow).
Reproduced from Beaman DN, Saltzman CL: Arthritis of the midfoot, in Mizel MS, Miller RA, Scioli (eds): *Orthopaedic Knowledge Update Foot and Ankle* 2. Rosemont, IL, American Academy of Orthopaedic Surgeons, 1998, p 294.

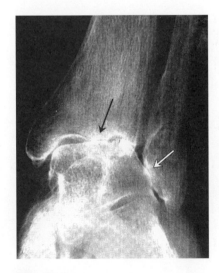

**Figure 3**
AP view of ankle showing ankle arthritis with loss of joint space (arrows).

SECTION 7 ■ FOOT AND ANKLE

## DIFFERENTIAL DIAGNOSIS

Charcot arthropathy (history of diabetes mellitus, swelling that is disproportionate to symptoms)

Gout (redness and swelling)

Tendinitis (normal radiographs)

## ADVERSE OUTCOMES OF THE DISEASE

Pain and difficulty with ambulation are common with untreated foot and ankle arthritis.

## TREATMENT

Initial therapy consists of shoe modifications, orthotic inserts, and NSAIDs.

A stiff-soled shoe with a rocker bottom will help relieve symptoms in patients with hallux rigidus.

Midfoot arthritis can be treated nonsurgically with a rigid custom orthotic insert or a steel shank inserted into the sole of the shoe. Patients with refractory symptoms will benefit from a surgical midfoot fusion.

Symptoms of talonavicular and subtalar arthritis can be improved with a medial longitudinal arch support or the more rigid UCBL (University of California Biomechanics Laboratory) orthoses. Corticosteroid injections and NSAIDs may be helpful. Predictable pain relief can be obtained with subtalar arthrodesis, or fusion, which retains ankle motion.

Ankle arthritis is treated initially with a custom-molded ankle-foot orthosis (AFO) and NSAIDs. Injection of a corticosteroid also may be beneficial (see Ankle Joint Injection, pp 601-602). In mild to moderate cases, débridement of the joint may defer the need for fusion. Ankle arthrodesis will benefit patients with refractory symptoms. Function is surprisingly good after an ankle fusion because midfoot dorsiflexion and plantar flexion increase. Total ankle replacement has shown great promise in recent studies.

## ADVERSE OUTCOMES OF TREATMENT

Infection, nonunion, and persistent pain may occur after foot and ankle fusions.

## REFERRAL DECISIONS/RED FLAGS

Persistent and disabling pain needs further evaluation. Chronic symptoms can be relieved by surgical débridement or fusion.

# PROCEDURE

## ANKLE JOINT INJECTION

### STEP 1

Wear protective gloves at all times during this procedure and use sterile technique.

### STEP 2

Cleanse the skin with a bactericidal skin preparation.

### STEP 3

Palpate the soft spot over the ankle joint just medial to the anterior tibial tendon (**Figure 1**). Using a 3-mL syringe with a 22-gauge needle, inject 2 mL of the 1% lidocaine anesthetic into the subcutaneous tissue of the soft spot.

### STEP 4

Advance the needle into the joint by directing it slightly laterally and superiorly. Inject the last 1 mL of the 1% lidocaine anesthetic. If the needle is in the joint, injection of the fluid should meet no resistance. Leave the needle in place and exchange the syringe.

### STEP 5

Inject 1 mL of 40 mg/mL corticosteroid preparation. Injection of the fluid should meet no resistance. Withdraw the needle.

### STEP 6

Dress the puncture wound with a sterile adhesive dressing.

### CPT Code

**20605**

Arthrocentesis, aspiration and/or injection; intermediate joint or bursa (eg, temporomandibular, acromioclavicular, wrist, elbow or ankle, olecranon bursa)

*Current Procedural Terminology* © 2004 American Medical Association. All Rights Reserved.

### MATERIALS

Sterile gloves

Bactericidal skin preparation solution

Two 3-mL syringes

One 22-gauge needle

3 mL of 1% lidocaine

1 mL of 40 mg/mL corticosteroid preparation without epinephrine

Sterile adhesive dressing

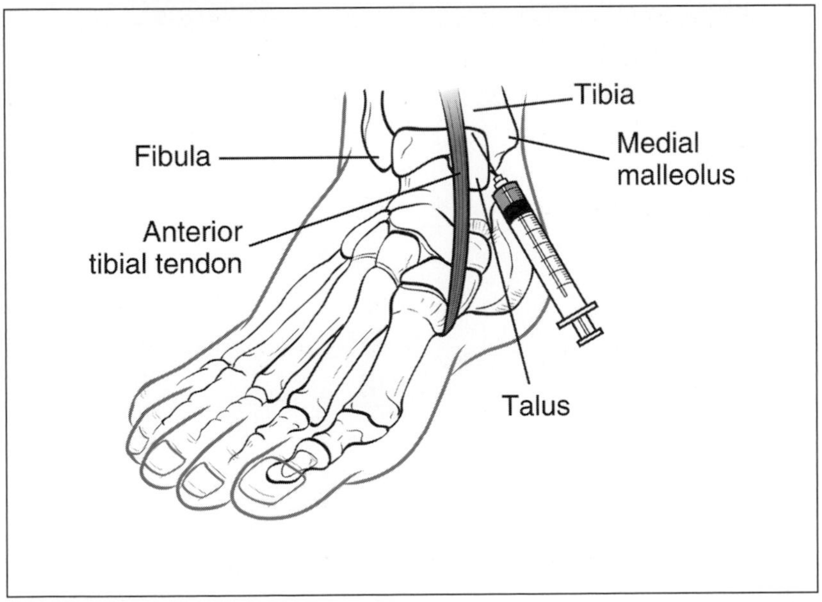

**Figure 1**
Proper location for ankle joint injection.

## ADVERSE OUTCOMES

Injury to the distal branch of the saphenous nerve is possible. Slow atrophy at the site of the injection is possible secondary to subcutaneous steroid deposition.

## AFTERCARE/PATIENT INSTRUCTIONS

Remind the patient that one third of patients experience a flare-up of symptoms, with increased joint pain for 1 to 2 days. NSAIDs or analgesics may be given during this period. Ice may be helpful for the first 24 hours.

# BUNIONETTE

## SYNONYM

Tailor's bunion

**ICD-9 Code**

**727.1**
Bunion

## DEFINITION

A bunionette, sometimes referred to as a tailor's bunion, is a deformity of the fifth metatarsophalangeal (MTP) joint that is analogous to a bunion (hallux valgus) deformity of the great toe. A bunionette is characterized by prominence of the lateral aspect of the fifth metatarsal head and medial deviation of the small toe. A bunionette is associated with frequent wearing of tight, narrow, pointed-toe shoes.

## CLINICAL SYMPTOMS

Patients report pain and problems finding comfortable shoes.

## TESTS

### Physical Examination

Deformity is evident on physical examination. An overlying hard corn is frequently present.

### Diagnostic Tests

Weight-bearing AP radiographs will show medial deviation of the fifth proximal phalanx and lateral deviation of the fifth metatarsal shaft and/or a prominence on the lateral aspect of the fifth metatarsal head (**Figure 1**). The joint usually is normal.

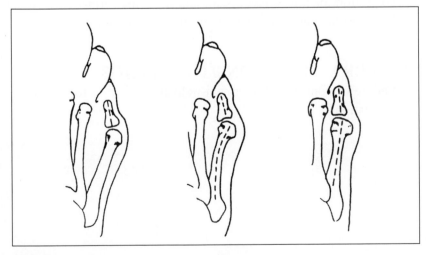

**Figure 1**

Typical deformities associated with a bunionette.

Reproduced with permission from Coughlin MJ: The bunionette deformity: Etiology and treatment, in Gould JS (ed): *Operative Foot Surgery*. Philadelphia, PA, WB Saunders, 1994, p 54.

SECTION 7 ■ FOOT AND ANKLE

# DIFFERENTIAL DIAGNOSIS

Cavovarus foot deformity (excessive weight bearing on the lateral side of the foot and pain over the fifth metatarsal noted on physical examination)

Inflammatory arthropathy (painful, swollen fifth MTP joint with deviation of the small toe often noted)

# ADVERSE OUTCOMES OF THE DISEASE

The most common problem is persistent pain aggravated by shoe wear. Patients also may have associated hard and soft corns, with possible ulceration and infection.

# TREATMENT

Patients should be advised to select proper shoes with a soft upper and a roomy toe box. A shoe repair shop can stretch the shoe in the area over the bunionette. A modified metatarsal pad also can help shift pressure off the fifth metatarsal head. Pads can be applied to the lateral aspect of the toe box to float the painful fifth metatarsal head (see Application of a Metatarsal Pad, p 605). A medial longitudinal arch support can help a patient who has a flexible flatfoot. This orthotic device rotates the forefoot slightly, which decreases direct pressure over the bunionette prominence.

With continued symptoms, surgical excision of the bunionette or realignment osteotomy of the fifth metatarsal may be required.

# ADVERSE OUTCOMES OF TREATMENT

Pain may persist despite the application of a metatarsal pad. Surgical risks include persistent pain, infection, incomplete correction, painful surgical scar, and neuroma formation from injury to the cutaneous nerves in the surgical field.

# REFERRAL DECISIONS/RED FLAGS

Failure of nonsurgical treatment indicates the need for further evaluation.

# PROCEDURE

## APPLICATION OF A METATARSAL PAD

### STEP 1

Ask the patient to mark the painful spot on the bottom of the foot with a material that transfers easily, such as lipstick or eyeliner (**Figure 1, A**). The mark should be approximately 0.5 cm square.

### STEP 2

Instruct the patient to stand in a shoe, without socks, to transfer the mark to the inside of the shoe.

### STEP 3

Place a metatarsal pad into the shoe about 5 mm proximal to (toward the heel), not directly under, the mark (**Figure 1, B**). This ensures that the painful area is suspended by the proximally placed pad. Prefabricated, off-the-shelf felt or gel pads are easy to use, inexpensive, and effective, and they come in different sizes to accommodate different-sized lesions and feet.

## AFTERCARE/PATIENT INSTRUCTIONS

If the pad is effective, continue the use of the pad and replace when worn. A custom-made orthosis also may be fabricated and can be transferred from shoe to shoe.

### MATERIALS

Felt, silicone, or gel metatarsal pad

Temporary marker (lipstick, eyeliner)

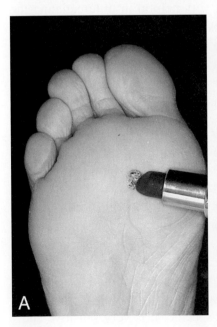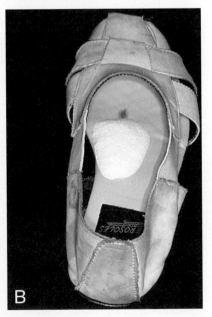

**Figure 1**
Application of a metatarsal pad. **A,** Marking the painful area.
**B,** Proper placement of the metatarsal pad in the shoe.

# CHRONIC LATERAL ANKLE PAIN

## DEFINITION

Chronic pain on the lateral aspect of the ankle is a common symptom that often follows an inversion injury. Several conditions may cause chronic lateral ankle pain after an inversion injury to the ankle, and they should be considered in the differential diagnosis.

## CLINICAL SYMPTOMS

Patients typically report pain on the lateral aspect of the ankle. Episodes of giving way and repeated sprains are typically associated with instability. Between sprains, however, the patient will have periods that are symptom free. In contrast, patients with a bone, cartilage, or tendon lesion often report constant, dull pain over the involved area.

## TESTS

### Physical Examination

Asking the patient to identify focal tenderness using one finger is the key element of the examination and can often identify the source of the problem. Identify any area of swelling. Range of motion should be assessed for both the ankle and subtalar joints. Assess laxity of the ankle and subtalar joints. Test sensation of the sural and superficial peroneal nerves.

Lidocaine injections can be very helpful in differentiating the source of a patient's symptoms. An intra-articular injection of 5 mL of 1% lidocaine into the ankle joint, for example, should provide transient pain relief in a patient with anterolateral impingement syndrome. Other common areas for differential injection include the subtalar joint and peroneal sheath.

### Diagnostic Tests

AP, lateral, and mortise radiographs of the ankle joint are obtained for suspected ankle pathology. AP, lateral, and oblique radiographs of the foot are obtained for suspected foot pathology. If ankle or subtalar joint laxity is suspected, stress radiographs (varus and anterior) are helpful and should often include comparison stress views of the opposite, uninjured side. If the radiographs are normal, and occult bony pathology is suspected, a technetium Tc 99m bone scan, limited to AP and lateral views of both feet and ankles, will identify the lesion. Although the bone scan is not specific, it is very sensitive and will detect most bony lesions, including occult fractures, arthritic changes, and tumors. If the bone scan is abnormal and an occult fracture is suspected, CT with thin cuts through the area in question should be diagnostic. If a soft-tissue or tendon injury is suspected (eg, tenosynovitis, a partial tear, or rupture of a tendon), MRI is appropriate. In these cases, the radiologist should be directed to the specific area of the tendon in question.

# DIFFERENTIAL DIAGNOSIS

## Anterolateral Impingement Syndrome

Anterolateral impingement of the talus with inversion (lateral gutter syndrome) occurs after an inversion ankle sprain. The borders of the lateral gutter of the ankle include the talus medially, the fibula laterally, and the tibia superiorly. Following a sprain, chronic scar tissue in the lateral gutter causes the anterolateral impingement. This condition is common in athletes, who often report pain and tenderness along the anterolateral aspect of the ankle. The pain is absent at rest and present with activities (especially dorsiflexion). These patients usually do not report buckling or giving way, or show any signs of instability. Examination reveals tenderness and swelling along the anterior talofibular ligament and lateral gutter. Radiographs, MRI scans, technetium Tc 99m bone scans, and CT scans appear normal, so this condition is often overlooked. An intra-articular injection of lidocaine will provide transient pain relief. Initial treatment should include an anti-inflammatory medication, physical therapy, and a possible steroid injection. Arthroscopic débridement of the lateral gutter provides definitive treatment.

## Chronic Ankle/Subtalar Instability

Following an inversion sprain, chronic instability of the ankle and/or the subtalar joint may develop. These patients report frequent "giving way" and generalized weakness in the ankle and an inability to return to full sports or daily activities. The cause may be inadequate rehabilitation or inadequate healing, with subsequent attenuation of one or more ligaments. After a moderate to severe inversion injury, a patient will often lose proprioception, range of motion, and muscle strength. A mild contracture of the Achilles tendon also may develop. Six weeks of physical therapy, directed specifically at increasing proprioception and range of motion, will often benefit these patients. The use of an ankle brace during sports activities also can be of significant benefit. If symptoms persist, further evaluation is required. The anterior drawer test (see p 483) and the varus stress test (see p 482) should be administered. Stress radiographs may be helpful. Surgical management options are reconstruction of the ligaments or checkrein tenodesis transfers.

SECTION 7 ■ FOOT AND ANKLE

## Nerve Injury

Injury by direct blow, stretch, entrapment, or even transection of the superficial peroneal or sural nerves may be a cause of chronic lateral ankle pain. Repetitive stretching or nerve compression typically causes symptoms over the site of a fascial band or bony ridge. Patients report diffuse, dull, achy pain on the lateral aspect of the ankle, and burning, tingling, or radiating pain in the nerve distribution. Plantar flexion and inversion of the ankle and foot will often aggravate the symptoms. Focal tenderness and radiating paresthesias with percussion over the site of nerve injury (Tinel sign) is diagnostic. A more generalized neurologic examination should include an evaluation of the L4, L5, and S1 nerve roots to rule out a proximal nerve lesion. Electromyography and nerve conduction velocity studies often are not helpful in the diagnosis of superficial peroneal or sural nerve lesions. Many of these injuries resolve spontaneously, but some require surgical intervention.

## Occult Bony Pathology

Routine radiographs identify most fractures in the foot and ankle, but osteochondral lesions of the talus, avulsion fractures of the calcaneus, lateral process fractures of the talus, and stress fractures of the fibula may not be obvious. A bone scan is an excellent initial study if these injuries are suspected. Once diagnosed, an occult bony lesion often can be treated with 4 to 6 weeks of immobilization. For persistent symptoms, excision of a loose bone fragment, arthroscopic débridement of an osteochondral lesion, or surgical fusion of an arthritic joint may be required.

## Peroneal Tenosynovitis/Peroneal Tendon Subluxation

A common cause of chronic lateral ankle pain is tenosynovitis from a tear or subluxation of one of the peroneal tendons. The peroneus brevis is most commonly affected by a tear, usually just posterior to the tip of the fibula. Patients report chronic retromalleolar swelling, pain, and tenderness. Recurrent subluxation of the peroneal tendons over the lateral ridge of the fibula also may be associated with this condition. MRI is helpful in the evaluation of peroneal pathology. A simple tenosynovitis may be treated with cast immobilization for 4 to 6 weeks. However, a tear or chronic subluxation of the tendon usually requires surgical treatment.

## Subtalar Joint Arthritis

Early arthritis of the subtalar joint may be difficult to identify. These patients present with chronic lateral ankle pain that is aggravated by standing and walking activities, particularly on uneven terrain. Examination reveals limited inversion and eversion. Special radiographic views and/or differential injections may be required to confirm early arthritis in this joint.

## Subtalar Joint Synovitis/Subtalar Impingement Lesion

Similar to anterolateral impingement syndrome, subtalar joint synovitis/subtalar impingement lesion (STIL) is characterized by a chronic synovitis of the subtalar joint, often following an inversion injury. The interosseous ligaments of the ankle that insert on the floor of the sinus tarsi tear, creating thick scar tissue and impinging in the subtalar joint. Examination reveals focal pain over the lateral entrance to the sinus tarsi, which is the lateral entrance to the subtalar joint. Patients often have slight restriction and discomfort with passive subtalar motion. Diagnostic studies usually are normal, although MRI may detect chronic inflammation or fibrosis within the subtalar joint. The treatment is similar to lateral gutter syndrome. Surgical débridement of the subtalar joint usually produces good results.

SECTION 7 ■ FOOT AND ANKLE

# CORNS AND CALLUSES

## SYNONYMS
Callosity
Clavus
Heloma durum
Heloma molle

## DEFINITION
A callus is a hyperkeratotic lesion of the skin that forms in response to excessive pressure over a bony prominence. When the callus forms on a toe, it is called a corn. When it forms elsewhere (as under a metatarsal head), it is called a callus (**Figure 1**). A persistent callus on the sole of the forefoot also is referred to as intractable plantar keratosis.

A callus usually occurs beneath the metatarsal heads and is associated with metatarsalgia, a general term for pain overlying one or several of the metatarsal heads. Pain may be caused by the callus itself or by some other manifestation of chronic pressure overload of the metatarsal head, such as synovitis of the joint, attritional tearing of the metatarsophalangeal (MTP) ligaments, or claw toe deformity. Pressure overload also may be secondary to a cavus foot, long toe (typically, the second), or wearing high-heeled shoes.

Corns usually occur from inappropriately tight footwear, with subsequent development of toe deformities (hammer toe, bunionette, claw toe). Hard corns (heloma durum) occur over exposed bony prominences, whereas soft corns (heloma molle) develop between the toes in the web space as well as over bony prominences (**Figure 2**). Periungual corns are small but painful

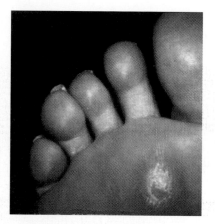

**Figure 1**
Clinical appearance of a diffuse callus beneath the second metatarsal head.

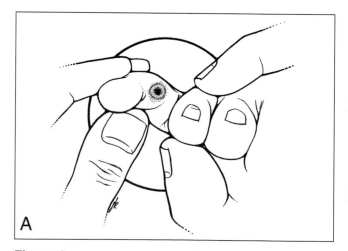

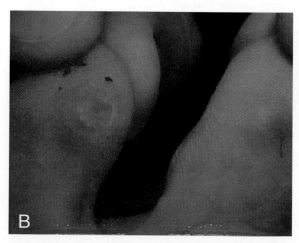

**Figure 2**
**A,** Soft interdigital corn on the medial aspect of the small toe. **B,** Corn on the plantar aspect of the small toe.

lesions that occur at the edge of a nail, often in association with a mallet toe or improper shoe fit.

## CLINICAL SYMPTOMS

Patients with corns and calluses typically report pain with walking or when wearing shoes.

## TESTS

### Physical Examination

The pared surface of a callus has a uniform, waxy appearance. Warts and calluses generally can be distinguished by palpation. Warts are tender when pinched from side to side, whereas corns and calluses are tender with direct pressure. Plantar warts usually do not develop over a bony prominence. Corns occur over or between the toes.

When tenderness exists over the dorsal surface of the MTP joint, perform the MTP instability test (see p 588) to assess joint instability.

### Diagnostic Tests

None

## DIFFERENTIAL DIAGNOSIS

Foreign body (history of penetrating wound)

Interdigital (Morton) neuroma (location between the third and fourth metatarsal heads or second and third metatarsal heads, no callus)

Plantar warts (occur on non–weight-bearing areas, may have a nearby satellite lesion, pared surface has multiple tiny points of hemorrhage near the base)

Synovitis of the MTP joint (tenderness over the dorsal MTP joint, no plantar callus, painful MTP instability test)

## ADVERSE OUTCOMES OF THE DISEASE

Persistent pain or ulceration of the skin may develop. Metatarsalgia, when caused by ligament tears or MTP synovitis, may result in gradual subluxation of the joint and deformity of the toe.

## TREATMENT

Paring and pressure relief are the principal treatment (see Trimming a Corn or Callus, p 613). Paring involves shaving the lesion layer by layer with a scalpel after the skin has been prepared with alcohol or iodine. The goal is to remove enough

SECTION 7 ■ FOOT AND ANKLE

of the avascular keratin to restore a more normal contour to the skin without drawing blood. When performed gradually and with care, this can be accomplished using a No. 15 blade, without anesthetic. Paring also provides excellent short-term pain relief. Patients then should be instructed in self-care, using a pumice stone or callus file to regularly débride the lesion after soaking the foot or after a shower.

Treatment of metatarsalgia includes use of a metatarsal pad (see Application of a Metatarsal Pad, p 605), trimming the callus/corn, and correction of associated problems, such as improper shoe fit and claw toe deformities. Pressure is relieved by wearing roomier shoes, using commercially available silicone cushions, or inserting small foam donut pads or metatarsal pads to shift pressure from the lesion. For soft corns, a small amount of lamb's wool or a silicone spacer between the toes can wick away moisture and help cushion the area.

When nonsurgical measures fail, surgical treatment to remove the underlying bony prominences is indicated. With soft corns, syndactylization (creating a partial webbing of the involved toes) may be required.

## ADVERSE OUTCOMES OF TREATMENT

Infection and bleeding can occur from excessively deep paring. Paring a soft corn can be especially difficult because of its awkward location in the web space. Medicated keratolytic corn pads often cause maceration and can result in infection; therefore, these pads are probably best avoided.

## REFERRAL DECISIONS/RED FLAGS

Failure to respond to nonsurgical treatment, presence of ulceration, and/or infection are indications for further evaluation of hyperkeratotic lesions. Deformity or persistent metatarsalgia also requires further evaluation.

# PROCEDURE

## TRIMMING A CORN OR CALLUS

### STEP 1
Wear protective gloves at all times during the procedure, and use excellent lighting and sterile technique.

### STEP 2
Anesthesia is not required to trim a corn or callus; however, prior to the procedure, the patient should soak the foot in water for several minutes to soften the skin.

### STEP 3
Holding the blade tangential to the lesion, shave the excess skin (**Figure 1**). Bleeding should not occur.

### STEP 4
Take special care with a corn on the toe because the skin is thin and may be fragile. Shell out several millimeters of the hard central core of a plantar callus with the sharp tip of the blade.

## ADVERSE OUTCOMES
Paring down a corn or callus too deeply may expose subcutaneous tissue. If bleeding occurs, the corn or callus has been trimmed too deeply. A wart, on the other hand, tends to bleed because of its hypervascularity.

## AFTERCARE/PATIENT INSTRUCTIONS
Instruct the patient to continue to pare down the lesion daily after a shower or bath with a pumice stone or nail file.

**CPT Code**

**11055**
Paring or cutting of benign hyperkeratotic lesion (eg, corn or callus); single lesion

*Current Procedural Terminology* © 2004 American Medical Association. All Rights Reserved.

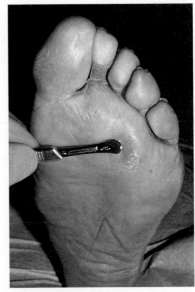

**Figure 1**
Trimming a callus.

SECTION 7 ■ FOOT AND ANKLE

# Dance Injuries to the Foot and Ankle

## Definition

Dancing emphasizes flexibility, repetition, and technique, and great demands are placed on the front part of the foot. Poor technique and overuse can lead to injury.

Most dancers are girls and young women. Although many of the physical demands placed on dancers are similar to those of other athletes, several are unique. Unique to dance are the demi-pointe, en-pointe, and turned-out positions of the foot. These positions place considerable stress on the anatomic structures of the foot and ankle and, particularly if improper technique is used or preexisting conditions exist, may lead to injuries and conditions commonly seen in dancers.

Management of injuries in dancers may be difficult because dancers are required to perform repetitive movements and move the joints through extreme ranges of motion as part of their training. Also, dancers often ignore injuries, especially during times of rehearsal or performance, until they become chronic.

Common injuries of the foot and ankle as seen in dancers are described in this chapter. For a more complete discussion of these conditions as seen in the general population, see the following chapters: Ankle Sprain, Hallux Rigidus, Hallux Valgus, Posterior Heel Pain, Sesamoiditis, and Stress Fractures of the Foot and Ankle.

## Hallux Valgus and Hallux Rigidus

Dancing en point does not cause hallux valgus, but it may cause an existing hallux valgus to progress. Similarly, hallux rigidus may be made worse by a dancer's efforts to rise into the demi-pointe position. A dancer with hallux rigidus will "sickle," or abduct the forefoot, while attempting to assume the demi-pointe position. The proper demi-pointe position will be difficult if not impossible to achieve because it requires the great toe to be capable of at least 90° of flexion. Treatment for hallux valgus is usually limited to symptomatic care, if possible, until the end of the dancer's career, as surgery may limit the range of motion of the great toe. Treatment for hallux rigidus may be successful in many dancers. Ballet dancers are an exception because a full range of motion is necessary for the demi-pointe position, and this will most likely not be achieved with surgery.

# SESAMOIDITIS

Sesamoiditis in dancers may result from poor technique when landing from jumps, which puts excessive stress on the sesamoids. An ideal landing in ballet includes a small plié (knees bent) to absorb the forces of landing, whereas a poor landing is usually audible. On examination, the dancer will have pain on palpation over the involved (usually the medial) sesamoid. With dorsiflexion of the great toe, the point of maximal tenderness will move with the sesamoids and their soft-tissue attachments. Treatment includes using proper landing technique. If it fits in the shoe, a small felt pad can be added to the ballet shoe to float the sesamoid.

# STRESS FRACTURES

The most common site of stress fractures of the foot is at the neck of the second metatarsal, followed by the base of the second metatarsal. The second metatarsal is the longest metatarsal and is where the body weight of a dancer is centered when in the demi-pointe position. Stress fractures also may occur at the distal fibula, the sesamoids, the talus, the calcaneus, and the navicular bone. On examination, the dancer with a stress fracture will have swelling and pain to palpation over the injured bone. Occasionally, crepitus will be present as well.

Treatment of stress fractures is conservative. Because dancers, like athletes, want to heal and return to participation as quickly as possible, non-weight bearing on crutches, followed by a gradual return to dance, may be recommended.

# OSTEOPHYTES AT THE ANTERIOR ANKLE

Extreme plantar flexion of the ankle places stress on the anterior joint capsule. This may result in thickening of the capsule or traction osteophytes off the distal tibia. The thickened capsule or the osteophytes impinge, limit range of motion, and cause pain with dorsiflexion. On examination, a dancer with anterior impingement of the ankle will have maximal tenderness over the anterior osteophytes or the hypertrophied anterior ankle joint capsule. Pain will be exaggerated with dorsiflexion of the ankle, and occasionally dorsiflexion will be limited on the involved side.

The condition is initially treated with rest and, if that fails, surgical débridement of the thick anterior capsule and/or anterior osteophytes.

SECTION 7 ■ FOOT AND ANKLE

## ANKLE SPRAIN

The most common acute injury in dancers is an inversion sprain of the ankle (lateral collateral ligament injury). If the sprain occurs while the dancer is in demi-pointe, the injury may be quite severe. Care should be taken to examine and perform a stress test on each ligament. It is extremely important in a dancer to perform comparison stress tests on the opposite, uninjured side, as a dancer's range of motion may be exceptional compared with that of the general population. Most ankle sprains are treated conservatively, with the dancer returning to dance 2 to 4 weeks postinjury.

## RETROCALCANEAL BURSITIS

The retrocalcaneal bursa may be compressed between the posterior aspect of the calcaneus and the Achilles tendon when the dancer rises up on the ball of the foot. Such compression results in the bursa becoming inflamed and painful. On physical examination, the patient will experience pain with side-to-side compression of the bursa, just anterior to the Achilles tendon. Most cases of retrocalcaneal bursitis resolve with rest, ice, NSAIDs, and a heel lift worn in street shoes. If the dancer ignores the pain, the problem may become chronic and require surgical excision of the bursa.

## POSTERIOR IMPINGEMENT SYNDROME

The posterior lateral tubercle of the talus (also known as Stieda's process) varies greatly in size and configuration. In 10% of people, the tubercle does not fuse with the body of the talus and is called the os trigonum, which projects into the posterior aspect of the ankle. Impingement of this bone on the soft tissue of the ankle, especially as the dancer assumes the en-pointe and demi-pointe positions, results in posterior impingement syndrome. This syndrome is characterized by pain at the back of the ankle when rising up on the toes. Examination reveals tenderness at the posterior aspect of the ankle, deep behind the flexor tendons. Pain increases as the foot is placed into plantar flexion, compressing the soft tissues at the posterior aspect of the ankle.

Conservative treatment includes rest, NSAIDs, and, if these measures do not relieve the pain, an injection of local anesthetic into the posterior aspect of the ankle. If these measures do not provide relief, surgical excision of the posterior lateral tubercle or os trigonum is recommended.

# TENDINITIS OF THE FLEXOR HALLUCIS LONGUS TENDON

For dance positions requiring a turned-out foot position, turnout should take place at the hip because when the femur is externally rotated the greater trochanter of the femur clears the pelvis, allowing the leg to abduct. Some dancers, however, using poor technique, turn out only the feet. This causes the feet to roll into an everted position and puts stress on the medial side of the foot, which can lead to tendinitis of the flexor hallucis longus (FHL) tendon.

The FHL tendon passes through a fibro-osseous tunnel posterior to the talus as it travels to its insertion at the great toe. With chronic overuse, inflammation and fibrosis of the tendon may result in a nodular thickening. The inflamed, thickened tendon may catch and cause the great toe to trigger. FHL tendinitis will cause pain and occasionally clicking over the course of the tendon. The pain may increase when the FHL travels through the fibro-osseous tunnel behind the talus. Pain may also increase when the dancer rises up on the toes or goes into a grand plié position, which puts tension on the FHL.

Examination should include palpating the entire course of the FHL while passively moving the great toe. Check for crepitus or a click in the fibro-osseous tunnel posterior to the talus.

Conservative treatment includes ice, NSAIDs, rest, and an injection of a local anesthetic agent into the fibro-osseous tunnel. If conservative treatment fails, surgical release of the fibro-osseous tunnel and a tenosynovectomy may be recommended.

# TESTS

Clinical and diagnostic tests depend on the specific condition. A lateral view of the ankle in plantar flexion is recommended to examine for posterior impingement syndrome of the ankle. This view will reveal not only the position and size of the posterior lateral process of the talus (and os trigonum) but also any visible impingement. A lateral view with the ankle in full dorsiflexion is also recommended to evaluate for anterior impingement.

# ADVERSE OUTCOMES OF THE DISEASE

Some conditions, such as hallux rigidus, may end a dancer's career because full range of motion of the great toe will most likely not be achieved, even with proper treatment.

SECTION 7 ■ FOOT AND ANKLE

## TREATMENT

The goal of treatment is to return the dancer to a preinjury level of dance. This usually includes a sequence of physical therapy, barre work, return to class, and then return to performance. This should be gradual and include consultation with the physical therapist, the dance instructor, and the dancer.

## REFERRAL DECISIONS/RED FLAGS

Further evaluation is indicated in any patient with an overuse injury that does not respond within 72 hours to ice, anti-inflammatory medication, and rest; an injury that is associated with a pop, click, or other audible sound; triggering of the great toe; any fracture; or any loss of range of motion.

# THE DIABETIC FOOT

## SYNONYMS
Charcot arthropathy
Neuropathic foot

**ICD-9 Code**
713.5
Arthropathy associated with
neurologic disorders

## DEFINITION
Diabetes is a group of metabolic disorders characterized by high
blood glucose levels. The four major categories are type 1
(insulin-dependent diabetes mellitus), type 2
(non–insulin-dependent diabetes mellitus), gestational diabetes
mellitus, and diabetes secondary to other conditions. Types 1 and 2
are the most common forms, with approximately 5% to 10% of all
cases of diabetes identified as type 1 and 85% to 90% as type 2.

Diabetic foot problems are a major health problem in the
United States and are a common cause of hospitalization and
amputation. Patients present with skin ulceration, infection,
and/or Charcot arthropathy. The primary etiology is peripheral
nerve impairment that results in loss of protective sensation,
autonomic dysfunction, and/or motor impairment. With
inadequate sensory feedback, skin breakdown results from
unperceived repetitive trauma. Vascular insufficiency also may
contribute to foot problems in patients with diabetes.

Patients with autonomic dysfunction have dry, scaly, and
cracking skin, a condition that predisposes the skin to
ulceration.

Motor neuropathy leads to weakness of the intrinsic muscles
of the foot, claw toe deformities, subluxation or dislocation of
the metatarsophalangeal (MTP) joints, abnormal plantar
positioning of the metatarsal heads, increased pressure on the
sole of the foot, skin breakdown, ulcers, deep infections, and
osteomyelitis. Extrinsic forces, such as tight shoes, may
contribute to skin breakdown.

Charcot arthropathy results from repetitive stress in a patient
in whom pain and proprioceptive sensation is not perceived
normally. The result is progressive disruption of joint stability
and severe bony deformities (**Figure 1**).

## CLINICAL SYMPTOMS
Patients may have no symptoms or they may report foot pain at
night, characterized as burning and tingling, secondary to
neuritis. With abnormal areas of pressure, skin breakdown
follows, leading to a painless ulcer. Deep infections and
osteomyelitis may subsequently develop, usually with a sudden
increase in swelling, redness, and drainage and sometimes pain.

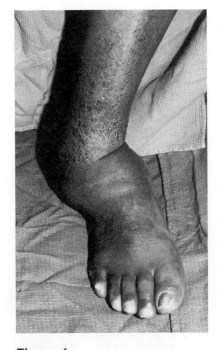

**Figure 1**
Severe deformity from Charcot
breakdown of the ankle joint.
Reproduced from Harrelson JM: The diabetic
foot: Charcot arthropathy. *Instr Course
Lect* 1993;42;141-146.

Patients with Charcot arthropathy have noticeable swelling, warmth, and redness, even though pain is only mild or absent. Charcot arthropathy may be misdiagnosed as cellulitis, osteomyelitis, or gout.

# TESTS

## Physical Examination

A thorough evaluation of the feet is essential when examining patients with diabetes. A significant number of amputations can be avoided by simple preventive measures and early treatment of skin lesions. Light touch should be tested. Protective foot care, including wearing well-cushioned shoes, is particularly necessary in patients below the protective sensation threshold, ie, those who cannot feel a 10-g (5.07-mm) nylon filament applied to the plantar aspect of the foot.

Diabetic ulcers are insensate and can be easily inspected and probed to determine depth and size. If bone can be probed, osteomyelitis is likely to be present.

Examination of a Charcot joint reveals a hot, red, swollen joint with intact skin. Pulses usually are strong in patients with Charcot arthropathy. A Charcot foot elevated above the heart for 1 minute will lose its redness, whereas a foot affected by cellulitis, soft-tissue abscess, and/or osteomyelitis will not.

## Diagnostic Tests

Plain radiographs are necessary to help rule out osteomyelitis and Charcot arthropathy (**Figure 2**). Vascular studies are appropriate when pulses are absent or when the patient has a

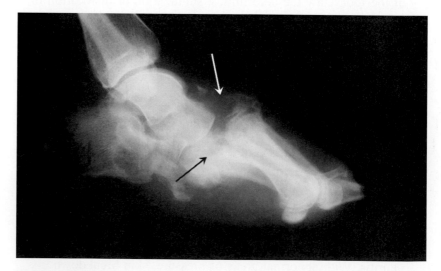

**Figure 2**

Lateral radiograph showing Charcot degeneration of the midfoot (arrows).

Reproduced from Harrelson JM: The diabetic foot: Charcot arthropathy. *Instr Course Lect* 1993;42;141-146.

nonhealing ulcer. MRI can help confirm a deep abscess or osteomyelitis but usually is not necessary. Combined technetium-iridium bone scans have been used in difficult cases to differentiate Charcot arthropathy from osteomyelitis.

## DIFFERENTIAL DIAGNOSIS

Cellulitis (most likely associated with skin breakdown)

Gout (painful lesion, increased serum uric acid)

Osteomyelitis (usually beneath an open skin ulcer)

Other neuropathies (Charcot-Marie-Tooth disease, alcoholic neuropathy, spinal cord neuropathy)

## ADVERSE OUTCOMES OF THE DISEASE

Skin ulceration, Charcot joint, chronic osteomyelitis, and gangrene all occur in the diabetic foot. Amputation may be necessary.

## TREATMENT

The goal of treatment is patient education and prevention (see Care of Diabetic Feet, pp 623-625). Good control of serum glucose is paramount. Once neuropathy occurs, it is irreversible. When a problem exists, aggressive treatment is needed to avoid a more serious and debilitating situation. A callus, which indicates a pressure point, is the first phase of a diabetic ulcer and signals the need for adaptive footwear (cushioned shoes and soft, molded insoles) and close follow-up.

Treatment of a diabetic ulcer requires removing the pressure causing the ulcer, allowing the ulcer to heal, and prescribing optimal footwear to prevent recurrence. Accommodative footwear, an orthotic device, and total contact casting may be used for superficial ulcerations. For deeper ulcerations, these measures are often inadequate, and surgery may be required. An associated equinus contracture should be corrected by serial casting or percutaneous heel cord lengthening.

Treatment of a deep infection must be aggressive and prompt. The infection is often polymicrobial. Skin swab cultures are inaccurate. Bone biopsy provides more definitive cultures to direct antibiotic therapy. Any abscess should be considered an emergency and drained surgically. Osteomyelitis can be treated surgically with débridement of the affected bone. Digit or ray (toe plus metatarsal) amputation is often needed to eradicate osteomyelitis of the toes or metatarsal heads.

In the initial stage of Charcot arthropathy, the foot and ankle need to be unweighted and stabilized, usually with a total contact cast. After the acute swelling and erythema have

SECTION 7 ■ FOOT AND ANKLE

subsided, the patient can begin bearing weight with continued use of a cast or a customized clamshell-type short leg brace. The patient must be advised that the period of immobilization may be lengthy, often up to 12 months, and that a permanent brace might be required for ambulation. When Charcot arthropathy is properly recognized and treated, acceptable limb salvage can be achieved. Occasionally, surgical reconstruction by arthrodesis is needed for severe deformity that cannot be treated with bracing.

## ADVERSE OUTCOMES OF TREATMENT

The adverse outcomes of treatment are the same as those for diabetes and, in addition, include surgical complications of infection, ischemia, and death.

## REFERRAL DECISIONS/RED FLAGS

Unexplained pain in a diabetic foot, sudden onset of swelling and pain, and nonhealing ulcerations all signal the need for further evaluation.

## ACKNOWLEDGMENT

Information regarding the sensory testing nylon filament was provided by the Filament Project, 5445 Point Clair Road, Caryville, LA 70721.

# PROCEDURE

## CARE OF DIABETIC FEET

*CARE OF THE FEET*

1. Never walk barefoot; always wear shoes or slippers.
2. Wash feet daily with mild soap and water.

   • Always test the water temperature with your hands or elbows before putting your feet in the water.

   • After washing, pat your feet dry; do not rub vigorously.

   • Use only one thickness of towel to dry your feet, especially between the toes.

   • Use a skin moisturizing lotion to prevent skin from getting dry and cracked; however, do not use these lotions between the toes.

3. Inspect your feet daily for puncture wounds, bruises, pressure areas and redness, and blisters.

   • Puncture wounds—Have you stepped on any nails, glass, or tacks?

   • Bruises—Feel for swelling.

   • Pressure areas and redness—Check the six major locations for pressure on the bottom of the foot:

     a. Tip of the big toe

     b. Base of the little toe

     c. Base of the middle toes

     d. Heel

     e. Outside edge of the foot

     f. Across the ball of the foot (metatarsal heads)

   • Blisters—Check the six major locations on the bottom of the foot for blisters, plus the tops of the toes and the back of the heel. *Never* pop a blister!

4. Seek treatment by a physician for any foot injuries or open wounds.

5. Do not use Lysol disinfectant, iodine, cresol, carbolic acid, kerosene, or other irritating antiseptic solutions to treat cuts or abrasions on your feet. These products will damage soft tissue.

6. Do not use sharp instruments, drugstore medications, or corn plasters on your feet. Always seek the advice of your physician for any condition that needs such care.

7. Protect your feet.

   • Wear loose bed socks while sleeping.

   • Avoid frostbite by wearing warm socks and shoes during cold weather.

   • Do not use a heating pad on your feet.

   • Do not place your feet on radiators, furnaces, furnace grills, or hot water pipes.

SECTION 7 ■ FOOT AND ANKLE

- Do not hold your feet in front of the fireplace, circulators, or heaters.
- Do not use a hair dryer on your feet.

8. Place thin pieces of cotton or lamb's wool between your toes if there is maceration of the skin between your toes or if your toes overlap.

9. Do not sit cross-legged; it can decrease circulation to your feet.

10. Take care of your toenails in the following manner:

- Soak or bathe feet before trimming nails.
- Make sure that you trim your nails under good lighting.
- Trim toenails straight across.
- Never trim toenails into the corner.
- If toenails are thick, see your physician and use a nail file or emery board for trimming.
- Consult your physician when there are any signs of an ingrown toenail. Do not treat an ingrown toenail with drug- store medications; however, you can place a thin piece of cotton or waxed dental floss under the toenail. (See Ingrown Toenail, pp 651-652)

## SOCKS AND STOCKINGS

1. Wear clean, dry socks daily. Make certain that there are no holes or wrinkles in your socks or stockings.

2. Wear thin, white, cotton socks in the summer; they are more absorbent and porous. Change them if your feet sweat excessively.

3. Wear square-toe socks; they will not squeeze your toes.

4. Wear pantyhose or stockings with a garter belt. It is important that you do not wear or use the following:

- Elastic-top socks or stockings, or knee-high stockings
- Circular elastic garters
- String tied around the tops of stockings
- Stockings that are rolled or knotted at the top

## SHOE WEAR

1. Always wear proper shoes. Check the following components daily to ensure that your shoes fit properly and will not damage your feet:

- Shoe width—Make sure that the shoes are wide and deep enough to give the joints of your toes breathing room. Shoes that are too narrow will cause pressure bruises and blisters on the inside and outside edges of your foot at the base of the toes.

# CARE OF DIABETIC FEET (CONTINUED)

- Shoe length—Shoes that are too short will cause pressure and blisters on the tops of your toes.
- Back of shoe—Looseness at the heel will cause blisters at your heels.
- Bottom of heel—Make sure there are no nails. The presence of holes indicates that there are nails in the heels.
- Sole—Make sure that the sole is not broken. A break in the sole will allow nails or other sharp objects to puncture the skin.

2. Be careful about the type of new shoes you purchase. Use the following guidelines when you look for new shoes:

- Buy new shoes in the evening to allow for swelling in your feet.
- Inspect your feet once an hour for the first few days. Look for red areas, bruises, and blisters.
- Do not wear your new shoes for more than a half day for the first few days.
- The following components in shoes are desirable:
  a. Laces or adjustable closure
  b. Soft leather tops (to allow feet to breathe; they mold to the feet)
  c. Crepe soles (to provide a good cushion for walking)
- Avoid the following components in shoes:
  a. Elastic across the tops of the shoes
  b. Pointed-toe styles (they constrict the toes)
  c. High heels
  d. Shoes made of plastic (retain moisture and do not allow the feet "to breathe")

3. Put your shoes on properly.

- Inspect the inside of each shoe before putting it on. Make sure to remove any small stones or debris. Be certain that the inside of the shoe is smooth.
- Loosen the laces before putting on or taking off your shoes. Make sure that the tongue is flat, with no wrinkles.
- Be certain that you do not tie your laces either too tightly or too loosely.

SECTION 7 ■ FOOT AND ANKLE

# FRACTURE-DISLOCATIONS OF THE MIDFOOT

## SYNONYM

Lisfranc fracture-dislocation

## DEFINITION

Fracture-dislocations of the midfoot, commonly called Lisfranc fracture-dislocations, are traumatic disruptions of the tarsometatarsal joints. Injury to these joints occurs as a result of significant trauma or from an indirect mechanism, as may occur in athletics or as a result of tripping. The critical injury involves the second tarsometatarsal joint. The second metatarsal wedges into a slot in the cuneiforms and is key to stabilizing the other tarsometatarsal joints.

## CLINICAL SYMPTOMS

Patients often report a "sprain." Pain is localized to the dorsum of the midfoot. The swelling may be relatively mild.

## TESTS

### Physical Examination

This injury is easily missed and is sometimes misdiagnosed as a foot or ankle sprain. Examination reveals maximum tenderness and swelling over the tarsometatarsal joint rather than the ankle ligaments. An acute injury to this joint usually presents with ecchymosis in the plantar arch.

During examination, stabilize the hindfoot (calcaneus) with one hand and rotate and/or abduct the forefoot with the other hand (**Figure 1**). This maneuver produces severe pain with a Lisfranc injury but only minimal pain with an ankle sprain.

### Diagnostic Tests

AP, lateral, and oblique radiographs of the foot should be obtained. Spontaneous reduction after complete dislocation may occur. Subtle injuries may be more apparent on weight-bearing radiographs. The medial aspect of the middle cuneiform should line up with the medial aspect of the second metatarsal on an AP radiograph (**Figure 2**). The oblique view should show the medial aspect of the fourth metatarsal aligned with the medial aspect of the cuboid. Comparison views of the uninjured foot may be helpful.

When the AP radiograph shows that the second metatarsal base has shifted laterally, even by only a few millimeters, a

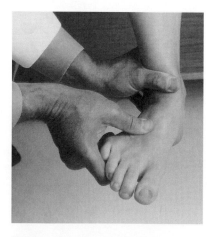

**Figure 1**
To test for a Lisfranc fracture-dislocation, stabilize the hindfoot with one hand and rotate and/or abduct the forefoot with the other.

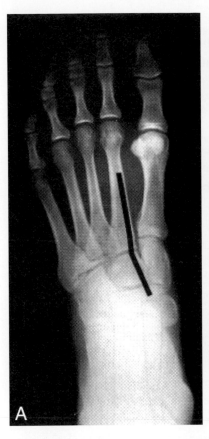

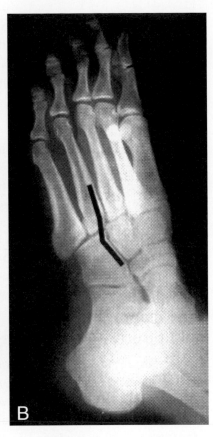

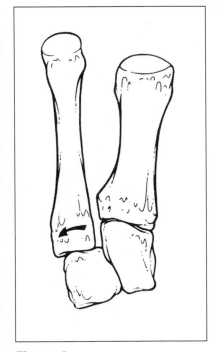

**Figure 3**
Lisfranc fracture-dislocation, with lateral shift of the second metatarsal.

Reproduced with permission from Alexander IJ (ed): *The Foot: Examination and Diagnosis.* New York, NY, Churchill Livingstone, 1990, p 131.

**Figure 2**
The normal radiographic relationship of the metatarsals and cuneiforms. **A,** AP view. Note the relationship of the second metatarsal and the middle cuneiform. **B,** Oblique view. Note the unbroken line at the medial fourth metatarsal base and the medial cuboid.

Reproduced from Lutter LD, Mizel MS, Pfeffer GP (eds): *Orthopaedic Knowledge Update: Foot and Ankle.* Rosemont, IL, American Academy of Orthopaedic Surgeons, 1994, p 261.

Lisfranc fracture-dislocation has occurred (**Figure 3**). A small avulsion fracture between the base of the first and second metatarsals indicates disruption of the ligament connecting the base of the second metatarsal and the medial cuneiform (Lisfranc ligament) and instability of the tarsometatarsal joints.

When radiographs are normal but physical examination suggests injury to the tarsometatarsal joints, stress radiographs of the midfoot under local anesthetic or sedation may be indicated. If confusion still exists, CT or MRI is helpful in confirming the diagnosis.

## DIFFERENTIAL DIAGNOSIS

Ankle fracture (bony tenderness over the malleolus)

Ankle sprain (focal tenderness over the lateral ankle ligament)

Metatarsal fracture (focal tenderness over the metatarsal)

Midfoot arthritis (chronic pain and tenderness, no recent history of trauma)

Navicular fracture (focal tenderness over the navicular)

SECTION 7 ■ FOOT AND ANKLE

## ADVERSE OUTCOMES OF THE DISEASE

Adverse outcomes include midfoot instability, deformity, and arthritis. Compartment syndrome with subsequent ischemic contracture, claw toes, and sensory impairment also can occur.

## TREATMENT

Nondisplaced injuries are treated by 6 to 8 weeks of non–weight-bearing cast immobilization, followed by use of a rigid arch support for 3 months. A fracture or fracture-dislocation with any displacement requires surgical stabilization.

## ADVERSE OUTCOMES OF TREATMENT

If the tarsometatarsal articulations are not well reduced, posttraumatic arthritis may develop.

## REFERRAL DECISIONS/RED FLAGS

Because these injuries are frequently missed, further evaluation and diagnostic testing is warranted if there is even a slight suspicion of their presence. Even a minimally displaced fracture-dislocation requires surgical reduction. Any possibility of compartment syndrome requires immediate surgical evaluation.

# FRACTURES OF THE ANKLE

## DEFINITION

Ankle fractures may injure the lateral malleolus (distal fibula), the medial malleolus, the posterior lip of the tibia (posterior malleolus), the collateral ligamentous structures, and/or the talar dome. Stable fractures involve only one side of the joint (eg, a fracture of the distal fibula without injury to the medial deltoid ligament) (**Figure 1**). Unstable ankle fractures involve both sides of the ankle joint and may be bimalleolar or trimalleolar. Bimalleolar injuries are either fractures of the lateral and medial malleolus, or a fracture of the distal fibula with disruption of the deltoid ligament. Trimalleolar injuries include a fracture of the posterior malleolus (**Figure 2**). Posterior dislocation of the

**ICD-9 Code**

**824.8**
Fracture of ankle; unspecified, closed

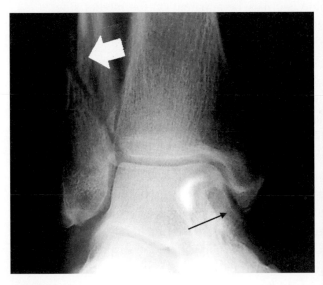

**Figure 1**
Minimally displaced fracture of the lateral malleolus (white arrow). Note small chip off medial malleolus (black arrow).

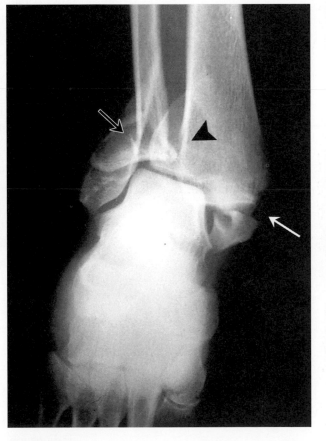

**Figure 2**
Displaced trimalleolar ankle fracture. Note the fracture of the lateral malleolus (black arrow), posterior malleolus (black arrowhead), and medial malleolus (white arrow). This fracture requires immediate reduction.

Reproduced from Grantham SA: Trimalleolar ankle fractures and open ankle fractures. *Instr Course Lect* 1990;39:105-111.

SECTION 7 ■ FOOT AND ANKLE

ankle also may be present with a trimalleolar fracture. This injury is described as a trimalleolar fracture-dislocation.

Stable injuries may be treated nonsurgically. Unstable injuries, however, are vulnerable for displacement and subsequent posttraumatic arthritis and usually require surgical management.

# CLINICAL SYMPTOMS

Patients usually report acute pain following trauma. The etiologies of ankle fractures are as varied as the circumstances, but usually some element of rotation or twisting has occurred.

# TESTS

## Physical Examination

Medial, lateral, and/or posterior swelling accompanies most ankle fractures. Marked tenderness is evident at the fracture site. A palpable gap may be apparent on the medial side. External rotation or lateral displacement of the foot from the tibia may be present as well.

A fracture of the distal fibula (lateral malleolus) with tenderness over the medial deltoid ligament is presumed to be an unstable bimalleolar injury.

Palpate the proximal fibula for tenderness because this, coupled with swelling of the medial ankle, may indicate a Maisonneuve fracture, an unstable external rotation injury that includes fracture of the proximal fibula, a tear of the medial deltoid ligament, and a disruption of the tibiofibular syndesmotic ligaments.

Assess circulatory status and posterior tibial, superficial peroneal, and deep peroneal nerve function distal to the fracture. Lacerations over the fracture site may indicate an open fracture and should be assessed carefully.

## Diagnostic Tests

AP, lateral, and mortise (AP view with the ankle internally rotated, usually 15°) views will reveal most fractures. The relationships of the tibia, fibula, and talus are clearest in the mortise view (**Figure 3**). AP and lateral views should include the proximal fibula and tibia when there is tenderness in that area.

Minimally displaced fractures may not be apparent on initial radiographs; therefore, when such a fracture is suspected, radiographs should be repeated in 10 to 14 days, when callus will usually be evident.

With a rotational injury, an osteochondral fracture of the lateral articular surface of the talus may occur. This is best seen on the mortise view. CT may be required for evaluation of complex fractures.

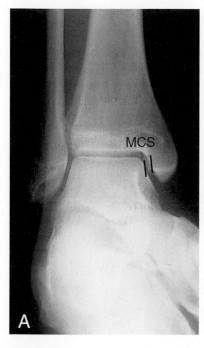
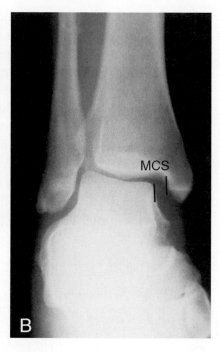

**Figure 3**

Mortise views of the ankle. **A,** Uninjured ankle demonstrates normal medial clear space (MCS). **B,** Ankle with lateral fibular fracture and deltoid disruption, resulting in widening of the MCS (> 5 mm).

Reproduced from Stiehl JB: Ankle fractures with diastasis. *Instr Course Lect* 1990;39:95-103.

## DIFFERENTIAL DIAGNOSIS

Ankle sprain (history of inversion injury, lateral tenderness, normal radiographs)

Charcot arthropathy (diffuse swelling, erythema, minimal tenderness)

Fracture of the base of the fifth metatarsal (focal tenderness)

Maisonneuve fracture (widening of syndesmosis, tenderness over the proximal fibula)

Osteochondral fracture of the talar dome, lateral process of the talus, or anterior process of the calcaneus (focal tenderness over the fracture site)

## ADVERSE OUTCOMES OF THE DISEASE

Posttraumatic arthritis, instability, deformity, complex regional pain syndrome, nerve injury, and compartment syndrome are possible.

## TREATMENT

Stable fractures of the distal fibula may be treated with a weight-bearing cast or brace for 4 to 6 weeks. Unstable but nondisplaced fractures require a non–weight-bearing short or long leg cast and more prolonged immobilization. Unstable,

SECTION 7 ■ FOOT AND ANKLE

displaced fractures require either closed or open reduction. In most cases, open reduction provides better restoration of joint function. Osteochondral fragments of the talus should be removed. If the fragment is large and there is viable bone on both the fragment and the base, the fracture may be reduced and pinned. The outcome of this procedure usually is good only in young patients. Concomitant dislocation should be reduced as soon as possible to relieve pressure on the skin and neurovascular structures. Open fractures require immediate surgical débridement. Physical therapy is indicated in elderly patients or if full range of motion and balance are not achieved by 3 months after the fracture has healed.

## ADVERSE OUTCOMES OF TREATMENT

Infection, nonunion, malunion, posttraumatic arthritis, and complex regional pain syndrome may occur.

## REFERRAL DECISIONS/RED FLAGS

Patients with unstable fractures or osteochondral fractures of the talus need further evaluation. All open fractures or open joint injuries require immediate evaluation.

# FRACTURES OF THE CALCANEUS AND TALUS

## SYNONYMS

Aviator's fracture (talus)

Heel fracture

### ICD-9 Codes

**825.0**
Fracture of calcaneus, closed

**825.20**
Fracture of talus

## DEFINITION

Fractures of the two bones of the hindfoot, the talus and calcaneus, usually occur as a result of severe trauma, such as a motor vehicle accident or a fall from a height. The two fractures seldom occur together, however. Most fractures of the talus or calcaneus involve the articular surface and are serious injuries.

## CLINICAL SYMPTOMS

Patients often report acute pain and inability to bear weight.

## TESTS

### Physical Examination

Examination reveals swelling and tenderness. Assess function of the superficial peroneal, deep peroneal, sural, and medial and lateral plantar nerves distal to the fracture. With swelling, the pulses might not be palpable. Check capillary refill of the toes.

Compartment syndrome is difficult to evaluate with calcaneal and talar injuries; however, notable swelling in the area of the arch is suggestive of a plantar compartment syndrome.

Falls that fracture the calcaneus or talus may be associated with a compression fracture of the lumbar spine. Palpate the spine for tenderness.

### Diagnostic Tests

AP and lateral radiographs of the hindfoot are indicated (**Figure 1**), along with AP and mortise views of the ankle. AP and lateral views of the spine should be obtained if there is spinal tenderness. CT may be necessary if further evaluation is needed.

## DIFFERENTIAL DIAGNOSIS

Ankle fracture (ankle swelling or deformity; evident on radiograph)

Associated lumbar spine fracture (pain and tenderness in the lower back)

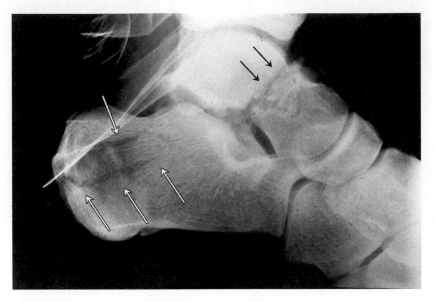

**Figure 1**

Lateral view of the hindfoot demonstrating fractures of both the talus (black arrows) and the calcaneus (white arrows).

Reproduced from Levine AM (ed): *Orthopaedic Knowledge Update: Trauma.* Rosemont, IL, American Academy of Orthopaedic Surgeons, 1996, pp 191-209.

Medial or lateral ankle ligament injury (swelling and tenderness over involved ligaments)

Talocalcaneal dislocation (deformity of the hindfoot)

## ADVERSE OUTCOMES OF THE DISEASE

The adverse outcomes of either type of fracture are potentially severe and disabling, and treatment is difficult. Fractures of the talus often interrupt the blood supply to the body of the talus and may lead to osteonecrosis. Chronic pain, posttraumatic arthritis, osteonecrosis of the talus, deformity, tarsal tunnel syndrome, complex regional pain syndrome, or plantar compartment syndrome may result from either a calcaneal or a talar fracture.

## TREATMENT

Immediate treatment consists of splinting with a well-padded posterior splint from the toe to the upper calf. The extremity should be elevated above the level of the heart and ice applied for 20 minutes every 1 to 2 hours.

Many of these fractures require surgical reduction and fixation to minimize later complications. Physical therapy to obtain range of motion of the subtalar joint is indicated after clinical healing of the fracture has occurred.

## ADVERSE OUTCOMES OF TREATMENT

Posttraumatic degenerative arthritis frequently occurs after these injuries. Nonunion, postoperative infection, and complex regional pain syndrome also are possible.

## REFERRAL DECISIONS/RED FLAGS

Patients with fractures of the calcaneus or talus or a dislocation of the talocalcaneal joint need further evaluation immediately upon diagnosis.

SECTION 7 ■ FOOT AND ANKLE

# FRACTURES OF THE METATARSALS

**ICD-9 Code**

**825.25**
Fracture of other tarsal and metatarsal bones, closed; metatarsal bone(s)

## SYNONYM
Forefoot fracture

## DEFINITION
Fractures of the metatarsal bones usually heal with nonsurgical treatment; however, a zone 2 fracture of the proximal diaphysis of the fifth metatarsal (classic Jones fracture) requires more extensive immobilization, and a zone 3 fracture of this bone may result in nonunion or delayed union (**Figure 1**).

## CLINICAL SYMPTOMS
Swelling and pain on weight bearing are common. Stress fractures usually occur after a sudden increase in activity, such as a new training regimen (increase in intensity or distance), change in running surface, or even prolonged walking.

## TESTS

### Physical Examination
Examination reveals swelling, ecchymosis, and tenderness over the fractured metatarsal.

### Diagnostic Tests
AP, lateral, and oblique radiographs of the foot may demonstrate the fracture. A stress fracture of a metatarsal may not show up on radiographs for 2 to 3 weeks. Follow-up radiographs are necessary if a stress fracture is suspected.

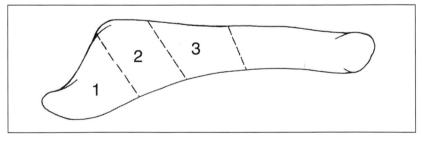

**Figure 1**
The three anatomic zones at the base of the fifth metatarsal. Zone 1 includes the articular surface of the fifth metatarsocuboid joint; zone 2 encompasses the articulation of the proximal fourth and fifth metatarsals; zone 3 extends 1.5 cm distal to zone 2.

Reproduced from Dameron TB, Jr, Fractures of the proximal fifth metatarsal: Selecting the best treatment option. *J Amer Acad Orthop Surg* 1995;2:110-114.

## DIFFERENTIAL DIAGNOSIS

Interdigital (Morton) neuroma (plantar pain and tenderness between the metatarsal heads)

Lisfranc dislocation or sprain (location at the tarsometatarsal joint)

Lisfranc fracture (location at the tarsometatarsal joint)

Metatarsalgia (plantar pain and tenderness over the metatarsal head)

## ADVERSE OUTCOMES OF THE DISEASE

Both malunion and nonunion are possible; however, nonunion is uncommon except in association with a fracture in zone 2 or 3 of the proximal fifth metatarsal. Malunion of a metatarsal shaft or neck fracture may result in metatarsalgia with a plantar callus. Compartment syndrome may develop after severe trauma or multiple metatarsal fractures.

## TREATMENT

Treatment of nondisplaced metatarsal neck and shaft fractures includes the use of a short leg cast, fracture brace, or wooden-soled shoe. The device that requires the minimum amount of immobilization while providing adequate comfort should be selected. Weight bearing is permitted as tolerated. In most cases, radiographs should be repeated after 1 week to identify any displacement, then again at 6 weeks to confirm healing. Tenderness at the fracture site will diminish as the fracture heals. A fracture of the first metatarsal is often the result of a high-impact injury and may require surgery (**Figure 2**).

Multiple metatarsal fractures and fractures with more than 4 mm of displacement or an apical angulation of more than 10° (seen on the lateral view) may require either closed or open reduction to reestablish a physiologic weight-bearing position of the metatarsal head.

Fractures of the proximal fifth metatarsal may be easy or difficult to manage. Avulsion fractures of the base of the fifth metatarsal (zone 1) or proximal metaphyseal fractures (zone 2) do well with nonsurgical treatment. Immobilization with an air stirrup, wooden-soled shoe, or fracture brace is continued until symptoms subside. Acute fractures in zone 2 are more difficult to treat. Most cases will heal with cast immobilization, but treatment of these injuries should start with non–weight-bearing ambulation in a short leg cast for 6 to 8 weeks. Early internal fixation may be considered for some patients, such as athletes. Fractures in zone 3 often resemble a stress fracture with prodromal symptoms suddenly exacerbated by an inversion injury. These need surgical intervention to avoid nonunion or delayed union.

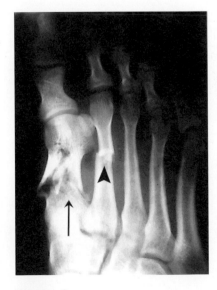

**Figure 2**

Radiograph showing fractures of the first metatarsal (arrow) and second metatarsal (arrowhead).

Reproduced from Shereff MJ: Fractures of the forefoot. *Instr Course Lect* 1990;39:133-140.

SECTION 7 ■ FOOT AND ANKLE

## ADVERSE OUTCOMES OF TREATMENT

Malunion with painful plantar callosities under the metatarsal heads or transfer lesions under the neighboring metatarsal heads may occur if there is displacement or shortening of the metatarsal.

## REFERRAL DECISIONS/RED FLAGS

Multiple metatarsal fractures, a metatarsal fracture with more than 4 mm of displacement or more than 10° of angulation, possible compartment syndrome, and/or proximal fifth metatarsal fracture in zones 2 or 3 are all indications for further evaluation. Displaced or comminuted fractures of the first metatarsal also require further evaluation. Open fractures require immediate surgical intervention.

# FRACTURES OF THE PHALANGES

## SYNONYM
Broken toe

## DEFINITION
Phalangeal fracture, commonly known as a broken toe, usually involves the proximal phalanx and is caused by direct trauma. These fractures rarely result in major disability. The fifth, or little, toe is the most commonly affected.

## CLINICAL SYMPTOMS
Patients have pain, swelling, or ecchymosis.

## TESTS

### Physical Examination
Examination may reveal deformity of the toe, but local bony tenderness, swelling, and ecchymosis are often the only principal findings.

### Diagnostic Tests
AP radiographs usually confirm the diagnosis.

## DIFFERENTIAL DIAGNOSIS
Freiberg infraction (osteonecrosis of the metatarsal head seen on radiographs)

Ingrown toenail/paronychia (inflammation of the fold of tissue around the toenail noted on physical examination)

Metatarsalgia (plantar tenderness over the metatarsal head)

Metatarsophalangeal (MTP) synovitis (tenderness over the MTP joint)

## ADVERSE OUTCOMES OF THE DISEASE
Permanent deformity is an uncommon possibility.

## TREATMENT
Phalangeal fractures are treated by buddy taping the fractured toe to an adjacent toe, usually the toe medial to the fractured one. A gauze pad may be placed between the toes to absorb moisture and prevent maceration of the skin from sweating. The tape and gauze should be changed as often as needed (**Figure 1**).

**ICD-9 Code**

**826.0**
Fracture of one or more phalanges of foot; closed

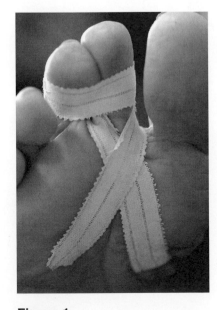

**Figure 1**
Buddy taping.

SECTION 7 ■ FOOT AND ANKLE

Closed reduction under a digital block or open reduction and pinning is rarely necessary but should be considered for markedly angulated fractures or for fractures involving the articular surface of the MTP joints of all toes or the interphalangeal joint of the great toe.

## ADVERSE OUTCOMES OF TREATMENT

Chronic swelling and deformity of the toe are possible.

## REFERRAL DECISIONS/RED FLAGS

Patients with an open fracture or a displaced intra-articular fracture (especially at the MTP joint) need further evaluation.

# FRACTURES OF THE SESAMOIDS

## DEFINITION

The first metatarsophalangeal (MTP) joint has two sesamoids, one medial and one lateral (**Figure 1**). The plantar aspect of each sesamoid is surrounded by the fibers of the flexor hallucis brevis and the plantar plate, and the dorsal aspect of the sesamoid has a facet that articulates with the metatarsal head. Because of its more protected position in the lateral soft tissues, the lateral, or fibular, sesamoid is less susceptible to fracture than is the medial sesamoid. Sesamoid fractures may occur secondary to avulsion forces, such as hyperdorsiflexion of the first MTP joint; repetitive stress; or, more commonly, from direct trauma. The repetitive stress from running or dancing can result in either a stress fracture or an avulsion fracture. Accessory sesamoids also may be found under any of the lesser metatarsal heads. The most common location is under the second metatarsal head on the tibial side. Although fractures of the sesamoids of the MTP joint (**Figure 2**) are the most common, sesamoids under any metatarsal head may fracture.

A bipartite sesamoid is a normal variant. It is important to distinguish this normal condition from a fracture (**Figure 3**)

## CLINICAL SYMPTOMS

Patients report pain under the first metatarsal head. Swelling and, rarely, ecchymosis may be present. The patient may have a history of direct trauma, a hyperdorsiflexion injury (resulting in

**ICD-9 Codes**

**733.99**
Other disorders of bone and cartilage

**825.20**
Fracture of unspecified bone(s) of foot (except toes), closed

SECTION 7 ■ FOOT AND ANKLE

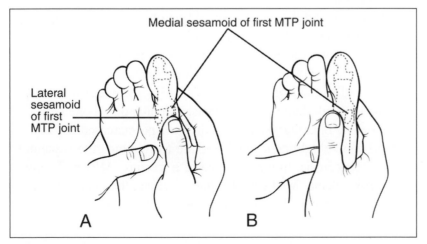

**Figure 1**
Palpating the sesamoids of the first MTP joint.

Reproduced with permission from Alexander IJ: *The Foot: Examination and Diagnosis.* New York, NY, Churchill Livingstone, 1990, p 65.

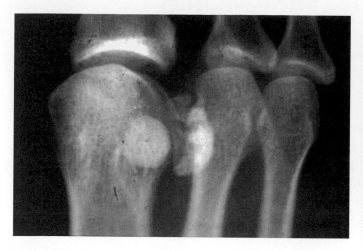

**Figure 2**
AP view of the foot showing a fracture of the lateral sesamoid of the MTP joint.

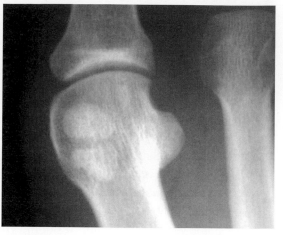

**Figure 3**
AP view of a right foot showing a bipartite lateral sesamoid.

an avulsion fracture), or a history of repetitive stress such as running, jumping, or dancing.

# TESTS

## Physical Examination
Patients report pain localized over the fractured sesamoid. The painful spot will move with the sesamoid as the great toe is flexed and extended. The pain may increase with dorsiflexion of the first MTP joint, as tension is applied to the flexor tendon complex. Range of motion of the first MTP joint may be restricted, especially in dorsiflexion, due to pain or guarding.

## Diagnostic Tests
AP, lateral, and axial views should be obtained to establish the diagnosis. The lateral sesamoid is best visualized on an internal oblique view. A technetium Tc 99m bone scan can help differentiate an acute fracture or stress fracture from a bipartite sesamoid and is considered to be 100% sensitive. A fractured sesamoid will demonstrate increased uptake on a bone scan, whereas a bipartite sesamoid will show no increased activity. MRI can help differentiate a fracture from a bipartite sesamoid or osteonecrosis. In the presence of a fracture, MRI will show marrow edema. MRI can also help evaluate the plantar plate, the intersesamoid ligament, and the flexor tendons.

## DIFFERENTIAL DIAGNOSIS

Bipartite sesamoid (smooth, sclerotic edges on radiographs; negative bone scan; may be bilateral)

Osteonecrosis (sclerotic appearance of entire sesamoid or irregularity with fragmentation seen on radiographs)

Plantar plate disruption (proximal migration of sesamoid noted on physical examination and radiographs)

## ADVERSE OUTCOMES OF THE DISEASE

The patient with an untreated sesamoid fracture will usually demonstrate pain and a limp. A nonunion may occur following an acute fracture.

## TREATMENT

The recommended treatment for an acute sesamoid fracture is a removable short leg fracture brace or a stiff-soled shoe with a rocker bottom. Usually at 4 weeks, as the symptoms improve, the patient is allowed to wear a stiff-soled shoe with a high toe box. Once the fracture is clinically healed, a felt pad to suspend the metatarsal head is recommended for 6 months.

## ADVERSE OUTCOMES OF TREATMENT

Healing of this fracture may take 6 to 12 months, resulting in limited dorsiflexion of the first MTP joint.

## REFERRAL DECISIONS/RED FLAGS

Persistent pain is an indication for further evaluation. In more severe cases, the fractured sesamoid may have to be removed surgically.

SECTION 7 ■ FOOT AND ANKLE

# PROCEDURE

# DIGITAL ANESTHETIC BLOCK (FOOT)

## CPT Code

**64450**

Injection, anesthetic agent; other peripheral nerve or branch

*Current Procedural Terminology* © 2004 American Medical Association. All Rights Reserved.

## MATERIALS

Sterile gloves

Bactericidal skin preparation solution

Ethyl chloride spray

10-mL syringe

18-gauge needle

25-gauge, 1½" needle

10 mL of 1% lidocaine or 0.5% bupivacaine, both without epinephrine

Adhesive dressing

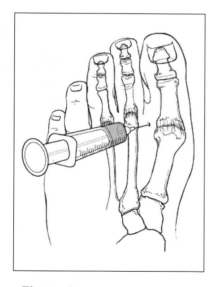

**Figure 1**
Location of needle insertion for a digital anesthetic block.

### STEP 1
Wear protective gloves at all times during the procedure and use sterile technique.

### STEP 2
Use the 18-gauge needle to draw 10 mL of the local anesthetic into the syringe, then switch to the 25-gauge needle to preserve sterility.

### STEP 3
Cleanse the dorsal surface of the foot with bactericidal solution on either side of the metatarsal heads.

### STEP 4
Freeze the dorsal skin with ethyl chloride spray.

### STEP 5
Insert the 25-gauge needle into the soft-tissue space on either side of the metatarsal head until it just begins to tent the plantar skin (**Figure 1**). Remember that the sensory nerves travel along the plantar side of the metatarsal.

### STEP 6
Withdraw the needle approximately 1 cm or until the tip rests at the level of the plantar aspect of the metatarsal head.

### STEP 7
Inject 3 mL of anesthetic, then an additional 2 mL while the needle is withdrawn. Make certain that some of the anesthetic is deposited subcutaneously around the dorsal sensory nerves.

### STEP 8
Repeat the procedure on the other side of the metatarsal of the toe that is to be anesthetized. Within 1 to 2 minutes, the involved toe should become numb.

### STEP 9
Dress the puncture wound with a sterile adhesive dressing.

## ADVERSE OUTCOMES
Although rare, infection is possible. Necrosis of a digit is possible if epinephrine is used in the anesthetic solution.

## AFTERCARE/PATIENT INSTRUCTIONS
Advise the patient that a collection of fluid on the plantar aspect of the foot may appear but that the fluid will dissipate within several hours after the block.

SECTION 7 ■ FOOT AND ANKLE

# HALLUX RIGIDUS

## SYNONYMS
Great toe arthritis
Hallux limitus

ICD-9 Code
**735.2**
Hallux rigidus

## DEFINITION
Hallux rigidus, or degenerative arthritis of the metatarsophalangeal (MTP) joint of the great toe, is the most common site of arthritis in the foot. The principal symptoms are pain and stiffness, especially as the toe moves into dorsiflexion. Hallux rigidus is the second most common malady of the great toe and affects approximately 2% of the population between the ages of 30 and 60 years.

## CLINICAL SYMPTOMS
Patients have pain in the great toe joint with activity, especially in the toe-off phase of gait as the MTP joint goes into extension. The osteophytes that develop on the dorsum of the toe may cause the overlying soft tissue to become red and irritated with shoe wear (**Figure 1**). The dorsal sensory nerves of the great toe may be irritated by the associated swelling.

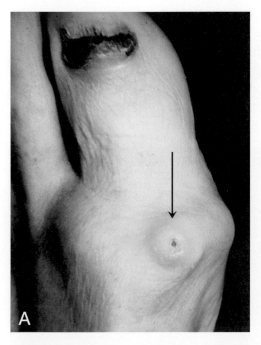
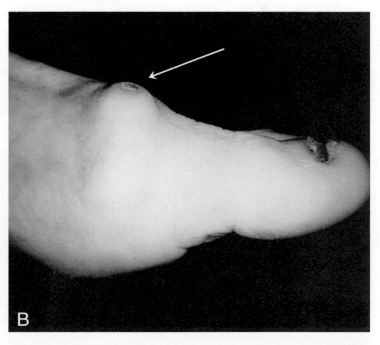

**Figure 1**
Foot with dorsal prominence from underlying bony osteophyte (arrow). **A,** Top view. **B,** Lateral view.
Reproduced from Mann RA: Hallux rigidus. *Instr Course Lect* 1990;39:15-21.

## TESTS

### Physical Examination

Stiffness of the great toe with loss of extension at the MTP joint is the hallmark of hallux rigidus. Osteophytes develop primarily on the dorsal portion of the first metatarsal head (**Figure 2**). The toe is usually in normal alignment.

### Diagnostic Tests

AP and lateral radiographs show narrowing of the MTP joint of the great toe and osteophytes, predominantly on the dorsal and lateral aspects of the great toe (**Figure 3**).

## DIFFERENTIAL DIAGNOSIS

Gout (recurrent episode of erythema and swelling, positive clinical history)

Hallux valgus (bunion and valgus angulation of the great toe)

Turf toe (history of injury, pain on the plantar aspect of MTP joint exacerbated by extension of the toe)

## ADVERSE OUTCOMES OF THE DISEASE

Pain aggravated by walking is common. Weight is transferred to the lateral side of the foot, especially during toe-off, causing increased stress and overuse on the lateral side of the foot.

## TREATMENT

Nonsurgical treatment consists of wearing a shoe with a large, soft toe box to decrease pressure on the toe. A stiff-soled shoe modified with a steel shank or rocker bottom limits dorsiflexion of the great toe and decreases pain caused by motion in the arthritic joint. Patients should be advised to avoid wearing high-heeled shoes. NSAIDs, ice, and contrast baths also can help

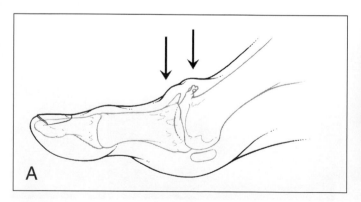 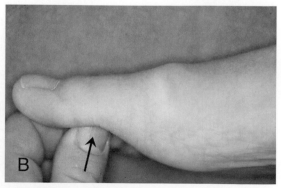

**Figure 2**

**A,** Hallux rigidus osteophytes (arrows). **B,** Loss of extension is the hallmark of this condition.

Reproduced with permission from Alexander IJ: *The Foot: Examination and Diagnosis.* New York, NY, Churchill Livingstone, 1990, p 65.

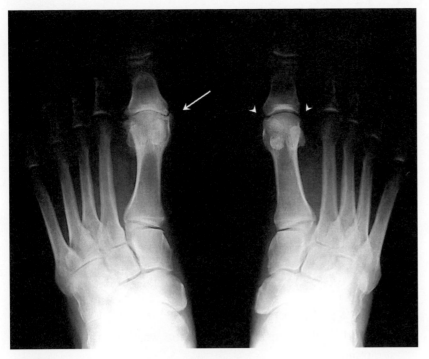

**Figure 3**
Weight-bearing AP radiograph of the feet of a patient with hallux rigidus.
Note the advanced arthritic changes in the left foot (white arrow) and
the small medial and lateral spurs (white arrowheads) in the right foot.

decrease inflammation and control symptoms for a short period
of time.

Surgical treatment consists of either excision of the dorsal
osteophytes or fusion of the joint (arthrodesis). Resection of the
joint may be indicated in some patients. An artificial joint
implant is not recommended.

# ADVERSE OUTCOMES OF TREATMENT

NSAIDs may cause gastric, renal, or hepatic complications. No
other adverse outcomes associated with treatment have been
found to occur, other than the usual surgical complications.

# REFERRAL DECISIONS/RED FLAGS

Failure of nonsurgical treatment is an indication for further
evaluation.

SECTION 7 ■ FOOT AND ANKLE

# Hallux Valgus

**ICD-9 Code**
**735.0**
Hallux valgus (acquired)

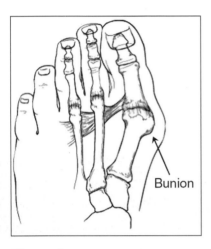

**Figure 1**

Anatomy of hallux valgus.

Adapted with permission from Pedowitz W: Bunion deformity, in Pfeffer G, Frey C (eds): *Current Practice in Foot and Ankle Surgery.* New York, NY, McGraw Hill, 1993, pp 219-242.

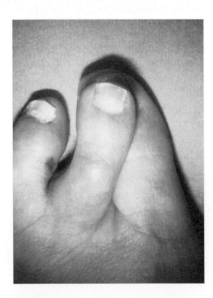

**Figure 2**

Severe hallux valgus with dislocation of the second toe.

## SYNONYMS

Bunion
Metatarsus primus varus

## DEFINITION

Hallux valgus is lateral deviation of the great toe at the metatarsophalangeal (MTP) joint that may lead to a painful prominence of the medial aspect of the first metatarsal head, known as a bunion (**Figure 1**). The female-to-male ratio of symptomatic hallux valgus occurrence is approximately 10:1.

## CLINICAL SYMPTOMS

Pain and swelling, aggravated by shoe wear, are the principal symptoms.

## TESTS

### Physical Examination

A hypertrophic bursa may occur over the medial eminence of the first metatarsal. The great toe may pronate (rotate inward), with resultant callus on the medial aspect. Irritation of the medial plantar sensory nerve may cause numbness or tingling over the medial aspect of the great toe. Assess the valgus angulation at the MTP joint (normal valgus at the MTP joint is < 15°). Measure the range of motion at the MTP joint. Most patients with hallux valgus have relatively normal MTP motion (60° to 90° of extension and 30° of flexion). Evaluate the lesser toes for associated deformities. A second toe that overrides the laterally deviated great toe is a frequent problem (**Figure 2**). Other lesser toe problems include corns, calluses, hammer toes, and bunionette (a bunion-like prominence on the lateral side of the fifth MTP joint).

## DIAGNOSTIC TESTS

The severity of a bunion deformity is graded by measuring forefoot angles on weight-bearing AP radiographs of the foot. The normal hallux valgus angle is < 15°, and a normal intermetatarsal (IM) angle is < 10° (**Figure 3**). Radiographs also are used to assess lateral subluxation of the sesamoids, the shape of the metatarsal head, degenerative changes in the MTP joint, valgus at the interphalangeal (IP) joint, and lesser toe

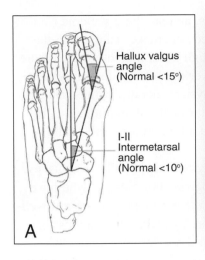
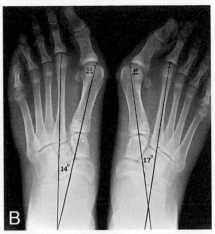

**Figure 3**

Hallux valgus severity is assessed by measuring the hallux valgus angle and the IM angle on a weight-bearing AP radiograph of the foot. **A,** Diagram showing the hallux valgus angle and the IM angle. **B,** AP radiograph of the feet of a patient with hallux valgus demonstrates valgus angulation of 14° in the left foot and 17° in the right foot.

Part A is adapted with permission from Pedowitz W: Bunion deformity, in Pfeffer G, Frey C (eds): *Current Practice in Foot and Ankle Surgery.* New York, NY, McGraw Hill, 1993, pp 219-242.

abnormalities. A weight-bearing lateral radiograph of the foot is less helpful but is important for evaluating any lesser toe subluxation or arthritic changes of the great toe MTP joint.

## DIFFERENTIAL DIAGNOSIS

Gout (articular and periarticular inflammation and tenderness on physical examination)

Hallux extensus (cock-up toe, or extension of the great toe) (seen on physical examination)

Hallux interphalangeus (lateral deviation of the great toe at the IP joint) (seen on physical examination or radiographs)

Hallux rigidus (osteoarthritis of the first MTP joint) (limited dorsiflexion of great toe)

Hallux varus (medial deviation of the great toe at the MTP joint seen on physical examination)

## ADVERSE OUTCOMES OF THE DISEASE

Chronic pain is a primary symptom and requires alterations in activity and shoe modifications (greater shoe width and minimal heel height).

## TREATMENT

The initial treatment is patient education and shoe wear modifications. Nonsurgical treatment is usually successful in mild to moderate cases. Recommended shoes have adequate width at the forefoot, soft uppers, and stitching patterns over the bunion. An orthotist or skilled shoemaker can stretch the shoe directly over the bunion. High heels increase the pressure under the ball of the foot and over the bunion deformity and, therefore, should be avoided. Physical therapy, splints, and bracing are not helpful, although a medial longitudinal arch support can decrease pressure on a bunion associated with a pronated flatfoot.

No treatment is needed for asymptomatic hallux valgus, even if the deformity continues to progress. For patients who have continued disability despite nonsurgical treatment, several well-established surgical procedures are available. Indications for different procedures are based on the severity of the hallux valgus, the IM angle, and joint congruity. Joint replacement is rarely indicated because of the high complication rate.

## ADVERSE OUTCOMES OF TREATMENT

Surgical treatment may result in recurrence, undercorrection, overcorrection (hallux varus), decreased function, stiffness, pain, malunion or nonunion of an osteotomy, and transfer lesions (metatarsalgia).

## REFERRAL DECISIONS/RED FLAGS

Persistent pain despite shoe modifications indicates the need for further evaluation. Patients with persistent pain may benefit from surgical correction.

# INGROWN TOENAIL

## SYNONYMS
Infected toenail
Onychocryptosis
Paronychia

**ICD-9 Code**
**703.0**
Diseases of nail; ingrowing nail

## DEFINITION
With an ingrown toenail, the distal margin of the nail grows into the adjacent skin, causing irritation, inflammation, and possibly secondary bacterial or fungal infection. The condition is virtually limited to the great toe. Ingrown toenails are associated with improper trimming of the toenail, tight shoes, hereditary predisposition, subungual pathology, congenital incurved nail, thickened nail, direct trauma, or any combination of these factors (**Figure 1**).

Unlike fingernails, toenails should not be cut in a curved fashion because this allows the sharp edge of the nail to grow into the more prominent skin margins (nail fold) found at the end of toenails. Properly trimmed toenails are cut straight across to keep the lateral margin of the toenail beyond the nail fold. Some people have toenails that have a naturally incurved shape. Ingrown toenails may occur in these patients even with proper trimming techniques. Soft-tissue hypertrophy over a normal nail plate secondary to trauma or tight shoes also may cause an ingrown toenail. Skin breakthrough creates a portal of entry for a secondary bacterial or fungal infection.

## CLINICAL SYMPTOMS
Stage I (inflammation) is characterized by induration, swelling, and tenderness along the nail fold. In stage II (abscess), the patient has purulent or serous drainage, increased tenderness, and increased erythema. In stage III (granulation), granulation tissue grows onto the nail plate, inhibiting drainage. This stage is less painful than stage II.

## TESTS

### Physical Examination
The diagnosis is clinical; visual inspection is the basis for staging the condition.

### Diagnostic Tests
Radiographs of stage II and stage III ingrown toenails may be obtained to rule out a subungual exostosis (cartilage-capped projection from bone) and osteomyelitis.

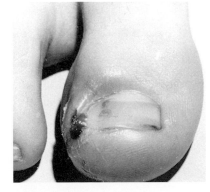

**Figure 1**
Ingrown toenail.

Reproduced from Lutter LD, Mizel MS, Pfeffer GB (eds): *Orthopaedic Knowledge Update: Foot and Ankle*. Rosemont, IL, American Academy of Orthopaedic Surgeons, 1994, p 54.

SECTION 7 ■ FOOT AND ANKLE

## DIFFERENTIAL DIAGNOSIS

Felon (deep abscess on the plantar aspect of the toe)
Onychomycosis (fungal infection of the nail)
Osteomyelitis (bone infection with changes on radiograph)
Paronychia (superficial abscess on the base of the toenail)
Subungual exostosis (osteochondroma beneath the nail, noted radiographically)

## ADVERSE OUTCOMES OF THE DISEASE

Progressive pain, paronychia, felon, nail plate deformity, and osteomyelitis are all possible. Hematogenous seeding of other organs may occur but is very uncommon.

## TREATMENT

Stage I: Warm soaks, proper nail trimming, accommodative shoe wear, and clean socks are recommended. With a blunt instrument, insert cotton or waxed dental floss beneath the nail to lift the edge of the nail from its embedded position. Exchange packing daily until the nail has grown out sufficiently. Nonconstrictive shoes or sandals prevent extrinsic irritation of the inflamed skin.

Stage II: Initial treatment should include foot soaks along with broad-spectrum oral antibiotics (cephalosporin). Partial excision of the nail under digital block should be performed when the patient has severe pain, when there is a risk of secondary infection to a prosthetic joint, or when a course of oral antibiotics fails to treat associated infection (see Digital Anesthetic Block [Foot], p 644). Partial nail excision is preferred (see Nail Plate Avulsion, pp 653-654). Complete nail excision increases the risk of deformity of the nail bed (clubbing). An avulsed nail requires 3 to 4 months to regrow.

Stage III: Partial or complete nail plate excision with or without ablation of the germinal matrix of the nail is indicated.

## ADVERSE OUTCOMES OF TREATMENT

Adverse outcomes include recurrence (50% to 70% with excision alone), nail plate deformity, upturned nail or clubbed nail after complete nail plate excision, and poor cosmetic result.

## REFERRAL DECISIONS/RED FLAGS

Failure of nonsurgical treatment or the presence of stage III disease is an indication for further evaluation.

# PROCEDURE
## NAIL PLATE AVULSION

### ANATOMY

A recurrent ingrown toenail or paronychial infection, which usually occurs in the great toe, makes it necessary to remove a portion of the nail plate. The lateral and/or medial margins of the nail may be involved.

Removal of the entire nail plate is described below. Partial removal involves undermining the lateral or medial third of the nail, vertically cutting the nail with strong small scissors or an anvil nail cutter at the junction of the lateral or medial third, and avulsing the small segment adjacent to the nail fold.

### STEP 1

Wear protective gloves at all times during the procedure and use sterile technique.

### STEP 2

Cleanse the toe with a bactericidal solution.

### STEP 3

Follow the steps in the procedure titled Digital Anesthetic Block (Foot) on p 644 to administer a digital block.

### STEP 4

Wrap a 1/4" Penrose drain or strip of rubber around the base of the toe to act as a tourniquet and control bleeding (optional).

### STEP 5

Using a small scissors or hemostat, elevate the nail plate from the underlying nail bed (**Figure 1**).

---

**CPT Codes**

**11730**
Avulsion of nail plate, partial or complete, simple; single

**11732**
Avulsion of nail plate, partial or complete, simple; each additional nail plate
(List separately in addition to code for primary procedure)

*Current Procedural Terminology* © 2004 American Medical Association. All Rights Reserved.

### MATERIALS

Sterile gloves

Bactericidal skin preparation solution

¼" Penrose drain or a strip cut from a rubber glove (optional)

Materials to administer a digital block (see Digital Anesthetic Block [Foot], p 644)

Strong small scissors or anvil nail cutter

Small hemostat

Nonadherent sterile gauze

Sterile dressing material

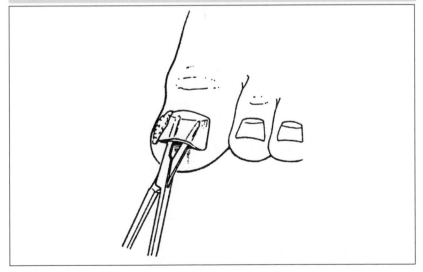

**Figure 1**
Nail plate avulsion: elevating the nail plate from the nail bed.

# Nail Plate Avulsion (continued)

### Step 6

Separate the proximal cuticle (nail fold) from the nail plate.

### Step 7

Grasp the free portion of the nail plate with a hemostat and avulse it (**Figure 2**), then palpate the nail bed to ensure that no spikes of nail tissue remain.

### Step 8

If a tourniquet was used, remove it and apply compression to stop local bleeding.

### Step 9

Apply nonadherent sterile gauze over the exposed nail bed and wrap the entire toe with a sterile dressing.

## Adverse Outcomes

Because of recurrence of ingrown toenails after nail plate avulsions, permanent ablation of the nail matrix may be required.

## Permanent Ablation

This procedure may be necessary and can be performed by curettage and/or phenol ablation of the nail matrix.

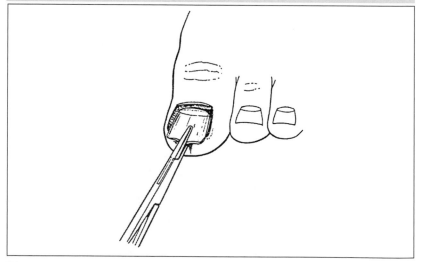

**Figure 2**
Nail plate avulsion: avulsing the nail plate.

# INTERDIGITAL (MORTON) NEUROMA

## SYNONYMS

Intermetatarsal neuroma
Morton neuroma
Plantar neuroma

**ICD-9 Code**

**355.6**
Mononeuritis of lower limb; lesion of
plantar nerve

## DEFINITION

A plantar interdigital neuroma, also referred to as a Morton neuroma, is not a true neuroma but rather a perineural fibrosis of the common digital nerve as it passes between the metatarsal heads. The fibrosis is secondary to repetitive irritation of the nerve. The condition most commonly occurs between the third and fourth toes (third web space) (**Figure 1**). Interdigital neuromas occur less frequently in the second web space (between the second and third toes) and rarely in either the first or fourth intermetatarsal space. The simultaneous occurrence of two neuromas is extremely uncommon. Interdigital neuroma has a female-to-male ratio of 5:1, probably related to compression of the nerve by tight shoes.

## CLINICAL SYMPTOMS

Plantar pain in the forefoot is the most common presenting symptom. Dysesthesias into the affected two toes or burning plantar pain that is aggravated by activity also is common. Occasionally, patients report numbness in the toes adjacent to the involved web space. Night pain is rare. Many patients state that they feel as though they are "walking on a marble" or that there is "a wrinkle in my sock." Relief often is obtained by removing the shoe and rubbing the ball of the foot. Symptoms are aggravated by wearing high-heeled or tight, restrictive shoes.

## TESTS

### Physical Examination
Isolated pain on the plantar aspect of the web space is consistent with an interdigital neuroma. Apply direct plantar pressure to the interspace with one hand and then squeeze the metatarsals together with the other hand. If an interdigital neuroma is present, this maneuver will cause increased tenderness and pain radiating to the toes.

Inspect the plantar surface for calluses, then palpate dorsally along the metatarsal shafts and plantarly over the metatarsal

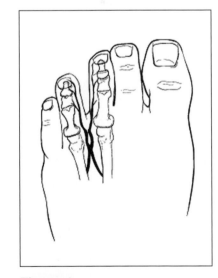

**Figure 1**
Interdigital neuroma between the metatarsal heads.

**Adapted with permission from McElvenny RT: The etiology and surgical treatment of intractable pain about the fourth metatarsophalangeal joint (Morton toe).** *J Bone Joint Surg Am* **1943;25:675-679.**

heads to evaluate for stress fractures or metatarsalgia, respectively. Evaluate sensory function of the digital nerves. Stress each tarsometatarsal joint by grasping the midfoot with one hand and moving each metatarsal dorsally and then plantarly to rule out midfoot arthritis. Similarly, grasp the metatarsal shaft and, while keeping the toe parallel to the metatarsal, try to displace the digit dorsally, then plantarly. Pain or excess motion with this maneuver indicates synovitis or inflammation of the metatarsophalangeal (MTP) joint.

### Diagnostic Tests

Radiographs are normal in patients with interdigital neuroma. MRI and ultrasound sometimes detect neuromas, but these modalities are unreliable for this purpose and their use is not commonly indicated.

## DIFFERENTIAL DIAGNOSIS

Hammer toe (flexion deformity of the proximal interphalangeal joint noted on physical examination)

Metatarsalgia (plantar tenderness over the metatarsal head noted on physical examination)

MTP synovitis (tenderness and swelling directly over the MTP joint noted on physical examination)

Stress fracture (dorsal metatarsal tenderness noted on physical examination)

## ADVERSE OUTCOMES OF THE DISEASE

Chronic, intermittent pain and the need for shoe and activity modifications are possible.

## TREATMENT

Patients should be advised to wear a low-heeled, well-cushioned shoe with a wide toe box. A well-cushioned sandal is also an option. In addition, pain relief may be obtained using metatarsal pads to spread the metatarsal heads and take pressure off the nerve (see also Procedure: Application of a Metatarsal Pad, p 605).

Locate the neuroma on the plantar aspect of the foot in the soft tissue between the involved metatarsal heads. Ask the patient to mark the painful spot on the bottom of the foot with a material that transfers easily, such as lipstick or eyeliner. Instruct the patient to stand, without socks, in a shoe to transfer the mark to the inside of the shoe. Place the pad in the shoe just proximal to the mark, to suspend the painful area. This also ensures that the metatarsal heads are kept apart and away from the neuroma when the patient is bearing weight. Felt or gel pads are inexpensive, effective, and come in different sizes to accommodate shoes and feet of different sizes. Advise the patient that if the pad is effective, a more permanent orthotic can be fabricated that can be transferred from shoe to shoe. Avoid using a rigid orthotic, as it may aggravate the neuroma.

A mixture of 1 to 2 mL of lidocaine without epinephrine and 1 mL (10 mg/mL) of corticosteroid injected just proximal to the metatarsal heads can be both diagnostic and therapeutic (see Interdigital (Morton) Neuroma Injection, pp 658-659). Multiple injections should be avoided.

If symptoms persist or recur, surgical excision of the neuroma or division of the transverse metatarsal ligament is indicated.

## ADVERSE OUTCOMES OF TREATMENT

Symptoms may persist or recur after nonsurgical treatment. Symptoms may recur or become worse after surgical excision of the neuroma if a painful stump of nerve develops.

## REFERRAL DECISIONS/RED FLAGS

Persistent pain despite shoe or insert modifications or injection of corticosteroid indicates the need for further evaluation.

SECTION 7 ■ FOOT AND ANKLE

# PROCEDURE

## INTERDIGITAL (MORTON) NEUROMA INJECTION

### CPT Code

**28899**
Unlisted procedure, foot or toes
*Current Procedural Terminology © 2004
American Medical Association. All Rights
Reserved.*

### MATERIALS

Sterile gloves

Bactericidal skin preparation
solution

Ethyl chloride spray

3-mL syringe

18-gauge needle

25-gauge, 1- to 1½″-needle

1 mL of 10 mg/mL corticosteroid
preparation

2 mL of 1% lidocaine or 0.5%
bupivacaine, both without
epinephrine

Adhesive dressing

### STEP 1

Wear protective gloves at all times during the procedure and
use sterile technique.

### STEP 2

Use the 18-gauge needle to draw 1 mL of the 10 mg/mL
corticosteroid preparation and 2 mL of the local anesthetic into
the syringe, then switch to the 25-gauge needle to preserve
sterility.

### STEP 3

Cleanse the dorsal skin between the metatarsal heads with
bactericidal solution.

### STEP 4

Freeze the dorsal skin with ethyl chloride spray.

### STEP 5

Place the needle in line with the metatarsophalangeal joint,
which is approximately 1 to 2 cm proximal to the web of the
toe (**Figure 1**).

### STEP 6

Insert the needle through the dorsal tissues until the tip barely
tents the skin of the plantar aspect of the foot. Withdraw the

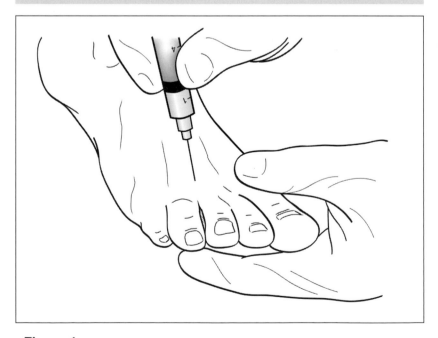

**Figure 1**
Proper location for injection for interdigital neuroma.

# Interdigital (Morton) Neuroma Injection (continued)

needle approximately 1 cm so that the tip is where the neuroma is found, at the level of the plantar metatarsophalangeal joint.

*Step 7*
Inject the corticosteroid-anesthetic mixture around the neuroma, taking care not to inject into the plantar fat pad.

# Metatarsalgia

**ICD-9 Code**

**726.70**
Enthesopathy of ankle and tarsus,
unspecified

## Synonym
Forefoot pain

## Definition
Metatarsalgia is a general term indicating forefoot pain localized under one or more of the lesser metatarsals. Abnormal metatarsal length with alteration of weight-bearing forces is one cause of metatarsalgia. Toe deformities such as claw or hammer toe also may lead to metatarsalgia by causing displacement of the plantar fat pad and loss of cushioning under the metatarsal heads. Callus formation occurs, and this thickened skin may be a major component of the patient's symptoms. A persistent callus on the sole of the foot is called intractable plantar keratosis.

## Clinical Symptoms
Activity-related pain is localized to the plantar aspect of the forefoot directly over the metatarsal heads. The patient may complain about the diffuse callus formation.

## Tests

### Physical Examination
Observe the alignment of the toes. Evaluate swelling, range of motion, and stability of the metatarsophalangeal (MTP) joints. Palpate for swelling or masses along the plantar and dorsal aspects of the metatarsals as well as adjacent interspaces. Note the extent of any callus and whether it is discrete or diffuse. A discrete callus is tender with direct pressure. Evaluate digital nerve function.

### Diagnostic Tests
Weight-bearing AP and lateral radiographs of the foot should be obtained to assess metatarsal and toe alignment.

## Differential Diagnosis
Claw toe-related pain (plantar displacement of the metatarsal heads and fat pad noted on physical examination)

Interdigital neuroma (numbness in the involved web space)

Intractable plantar keratosis (persistent callus on sole of foot)

Metatarsal stress fracture (localized tenderness over the fracture site, radiographic findings)

MTP synovitis (swelling of the joint, dorsal tenderness)

Plantar wart (tender with circumferential pressure)

## ADVERSE OUTCOMES OF THE DISEASE

Patients may experience progressive pain and difficulty walking.

## TREATMENT

Accommodative shoes, a metatarsal pad (see Application of a Metatarsal Pad, p 605), or an orthotic device is the key to treatment. A thickened callus can be shaved (see Corns and Calluses, pp 610-612, and Trimming a Corn or Callus, p 613). Nonsurgical treatment usually is successful, but if these measures fail, surgery to realign the toes and/or metatarsal head may be considered. Removal of the metatarsal head should be avoided.

## ADVERSE OUTCOMES OF TREATMENT

Inadequate pain relief, delayed union, nonunion, and transfer lesions (stress with resultant pain transferred to the adjacent metatarsal) are possible complications of surgical treatment.

## REFERRAL DECISIONS/RED FLAGS

Symptoms that persist despite nonsurgical care indicate the need for further evaluation.

SECTION 7 ■ FOOT AND ANKLE

# NAIL FUNGUS INFECTION

**ICD-9 Code**

**110.1**
Dermatophytosis, of nail

## SYNONYMS

Dermatophytic onychomycosis

Tinea ungulum

## DEFINITION

Fungal infection of the nail (onychomycosis) occurs four times more frequently in the toes than in the fingers. *Trichophyton rubrum* and *T mentagrophytes* cause 90% of the infections. Approximately 50% of patients are older than 70 years. The problem may be primarily cosmetic, or the nail may become so hypertrophic that it interferes with shoe wear and is painful.

## CLINICAL SYMPTOMS

Patients report discoloration, thickening, and difficulty in trimming the nails.

## TESTS

### *Physical Examination*

Thickening and chalky yellow or white discoloration of the nail is observed (**Figure 1**).

### *Diagnostic Tests*

Diagnosis is made by microscopic examination of nail scrapings and potassium hydroxide slide preparation.

## DIFFERENTIAL DIAGNOSIS

Onychogryphosis (severe nail deformity, curling at the edge of the nail)

Repetitive trauma (ridges and cracking of the nail with thickening)

## ADVERSE OUTCOMES OF THE DISEASE

A thickened nail can make shoe wear difficult.

## TREATMENT

Treatment options include observation with periodic trimming of the thickened nail, removal of the nail, and/or medications. Topical medications are less effective than oral agents because topical medications cannot penetrate the thickened nail. Recently developed oral agents such as itraconazole,

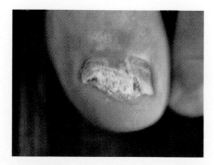

**Figure 1**
Toenail with fungal infection.

fluconazole, ketoconazole, and terbinafine have been shown to be effective in the treatment of onychomycosis. For example, itraconazole 200 mg per day given continuously or as a pulse dose (200 mg twice daily for 1 week per month for 3 consecutive months) has been reported to achieve a mycologic cure of 64% at 12 months, with 88% of patients showing marked improvement.

## ADVERSE OUTCOMES OF TREATMENT

Oral therapy is costly and may elevate hepatic enzyme levels. These levels should be tested periodically (especially in patients with a history of hepatic dysfunction). Rare cases of hepatobiliary dysfunction have been reported.

SECTION 7 ■ FOOT AND ANKLE

# ORTHOTIC DEVICES

## DEFINITION

Proper shoe fit, shoe modifications, inserts, pads, and orthoses can significantly relieve symptoms caused by common foot problems. An orthosis can support an area of collapse, cushion an area of pressure, accommodate fixed deformity, limit motion, equalize limb length, and reduce shear of the foot in the shoe. The appropriate use of shoe orthoses, commonly referred to as "orthotics," depends on an adequate physical examination and a basic understanding of foot alignment and functions.

## FOOT TYPES AND FUNCTIONS

During gait, the normal foot changes from a supple, shock-absorbing structure to a rigid lever for push-off. At heel strike, the foot is supple, allowing shock absorption and accommodations to uneven ground. During midstance, the foot is converted to a rigid lever that supports full body weight while allowing continued progression of the limb (rollover).

A cavus (highly arched) foot is rigid, cannot unlock during early stance, and lacks shock absorption. A pes planus (flatfoot) foot is extremely supple and often does not effectively supinate to form a rigid lever for push-off.

Many types of simple orthotic devices can be dispensed directly from the physician's office or are available at drugstores, sporting goods stores, and shoe stores. Custom orthoses are used for more complex problems or after off-the-shelf devices fail to correct the problem (**Figure 1**).

## TYPES OF ORTHOTIC DEVICES

### *Pads/Inserts*

1. Full-contact (full-length) insert: A prefabricated rubber or silicone insert that reduces shock by absorbing normal and shear forces.

2. Full-contact orthosis: An orthosis that is molded to the shape of the patient's foot. These are often posted with a wedge that redistributes weight to improve foot alignment and biomechanics, accommodate a deformity, and/or cushion the foot.

3. Soft orthosis: An orthosis that is used primarily for cushioning but offers little control of foot motion.

4. Semirigid orthosis: The most common type of orthosis; it provides reasonable strength and durability and is made to help control alignment of the foot during gait.

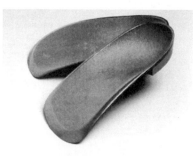

**Figure 1**

Custom orthoses.

Reproduced with permission from Prolab, San Francisco, CA.

5. Rigid orthosis: An orthosis that offers maximum durability and support but requires a precise fit because it provides little flexibility.

6. Heel insert (eg, felt, foam, gel, rubber, or silicone): Prefabricated, shock-absorbing device available over the counter (**Figure 2**).

7. Heel wedge: A device that is tapered to support varus or valgus hindfoot.

8. Scaphoid pad (arch cookie): A medial longitudinal arch pad that provides support for a flatfoot.

9. Metatarsal pad: A pad that is fixed to an insert or the bottom of the shoe (**Figure 3**).

10. Toe crest: An insert that elevates a toe to relieve pressure at the tip (for mallet toe).

11. Toe separator: A pad that is placed between toes to decrease friction. It is used for calluses and corns.

12. UCBL (University of California Biomechanics Laboratory) orthosis: A type of full-contact orthosis that stabilizes the hindfoot by using medial and lateral vertical supports. Custom molded by a certified pedorthotist, this is used for subtalar arthrosis, midfoot plantar fasciitis, or a moderate pes planovalgus foot (**Figure 4**).

## *Shoes/Modifications*

1. Extra-depth shoe: A shoe with increased depth that accommodates forefoot problems, such as a hammer toe, and allows room for inserts.

2. Shoe lift: A device that partially or fully corrects limb-length discrepancy. Typically, ¼″ of lift can be accommodated inside the shoe. Any elevation of ½″ or more must be added to the outside of the shoe.

3. Metatarsal bar: An internal or external transverse bar that unloads the forefoot (for metatarsalgia).

4. Rocker bottom sole: Sole of shoe that is contoured to simulate the rollover phase of gait and therefore reduce forces on the plantar surface of the foot during walking (**Figure 5**).

5. Solid Ankle–Cushion Heel (SACH): Soft material that replaces the posterior portion of the shoe's heel to reduce shock at heel strike.

6. Running shoes: Shoes that are designed for shock absorbency. Typically, 50% of shock absorbency is lost at 300 to 500 miles, so running shoes should be replaced at least every 6 months.

7. Shoe fit: Measure the foot by tracing the width of the forefoot while standing barefoot. The forefoot width of the shoe should be wider than this measurement. The end of the longest toe should be about ½″ from the end of the shoe.

8. Thomas heel: Medial extension of the heel to support flatfoot.

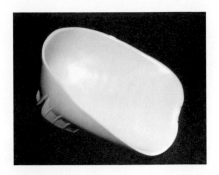

**Figure 2**
Heel insert.

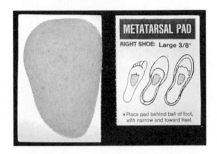

**Figure 3**
Metatarsal pad.
Reproduced with permission from Hapad, Inc, Bethel Park, PA.

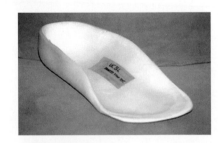

**Figure 4**
UCBL orthosis.

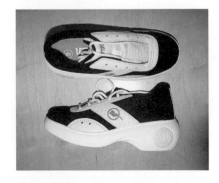

**Figure 5**
Over-the-counter shoe with rocker bottom sole.

SECTION 7 ■ FOOT AND ANKLE

# APPLICATION OF ORTHOTIC DEVICES AND SHOE MODIFICATIONS

**Table 1** lists the types of orthotic therapy recommended for specific foot conditions.

### Table 1   Recommended Orthotic Treatment for Specific Diagnoses

| Diagnosis | Orthotic Therapy |
|---|---|
| Bunions and/or bunionettes | Wide toe box, stretch shoes, soft seamless uppers, "bunion shield" type pad |
| Cavus foot (rigid) | Soft orthotic cushions to distribute pressures evenly |
| Flatfoot (adult) | Asymptomatic: No special orthotic or shoe treatment indicated |
|  | Symptomatic: Semiflexible insert or longitudinal arch pad, medial heel wedge, extended medial heel counter |
| Flatfoot (child) | No special orthotic or shoe treatment indicated; normal in infancy, with more than 97% correcting spontaneously |
| Hallux rigidus | Full-length prefabricated stiff insert, Morton extension inlay, rocker bottom sole, stiff (stable) midsole |
| Hammer toe or claw toe | Accommodative shoe wear, toe crest |
| Interdigital (Morton) neuroma | Wide toe box, metatarsal pad with neuroma positioning |
| Metatarsalgia | Wide shoes, metatarsal pads, metatarsal bars, or rocker bottom sole; wide toe box, metatarsal pad with neuroma positioning |
| Neuropathic ulceration | Full-contact cushioned orthosis, extra-depth or custom shoes, rocker bottom sole to unload forefoot |
| Plantar fasciitis | Prefabricated heel insert (silicone, rubber, or felt) |
| Runner's painful knee | Full-length, soft, prefabricated (decreases pronation and stress) medial longitudinal arch support |

# Plantar Fasciitis

## Synonyms

Heel pain syndrome
Heel spur
Plantar heel pain

**ICD-9 Code**
**728.71**
Plantar fascial fibromatosis

## Definition

The plantar fascia arises from the medial tuberosity of the calcaneus and extends to the proximal phalanges of the toes (**Figure 1**). The plantar fascia provides support to the foot, and as the toes extend during the stance phase of gait, the plantar fascia is tightened by a windlass mechanism, resulting in elevation of the longitudinal arch, inversion of the hindfoot, and a resultant external rotation of the leg.

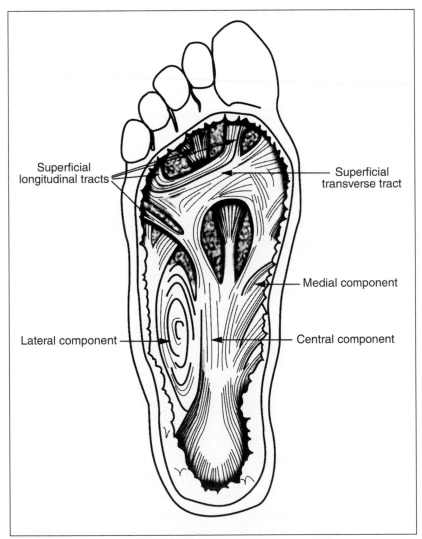

Superficial longitudinal tracts

Superficial transverse tract

Medial component

Lateral component

Central component

**Figure 1**
Anatomy of the plantar fascia.

Plantar fasciitis is the most common cause of heel pain in adults. The etiology is probably a degenerative tear of part of the fascial origin from the calcaneus, followed by a tendinosis-type reaction. Chronic degenerative changes in the fibers of the plantar fascia are the predominant histologic finding. Plantar fasciitis affects women twice as often as men and is more common in overweight persons. It is not associated with a particular foot type.

## CLINICAL SYMPTOMS

Onset of symptoms is usually insidious and not related to a fall or twisting injury. Patients report focal pain and tenderness directly over the medial calcaneal tuberosity and 1 to 2 cm distally along the plantar fascia. Pain is usually most intense when the patient rises from a resting position, especially in the morning. This occurs because the foot is usually in plantar flexion during rest and the first few steps stretch the plantar fascia. Prolonged standing and walking also increase the pain. Sitting typically relieves symptoms.

## TESTS

### Physical Examination

Examination reveals tenderness directly over the plantar medial calcaneal tuberosity and 1 to 2 cm distally along the plantar fascia. Often, considerable pressure must be applied to this area during the examination to reproduce weight-bearing stress and the patient's symptoms. Patients may have tightness in the Achilles tendon. Passive dorsiflexion of the toes (windlass mechanism) may cause increased pain.

### Diagnostic Tests

Radiographs are not necessary as part of the initial evaluation if the patient's history and examination are consistent with a diagnosis of plantar fasciitis. Weight-bearing lateral radiographs should be obtained before an injection of corticosteroid or for patients who continue to have symptoms after 6 to 8 weeks of nonsurgical treatment. Weight-bearing lateral radiographs also may be indicated for patients with systemic symptoms or pain at rest.

A heel spur (osteophyte) develops in the origin of the flexor brevis muscle just superior to the plantar fascia in approximately 50% of patients with plantar fasciitis (**Figure 2**). However, the spur is not a source of pain and is present in 20% of similar-age adults who do not have plantar fasciitis.

Although not necessary for diagnosis, a bone scan may show increased uptake at the medial calcaneal tuberosity. MRI, which

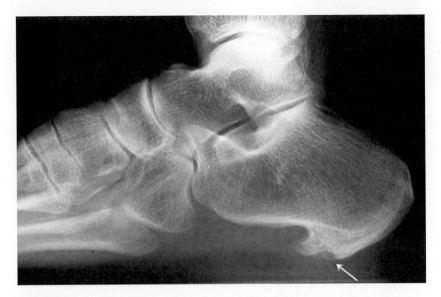

**Figure 2**
Radiographic appearance of a plantar heel spur (arrow).

also is not necessary for diagnosis or treatment, will often show thickening of the origin of the plantar fascia, as well as marrow edema in the calcaneal tuberosity.

# DIFFERENTIAL DIAGNOSIS

Acute traumatic rupture of the plantar fascia (ecchymosis, tenderness, swelling over the proximal plantar fascia)

Calcaneal stress fracture (rare, tenderness with medial and lateral pressure of the calcaneus)

Calcaneal tumor (rare, pain at rest, night pain)

Fat pad atrophy/contusion (tenderness over an abnormally prominent calcaneal tuberosity)

Sciatica (radicular symptoms)

Seronegative spondyloarthropathy (typically bilateral enthesitis of the plantar fascia, other sites of enthesitis, arthralgic joints involved)

Tarsal tunnel syndrome (paresthesias and numbness on the plantar aspect of the foot)

# ADVERSE OUTCOMES OF THE DISEASE

Patients may experience chronic heel pain and a significant alteration in daily activities. Altered gait may aggravate forefoot, knee, hip, or back problems.

# TREATMENT

More than 95% of patients with plantar fasciitis can be managed satisfactorily with nonsurgical treatment. Patients should be informed that it commonly takes 6 to 12 months for

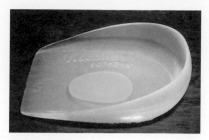

**Figure 3**
Orthotic heel pad.

symptoms to resolve. Avid walkers and joggers should be counseled concerning alternative exercise regimens, such as use of a stationary bike.

Initial treatment should include an over-the-counter orthotic device, such as a silicone, rubber, or felt heel pad (**Figure 3**), along with a home program of stretching exercises. To stretch the Achilles tendon, the patient should lean forward against a wall with the affected leg straight and the other leg slightly bent. As the patient lowers the hips toward the wall, he or she should feel the calf muscles stretch. The stretch should be held for 30 seconds. Patients should perform the exercise 4 times, 2 to 3 times each day.

Some studies suggest that a night splint should be used as part of initial treatment if the patient experiences increased pain on rising from a resting position in the morning. The night splint holds the ankle and foot in slight extension, which maintains the Achilles tendon and plantar fascia in a stretched position during sleep.

Contrast baths, ice, NSAIDs, and/or shoes with shock-absorbing soles also can be used to decrease inflammation in the painful heel.

If symptoms persist despite attempts at conservative management, injection of corticosteroid into the heel may be indicated (see Plantar Fasciitis Injection, pp 673-674). A formal physical therapy consultation may be necessary to help direct the patient's continued stretching program.

If symptoms persist, the use of a nonremovable cast or custom orthotic device should be considered. Surgical treatment typically consists of partial release of the plantar fascia.

## PHYSICAL THERAPY PRESCRIPTION

Early rehabilitation is directed at controlling pain and increasing the range of motion of the ankle. Heel cord stretching is an important part of a home exercise program (see p 672). Use of a night brace and limited weight bearing are also important. If the symptoms do not respond to these measures, formal physical therapy may be ordered. The prescription should include evaluation of the foot and ankle mechanics during gait. If overpronation is present, the use of foot orthotics may result in significant improvement. Continued stretching and pain-relieving modalities such as iontophoresis or laser therapy may be ordered.

## ADVERSE OUTCOMES OF TREATMENT

NSAIDs may cause gastric, renal, or hepatic complications. Fat pad necrosis or rupture of the plantar fascia may develop from improper injection of corticosteroids. Surgical treatment may

not improve symptoms and also may cause complete disruption
of the plantar fascia.

## REFERRAL DECISIONS/RED FLAGS

Patients whose symptoms do not respond to nonsurgical
treatment need further evaluation. Surgical release should be
considered only after 6 to 12 months of intense nonsurgical
management. Preliminary data indicate that radial or focal
shock wave treatment may be a good treatment option in some
patients whose symptoms do not respond to nonsurgical
treatment.

SECTION 7 ■ FOOT AND ANKLE

# HOME EXERCISE PROGRAM FOR PLANTAR FASCIITIS

Apply moist or dry heat to the painful area of the foot during the exercise. To prevent inflammation, apply a bag of crushed ice or frozen peas to the heel for 20 minutes after performing the exercise. You should not experience pain with the exercise. If you are unable to perform the exercise because of pain or stiffness or if your symptoms do not improve after performing the exercise for 3 to 4 weeks, call your doctor.

| Exercise | Muscle Group | Number of Repetitions/Sets | Number of Days per Week | Number of Weeks |
|---|---|---|---|---|
| Heel cord stretch | Gastrocnemius-soleus complex | 4 repetitions/2 or 3 sets | Daily | 3 to 4 |

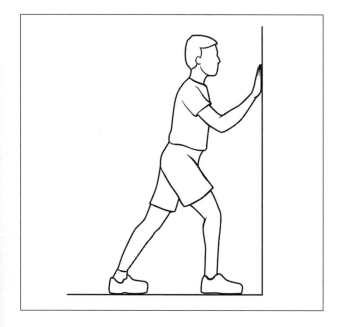

## Heel Cord Stretch

Stand facing a wall with the knee of the unaffected limb bent, the affected limb straight, and the toes pointed in slightly. Keeping the heels of both feet flat on the floor, lower your hips toward the wall. Hold the stretch for 30 seconds and then relax for 30 seconds. Repeat 4 times. Perform this exercise daily, 2 or 3 times a day.

# PROCEDURE

## PLANTAR FASCIITIS INJECTION

### STEP 1

Wear protective gloves at all times during the procedure and use sterile technique.

### STEP 2

Use the 18-gauge needle to draw 1 mL of 40 mg/mL corticosteroid preparation and 4 mL of the local anesthetic into the syringe, then switch to the 21-gauge needle to preserve sterility.

### STEP 3

Prepare the medial aspect of the heel.

### STEP 4

Spray ethyl chloride onto the heel to freeze the skin.

### STEP 5

Measure the soft-tissue thickness beneath the calcaneus directly on the radiograph.

### STEP 6

Using the measurement from the radiograph as a guide, palpate the calcaneus medially where it begins to curve upward. Insert the 21-gauge needle into this area, which is approximately 2 cm from the plantar surface of the foot (**Figure 1**).

**CPT Code**

**20550**

Injection(s); single tendon sheath, or ligament, aponeurosis (eg, plantar "fascia")

*Current Procedural Terminology* © 2004 American Medical Association. All Rights Reserved.

### MATERIALS

Sterile gloves

Bactericidal skin preparation solution

Ethyl chloride spray

Lateral radiograph of the heel

5-mL syringe

18-gauge needle

21-gauge, 1- to 1½″ needle

Mixture of 1 mL of 10 to 40 mg/mL of corticosteroid preparation and 4 mL of 1% lidocaine, without epinephrine

Adhesive dressing

**SECTION 7 ■ FOOT AND ANKLE**

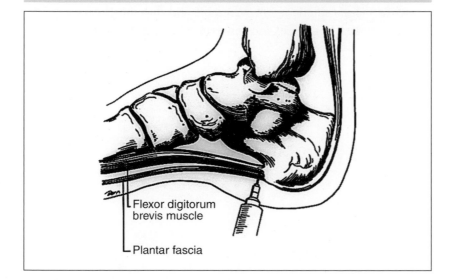

Flexor digitorum brevis muscle

Plantar fascia

**Figure 1**
Proper location for injection for plantar fasciitis.

## Step 7

Advance the needle down to the calcaneus until it hits the bone. Walk the tip of the needle distally along the bone to the plantar surface of the calcaneus. The needle should be immediately superior (deep) to the plantar fascia.

## Step 8

Advance the needle to its hilt and inject 3 mL of the anesthetic-corticosteroid mixture. Inject the remaining 2 mL of the preparation while withdrawing the needle 2 cm, then withdraw the needle completely. Make certain that you do not inject the anesthetic-corticosteroid preparation into the medial subcutaneous tissue or the fat pad of the heel that is superficial to the plantar fascia.

## Step 9

Dress the puncture wound with a sterile adhesive bandage.

## Adverse Outcomes

Injection of a corticosteroid into the superficial fat pad may cause fat necrosis, with loss of cushioning of the plantar heel. The injection may cause rupture of the plantar fascia.

## Aftercare/Patient Instructions

Advise the patient that transient numbness of the heel may occur. Also explain that heel pain might return in a few hours when the anesthetic agent wears off and that the corticosteroid might take a few weeks to have an effect on the symptoms.

# PLANTAR WARTS

## SYNONYM
Verruca vulgaris

## DEFINITION
Plantar warts are hyperkeratotic lesions on the sole of the foot caused by human papillomavirus. The peak incidence is in the second decade of life. Plantar warts are more commonly observed in athletic youngsters.

## CLINICAL SYMPTOMS
Patients have painful, slightly raised lesions on the sole of the foot. These lesions may occur in clusters known as "mosaic warts."

## TESTS

### Physical Examination
Warts usually appear on non–weight-bearing areas on the sole of the foot. Normal papillary lines of the skin (fingerprint pattern) cease at the margin of the lesion (**Figure 1**). The lesions usually are very tender if pinched side to side, a finding not observed with a corn or callus. By contrast, a corn is tender with direct pressure. A plantar wart may occur anywhere on the sole, whereas a callus is associated with a bony prominence. Superficial paring of a wart with a scalpel reveals punctate hemorrhage and a fibrillated texture. A callus is avascular and on paring has a uniform texture that resembles yellow candle wax.

### Diagnostic Tests
When doubt exists, histopathologic examination of a specimen confirms the diagnosis. However, this type of testing is seldom necessary, given the characteristic gross appearance after superficial paring.

## DIFFERENTIAL DIAGNOSIS
Callus (hyperkeratotic lesion that forms in response to a bony prominence)

Foreign body (history and examination)

Plantar fibromatosis (location beneath the skin)

**ICD-9 Code**
**078.19**
Viral warts, unspecified; other specified viral warts

SECTION 7 ■ FOOT AND ANKLE

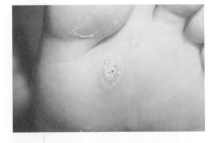

**Figure 1**
Clinical appearance of a plantar wart.
**Reproduced with permission from California Pacific Medical Center, San Francisco, CA.**

## ADVERSE OUTCOMES OF THE DISEASE

Plantar warts are often persistent; they can spread to other areas of the foot, grow larger, and leave scars on the sole of the foot.

## TREATMENT

Most lesions resolve spontaneously within 5 to 6 months, so aggressive treatment should be reserved for unusually large, painful, or persistent lesions. Initial treatment commonly includes superficial paring, followed by the use of a keratolytic agent, such as salicylic acid in liquid or salve form. The lesion should then be covered with occlusive tape to ensure that the medication stays within the desired area and débrides the necrotic layers of tissue upon removal of the tape. Medication should be applied twice daily for 1 month.

Warts that are resistant to initial treatment will sometimes respond to intralesional injection of approximately 1 mL of local anesthetic with epinephrine. Electrocautery, cryotherapy with liquid nitrogen, laser ablation, or curettage may be performed under local anesthetic. Care should be taken to avoid causing necrosis of the deep dermis, which may produce intractable, painful scarring on the sole of the foot. In curettage, for example, the subcutaneous fat should not be visible when the procedure is finished. Intralesional injections of bleomycin and radiation therapy also have been described for severe, recalcitrant lesions, but these options are best performed by specialists with experience in their use.

## ADVERSE OUTCOMES OF TREATMENT

Secondary infection may occur after treatment. Intractable scarring from excessively deep ablation is also a significant risk.

## REFERRAL DECISIONS/RED FLAGS

Persistent or recurring warts warrant further evaluation.

# POSTERIOR HEEL PAIN

## SYNONYMS
Achilles tendinosis
Haglund syndrome
Insertional Achilles tendinitis
Pump bump

**ICD-9 Code**
**726.71**
Achilles bursitis or tendinitis

## DEFINITION
Pain in the posterior heel around the insertion of the Achilles tendon may originate from one or more of the following structures: the insertion of the Achilles tendon onto the calcaneus (insertional Achilles tendinosis); the retrocalcaneal bursa (retrocalcaneal bursitis); a prominent process of the calcaneus impinging on the retrocalcaneal bursae and/or Achilles tendon (Haglund syndrome); or inflammation of the bursa between the skin and the Achilles tendon (pre-Achilles bursitis). The exact etiology may be confusing because frequently more than one of these areas is involved (**Figure 1**).

## CLINICAL SYMPTOMS
Patients with a prominent process of the calcaneus initially develop a bursa that is irritated by shoe wear and causes a pump bump (**Figure 2**). In older patients, insertional tendinosis with enthesopathy, calcification, and degenerative tears of the Achilles tendon are most often seen. A limp and pain with

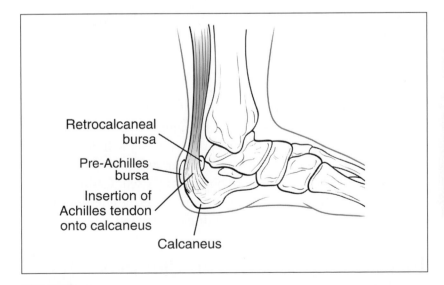

**Figure 1**
Sites of posterior heel pain.

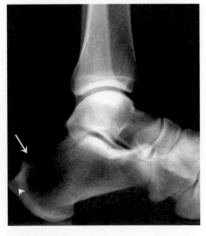

**Figure 2**
Prominent superior process of calcaneus (white arrow) with calcification of tendon (white arrowhead).

SECTION 7 ■ FOOT AND ANKLE

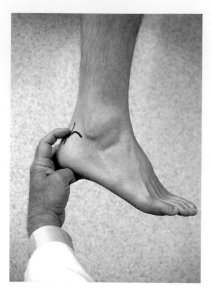

**Figure 3**
Pain on palpation on either side of the retrocalcaneal bursa, anterior to the Achilles tendon insertion, is indicative of retrocalcaneal bursitis.

start-up or activity are common. Shoe wear may be difficult because of the direct pressure on the posterior heel prominence.

# TESTS

## Physical Examination

Examination reveals swelling and tenderness at the posterior heel. If a calcaneal prominence is present, it is usually larger on the lateral side of the heel. A superficial bursa (pump bump) may be present and may be inflamed by shoe wear.

If Achilles tendinosis is present, pain is present directly over the Achilles tendon and is increased by squeezing the tendon. The tendon may be thickened and have a nodule. Retrocalcaneal bursitis can cause pain anterior to the Achilles tendon that is increased by squeezing the bursa from side to side and just anterior to the Achilles tendon (**Figure 3**).

## Diagnostic Tests

Lateral radiographs of the heel may show calcification of the Achilles tendon and spur formation. A prominent posterosuperior process of the calcaneus also might be apparent.

# DIFFERENTIAL DIAGNOSIS

Achilles tendon avulsion (palpable defect in the tendon, positive Thompson test)

Os trigonum syndrome (posterolateral pain increased with forced dorsiflexion)

Plantar fasciitis (pain below the calcaneus)

Stress fracture of the calcaneus (midcalcaneal bony tenderness)

# ADVERSE OUTCOMES OF THE DISEASE

Difficulty with shoe wear and sports activities may result, as well as chronic pain and limping.

# TREATMENT

A heel lift or open-back shoes will minimize pressure on the inflamed area. Ice massage and contrast baths will decrease inflammation. Achilles tendon stretching exercises should be started after the inflammatory phase has passed. Casting for 4 to 6 weeks may alleviate symptoms. Surgical intervention will remove the prominent bone and diseased tendon.

# PHYSICAL THERAPY PRESCRIPTION

A home exercise program of heel cord stretching with the toe pointing in and the knee bent (see p 680) will isolate and stretch the soleus muscle. A heel lift in the shoe may be helpful in resting the tendon. If these measures are not successful, formal physical therapy may be ordered. The prescription should include a biomechanical evaluation of the foot and ankle during ambulation. If overpronation is present, foot orthotics may be very helpful in relieving the symptoms. In addition, pain-relieving modalities such as phonophoresis, ice, or laser therapy may be ordered.

## ADVERSE OUTCOMES OF TREATMENT

Surgical removal of bone and débridement of the Achilles tendon may predispose the tendon to rupture.

## REFERRAL DECISIONS/RED FLAGS

Recalcitrant pain or failure to respond to nonsurgical management indicates the need for further evaluation.

SECTION 7 ■ FOOT AND ANKLE

# Home Exercise Program for Posterior Heel Pain

Apply moist or dry heat to the heel while exercising, and to prevent inflammation, apply a bag of crushed ice or frozen peas to the heel for 20 minutes after performing the exercise. You should not experience pain with the exercise. If your symptoms do not improve after performing the exercise for 3 to 4 weeks, call your doctor.

| Exercise | Muscle Group | Number of Repetitions/Sets | Number of Days per Week | Number of Weeks |
|---|---|---|---|---|
| Heel cord stretch with knee bent | Soleus | 4 repetitions/2 or 3 sets | Daily | 3 to 4 |

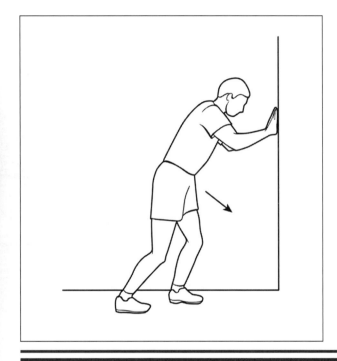

## Heel Cord Stretch With Knee Bent

Stand facing a wall with the unaffected limb in front and with the knee bent for support, the affected limb in back and with the knee also bent, and the toes pointed in slightly. Keeping the heels of both feet flat on the floor, lower your hips toward the wall. Hold the stretch for 30 seconds and then relax for 30 seconds. Perform 2 or 3 sets of 4 repetitions daily.

# POSTERIOR TIBIAL TENDON DYSFUNCTION

**ICD-9 Code**
**726.72**
Posterior tibial tendinitis

## SYNONYMS

Acquired flatfoot
Posterior tibial tendon insufficiency
Posterior tibial tendon rupture

## DEFINITION

The posterior tibial tendon is one of the main supporting structures of the medial ankle and arch. Posterior tibial tendon dysfunction is the primary cause of medial ankle pain in the middle-aged patient. Demographically, the classic presentation is an overweight woman over 55 years of age. Steroid injections, diabetes mellitus, hypertension, and/or previous injury to the foot are other risk factors. The posterior tibial tendon is thickened and shows degenerative changes. As a result, the posterior tibialis muscle is ineffective and its function of supporting the medial longitudinal arch is lost. As a result, a flatfoot develops. Initially the foot is flexible, but over time the deformity becomes fixed and arthritic changes may occur in the hindfoot.

## CLINICAL SYMPTOMS

Pain and swelling on the medial aspect of the ankle are the most common symptoms. Usually patients state that they have lost the arch and that the ankle rolls in. The onset of symptoms is insidious, and there is usually no history of trauma. Although pain and tenderness initially occur along the medial aspect of the foot, lateral pain ultimately develops as the collapsed flatfoot abuts the fibula or causes impingement in the sinus tarsi.

## TESTS

### Physical Examination

Both feet should be examined from the knee down with the patient standing. Examination shows swelling and tenderness posterior and inferior to the medial malleolus, along the course of the posterior tibial tendon. The medial arch is decreased or completely flattened. The heel shows increased valgus, and with advanced changes, the forefoot is in abduction. When viewed from behind, more than two toes will be visible on the affected foot (the "too many toes" sign) because of the forefoot abduction and hindfoot

SECTION 7 ■ FOOT AND ANKLE

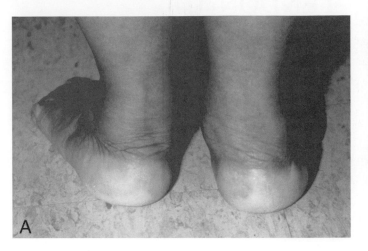
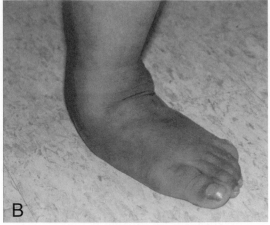

**Figure 1**

**A,** "Too many toes" sign in the left foot, caused by forefoot abduction and hindfoot valgus typical of posterior tibial tendon dysfunction. **B,** Patient is unable to rise up on the toes of the affected foot.

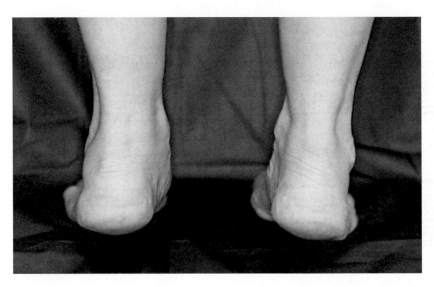

**Figure 2**

In this patient with posterior tibial tendon dysfunction of the left foot, the left heel does not rotate inward (varus) when the patient stands on her toes.

valgus (**Figure 1, A**). Also, the patient will not be able to rise on the toes of the affected foot (**Figure 1, B**).

Posterior tibial tendon strength is decreased on both manual muscle testing as well as functional maneuvers. Normally a patient with both hands placed on a wall can perform a toe rise on one leg, and during this maneuver, the posterior tibial tendon will pull the heel into inversion. Patients with dysfunction or rupture of the posterior tibial tendon cannot perform a complete heel rise on the affected leg, and when this test is performed while standing on both legs, normal inversion of the heel does not occur (**Figure 2**).

## *Diagnostic Tests*

Weight-bearing AP and lateral radiographs of the foot reveal a flatfoot, with alignment changes at the talonavicular and other joints. MRI of the posterior tibial tendon may be useful in equivocal situations.

# Differential Diagnosis

Congenital pes planus (bilateral, present since childhood)

Lisfranc fracture-dislocation (history of trauma, pain in the midfoot)

Medial ankle laxity (rare, abnormal ankle radiographs)

Medial malleolus stress fracture (focal bony tenderness)

Tarsal coalition (fixed deformity, onset as adolescent or young adult)

# Adverse Outcomes of the Disease

A progressive, painful flatfoot with gait disturbance is common. A severe flatfoot makes shoe wear or even bracing difficult.

# Treatment

Tenosynovitis of the tendon without a flatfoot should be treated with a short leg cast or cast brace for 4 weeks, NSAIDs, and activity limitation. After the cast is removed, a molded ankle-foot orthosis may be used as the tendinitis resolves. A custom orthotic device with a medial longitudinal arch support and medial internal heel wedge is often recommended to help decrease the excursion of the tendon. An injection of corticosteroid may weaken the already pathologic tendon and is not recommended. When nonsurgical treatment fails, surgical débridement of the tendon may be indicated.

If a flexible flatfoot develops, use of a custom orthotic device or ankle brace should be continued. A UCBL (University of California Biomechanics Laboratory) orthotic insert can also be effective. Often surgery is required. If the deformity is flexible, a tendon transfer combined with a realignment osteotomy is usually recommended. However, once a rigid flatfoot develops, stabilization of the hindfoot by arthrodesis is the better alternative.

# Adverse Outcomes of Treatment

Tendon transfer surgery may fail, requiring an arthrodesis of the hindfoot.

Section 7 ■ Foot and Ankle

## REFERRAL DECISIONS/RED FLAGS

Patients with unexplained medial ankle pain require further evaluation because a medial ankle sprain is rare and therefore other, more serious, conditions must be considered. Patients with a recent onset of flatfoot deformity also require further evaluation.

# Rheumatoid Foot And Ankle

## Definition

Ninety percent of patients with rheumatoid arthritis are estimated to have symptoms that are related to the foot or ankle. The presence and severity of symptoms correlates with the longevity of the disease. Ninety percent of patients report symptoms in the forefoot and midfoot, and 67% report symptoms in the ankle and hindfoot. Chronic synovitis leads to stretching of the capsule and ligaments of the joints with subsequent malalignment of the joints, and ultimately to structural deformities such as hallux valgus, claw toes with subluxated or dislocated metatarsophalangeal (MTP) joints, and end-stage arthritis of the ankle or subtalar joint.

## Clinical Symptoms

Patients present with loss of motion and pain on weight bearing. Metatarsalgia commonly occurs with subluxation/ dislocation of the lesser toe MTP joints, claw toes, and distal migration of the fat pad (**Figure 1**). Severe hallux valgus often accompanies lesser toe deformities (**Figure 2**).

In the hindfoot, tenosynovitis of the posterior tibial tendon may produce medial ankle pain and swelling. Early arthritis of the talonavicular or subtalar joint also is common and typically occurs before ankle involvement.

The ankle is usually one of the last joints to be involved in rheumatoid arthritis.

## Tests

### Physical Examination

MTP synovitis, with focal pain and swelling over the MTP joints, may be the presenting symptom in patients with rheumatoid arthritis. Bilateral symptoms, multiple joint involvement, and the presence of nodules should lead to clinical suspicion of rheumatoid arthritis.

### Diagnostic Tests

Laboratory tests reveal an elevated erythrocyte sedimentation rate and positive rheumatoid factor. Radiographs reveal soft-tissue swelling, osteopenia, subchondral erosions, and malalignment. Lateral drift occurs at the MTP joints and at the talonavicular joint (**Figure 3**).

**ICD-9 Code**

**714.0**
Rheumatoid arthritis

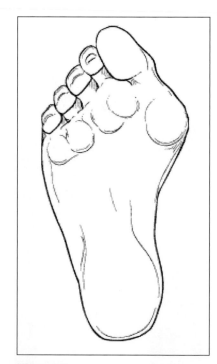

**Figure 1**
Metatarsalgia develops as the fat pad is pulled distally and the metatarsal heads become more prominent.

SECTION 7 ■ FOOT AND ANKLE

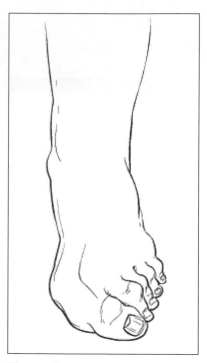

**Figure 2**

Hallux valgus and lesser toe deformities are associated with rheumatoid arthritis.

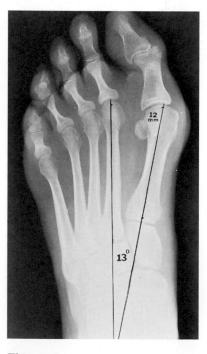

**Figure 3**

AP radiograph of foot showing severe hallux valgus.

# DIFFERENTIAL DIAGNOSIS

Posterior tibial tendon dysfunction (swelling and tenderness over the posterior tibial tendon)

Seronegative spondyloarthropathies (enthesitis present on physical examination with pain at the insertion sites of the plantar fascia and Achilles tendon)

Traumatic arthritis (history of preceding trauma)

# ADVERSE OUTCOMES OF THE DISEASE

Pain, progressive deformity, and metatarsalgia with plantar ulcerations are common if the condition remains untreated.

# TREATMENT

Medical management can improve symptoms and slow the progression of disease. Disease-modifying agents (such as methotrexate) have been shown to decrease synovitis and slow progression of the disease. Corticosteroid injections may be helpful for inflamed joints and significant tenosynovitis.

An extra-depth accommodative shoe with a molded insole and rocker bottom sole often relieves metatarsalgia. A UCBL (University of California Biomechanics Laboratory) orthosis may provide significant pain relief for a patient who has a flexible hindfoot deformity. A molded ankle-foot orthosis may be used for more extensive disease involvement. (See Orthotic Devices, pp 664-666, for a discussion of various orthoses.)

The most reliable surgery for forefoot deformity involves fusion of the first MTP joint with metatarsal head resections. Implant arthroplasty of the great toe is rarely indicated.

Tenosynovectomy is only a temporizing procedure and is rarely indicated. Most patients with severe arthritis of the hindfoot joints require arthrodesis of the talocalcaneal, talonavicular, and/or calcaneocuboid joints. Patients still have dorsiflexion and plantar flexion through the ankle joint after a hindfoot arthrodesis.

Significant ankle arthritis may require arthrodesis. Patients with rheumatoid arthritis who have severe ankle destruction often have subtalar joint involvement. Injections into the joints may help determine which is more symptomatic. When both joints are involved, a pantalar (tibiotalocalcaneal) fusion should be performed. Although new results are encouraging, total ankle replacement in patients with rheumatoid arthritis remains investigational.

## ADVERSE OUTCOMES OF TREATMENT

Foot deformities may progress even with optimal medical management.

## REFERRAL DECISION/RED FLAGS

Persistent pain despite medical management signals the need for further evaluation.

SECTION 7 ■ FOOT AND ANKLE

# SESAMOIDITIS

## SYNONYM
Dancer's toe

## DEFINITION
The sesamoid bones are embedded in the flexor hallucis brevis tendon beneath the first metatarsal head (plantar surface) (**Figure 1**). Although less common, sesamoids under any of the metatarsal heads may occur. Sesamoid disorders include inflammation, fracture, and arthritis. Sesamoiditis occurs from repeated stress of the sesamoid and the subsequent inflammation.

## CLINICAL SYMPTOMS
Pain under the first metatarsal head is noted, with or without swelling and ecchymosis. The usual stresses involve dancing or running, but sesamoiditis also can be caused by trauma from falls or more commonly by forced dorsiflexion of the great toe with acute onset of pain.

## TESTS

### Physical Examination
With both sesamoiditis and sesamoid fractures, examination reveals focal tenderness at the sesamoid bone directly beneath the metatarsal head. The tender spot will move with the sesamoid as the great toe is flexed and extended. Dorsiflexion of the toe is painful, and range of motion may be restricted.

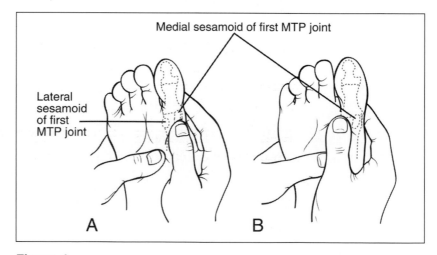

**Figure 1**
**A,** Location of the medial sesamoid. **B,** Location of the lateral sesamoid.
Reproduced with permission from Alexander IJ: *The Foot: Examination and Diagnosis.* New York, NY, Churchill Livingstone, 1990, p 65.

## *Diagnostic Tests*

AP, lateral, and axial radiographs of the sesamoid bones are indicated. An oblique view of the sesamoid also may be helpful in visualizing the entire bone and to rule out a fracture. Bipartite or multipartite sesamoid bones are common, occurring in 25% of the population. These normal variants have smooth margins and should not be confused with fractured sesamoids, which have irregular margins. Comparison views of the opposite foot or a bone scan may be helpful.

# DIFFERENTIAL DIAGNOSIS

Hallux rigidus (limited dorsiflexion, dorsal spur, dorsal tenderness)

Hallux valgus (pain medially, lateral deviation of the great toe)

Metatarsalgia (tenderness over the plantar aspect of a lesser metatarsal)

Neuroma (pain and tenderness over the medial sensory nerve)

# ADVERSE OUTCOMES OF THE DISEASE

Without treatment, the patient may have pain and a limp.

# TREATMENT

Patients with sesamoiditis should be advised to avoid wearing high-heeled shoes. For more severe symptoms, relieving pressure on the sesamoids by taping the great toe in plantar flexion, using sesamoid pads (a felt pad used to relieve pressure on the sesamoid bone), wearing a stiff-soled or rocker bottom shoe, or wearing a removable short leg fracture brace for 4 to 6 weeks may decrease inflammation. If these measures fail, excision of the sesamoid may be required.

# ADVERSE OUTCOMES OF TREATMENT

Hallux valgus or varus is rare but may develop following removal of a sesamoid.

# REFERRAL DECISIONS/RED FLAGS

Persistent pain is an indication for further evaluation.

SECTION 7 ■ FOOT AND ANKLE

# SHOE WEAR

Shoes protect and cushion the feet and in many cases serve a cosmetic purpose. Improperly fitted or improperly manufactured shoes are the cause of many foot deformities. Women who consistently wear high-heeled shoes with a narrow toe box have an increased incidence of bunions, hammer toes, corns, and—ultimately—foot surgery (**Figure 1**). Foot size increases with age, but many men and women continue to buy the same size shoe throughout their adult lives without having their foot measured. Patients need instruction about the proper fitting of shoes.

## SHOE DESIGN AND LASTING TECHNIQUES

The seven basic shoe styles are pump, Oxford, sandal, mule, boot, clog, and moccasin. Shoe designers create many variations of these styles, and unfortunately the design of some fashionable footwear indicates little regard for proper shoe function.

The three-dimensional form (either straight or curved) on which the base of the shoe is made is called the last. The shape of the toe box and instep and the curve of the shoe is determined by the last. The straighter the last, the straighter the shoe and the more medial support the shoe can provide.

Common methods of lasting include slip lasting, board (or flat) lasting, and combination lasting. A slip-lasted shoe is constructed by sewing together the upper, like a moccasin, then gluing it onto the sole. This method makes a lightweight, flexible shoe with no torsional rigidity.

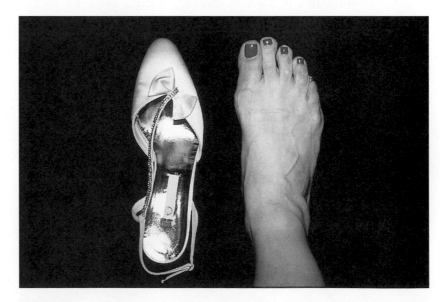

**Figure 1**

The foot takes the shape of the shoe. Common deformities include hallux valgus, hammer toes, corns, and calluses.

With board-lasting or flat-lasting techniques, the upper is fastened to the insole with tacks or staples. This construction makes a stable but less flexible shoe.

Combination lasting uses more than one technique for the same shoe. Shoes made in this way are typically board-lasted in the rear for stability and slip-lasted in the forefoot for flexibility.

## SHOE ANATOMY

The anatomy of several types of shoe is illustrated in **Figure 2**.

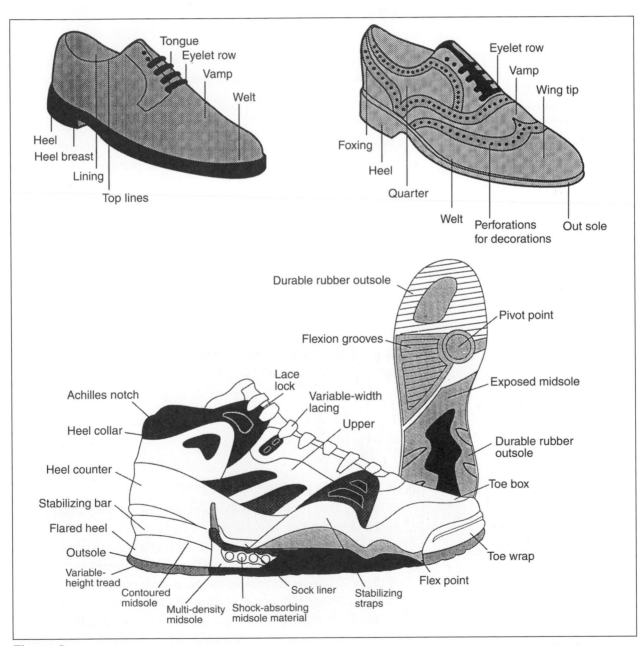

**Figure 2**

Anatomy of several types of shoe.

SECTION 7 ■ FOOT AND ANKLE

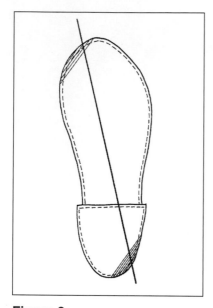

**Figure 3**

Normal wear pattern.

Reproduced from Yodlowski ML, Femino JE: Shoes and orthoses, in Mizel MS, Miller RA, Scioli MW (eds): *Orthopaedic Knowledge Update: Foot and Ankle 2*. Rosemont, IL, American Academy of Orthopaedic Surgeons, 1998, pp 55-64.

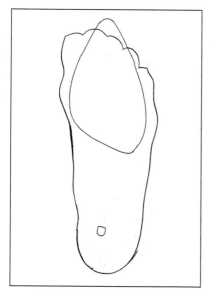

**Figure 4**

A large mismatch between the contour of a patient's foot and the shoe being worn is common. Note the compression of the forefoot and the very small contact area of the high heel. Such a tracing can often disclose the cause of a patient's foot pain.

## Outsole

The outsole makes contact with the ground and usually is attached to the midsole. Most athletic shoes have outsoles made of hard carbon rubber or blown rubber compounds. The outsole provides pivot points and may be designed with a herringbone pattern, suction cups, radial edges, or asymmetric studs. These design patterns enhance stability and traction.

## Midsole and Heel Wedge

The midsole and the heel wedge are located between the inner sole and the outsole and are attached to both. These components provide cushioning, shock absorption, lift, and control.

## Heel Counter

The heel counter is a firm cup built into the rear of the shoe that holds the heel in position and helps control excessive foot motion.

## Toe Box

The toe box may include a stiff material inserted between the lining and outer surface in the toe area to prevent collapse and protect the toes.

## Tongue

The tongue is designed primarily to protect the dorsum of the foot from dirt, moisture, and pressure.

## Sock Liners, Arch Supports, and Inserts

The sock liner covers the insole and provides comfort and appearance. This liner acts primarily as a buffer zone between the shoe and the foot. Arch supports, heel cups, and other types of padding provide additional support, cushioning, and motion control.

## Welt

The welt is a strip of leather or other material that joins the upper with the outer sole.

# SHOE ANALYSIS AND FIT

With any foot or ankle problem, evaluation of the patient's shoes should be an integral part of the examination. Wear patterns are generally predictable, with the normal wear pattern on the outsole slightly medial at the toe and lateral at the heel (**Figure 3**). Abnormalities in the wear pattern indicate problems with alignment and gait. A tracing of the weight-bearing foot should be compared with a tracing of the shoe (**Figure 4**).

Shoe manufacturers have added extra eyelets to many shoes so that they can be laced for a custom fit. Most people can use a conventional technique, where the laces criss-cross to the top of the shoe, aiming for a snug but comfortable fit. If foot or fit problems are present, other lacing techniques may be used (**Figure 5**).

Although proper fitting of shoes is not an exact science, relying on a number of easy-to-follow guidelines can help. Shoes always should be fit to the weight-bearing foot at the end of the day, when feet are at their largest. Shoes cannot be stretched to the shape of the foot. The upper should not wrinkle with flexion, and the foot should not bulge over the welt. The end of the longest toe of the larger foot should be within 3/8″ to 1/2″ of the end of the toe box. The forefoot should not be crowded, and the toes should easily extend. The shoe should

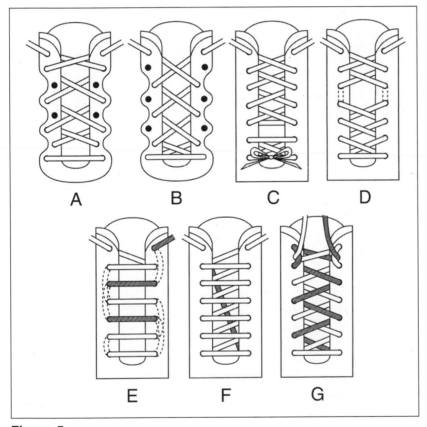

**Figure 5**

Lacing patterns. **A,** For narrow feet, use the eyelets set wider apart to bring up the sides of the shoe for a tighter fit. **B,** For wide feet, use the eyelets set closer to the tongue of the shoe. This has the same effect as letting out a corset. **C,** For a narrow heel and wide forefoot, use both sets of eyelets to achieve a custom fit. **D,** For dorsal pain from a bump on the top of the foot, a high arch, or pain from a dorsal nerve or tendon, leave a space in the lacing to alleviate pressure. **E,** For a high arch, avoid the normal criss-cross pattern to avoid pressure points. **F,** For hammer toes, claw toes, corns, or toenail problems, lace as shown to allow the toe box to be lifted by pulling on the lace that runs from the toe to the throat of the shoe. **G,** For heel blisters, lock the laces at the throat of the shoe to prevent excess motion of the heel in the shoe.

provide a relatively snug grip at the counter above the heel. High heels should be avoided because this style exerts excessive pressure on the front of the foot. Above all else, shoes should be comfortable from the moment they are tried on.

## ADVERSE OUTCOMES FROM POOR SHOE FIT

Bunions, hammer toes, neuromas, corns and calluses, and ingrown toenails are all possible.

SECTION 7 ■ FOOT AND ANKLE

# Soft-Tissue Masses of the Foot and Ankle

## Synonyms

Fibromatosis
Ledderhose disease
Mucoid cyst
Nodular fasciitis
Plantar fibromas

**ICD-9 Codes**

**727.43**
Ganglion and cyst of synovium, tendon, and bursa, unspecified

**728.71**
Plantar fascial fibromatosis

## Definition

Ganglia and plantar fibromas are the most common soft-tissue tumors in the foot and ankle. Other lesions are not included in this chapter.

A ganglion is a cystic tumor that contains gelatinous fluid and arises from a joint capsule or tendon sheath (**Figure 1**). Ganglia of the foot or ankle usually are small, 2- to 3-cm masses that arise on the top or side of the foot. A common site is the lateral aspect of the foot or ankle, with the ganglion cyst arising from the subtalar or ankle joint.

A plantar fibroma is a benign thickening of the plantar fascia that may vary in size from 1 to 6 cm in diameter. Plantar fibromas may evolve to plantar fibromatosis (nodular fasciitis of the plantar fascia), a condition that is similar histologically to Dupuytren disease of the palmar fascia. Compared with Dupuytren disease, plantar fibromatosis is less likely to cause severe deformities.

## Clinical Symptoms

A ganglion cyst typically is a painless, soft nodule, but it may cause problems with aching, nerve compression, or shoe wear. A plantar fibroma is a firm mass on the bottom of the foot that may be painful and is more likely to interfere with shoe wear.

## Tests

### Physical Examination

A ganglion cyst is a discrete mass that is usually movable with side-to-side pressure. A plantar fibroma may be focal or may have multiple, discrete masses that are hard (rubbery) and are part of the plantar fascial band.

### Diagnostic Tests

Plain radiographs are typically normal. Aspiration of a ganglion with an 18-gauge needle will return a straw-colored, gelatinous material. Sophisticated diagnostic imaging generally is not necessary for either a ganglion cyst or a plantar fibroma.

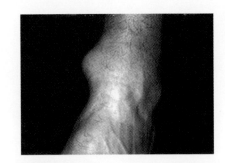

**Figure 1**
Ganglion cyst of the medial ankle.

## Differential Diagnosis

Giant cell tumor of the tendon sheath (solid mass, inability to aspirate soft core)

Lipoma (subcutaneous fatty deposit, pathology diagnosis)

Malignant sarcoma (synovial sarcoma, fibrosarcoma) (pathology diagnosis)

Neurofibroma (often tubular along the course of the nerve, pathology diagnosis)

## Adverse Outcomes of the Disease

Patients may report persistent discomfort and difficulty with shoe wear. Malignant degeneration of a plantar fibroma is possible, but the risk is small.

## Treatment

Pierce the wall of the ganglion three or four times with an 18-gauge needle to release the gelatinous core and promote complete collapse of the cyst. Care should be taken to avoid an overlying sensory nerve. If the ganglion recurs and continues to be symptomatic, it should be excised. The efficacy of corticosteroid injection into a ganglion has not been proved.

A plantar fibroma is best treated with shoe modifications and an orthotic device. The orthotic device should be cushioned and designed to float the fibroma. Surgical excision is indicated in patients with significant persistent symptoms or if the fibroma has increased significantly in size.

## Adverse Outcomes of Treatment

Surgical excision of a plantar fibroma should be avoided, if possible, because of the high rate of recurrence and potential for a painful plantar surgical scar.

## Referral Decisions/Red Flags

If the diagnosis of the mass is not clear based on anatomy, examination, radiographs, and aspiration, further evaluation is needed to rule out other etiologies. Recurrence of a ganglion following aspiration usually requires surgical excision.

# Stress Fractures of the Foot and Ankle

## Synonyms
Insufficiency fracture
March fracture

### ICD-9 Codes
**824**
Fracture of ankle

**825.2**
Fracture of tarsal and metatarsal bones

## Definition
A stress fracture is caused by repetitive overloading. The bone fails when the fatigue process exceeds the reparative process. Stress fractures often result from an increased level of activity or after beginning a different type of activity, such as military training or exercise walking. Conditions that weaken the bone predispose patients to stress fractures; therefore, these injuries are sometimes referred to as insufficiency fractures. Young, athletic women are at risk because of the female athlete triad of amenorrhea, osteopenia, and disordered eating. Older women are at risk because of osteoporosis.

The metatarsals (especially the second metatarsal) are the most common site of a stress fracture, but these fractures also can be seen in other bones of the foot and ankle including the navicular, calcaneus, and fibula (**Figure 1**) . Theoretically, any bone exposed to repetitive stress can sustain a stress fracture.

## Clinical Symptoms
Patients present with the insidious onset of pain and swelling. The pain increases with weight-bearing activity and is relieved by rest. Metatarsal fractures present with a diffusely swollen dorsal forefoot, whereas fibula fractures produce a swollen lateral ankle. Some patients report hearing a crack or pop when the incomplete stress fracture became a complete break.

## Tests

### Physical Examination
Localized point tenderness and concomitant swelling directly over the fracture site are the most reliable physical signs. Ecchymosis occasionally is observed.

### Diagnostic Tests
Early radiographs (less than 2 weeks from onset of symptoms) may be normal, but after 3 to 4 weeks, radiographs show healing callus at the fracture site. A bone scan is more sensitive than a radiograph and may be positive by 5 days postinjury (**Figure 2**). MRI can confirm the diagnosis but is not routinely used.

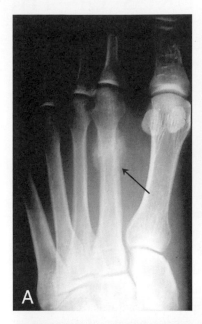
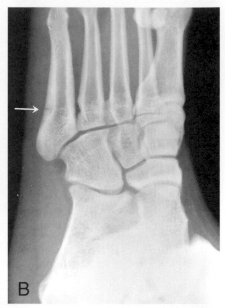
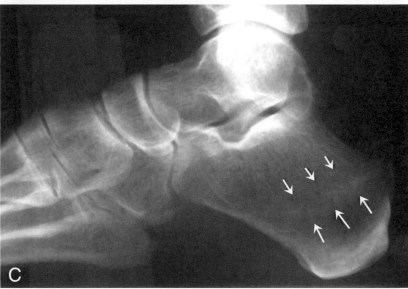

**Figure 1**

Radiographs showing stress fractures. **A,** AP radiograph showing a healed stress fracture of the second metatarsal (arrow). **B,** Stress fracture of the fifth metatarsal (arrow). **C,** Calcaneal stress fracture seen as an area of increased density (between arrows).

# DIFFERENTIAL DIAGNOSIS

Gout (redness, erythema)

Interdigital (Morton) neuroma (pain and tenderness in the intermetatarsal space)

Metabolic bone disorders (multiple stress fractures)

Neoplasm (pain at night or at rest)

Synovitis of the second metatarsophalangeal joint (swelling and tenderness of the joint)

**Figure 2**

Bone scan shows area of increased uptake, indicative of a stress fracture of the third metatarsal.

## ADVERSE OUTCOMES OF THE DISEASE

Chronic stress fractures may require prolonged immobilization to heal. Displacement of fractures with continued unprotected activity may lead to malunion or nonunion that requires surgical procedures. This is more likely with fifth metatarsal (Jones fracture) and navicular stress fractures.

## TREATMENT

Treatment for most patients is based on reduced activity and protective footwear. For metatarsal stress fractures, a stiff-soled shoe, wooden-soled postoperative sandal, or removable short leg fracture brace shoe is sufficient. Most patients with calcaneal and fibular fractures benefit from 2 to 4 weeks of immobilization in a short leg walking cast. Because of the high rate of nonunion, navicular and fifth metatarsal fractures both should be casted, and the patient should use crutches and avoid bearing weight on the involved limb. Internal fixation is often a better alternative for a stress fracture of the fifth metatarsal. Patients may resume activity when they are asymptomatic and show healing radiographically. Time to healing is variable, depending on the bone involved.

## ADVERSE OUTCOMES OF TREATMENT

Metatarsal stress fractures may displace in the sagittal plane and lead to a painful callus. NSAIDs may retard osteogenesis and should be avoided during fracture healing.

## REFERRAL DECISIONS/RED FLAGS

Navicular, fifth metatarsal, and all fibular stress fractures require further evaluation early after diagnosis. Failure to heal by 4 to 6 weeks or recurrent fractures suggest the need for a metabolic workup.

SECTION 7 ■ FOOT AND ANKLE

# TARSAL TUNNEL SYNDROME

**ICD-9 Code**

**355.5**
Tarsal tunnel syndrome

## SYNONYM

Tibial nerve entrapment

## DEFINITION

Tarsal tunnel syndrome describes the symptom complex associated with compression neuropathy of the tibial nerve or its branches posterior to the medial malleolus (**Figure 1**). Although an analogy to carpal tunnel syndrome of the upper extremity has been suggested, the only real similarity is the name. In contrast with carpal tunnel syndrome, tarsal tunnel syndrome is much less common, its symptoms are more vague and intermittent, and its diagnosis is more difficult. Numerous causes of tarsal tunnel syndrome have been reported, including compression from a ganglion or bony lesion, but most cases are of unknown etiology.

## CLINICAL SYMPTOMS

Most patients report diffuse, poorly localized pain along the medial ankle. Paresthesias (tingling) or dysthesias (burning) along the medial ankle and into the arch are a common component of the symptom complex. The pain is often worse after walking or other exercise and also may occur at night.

## TESTS

### Physical Examination
The physical examination reveals tenderness over the tarsal tunnel just posterior to the medial malleolus (**Figure 2**).

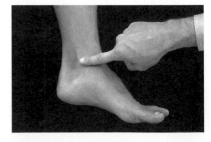

**Figure 2**
Tenderness over the tarsal tunnel just posterior to the medial malleolus may be indicative of tarsal tunnel syndrome.

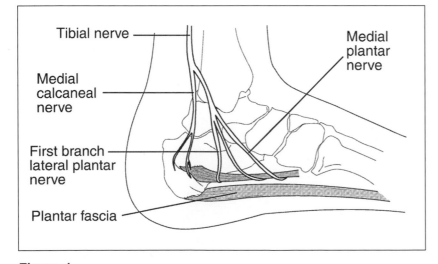

Tibial nerve

Medial
plantar
nerve

Medial
calcaneal
nerve

First branch
lateral plantar
nerve

Plantar fascia

**Figure 1**
Anatomy of the tarsal tunnel.

Percussion over the tibial nerve (Tinel sign) should reproduce the symptoms. Decreased sensation in the distribution of the tibial nerve on the plantar aspect of the foot also may be present.

## Diagnostic Tests

Radiographs of the foot and ankle are necessary to rule out bony pathology, but the radiographs are usually normal. MRI can be useful for determining an etiology such as a ganglion, but the MRI scan usually is normal. Electrodiagnostic testing may identify tibial nerve entrapment, but, at the ankle level and below, the test is not as accurate as in the upper extremity. Furthermore, a positive or negative test does not always correlate with intraoperative findings or clinical outcomes.

# DIFFERENTIAL DIAGNOSIS

Complex regional pain syndrome (discoloration of foot, skin and temperature changes)

Diabetic neuropathy (history of diabetes, bilateral loss of nerve function in a stocking distribution)

Herniated lumbar disk (leg and thigh pain)

Peripheral neuropathy (stocking distribution)

Posterior tibial tendon dysfunction (pain associated with pes planus)

# ADVERSE OUTCOMES OF THE DISEASE

Persistent pain and numbness are possible, and severe numbness may lead to plantar ulcers. Complex regional pain syndrome also may develop.

# TREATMENT

For patients with flatfeet and significant pronation, an orthotic device used to support the medial arch and decrease stretch along the tibial nerve may alleviate symptoms. Review of the surgical results shows a lower success rate for tarsal tunnel release than for carpal tunnel release.

# ADVERSE OUTCOMES OF TREATMENT

Symptoms may not resolve completely if permanent nerve damage has occurred. Surgical nerve release may lead to increased scarring and increased symptoms. The results of revision tarsal tunnel surgery are extremely poor, especially when an adequate decompression of the nerve was performed during the initial procedure.

SECTION 7 ■ FOOT AND ANKLE

## REFERRAL DECISIONS/RED FLAGS

Further evaluation is needed for patients who have one or more of the following conditions: severe or progressive symptoms; loss of motor strength; pain that radiates above the knee, which may indicate a herniated disk; or severe pain to light touch, which may indicate complex regional pain syndrome.

# TOE DEFORMITIES

## SYNONYMS

Claw toe
Hammer toe
Mallet toe

## DEFINITION

Deformities of the lesser toes are categorized as three types: hammer toes, claw toes, and mallet toes. These deformities are most commonly caused by tight, improperly fitting shoes. They also are caused by an imbalance of the intrinsic (arising from the foot) and extrinsic (arising from the leg) muscles.

A claw toe has fixed extension of the metatarsophalangeal (MTP) joint and flexion of the proximal interphalangeal (PIP) joint (**Figure 1**). A flexion contracture of the distal interphalangeal (DIP) joint may be present as well. Claw toes usually affect all of the lesser toes of the foot and often are secondary to a neurologic disorder such as Charcot-Marie-Tooth disease or an inflammatory arthritis such as rheumatoid arthritis. Patients with diabetes mellitus who have a peripheral neuropathy commonly develop claw toes.

A hammer toe has a flexion deformity of the PIP joint with no significant deformity of the DIP or MTP joints (**Figure 2**). The flexion deformity of the PIP joint may cause some passive extension of the MTP joint when the patient is standing, but the MTP joint is in neutral alignment when the foot is examined in a non–weight-bearing position.

A mallet toe has a flexion deformity at the DIP joint with relatively normal alignment of the PIP and MTP joints (**Figure 3**). Hammer toes and mallet toes may be isolated to a single toe and are often caused by improper shoe wear. The second toe, especially if longer than the great toe, is most commonly affected.

## CLINICAL SYMPTOMS

Pain, deformity, and difficulty with shoe wear are the common symptoms of patients with lesser toe deformities. A corn may develop on the dorsum of the PIP joint or the tip of the toe. These calluses are painful and may become infected. In patients with hyperextension of the MTP joint, the metatarsal head is displaced plantarly with resultant increased pressure, callus, and pain on the plantar side of the forefoot.

| ICD-9 Codes |
| --- |
| **734.8** |
| Claw toe (acquired) |
| **735.4** |
| Hammer toe (acquired) |
| **735.8** |
| Other acquired deformities of toe |

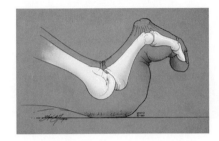

**Figure 1**
Clinical appearance of a claw toe.

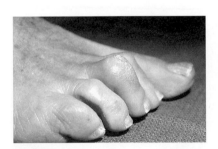

**Figure 2**
Clinical appearance of a hammer toe.

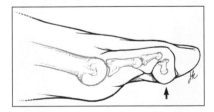

**Figure 3**
Clinical appearance of a mallet toe.

SECTION 7 ■ FOOT AND ANKLE

## TESTS

### Physical Examination

Examine the patient in both standing and sitting positions. Note alignment, the presence of corns, and flexibility and stability of the MTP, PIP, and DIP joints. Evaluate alignment and mobility of the ankle and hindfoot joints. Look for a cavus foot, which is associated with neurologic disorders. Evaluate sensory and motor function of the foot and lower extremities.

### Diagnostic Tests

Radiographs are helpful only in planning surgery and to rule out osteomyelitis when ulceration of the toe has occurred. A neurologic workup may be indicated in patients with claw toes and a high arch.

## DIFFERENTIAL DIAGNOSIS

Neurologic or rheumatologic disorder (claw toes) (noted on physical examination)

## ADVERSE OUTCOMES OF THE DISEASE

Without treatment, patients have difficulty with shoe wear and with persistent, painful corns and calluses. Ulceration may lead to infection and possible osteomyelitis.

## TREATMENT

A shoe with a soft, roomy toe box to accommodate the deformity is the mainstay of treatment. A shoe repair shop can help by stretching shoes to accommodate single hammer and mallet toe deformities. Athletic shoes usually provide enough room to accommodate the deformity. Shoes with heels higher than 2 1/4″ should be avoided. Protective cushions sold over the counter are helpful when corns develop.

Commercially available splints to hold the toes in place may provide symptomatic relief (**Figure 4**). In addition, the patient can tape the toe into flexion at the MTP joint. With a narrow strip of tape, begin on the plantar aspect of the foot under the metatarsal head, looping over the dorsum of the proximal phalanx and crossing back to the starting point while holding the toe flexed at the MTP joint.

Stretching and strengthening of the toes helps to preserve flexibility. The toe strengthening program on p 706-707 can be done at home.

Surgical correction may be necessary for fixed deformities. The goal of surgery is not cosmetic but the proper alignment of the toes to comfortably accommodate shoe wear. Surgical

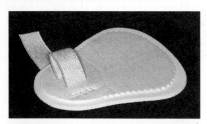
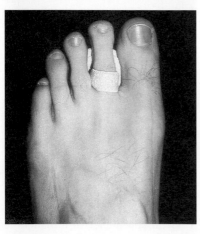

**Figure 4**

Type of splint used for a claw toe.

correction usually achieves toes that sit flat but that do not have normal range of motion. Postoperative swelling tends to last for several months.

## ADVERSE OUTCOMES OF TREATMENT

Continued pain, corns, and recurrent deformity are possible.

## REFERRAL DECISIONS/RED FLAGS

Failure of nonsurgical treatment or persistent ulceration requires further evaluation. Patients with vascular insufficiency are poor candidates for surgical treatment.

SECTION 7 ■ FOOT AND ANKLE

## Toe Strengthening Program

| Exercise | Recommended for | Repetitions or Duration |
|---|---|---|
| Toe squeeze | Hammer toes, toe cramps | 10 |
| Big toe pulls | Bunions, toe cramps | 10 |
| Toe pulls | Bunions, hammer toes, toe cramps | 10 |
| Golf ball roll | Plantar fasciitis, arch strain, foot cramps | 2 minutes |
| Marble pick-up | Pain in ball of foot, hammer toes, toe cramps | Until all marbles have been picked up |
| Towel curls | Hammer toes, toe cramps, pain in ball of foot | 5 |

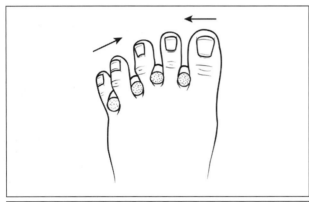

### Toe Squeeze
Place small sponges or corks between the toes and hold a squeeze for 5 seconds. Repeat 10 times.

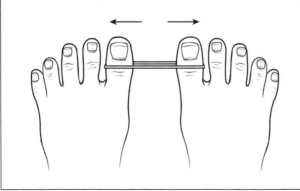

### Big Toe Pulls
Place a thick rubber band around both big toes and pull the big toes away from each other and toward the small toes. Hold for 5 seconds. Repeat 10 times.

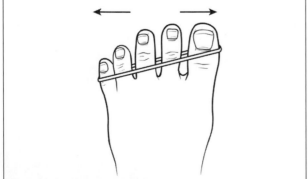

### Toe Pulls
Put a thick rubber band around all your toes and spread them. Hold this position for 5 seconds. Repeat 10 times.

Figures adapted from Brochure. *Bunion Surgery*. Rosemont, IL, American Academy of Orthopaedic Surgeons, 1995.

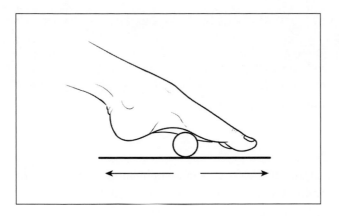

## Golf Ball Roll

Roll a golf ball under the ball of your foot for 2 minutes to massage the bottom of the foot.

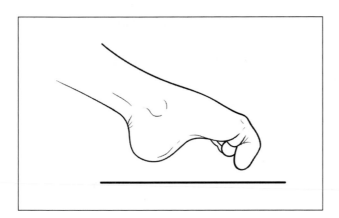

## Marble Pick-up

Place 20 marbles on the floor. Pick up one marble at a time and put it in a small bowl. Repeat until you have picked up all 20 marbles.

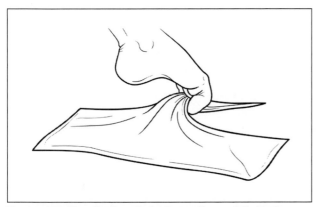

## Towel Curls

Place a small towel on the floor and curl it toward you, using only your toes. You can increase the resistance by putting weight on the end of the towel. Relax and repeat 5 times.

**Figures adapted from Brochure: *Bunion Surgery.* Rosemont, IL, American Academy of Orthopaedic Surgeons, 1995.**

SECTION 7 ■ FOOT AND ANKLE

# TURF TOE

**ICD-9 Code**

**845.12**
Sprains and strains of ankle and foot; metatarsophalangeal (joint)

## SYNONYM
First metatarsophalangeal joint sprain

## DEFINITION
Turf toe is a sprain of the first metatarsophalangeal (MTP) joint that most commonly occurs with hyperextension but may occur with any forced range of motion. The term "turf toe" was coined because the incidence of these injuries increased with the use of artificial turf on athletic playing fields. Turf toe injuries are associated with significant morbidity, and in some studies these injuries accounted for more missed playing time than did ankle sprains.

## CLINICAL SYMPTOMS
Patients usually report swelling, tenderness, and limited motion of the first MTP joint. A grade 1 sprain is a stretch injury of the capsule, with the athlete usually able to participate in sports with mild symptoms. A grade 2 sprain is a partial tear of the plantar ligamentous complex of the MTP joint. These patients have moderate swelling, ecchymosis, and decreased range of motion. A grade 3 sprain is a complete tear of the MTP ligamentous complex. Marked swelling, bruising, and limited motion occur with grade 3 injuries. The patient can neither compete athletically nor walk normally.

## TESTS

### Physical Examination
Assess the degree of swelling, ecchymosis, range of motion, and gait.

### Diagnostic Tests
Radiographs are useful to detect associated avulsion fractures, evaluate joint congruity, and rule out preexisting arthritic changes. When the diagnosis is in question, a bone scan or MRI can help exclude other possibilities such as sesamoid or metatarsal fractures.

## DIFFERENTIAL DIAGNOSIS
Hallux rigidus (limited range of motion of the first MTP joint)
Sesamoid stress fracture (focal pain over the sesamoid)

## Adverse Outcomes of the Disease

Instability and arthritis (hallux rigidus) of the first MTP joint may develop. Symptomatic loose bodies and osteochondritic lesions may occur.

## Treatment

Nonsurgical treatment with rest, ice, compression, and elevation (RICE) usually is sufficient. Early range of motion is started as symptoms allow. After a grade 1 or 2 sprain, a stiff-soled or rocker bottom shoe is recommended to restrict MTP joint motion and alleviate symptoms. Grade 3 injuries require protected weight bearing or immobilization for 1 to 2 weeks, with a 4- to 6-week period of rest from athletics. Taping, orthotic devices, or a stiff-soled or rocker bottom sole are then recommended. Surgical intervention is seldom necessary except in the case of displaced intra-articular or avulsion fractures.

## Adverse Outcomes of Treatment

Delayed return to sports activities, hallux rigidus, and acquired hallux varus or valgus may occur.

## Referral Decisions/Red Flags

Intra-articular fractures may require open reduction or excision. Urgent surgical intervention is necessary for an irreducible dislocation. Osteochondral lesions or loose bodies also require further evaluation.

Section 7 ■ Foot and Ankle

# PAIN DIAGRAM—SPINE

Cervical strain (acute)
Fracture of the cervical spine

Cervical spondylosis

Fractures of the thoracic
or lumbar spine

DISH
*(see General Orthopaedics)*

Cervical radiculopathy

Low back pain

Cauda equina syndrome
Lumbar degenerative disk disease
Spondylolisthesis
Lumbar spinal stenosis

Lumbar herniated disk
(sciatica)

**Note:** Also refer to
the more detailed
pain diagrams in
the chapters on
individual conditions.

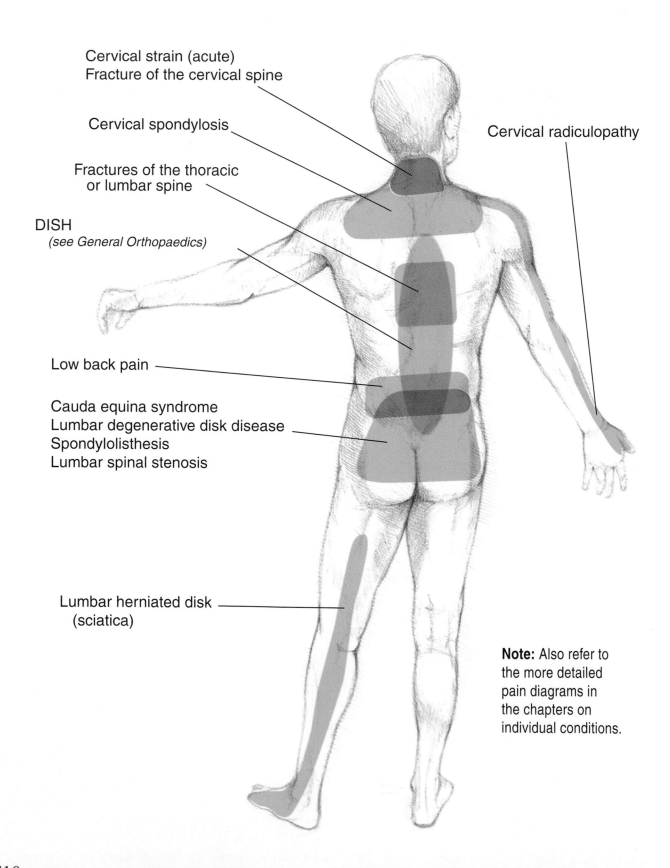

# SPINE

**Section Editor**
Dan M. Spengler, MD
Professor and Chair
Department of Orthopaedics and Rehabilitation
Vanderbilt Orthopaedic Institute
Nashville, Tennesee

Robert Donatelli, PhD, PT, OCS
National Director of Sports Rehabilitation
Physiotherapy Associates
Las Vegas, Nevada

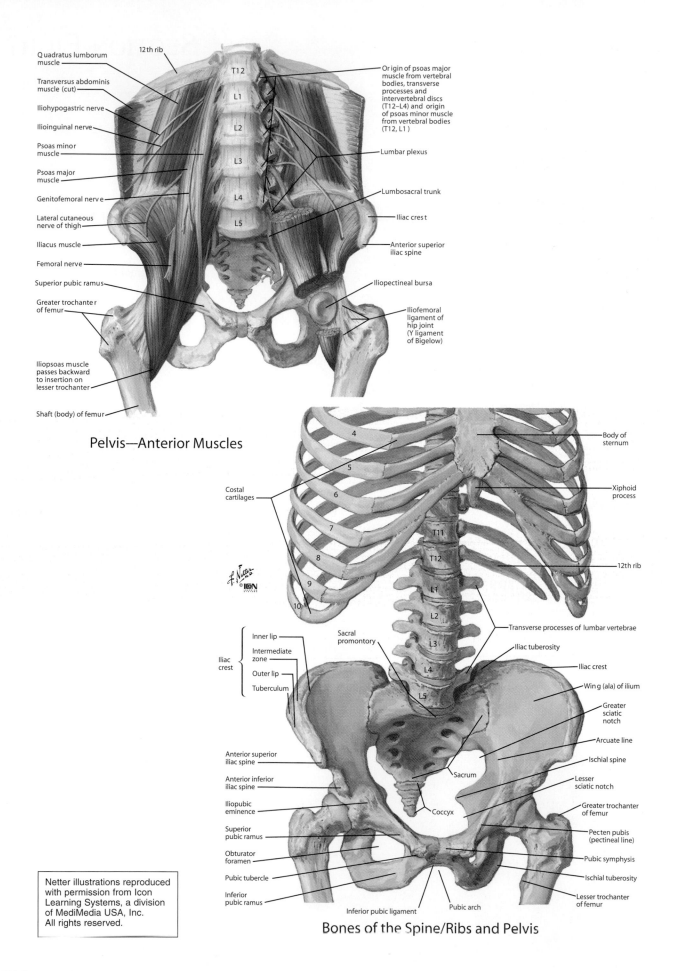

**Pelvis—Anterior Muscles**

12th rib

Quadratus lumborum muscle

Transversus abdominis muscle (cut)

Iliohypogastric nerve

Ilioinguinal nerve

Psoas minor muscle

Psoas major muscle

Genitofemoral nerve

Lateral cutaneous nerve of thigh

Iliacus muscle

Femoral nerve

Superior pubic ramus

Greater trochanter of femur

Iliopsoas muscle passes backward to insertion on lesser trochanter

Shaft (body) of femur

T12

L1

L2

L3

L4

L5

Origin of psoas major muscle from vertebral bodies, transverse processes and intervertebral discs (T12–L4) and origin of psoas minor muscle from vertebral bodies (T12, L1)

Lumbar plexus

Lumbosacral trunk

Iliac crest

Anterior superior iliac spine

Iliopectineal bursa

Iliofemoral ligament of hip joint (Y ligament of Bigelow)

**Bones of the Spine/Ribs and Pelvis**

4

5

6

7

8

9

10

Costal cartilages

Iliac crest
- Inner lip
- Intermediate zone
- Outer lip
- Tuberculum

Sacral promontory

Anterior superior iliac spine

Anterior inferior iliac spine

Iliopubic eminence

Superior pubic ramus

Obturator foramen

Pubic tubercle

Inferior pubic ramus

Inferior pubic ligament

Sacrum

Coccyx

Pubic arch

T11

T12

L1

L2

L3

L4

L5

Body of sternum

Xiphoid process

12th rib

Transverse processes of lumbar vertebrae

Iliac tuberosity

Iliac crest

Wing (ala) of ilium

Greater sciatic notch

Arcuate line

Ischial spine

Lesser sciatic notch

Greater trochanter of femur

Pecten pubis (pectineal line)

Pubic symphysis

Ischial tuberosity

Lesser trochanter of femur

# SPINE—OVERVIEW

Low back pain affects 60% to 70% of the adult population at some time in their lives, with up to 15% to 30% of the population affected at one time. Low back pain may be more a reflection of physiologic aging than a true disease process. Many pathologic disorders associated with low back pain, however, do adversely affect the quality of life of patients in their peak productive years. Low back pain and back injury are common in employees between 30 and 60 years of age and are a primary cause of absenteeism from work. In 1988, about 22.4 million people (17.6% of all US workers) missed an estimated 149 million work days as a result of low back pain. More than 30 million visits were made to physicians' offices in 2002 because of back problems.

Most individuals with low back pain experience pain for only a brief time, with near-complete resolution of symptoms within 30 days, but some patients experience persistent symptoms that progress to chronic pain, usually lasting longer than 90 days. In other patients, symptoms resolve, but the patients then experience bouts of recurrent pain.

It is essential that patients with low back pain symptoms provide a complete medical history and undergo a thorough physical examination. In the absence of red flags or significant physical findings, nonsurgical treatment may begin with anti-inflammatory medications and/or physical therapy. Initial treatment efforts should be directed toward diminishing symptoms. Later treatment (eg, physical therapy) should be initiated as symptoms resolve. Physical therapy is not initially effective in patients with marked paraspinous dysrhythmia, limited mobility, and marked pain. Following symptom resolution, however, active physical therapy is the best choice to reduce recurrence.

Most patients should be able to return to work quickly, depending on pain severity, but work modifications may be required initially. Patients unable to return to work quickly should undergo more extensive evaluation, including laboratory tests and advanced imaging studies to exclude lumbar infections, lumbar disk herniations, or other causes of nerve irritation. Other factors, such as litigation and workers' compensation claims, may significantly affect pain behavior and impact the motivation to return to work rapidly. These issues become clear over time. Patient education is important and requires time and patience on the part of the physician and other health care providers.

The differential diagnosis for low back pain is wide-ranging and must be considered carefully to ensure that no identifiable cause for the pain is overlooked (**Table 1**). Diagnoses to consider include inflammation, infection, degenerative disorders, neoplasms (primary and metastatic), trauma, metabolic disorders, developmental defects, neurologic disorders, referred pain, psychological problems, and various unusual conditions. Cauda equina syndrome is one of the more ominous conditions that should be considered because early recognition and treatment are critical to provide the best chance for recovery. **Table 2** lists and compares several conditions commonly associated with back pain.

## Table 1  Common Presentations of Spinal Problems

| Problem | Associated Signs and Symptoms | Possible Diagnosis |
|---|---|---|
| Neck pain | Paravertebral discomfort relieved with rest and aggravated with activity | Acute neck sprain<br>Upper cervical disk herniation |
| | Limited motion or morning stiffness | Cervical spondylosis |
| Neck and arm pain | A younger patient with an abnormal upper extremity neurologic examination | Cervical radiculopathy due to herniated nucleus pulposus |
| | An older patient with limited motion and pain on extension | Cervical radiculopathy due to cervical spondylosis |
| | Urinary dysfunction with global sensory changes, weakness, and an abnormal gait | Cervical myelopathy secondary to cervical spondylosis or trauma<br>Demyelinating disorder |
| | Shoulder pain and a positive impingement sign | Shoulder pathology<br>Superior sulcus tumor of lung (uncommon) |
| | Positive Tinel sign and nondermatomal distribution of symptoms | Peripheral nerve entrapment |
| Back pain | Paravertebral discomfort relieved with rest and aggravated with activity | Acute low back sprain |
| | Limited motion or stiffness | Degenerative disk disease, ankylosing spondylitis |
| | Unrelenting night pain and weight loss | Tumor<br>Infection |
| | Fevers, chills, and sweats | Infection or intervertebral disk infection |
| Back and leg pain | A younger patient with an abnormal lower extremity neurologic examination | Lumbar radiculopathy due to herniated nucleus pulposus |
| | An older patient with poor walking tolerance and a stooped gait | Spinal stenosis |
| | Tenderness over the lateral hip and discomfort at night | Trochanteric bursitis |

**Table 2   Conditions Commonly Associated With Back Pain**

| Condition | Age of Onset (years) | Sex Primarily Affected | Level Affected | Radiographic Findings | MRI Results |
|---|---|---|---|---|---|
| Spondylolysis | < 20 | Male | L5, L4, L3 | Defect in pars interarticularis (unilateral or bilateral) | Negative |
| Spondylolisthesis (Isthmic) | < 20 | Male | L5-S1 | Defects in L5 pars; slip of L5 anterior to S1 | May be positive if associated stenosis |
| Spondylolisthesis (Degenerative) | > 40 | Female | L4-L5 | No defect in pars; slip of L4 anterior to L5 | May be positive if associated stenosis |
| Disk herniation | 35 | Male | L5-S1/ L4-L5 | Normal for age | Positive |
| Stenosis | > 50 | Both | L4-L5/ L3-L4 | Aging changes | Positive |
| DISH | > 50 | Male | Multiple lumbar levels | Confluent anterior osteophytes, > 3 lumbar levels | Negative |

## TYPES OF PAIN

Night pain that interrupts or prevents sleep, along with fever and weight loss, may indicate a malignancy or infection. Night pain also may be experienced by patients with significant lumbar spinal stenosis. Thus, complete information must be gleaned before linking night pain to an ominous diagnosis, although malignancy and infection must be considered. Acute posttraumatic pain may indicate a fracture. Patients with advanced osteoporosis may experience acute pain and exhibit a vertebral compression fracture with no history of trauma. Low back pain is uncommon in children and always warrants a thorough evaluation.

## LOCATION OF PAIN

### Neck Pain

Pain located in the neck, trapezial, and interscapular areas most commonly occurs in association with degeneration or herniation of an intervertebral disk. If the herniation occurs above the C5-6 level, the patient may not experience radiculopathy but will report only neck, trapezial, and/or interscapular pain. Pain from an acute cervical sprain (flexion-extension or whiplash injury) is usually self-limiting but may lead to chronic pain, depending on the severity of the injury. When the injury results from a motor vehicle accident, one way to approximate the degree of injury is to ask questions regarding the cost of damages to the patient's vehicle. Minimal damage to the vehicle with maximal symptoms may suggest symptom amplification, although this diagnosis requires evaluation of the cervical spine with plain radiographs as well as a cervical MRI scan or possibly a cervical myelogram followed by a CT scan. Other causes of neck pain that should be considered include brachial plexopathy, such as burners or stingers. With brachial plexopathy, MRI scans are usually normal, but electromyographic tests are often positive.

## Neck and Radicular Arm Pain

When accompanied by pain that radiates into the arm, neck pain may be the result of an entrapment of a cervical nerve root by a herniated disk or an osteophyte. For screening diagnostic information, see **Figure 1**. Many patients with a herniated cervical disk are more comfortable when they place the hand of the symptomatic arm on their head, because this position reduces the tension on the nerve. In contrast, patients with intrinsic shoulder problems feel more comfortable with their arms at their sides. With peripheral nerve entrapment syndromes, such as carpal tunnel syndrome, patients may report arm pain and a lesser degree of neck pain. Other less common disorders may also cause neck and arm pain. For example, a superior sulcus tumor of the lung (Pancoast tumor) may cause neck, shoulder, and arm pain, typically in the distribution of the ulnar nerve. Clues to this less common condition include intrinsic hand weakness, Horner syndrome, and a long history of cigarette smoking.

## Low Back Pain

Several diagnostic categories commonly applied to patients with low back pain are unclear and are not supported by the literature. For example, patients with low back pain are often diagnosed as having "mechanical low back pain," "facet syndrome," or "sacroiliac joint dysfunction," although no clear distinction can be made among these diagnoses. It is true that some patients—such as those with ankylosing spondylitis, infection, or traumatic instability—may demonstrate involvement of the sacroiliac joint; however, the term sacroiliac joint dysfunction is generally used as a "wastebasket diagnosis," without clear, objective evidence of the particular pathology involved. In discussing low back pain in this section, a condition will be regarded as a specific diagnosis only if it can be clearly recognized as a discrete entity through patient history, physical examination, imaging studies, or pathologic

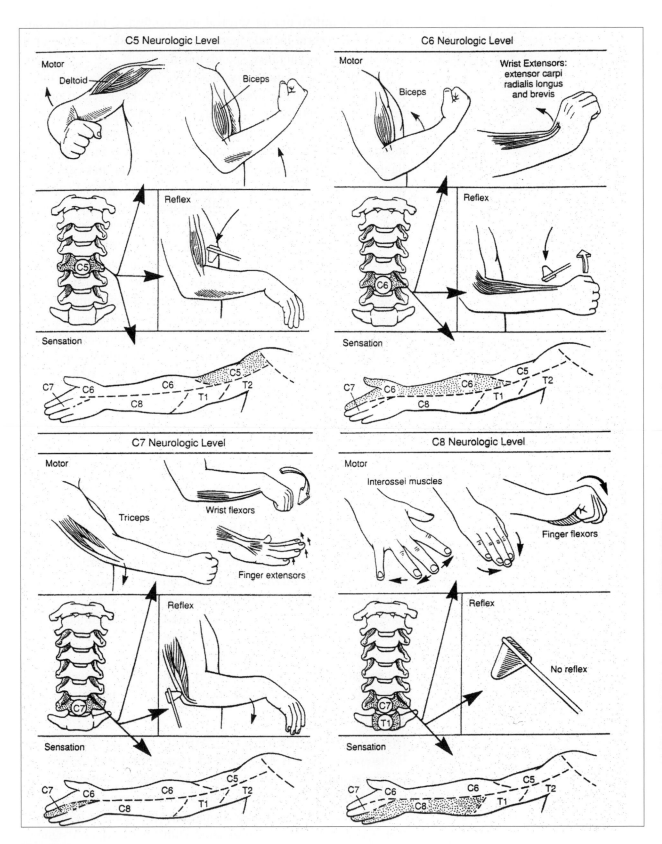

**Figure 1**

Neurologic evaluation of the upper extremity (C5, C6, C7, C8).

Reproduced with permission from Klein JD, Garfin SR: History and physical examination, in Weinstein JN, Rydevik BL, Somtag VKH (eds): *Essentials of the Spine*. New York, NY, Raven Press, 1995, pp 71-95.

SECTION 8 ■ SPINE

changes identified during surgical intervention. Conditions that meet these criteria include herniated lumbar disk, lumbar spinal stenosis, and degenerative spondylolisthesis.

Low back pain typically occurs in the midline at about the L4 or L5 level and may radiate to the buttocks. Back disorders that affect patients between the ages of 20 and 40 years are often related to sprains (affecting ligaments) or strains (affecting muscles) of the soft-tissue structures of the back, including the ligamentous support portion of the intervertebral disk, the anulus fibrosus. The anulus may weaken with repeated small tears, leading to herniations of the lumbar disk at a later time. Young adults with spondylolysis and spondylolisthesis often report recalcitrant back pain that may require further evaluation and treatment. Although nonsurgical treatment should be tried initially, many of these patients ultimately require surgical treatment. Job modifications may also be required, although many patients experience resolution of their symptoms and are able to continue rigorous physical work. With seronegative spondyloarthropathies (such as ankylosing spondylitis), patients often have back pain with morning stiffness that lasts longer than 30 minutes.

With aging and degeneration of the intervertebral disk, associated arthritis may develop in the facet joints and contribute to back pain in patients older than 40 years. Nevertheless, most patients with physiologic aging of the spine do not develop significant symptoms that adversely impact their quality of life. Back pain, with or without radiculopathy, may be associated with spinal stenosis. These symptoms are usually aggravated by spinal extension (standing or walking upright or sleeping supine). Diffuse idiopathic skeletal hyperostosis (DISH), which primarily affects men, often becomes symptomatic after age 50 years. (See pp 53-54, Diffuse Idiopathic Skeletal Hyperostosis, in the General Orthopaedics section.)

Extraspinal causes of back pain include pancreatitis, inflammatory bowel disease, kidney stones, pelvic infections, retroperitoneal lesions, aortic aneurysms, and tumors or cysts of the reproductive tract.

## Back and Radicular Leg Pain

Unilateral leg pain is common with herniation of an intervertebral disk, usually at the L4-5 or L5-S1 vertebral levels. Herniations at the L3-4 level generally cause pain that radiates into the thigh and/or groin area. This pain is typically worse with sitting and is associated with sciatic tension signs (straight-leg raising test, supine and seated) as well as altered sensation, motor strength, and reflexes in the lower extremity (**Figure 2**). Patients with an L3-4 disk herniation exhibit a

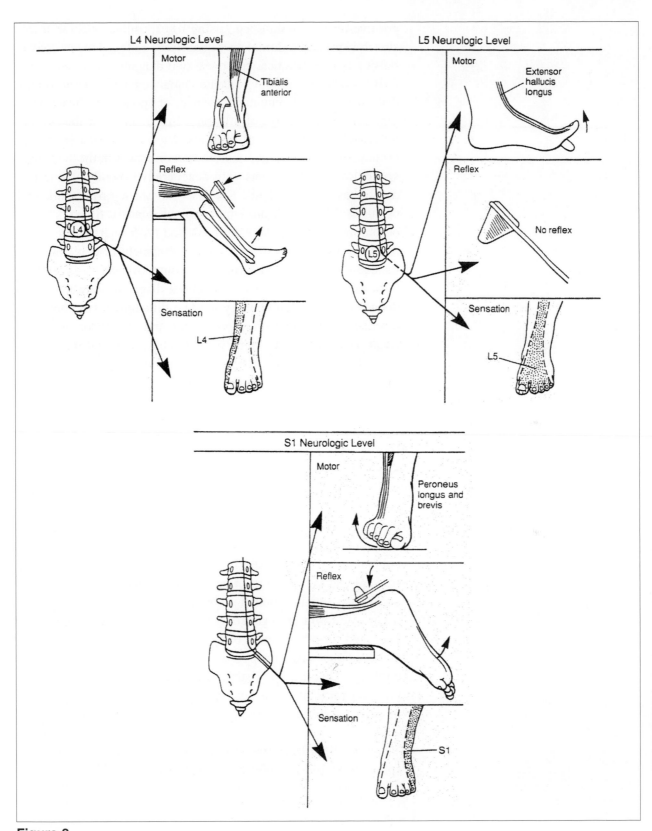

**Figure 2**

Neurologic evaluation of the lower extremity (L4, L5, S1).

Reproduced with permission from Klein JD, Garfin SR: History and physical examination, in Weinstein JN, Rydevik BL, Somtag VKH (eds): *Essentials of the Spine.* New York, NY, Raven Press, 1995, pp 71-95.

positive reverse straight-leg raising test (positive femoral nerve stretch sign) and a diminished quadriceps reflex. Trochanteric bursitis mimics sciatica, and these two diagnoses may coexist.

Bilateral leg pain may indicate spinal stenosis, a large central disk rupture, cauda equina syndrome, or spondylolisthesis, especially after the age of 40 years. In patients over the age of 40 years who present with back and leg pain, degenerative spondylolisthesis is much more common than isthmic spondylolisthesis. Patients with degenerative spondylolisthesis do not have spondylolysis. Exercise-induced leg pain (unilateral or bilateral) may indicate lumbar spinal stenosis. Spinal stenosis occurs most commonly at the L3-4 and L4-5 interspaces.

Extraspinal causes of nerve root entrapment or irritation include hip disease, pyriformis syndrome, ovarian cysts, and retroperitoneal lesions. The differential diagnosis between a hip disorder and a spinal etiology may be difficult because both disorders occur in an aging population and both disorders frequently occur in the same patient. Thus, a careful physical examination and appropriate radiographs are important. Not infrequently, both conditions require surgical management after nonsurgical management fails.

## DEFORMITY

Kyphotic deformities of the spine are best seen from the side with the patient bending forward. These deformities may occur in any segment of the spine but are more common in the thoracolumbar spine. Scoliosis, on the other hand, is associated with a coronal plane and rotatory deformity of the spinal column that is more easily recognized when the patient bends forward and is viewed from behind. In younger patients, scoliosis is usually idiopathic, but in older patients it may also occur as a result of degenerative changes. Patients should be evaluated for other causes of spinal deformity such as neurofibromatosis, spinal cord lesions, and a tethered spinal cord. Spondylolisthesis (isthmic) usually occurs at the lumbosacral joint and is accompanied by tight hamstring muscles (inability to toe-touch). Onset of a spinal deformity in adulthood suggests spinal instability, osteopenia, or a neoplasm. These conditions may be accompanied by compromise of the spinal nerve roots and/or the spinal cord.

## TRAUMA

All patients who sustain spinal trauma must be thoroughly evaluated with appropriate radiographs. Some bony injuries may be subtle, especially in the cervical spine. Flexion-distraction injuries of the thoracolumbar spine may also be missed on radiographs because ligamentous injuries may occur without any bony injury. These injuries are very unstable and early recognition is essential. The potential consequences of misdiagnosed spinal injuries can be devastating and include progressive deformities with or without neurologic deficits. Injuries to the spine are often associated with other life-threatening visceral, head, or skeletal injuries. For many reasons, some spinal injuries may be missed initially in the multiply injured patient, even after an appropriate evaluation. Special imaging of the spine should be deferred to the specialist to avoid duplication of these expensive tests.

## INCIDENCE BY SEX

Women have an increased incidence of the following spinal conditions: scoliosis in adolescence, metastatic breast cancer, trochanteric bursitis in later adulthood, and osteoporosis with vertebral body fractures that may lead to an increased kyphosis following menopause.

Men have an increased incidence of the following spinal conditions: kyphosis in adolescence, ankylosing spondylitis in adulthood, and multiple myeloma and DISH in later adulthood. The most common metastatic spinal lesions in men include prostate and lung cancers.

SECTION 8 ■ SPINE

# PHYSICAL EXAMINATION
# SPINE

This examination is for patients who present with low back pain with or without radiculopathy.

## STANDING EXAMINATION

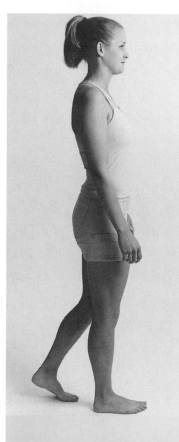

### Gait

Ask the patient to walk across the room as you observe the patient's gait. Watch for a Trendelenburg lurch. If myelopathy is suspected, ask the patient to perform a tandem (heel-to-toe) walk.

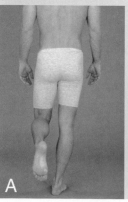
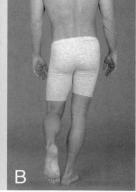

### Trendelenburg test

This tests strength of the gluteus medius muscle, which is an L5-innervated muscle. Ask the patient to stand on one leg. With normal gluteus medius strength, the pelvis will stay level (A). If the gluteus medius is weak on the stance limb side, the pelvis will drop, with the iliac crest becoming lower on the opposite side (B). This is a positive Trendelenburg test, which may also suggest hip problems. Repeat the test on the other side.

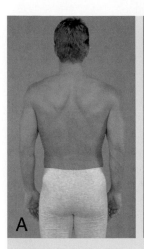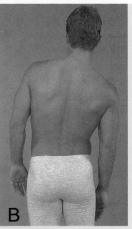

### Posterior view

Inspect the spine for normal, straight alignment (**A**). Moderate to severe scoliosis will be obvious. Also inspect for muscle atrophy. A lumbar list (**B**) might be present in association with a herniated disk or other condition in which the patient will lean to one side to alleviate nerve root compression. In men younger than 40 years, measure chest expansion. Expansion of less than 1 inch suggests ankylosing spondylitis.

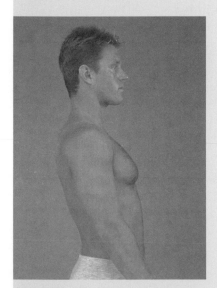

### Lateral view

With the patient standing, inspect for deviations in normal cervical lordosis, thoracic kyphosis, and lumbar lordosis. Loss of cervical lordosis or lumbar lordosis may occur with painful conditions such as acute sprains, fractures, or infectious or neoplastic processes.

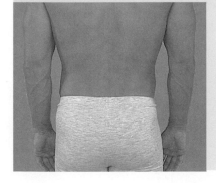

### Pelvic tilt

Observe the patient standing with the feet together and the knees straight. Inspect or palpate the top of the iliac crests. A pelvis that is not level may indicate a limb-length inequality, or it may be secondary to a spinal deformity.

SECTION 8 ■ SPINE

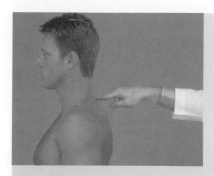

### Spinous process

Palpate the spinous processes to define the alignment of the spine. The examiner in the photograph is palpating C7, the most prominent cervical spinous process. The top of the thyroid cartilage is at the level of the C4 vertebral body, and the cricoid cartilage is parallel to the C6 vertebral body.

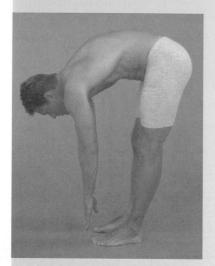

### Flexion, visual estimation

The Zero Starting Position is with the patient standing with the hips and knees straight and the trunk in line with the lower extremities. The feet should be comfortably apart to facilitate movement of the spine, and the arms should hang in a relaxed, extended position. With the spine at maximum flexion, measure the distance between the fingertips and the floor. If at maximum flexion the fingertips are more than 10 cm from the floor, paraspinous spasm, hamstring tightness, nerve root compression, and/or symptom amplification should be considered. Pain reported on flexion is consistent with nerve root irritation from a disk herniation.

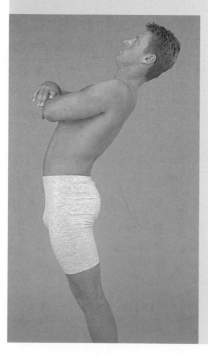

### Extension, visual estimation

Lumbar extension can be estimated visually. Pain on extension suggests spinal stenosis and/or spondylolisthesis.

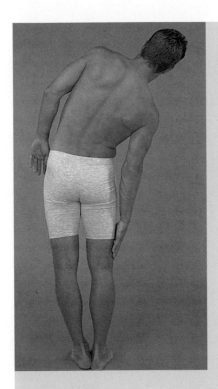

### Lateral bending

Ask the patient to bend to the right and to the left. Estimate the maximum lateral bend on each side.

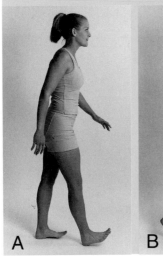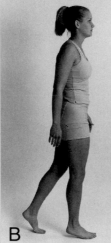

A        B

### Heel walking and toe walking

Ask the patient to walk first on the heels (**A**) and then on the toes (**B**) for a quick screen of the dorsiflexors (L4/L5 innervation) and plantar flexors (S1 innervation).

# SEATED EXAMINATION

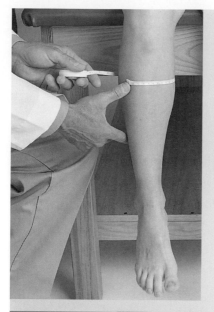

## *Calf and thigh circumference*

Measure the circumference of the thigh approximately one hand breadth above the patella and the circumference of the calf approximately one hand breadth below the patella to evaluate for circumferential atrophy. Atrophy may indicate chronic radiculopathy or disuse atrophy from a painful adjacent joint (knee or ankle).

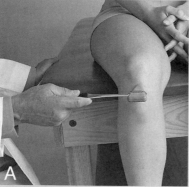

A

## *Deep tendon reflexes*

Assess deep tendon reflexes at the knee (**A**) and the ankle (**B**). A decreased knee reflex is consistent with L3 or L4 nerve root compression. The ankle reflex may be diminished or absent with a decrease in function of the S1 root.

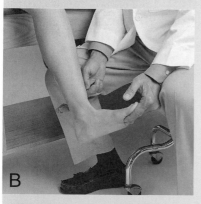

B

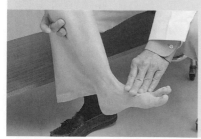

## *Dorsiflexion strength testing*

To assess the strength of the dorsiflexors, resist the patient's attempt to dorsiflex the ankle. Weakness may indicate L4 nerve compression.

SECTION 8 ■ SPINE

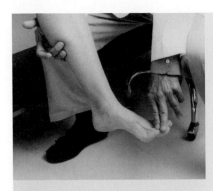

### Extensor hallucis longus strength testing

Stabilize the foot in a neutral position with one hand and ask the patient to extend the great toe as you apply resistance. The extensor hallucis longus is an L5-innervated muscle.

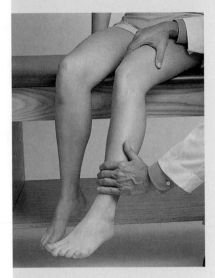

### Quadriceps testing

Ask the patient to extend the knee as you apply resistance. Weakness may indicate compression on the L3 or L4 nerve root or perhaps pain inhibition from a knee disorder.

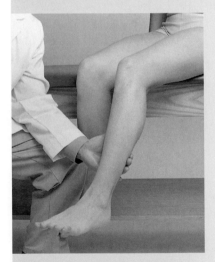

### Hamstrings testing

Ask the patient to pull the leg toward the table as you apply resistance. Weakness may indicate lumbar nerve root compression (nonspecific) or pain inhibition from a knee injury.

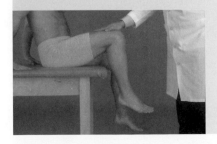

### Iliopsoas testing

Ask the patient to flex the hip as you apply resistance. Weakness may indicate a primary hip disorder or an upper lumbar nerve root compression.

SECTION 8 ■ SPINE

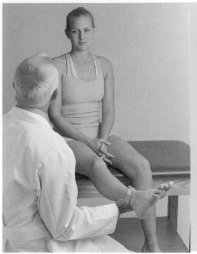
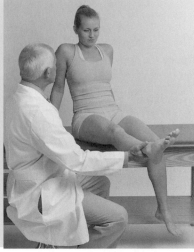

### Seated straight-leg raising test

Distract the patient's attention away from the back by asking whether he or she has knee problems and then lift the foot and extend the knee. If straightening the knee to full extension on both sides does not cause the patient to lean back, no significant sciatic tension is present.

# SUPINE EXAMINATION

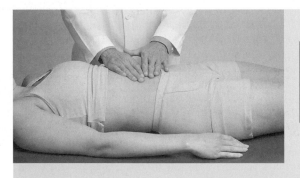

### Palpation of abdomen

Examine the patient's abdomen for tenderness, masses, or enlarged organs. Consider referring female patients to a gynecologist for a pelvic examination, especially for chronic pain.

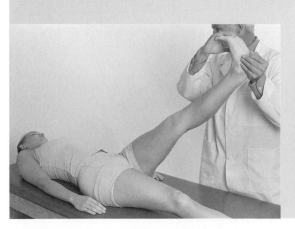

### Supine straight-leg raising test

Elevate the leg until either the knee begins to bend or the patient reports severe pain in the buttock or back. Pain on the symptomatic side when the leg on the asymptomatic side is raised is highly suggestive of lumbar disk herniation. A markedly positive test at 20° of elevation with a negative seated straight-leg raising test is suggestive of symptom amplification rather than a true pathologic process.

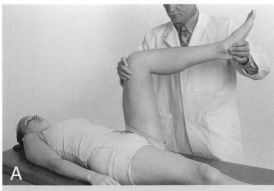

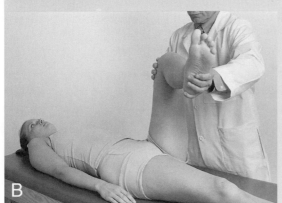

### Internal-external hip rotation in flexion

Flex the hip and knee to 90°, with the thigh held perpendicular to the transverse line across the anterior superior iliac spines. For internal rotation, rotate the tibia away from the midline of the trunk (**A**), thus producing inward rotation of the hip. For external rotation, rotate the tibia toward the midline of the trunk (**B**), thus producing external rotation of the hip. Pain in the groin or buttocks with this maneuver suggests hip irritability.

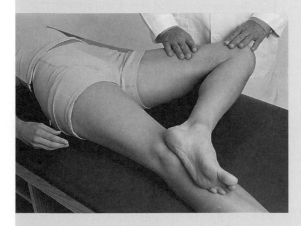

### FABER test

The FABER (flexion-abduction-external rotation) test, sometimes called the figure-of-4 test, is a stress maneuver to detect hip and sacroiliac pathology. Place the hip in flexion, abduction, and external rotation, and then place the patient's foot on the opposite knee. Press down on the flexed knee. If the maneuver is painful, the hip or sacroiliac region may be affected. Increased pain with this test also may be a nonorganic finding.

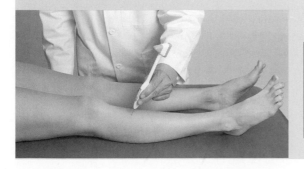

### Sensory Examination

Test for pin prick sensation over the lateral thigh and medial femoral condyle (L3 innervation), the medial leg and medial ankle (L4 innervation), the lateral leg and dorsum of the foot (L5 innervation), and the sole of the foot and lateral ankle (S1 innervation).

SECTION 8 ■ SPINE

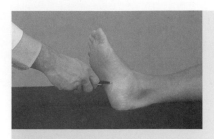

### Babinski sign (flexor plantar response)

Stroke lightly upward on the plantar surface of the foot and look for great toe extension (withdrawal response) and fanning of the lesser toes as a sign of long-tract spinal cord involvement.

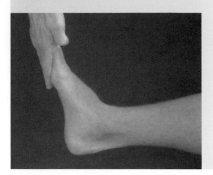

### Ankle clonus

Dorsiflex the ankle suddenly and observe for rhythmic beating (clonus), noting the duration of and the number of "beats." This is another sign of long-tract spinal cord involvement.

# PRONE EXAMINATION

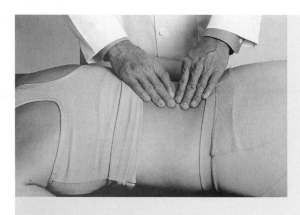

### Palpation of lower lumbar area

Palpate the tissues over the lower lumbar area, looking for areas of tenderness, swelling, or ecchymosis.

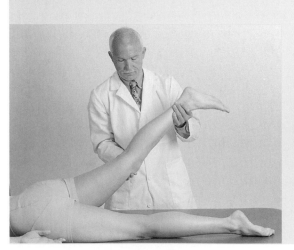

### Reverse straight-leg raising test

The reverse straight-leg raising test is a traditional way to place the L1-4 nerve roots under tension. With the patient prone, lift the hip into extension while keeping the knee straight. Pain over the anterior thigh suggests an upper lumbar disk problem, usually above L4-5. This test would also be markedly positive in a patient with a condition that involves inflammation of the iliopsoas, such as appendicitis.

SECTION 8 ■ SPINE

# INAPPROPRIATE FINDINGS (WADDELL SIGNS)

The four tests shown below comprise the Waddell signs. In addition, the examiner should make a subjective evaluation of the entire history and physical examination to decide if the patient's pain behavior seems to be excessive. If the results of two or more of these tests, including the subjective evaluation, are positive, the examiner should be concerned that issues other than peripheral nociception are creating pain behavior.

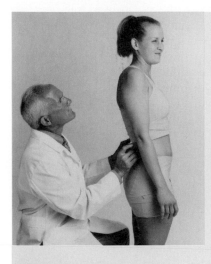

### Nonorganic tenderness

With the patient standing, lightly touch the tissues over the lower lumbar spine. This procedure should not cause pain. Marked pain behavior is a positive test.

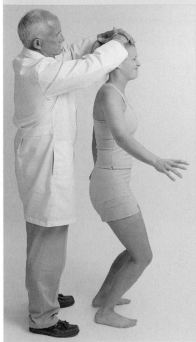

### Axial simulation

With the patient standing, apply light downward pressure on the patient's head. This maneuver should not cause pain in the lumbar spine. If the patient grimaces and moves, reporting pain, the test is positive.

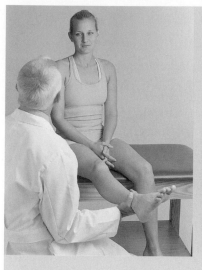
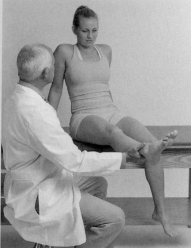

### Seated straight-leg raising test

Distract the patient's attention away from the back by asking whether he or she has knee problems and then lift the foot and extend the knee. If straightening the knee to full extension on both sides does not cause the patient to lean back, no significant sciatic tension is present.

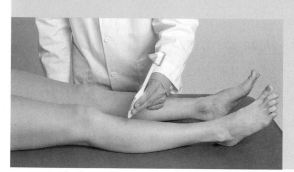

### Sensory examination

Results of a sensory examination that do not follow a dermatomal pattern constitute a positive sign.

# CERVICAL SPINE—RANGE OF MOTION

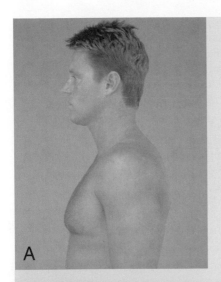

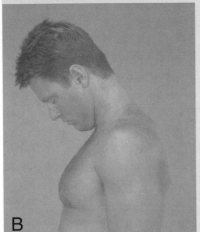

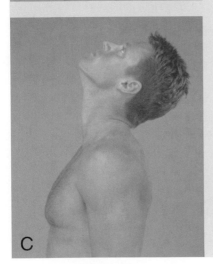

### *Flexion and extension: Zero Starting Position*

The Zero Starting Position is with the neck aligned with the trunk (**A**). Stabilize the trunk so that motion does not occur in the thoracic spine. Assess flexion with forward bending of the cervical spine (**B**) and extension with posterior inclination (**C**). Flexion and extension are typically estimated visually in degrees; however, limited flexion may also be measured as the distance between the chin and the sternum at maximum cervical flexion.

SECTION 8 ■ SPINE

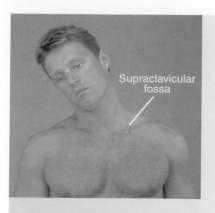

Supraclavicular fossa

### Lateral bend

The Zero Starting Position is with the nose vertical and in line with the axis of the trunk. Stabilize the trunk so that motion occurs only at the neck. Right lateral bend is with the head inclined toward the patient's right shoulder, and left lateral bend is inclination in the opposite direction. The degree of motion is the angle between the vertical axis and the mid-axis of the face.

Inspect and palpate the supraclavicular fossae for tenderness and/or masses. Superior sulcus tumors of the lung (Pancoast tumors) sometimes present as neck pain and pain in the ulnar distribution.

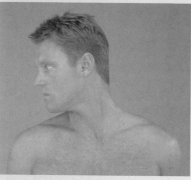

### Rotation

The Zero Starting Position is the same as that for lateral bend. Rotation is estimated in degrees. To estimate upper cervical vertebral rotation, measure rotation with the neck in maximum flexion.

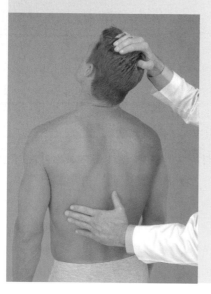

### Spurling test

Ask the patient to extend the neck while gently tilting the head to the side. This maneuver narrows the neural foramen and will increase or reproduce radicular arm pain associated with cervical disk herniations or cervical spondylosis.

**Note:** Performing this maneuver with incorrect technique can be harmful to the patient. You should perform the Spurling test only if you are confident in your ability to perform it correctly.

# CERVICAL SPINE—MUSCLE TESTING

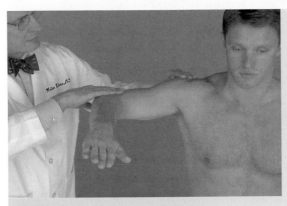

### C5–Deltoid muscle

With the patient seated, abduct the shoulder to 90°. Push down on the arm to resist activity of the deltoid. A ratchety, giving way motion more than likely is a nonorganic sign. Patients with true weakness exhibit a uniform ability to sustain resistance throughout the range of motion.

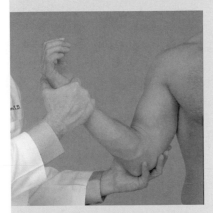

### C5–Biceps

With the patient seated, ask the patient to flex the elbow in a supinated position as you apply resistance. The biceps also is innervated by C6, but if C5 is intact, biceps strength should be at least grade 3. Test C5 sensation by assessing light touch on the lateral aspect of the arm.

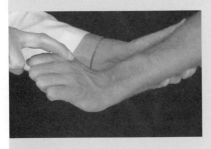

### C6–Radial wrist extensors

Flex the patient's fingers to eliminate wrist extension activity by the finger extensor muscles, and then ask the patient to extend the wrist in a radial direction as you apply resistance. Test C6 sensation by assessing light touch on the volar aspect of the thumb.

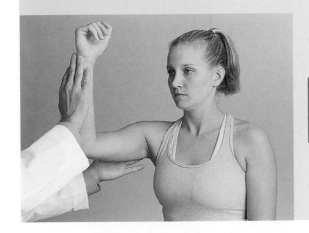

### C7–Triceps

With the patient seated and the shoulder flexed approximately 90°, ask the patient to extend the elbow as you apply resistance.

SECTION 8 ■ SPINE

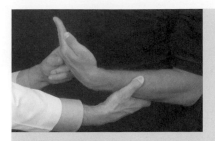

### C7–Flexor carpi radialis

With the patient seated, place the fingers in extension to eliminate wrist flexor activity by the finger flexor muscles, and then ask the patient to flex the wrist in a radial direction as you apply resistance. Test C7 sensation by assessing light touch on the volar aspect of the long finger.

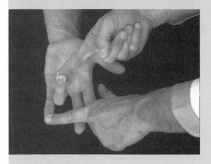

### C8–Flexor digitorum sublimus to ring finger

Stabilize the long, index, and little fingers in extension and ask the patient to flex the fingers as you apply resistance. Test C8 sensation by assessing light touch on the volar aspect of the little finger.

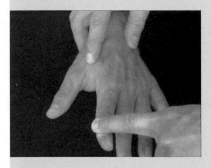

### T1–First dorsal interosseous

Ask the patient to abduct the index finger as you apply resistance. Palpate the muscle belly of the first dorsal interosseous muscle to confirm activity. Test T1 sensation by assessing light touch on the medial aspect of the arm proximal to the elbow.

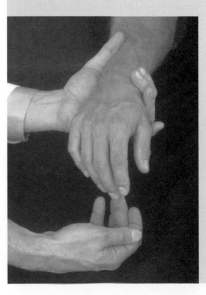

### Hoffmann reflex

With the patient seated and the patient's relaxed hand cradled in yours, flick the long fingernail and look for index finger and thumb flexion as a sign of long-tract spinal cord involvement in the neck.

SECTION 8 ■ SPINE

# CAUDA EQUINA SYNDROME

**ICD-9 Code**
**344.60**
Cauda equina syndrome, without
mention of neurogenic bladder

## DEFINITION

The distal end of the spinal cord, the conus medullaris, terminates at the L1-2 level. Below this, the spinal canal is filled with the L2-S4 nerve roots, known as the cauda equina. Compression of roots distal to the conus causes paralysis without spasticity.

The cauda equina syndrome results from a relatively sudden reduction in the volume of the lumbar spinal canal that causes compression of multiple nerve roots and leads to muscle paralysis. The sacral roots that control bladder and anal function (S2 to S4) are midline and are particularly vulnerable. Causes for cauda equina syndrome include central disk herniation, epidural abscess, epidural hematoma, and trauma to the spine with retropulsion of a portion of a vertebral burst fracture. Onset may be immediate (with a fracture) or may occur over a few hours or days (with other conditions). Cauda equina syndrome usually requires emergency surgery to relieve nerve root compression and to stop progression of neurologic deficit. Even with prompt recognition and immediate decompression, recovery of neurologic function is often incomplete and bowel and bladder function are often unimproved.

## CLINICAL SYMPTOMS

Radicular pain and numbness typically involve both legs; however, symptoms are often more severe in one extremity. The presence of perineal numbness in a saddle distribution is typical for most patients with cauda equina syndrome (**Figure 1**). Lower extremity pain may diminish as the paralysis progresses. Leg weakness may present as a stumbling gait, difficulty rising from a chair, or foot drop that is often symmetric. Patients often report difficulty voiding or loss of urinary and anal sphincter control.

Patients may have a history of preexisting spinal stenosis with a sudden increase in symptoms, or the history may reveal sudden onset of pain following lifting, or recent spine surgery with subsequent onset of fever, chills, and increased back and leg pain.

## TESTS

### Physical Examination

Watch the patient walk. Inability to rise from a chair without the assistance of armrests (quadriceps and/or hip extensor weakness) and inability to walk on the heels or toes (ankle dorsiflexor and plantar flexor weakness) suggest multiple nerve root dysfunction. Evaluate motor and sensory function of the

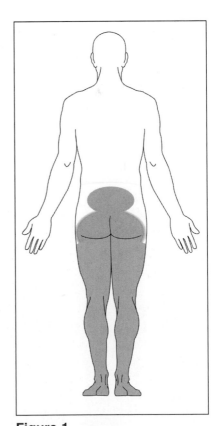

**Figure 1**
Pain diagram for cauda equina syndrome.

lumbosacral nerve roots, including anal sphincter tone and/or perianal numbness. Patients seen in the emergency department for acute back pain may receive an injection of narcotics that may cause acute urinary retention and confuse the diagnosis of cauda equina syndrome.

## Diagnostic Tests

Significant compression of the thecal sac seen on MRI of the lumbar spine or CT/myelogram will confirm the diagnosis of cauda equina syndrome. AP and lateral radiographs of the lumbar spine are important to identify structural problems such as a fracture and spondylolisthesis. A complete blood count (CBC), C-reactive protein, and erythrocyte sedimentation rate can assist with the diagnosis of a suspected infection.

# DIFFERENTIAL DIAGNOSIS

Guillain-Barré syndrome (intact sensation possible, normal MRI scan)

Herniated lumbar disk (unilateral radicular symptoms and motor weakness, normal rectal tone and perineal sensation)

Metastatic tumor (lymphoma or leukemia) (abnormal blood studies, pathologic fracture)

Multiple sclerosis (no history of trauma, patchy numbness, diplopia, facial and/or upper extremity numbness)

Spinal cord tumor (positive Babinski sign, patchy numbness above L2, spasticity)

# ADVERSE OUTCOMES OF THE DISEASE

Permanent paralysis and loss of sphincter function (urinary and anal) are possible. A possible error would be to relate the bladder symptoms to age-related conditions or female cystocele or male prostatism without considering the possibility of sphincter paralysis.

# TREATMENT

Cauda equina syndrome is a surgical emergency. Immediate decompression is almost always necessary once the anatomic lesion is defined.

# ADVERSE OUTCOMES OF TREATMENT

Wound infection and postoperative hematoma are possible.

# REFERRAL DECISIONS/RED FLAGS

Any unexplained neurologic deficit, loss of normal bowel or bladder function, increasing pain not controlled by simple analgesics, or decreasing pain in the face of increasing neurologic deficit is cause for concern.

# Cervical Radiculopathy

## Synonym
Herniated cervical disk

## Definition
Cervical radiculopathy is referred neurogenic pain in the distribution of a cervical nerve root or roots, with or without associated numbness, weakness, or loss of reflexes. The usual cause in young adults is herniation of a cervical disk that entraps the root as it enters the foramen. In older patients, a combination of foraminal narrowing due to vertical settling of the disk space and arthritic involvement of the uncovertebral joint is the most common cause of lateral nerve root entrapment.

## Clinical Symptoms
Neck pain and radicular pain with associated numbness and paresthesias in the upper extremity in the distribution of the involved root are common (**Figure 1**). Muscle spasms, or fasciculations, in the involved myotomes may occur. Other symptoms may include weakness, lack of coordination, changes in handwriting, diminished grip strength, dropping objects from the hand, and difficulty with fine manipulative tasks. Occipital headaches and pain radiating into the paraspinal and scapular regions also may occur.

Symptoms indicative of cervical myelopathy, such as trunk or leg dysfunction, gait disturbances, bowel or bladder changes, and signs of upper motor neuron involvement, occur more commonly with stenosis of the cervical spinal canal.

Patients may state that they can relieve the pain by placing their hands on top of their head, as this decreases tension on the involved nerve root.

## Tests

### Physical Examination
Cervical lordosis may be reduced and the range of neck motion may be mildly restricted. Extension and axial rotation will often cause pain in the arm or shoulder. Assess motor and sensory function of the C5-T1 nerve roots as well as upper extremity reflexes and other upper motor neuron signs. Careful examination for signs of shoulder pathology, vascular disturbances, and peripheral nerve entrapment is necessary. A complete neurologic examination should be performed (**Table 1**).

Signs of upper motor neuron involvement suggest spinal cord compression.

### ICD-9 Codes
**722.0**
Displacement of cervical intervertebral disk without myelopathy

**723.4**
Other disorders of cervical region, brachial neuritis or radiculitis

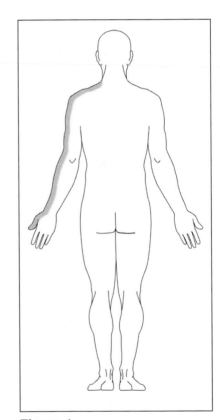

**Figure 1**
Typical pain diagram for a patient with cervical radiculopathy. Patients with root pressure above C5 may report scapular and interscapular pain with no extremity radiation.

SECTION 8 ■ SPINE

## Table 1  Clinical Features of Common Cervical Syndromes

| Disk | Pain | Sensory Change | Motor Weakness Atrophy | Reflex Change |
|------|------|----------------|------------------------|---------------|
| C4-5 (C5 root) | Base of neck, shoulder, anterolateral aspect of arm | Numbness in deltoid region | Deltoid, biceps | Biceps |
| C5-6 (C6 root) | Neck, shoulder, medial border of scapula, lateral aspect of arm, radial aspect of forearm | Dorsolateral aspect of thumb and index finger | Biceps, wrist extensors pollicus longus | Biceps, brachioradialis |
| C6-7 (C7 root) | Neck, shoulder, medial border of scapula, lateral aspect of arm, dorsum of forearm | Index, long fingers, dorsum of hand | Triceps and/or finger extensors | Triceps |

## Diagnostic Tests

Plain radiographs may identify regions of spondylosis or degenerative involvement of the disk and the facet joint. MRI or CT with intrathecal contrast (myelogram) confirms the diagnosis (**Figure 2**). Advanced imaging studies are necessary in patients who have not responded to nonsurgical management, in patients with profound neurologic deficits, or in patients who are considering surgical management. Electromyography and nerve conduction velocity studies help in some instances to identify the location of neurologic dysfunction. These studies are valuable to differentiate radiculopathy from peripheral

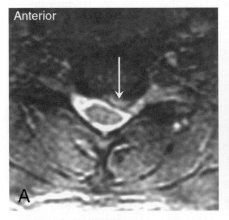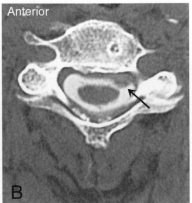

**Figure 2**

**A,** Axial MRI scan of a cervical disk herniation (arrow) in a younger patient. **B,** Axial CT scan with intrathecal contrast of a cervical disk herniation (arrow) in a younger patient.

neuropathy and various nerve compressions syndromes, such as carpal tunnel syndrome.

# DIFFERENTIAL DIAGNOSIS

Adhesive capsulitis (restricted passive and active motion of the shoulder)

Demyelinating conditions (varying symptoms, intensity, and location)

Myocardial ischemia (abnormal ECG or stress tests)

Peripheral nerve entrapment (positive Phalen test, positive Tinel sign at elbow or wrist)

Rotator cuff disease (painful wince with active shoulder abduction and circumduction movements)

Thoracic outlet syndrome (distinctly uncommon; decrease in radial pulse with shoulder abduction and external rotation may be observed)

# ADVERSE OUTCOMES OF THE DISEASE

Muscle paralysis, weakness, or chronic pain syndromes may develop. Rarely, the condition may progress to a myelopathy with spinal cord involvement.

# TREATMENT

Spontaneous resolution of all or most symptoms occurs within 2 to 8 weeks in most patients. With radicular pain, a short course of anti-inflammatory medication coupled with cervical traction in a head halter is usually beneficial. Referral to a physical therapist for cervical traction is more effective than simply providing a patient with a traction unit. Narcotic medication is best avoided and seldom warranted. Manipulation of the cervical spine should also be avoided.

# ADVERSE OUTCOMES OF TREATMENT

Quadriparesis, herniation of an intervertebral disk, stroke, or vertebral fracture may follow manipulation of the cervical spine.

# REFERRAL DECISIONS/RED FLAGS

Patients in whom nonsurgical treatment fails or who develop atrophy, motor weakness, or signs of myelopathy may require surgical evaluation. Patients with any signs that suggest a demyelinating condition, infection, or tumor require further evaluation. If radicular symptoms are accompanied by intolerable pain, early specialty evaluation should be obtained.

SECTION 8 ■ SPINE

# CERVICAL SPONDYLOSIS

**ICD-9 Codes**

**721.0**
Cervical spondylosis without myelopathy

**721.1**
Cervical spondylosis with myelopathy

**723.0**
Spinal stenosis in cervical region

## SYNONYMS

Cervical arthritis
Degenerative disk disease of the cervical spine

## DEFINITION

Cervical spondylosis is the nomenclature for degenerative disk disease in the cervical spine. This condition is produced by ingrowth of bony spurs, buckling or protrusion of the ligamentum flavum, and/or herniation of disk material. These anatomic alterations may result in narrowing of the neural foramen and stenosis of the cervical spinal canal. Cervical spondylosis may cause neck pain, cervical radiculopathy, and/or cervical myelopathy.

## CLINICAL SYMPTOMS

The most common symptoms are limited mobility of the cervical spine and chronic neck pain that worsens with upright activity. Paraspinous muscle spasm may occur, as may headaches that appear to originate in the neck. Increased irritability, fatigue, sleep disturbances, and impaired work tolerance also may develop. Radicular symptoms and pain may occur in the upper extremities with lateral recess stenosis and nerve root entrapment (**Figure 1**). Radiographs are of minimal value because many radiographic changes of spondylosis occur in patients who report no significant symptoms. Therefore, careful clinical evaluations are warranted to ensure that symptoms are linked to pathologic processes and not simply physiologic changes of aging.

Narrowing of the spinal canal and resultant myelopathy are more common in older men. Typical symptoms of early cervical myelopathy may include palmar parathesias in the upper extremities; difficulty with upper extremity dexterity, such as buttoning a shirt or blouse; and subtle gait disturbances that can usually be highlighted by asking the patient to perform a tandem walk (heel-to-toe walking). Urinary function may be abnormal as well. Loss of vibration and position sense (posterior column deficits) is more common in the feet than in the upper extremities. A concomitant radiculopathy in the upper extremity may obscure the diagnosis of cervical myelopathy. Additionally, because pain is frequently absent in patients with early cervical myelopathy, the subtle gait changes may be related to the lumbar spine, with the myelopathy being totally

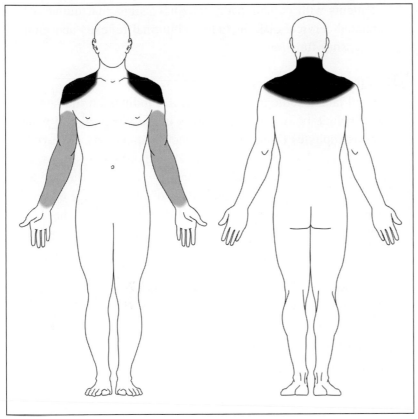

**Figure 1**
Typical pain diagram for a patient with cervical spondylosis.

overlooked. The key physical findings in these patients include the presence of long-tract signs (signs that indicate an upper motor neuron lesion), subtle gait disturbances, and alterations in upper extremity dexterity. These changes are not related to the common stenosis that is seen in the lumbar spine because peripheral nerves and not the spinal cord would be involved in lumbar stenosis unless the L1-L2 area is involved.

# TESTS

## *Physical Examination*
Examination may reveal tenderness along the lateral neck or along the spinous processes posteriorly. Motion may be limited or painful. Assess sensory and motor function of the upper (C5-T1) and lower (L1-S1) nerve roots. Evaluate gait and tandem walking as well as bowel and bladder function. With myelopathy, flexion may produce electric shocks that travel down the spine, arms, or legs. A Hoffmann reflex, clonus, hyperreflexia, and the Babinski sign (an extensor toe response) are possible, as are gait disturbances and global weakness.

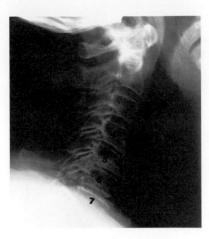

**Figure 2**

Lateral radiograph demonstrating advanced cervical spondylosis.

Patients with radiculopathy may have signs that mimic a herniated cervical disk, including abnormal reflexes and motor and sensory function.

# DIAGNOSTIC TESTS

AP and lateral radiographs are useful. Findings on the lateral view include bony reactive changes in the vertebral end plates, with osteophytes (bone spurs) projecting anteriorly (**Figure 2**). Osteophytes that emerge from the zygoapophyseal joints may also project into the neural foramina. In addition, osteophytes may develop on the posterior portion of the vertebral body and encroach into the spinal canal, producing stenosis of the cervical canal (**Figure 3**). Anterior subluxation of one vertebra onto the vertebra below (**Figure 4**) increases the likelihood of cervical stenosis and associated neurologic findings. Degenerative findings occur most commonly at the C5-6 and C6-7 disk spaces.

# DIFFERENTIAL DIAGNOSIS

Metastatic tumor (night pain that prevents sleep)

Soft cervical disk herniation (generally seen in younger patients)

Spinal cord tumor (extradural/metastatic, intradural/primary) (physical examination findings, confirmed by MRI and/or CT myelogram)

Syringomyelia (loss of superficial abdominal reflexes, insensitivity to pain)

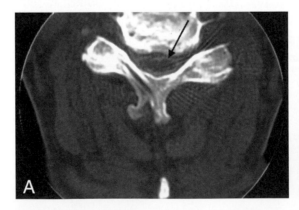
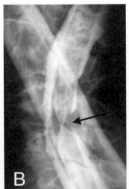

**Figure 3**

**A,** Axial CT myelogram through the midcervical spine demonstrating marked cervical spinal stenosis. Note the paucity of contrast material surrounding the deformed spinal cord (arrow). AP dimension of the cervical spinal canal and the AP dimension of the cervical cord are both reduced. **B,** Lateral radiograph of a 70-year-old man with significant cervical spinal stenosis, with symptoms of cord compression and myelography found on examination. Note the marked narrowing of the column of contrast material (arrow).

Vertebral subluxation (in patients with advanced spondylosis or rheumatoid arthritis or following trauma)

# ADVERSE OUTCOMES OF THE DISEASE

Chronic pain, myelopathy, or mixed myeloradiculopathy is possible. Note that these sequelae of cervical spondylosis occur more commonly when the anatomic changes are more advanced.

# TREATMENT

Supportive treatment and reassurance may be adequate, but symptoms may last several months or become chronic. NSAIDs are often adequate. Doxepin or amitriptyline, in minimal doses, may also be useful to help with sleep. Narcotic medication should be avoided. Management should also include a cervical pillow or cervical roll and physical therapy.

Surgical decompression and fusion may be necessary for patients with intractable pain, progressive neurologic findings, or symptoms of cervical myelopathy and spinal cord compression.

# ADVERSE OUTCOMES OF TREATMENT

NSAIDs may cause gastric, renal, or hepatic complications. Sedation from tricyclic antidepressants may occur, and adverse reactions to monoamine oxidase inhibitors are possible. Narcotic dependence is also possible, especially with the early and prolonged use of stronger narcotic medication. Monoparesis or loss of specific nerve root function may occur, and, although uncommon, quadriparesis or quadriplegia may result from progressive cervical stenosis with spinal cord compression.

# REFERRAL DECISIONS/RED FLAGS

Intractable neck pain that is not responsive to treatment, neurologic symptoms that affect either the upper or lower extremities, lack of coordination, gait disturbances, and radicular symptoms related to neck motion all indicate the need for further evaluation and referral to a specialist.

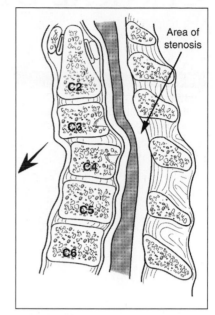

**Figure 4**
Degenerative disk changes and degenerative subluxations causing canal stenosis. The arrow on the left indicates the forward slippage of C3 on C4.

Adapted with permission from Bohlmann HH: Cervical spondylosis with moderate to severe myelopathy. *Spine* 1977;2:151-162.

SECTION 8 ■ SPINE

# CERVICAL STRAIN

**ICD-9 Code**

**847.0**
Sprains and strains of other and unspecified parts of back, neck

SECTION 8 ■ SPINE

## SYNONYM
Neck sprain

## DEFINITION
Cervical strain is a common condition that is usually self-limiting. By strict definition, an acute cervical strain is a muscle injury in the neck, whereas the term sprain generally refers to a ligamentous stretching-type injury. These terms are often used interchangeably, however, by both the medical profession and the lay public. Moreover, because neither physical examination nor imaging can distinguish between muscle and ligament injuries in the deeply located soft-tissue structures of the neck, the term cervical strain includes ligamentous injuries of the facet joints and/or intervertebral disks. Regardless of which soft-tissue structures have been injured, the diagnostic and treatment protocols are similar: evaluate the patient to identify unstable injuries and/or neurologic deficits, then provide appropriate treatment.

A whiplash mechanism (acceleration-deceleration of the neck with rapid flexion-extension) occurs commonly as a result of motor vehicle accidents. The classic situation is a stopped car that is struck from behind by another vehicle. These injuries may cause prolonged disability despite no apparent pathologic process. The cause may be a combination of a ligament/muscle injury and symptom amplification. On occasion, severe injuries result in definite instability patterns and/or cervical disk displacements. The concept of symptom amplification should not be advanced until after a thorough history, physical examination, and appropriate imaging studies have been performed.

## CLINICAL SYMPTOMS
Cervical pain may follow an incident of trauma or may be spontaneous in onset. Nonradicular, nonfocal neck pain, noted anywhere from the base of the skull to the cervicothoracic junction, is most common (**Figure 1**). Patients may also have pain in the region of the sternocleidomastoid muscles and/or the trapezius muscles. Pain is often worse with motion and may be accompanied by paraspinal spasm. Occipital headaches may occur in the early phase and may persist for months. Pain following trauma often persists longer than pain following strains or sprains of spontaneous onset. Patients may report

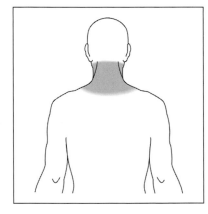

**Figure 1**
Typical pain diagram for a patient with an acute cervical strain.

increased irritability, fatigue, sleep disturbances, and difficulty concentrating. Work tolerance may be impaired.

## TESTS

### Physical Examination

Examination may reveal areas of tenderness in the paraspinous muscles, trapezii, sternocleidomastoid muscles, spinous processes, interspinous ligaments, and/or the medial border of the scapula. Limited motion is common and may involve rotation, lateral bending, and/or flexion and extension. Pain is often noted at the extremes of motions. The neurologic examination is usually normal.

### Diagnostic Tests

AP, lateral, and open mouth (odontoid) radiographs are necessary if the patient has a history of trauma or associated neurologic deficit or if the patient is elderly. All seven cervical vertebrae must be seen. Anterior displacement of the pharyngeal air shadow indicates soft-tissue swelling that may develop following injury to the intervertebral disk, anterior longitudinal ligament, occipital-cervical level, or spinal fracture. The presence of precervical swelling mandates a specialty consultation to assess the numerous possible causes. In normal adults, the width of the prevertebral soft tissue at the level of C3 should not exceed one third the width of the C3 vertebral body. The normal lordotic curve of the cervical spine may be straightened or reversed as a result of muscle spasm, but this finding is also observed in approximately 10% of normal adults. Preexisting degenerative changes may be noted; they are most commonly age related and occur most frequently at C5-6 or C6-7.

If the patient has severe pain, the screening radiographs should be examined for signs of instability that include translation of a vertebral body of more than 3.5 mm and/or more than 11° of angulation of adjacent vertebrae. Routine flexion-extension radiographs of the cervical spine should not be ordered until the patient has been evaluated by a specialist because of the risk of increased neurologic damage from the maneuvers.

## DIFFERENTIAL DIAGNOSIS

Cervical disk herniation (neurologic abnormality and radicular pain)

Cervical spine tumor or infection (night pain, weight loss, history, fever, chills, sweats)

SECTION 8 ■ SPINE

SECTION 8 ■ SPINE

Dislocation or subluxation of the spine (usually evident on radiographs; however, on occasion a spontaneous reduction occurs, masking the severity of the injury)

Inflammatory conditions of the cervical spine (rheumatoid arthritis with abnormal radiographs)

Spinal fracture (abnormal radiographs)

Symptom amplification/secondary gain (inconsistent or exaggerated findings)

## ADVERSE OUTCOMES OF THE DISEASE

Symptoms resolve completely in most patients within the first 4 to 6 weeks. With whiplash, resolution typically is delayed, but most symptoms resolve within 6 to 12 months with few residual symptoms.

Patients with subtle disk injuries superimposed on existing degenerative conditions of the cervical spine may have intractable pain. In some instances, radiculopathy due to lateral nerve root entrapment or myelopathy due to central spinal stenosis may develop.

## TREATMENT

Providing the patient with reassurance about the natural history of these disorders represents an important first step. Acute care (1 to 2 weeks) involves a soft cervical collar and appropriate pain medications and/or short-term NSAIDs. Muscle relaxants may help if the patient has spasm. Commercially available cervical pillows help with reestablishing a normal sleep pattern.

Massage, cervical traction, and ultrasound and other modalities may help, especially in the first 4 weeks. Mild narcotic medication may be useful initially but should be restricted to the first week or two following the injury. Doxepin or amitriptyline may also be helpful for sleep. Manipulation of the cervical spine is contraindicated in patients with acute cervical injuries.

Aerobic activities, such as walking, should be initiated as soon as possible. Add isometric exercises as the patient's comfort improves, preferably in the first 2 weeks. Encourage an early return to normal activities and work.

## PHYSICAL THERAPY PRESCRIPTION

Cervical strains secondary to limited mobility or tight muscles respond the best to stretching and strengthening exercises. A home program of exercises (see p 750) should include pain-free range-of-motion exercises such as head rolls in all directions. In addition, an upper back stretch helps to relieve tension and increase range of motion of the cervical spine. If the symptoms do not respond to the home program within 3 to 4 weeks, formal physical therapy may be ordered. The prescription should include an evaluation to determine specific segmental limitations and muscle involvement. The physical therapist may order cervical spine traction and mobilization of the restricted segments.

## ADVERSE OUTCOMES OF TREATMENT

NSAIDs may cause gastric, renal, or hepatic complications. If the patient's condition fails to improve, depression may develop. Chronic pain syndrome and drug dependence also may develop in these patients.

## REFERRAL DECISIONS/RED FLAGS

Patients with pain refractory to treatment, nerve root deficits, or myelopathy or who present a diagnostic dilemma must be evaluated thoroughly.

SECTION 8 ■ SPINE

# HOME EXERCISE PROGRAM FOR CERVICAL STRAIN

Perform the exercises in the order listed. Apply heat to the painful area for 20 minutes before performing the exercises. If the pain worsens or does not improve, call your doctor.

| Exercise Type | Area Targeted | Number of Repetitions/Sets | Number of Days per Week | Number of Weeks |
|---|---|---|---|---|
| Head rolls | Cervical spine | 3 repetitions (all directions)/ 3 sets | Daily | 3 to 4 |
| Cat back stretch | Upper back | 10 repetitions | Daily | 3 to 4 |

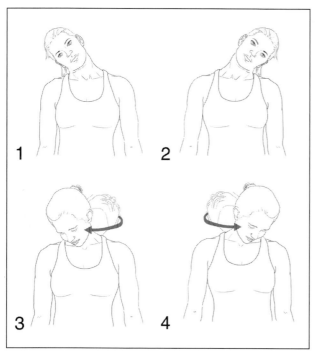

## Head Rolls

Sit in a chair or stand with your weight evenly distributed on both feet. Begin by gently bowing your head toward your chest, then stretching your right ear toward your right shoulder (**1**), then your left ear toward your left shoulder (**2**). (**3**) Next, gently roll your head in a clockwise circle three times. (**4**) Switch directions and gently roll your head in a counterclockwise circle three times.

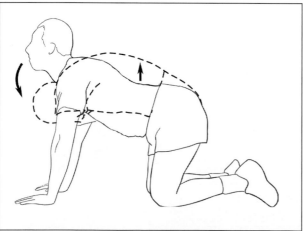

## Cat Back Stretch

Kneel on your hands and knees in a relaxed position. Raise your back up like a cat and hold for 5 seconds. Repeat 10 times.

# FRACTURES OF THE CERVICAL SPINE

## DEFINITION

Cervical spine fractures and associated ligamentous injuries occur commonly as the result of high-energy trauma, such as a motor vehicle accident, a fall from a height, or a diving accident. These fractures must be suspected and either identified or excluded in all trauma patients who report neck pain. In addition, because in unconscious or intoxicated patients the history and physical examination are compromised, such patients must have appropriate imaging studies to evaluate the cervical spine. Most missed spinal injuries occur in patients who are obtunded from a closed head injury, unconscious, and/or intoxicated.

**ICD-9 Code**

**805.0**
Fracture of vertebral column without mention of spinal cord injury, cervical, closed

## CLINICAL SYMPTOMS

Severe neck pain, paraspinous muscle spasm, and/or point tenderness are the most common presenting symptoms. Pain that radiates into the shoulder or arm with associated numbness or tingling suggests nerve root impingement. Global sensory or motor deficits suggest spinal cord injury. In patients who have sustained multiple trauma, associated injuries may be so painful that the patient may not report every area of the body that is painful. Therefore, in these patients, the absence of neck pain on initial examination does not "clear" the patient or eliminate the possibility of a cervical spine injury.

## TESTS

### Physical Examination

Inspect for swelling and contusions. Palpate for tenderness and paraspinal spasm. A gap or a step-off between spinous processes suggests an injury to the posterior ligamentous complex that is generally quite unstable. Evaluate motor and sensory function of the upper and lower extremities as well as the sensory status of the thoracic dermatomes. Perianal sensation, sphincter tone, and the bulbocavernosus reflex also should be assessed in any patient who is suspected of having a spinal injury.

### Diagnostic Tests

Radiographs of the cervical spine should include an AP and lateral view as well as an open mouth view of the odontoid (C2). In a multiply injured patient, however, the most important view is the cross-table lateral view of the cervical spine, to include C1 through T1. In large patients, CT and/or MRI might be required to completely evaluate the cervical spine. The most commonly missed injuries are those at the upper and lower portions of the cervical spine. Lateral radiographs must include the occiput superiorly and the top of T1 inferiorly. Occasionally, a swimmer's view is required to visualize the cervicothoracic junction, although this region can usually be assessed with CT reconstructions or with MRI.

The lateral radiograph should be evaluated for anterior soft-tissue swelling, height of the vertebral body, and alignment of the vertebral bodies, facet joints, and spinous processes. The odontoid view should be checked for odontoid fracture (often subtle), C1 lateral mass widening, and the position of the occipital condyles. The AP radiograph can show subtle malalignment of the spinous processes. This finding may indicate rotational malalignment secondary to facet fracture or dislocation.

If no fracture is seen, the radiographs should be carefully evaluated for other signs of instability, including translation of a vertebral body of more than 3.5 mm or more than 11° of angulation of adjacent vertebral bodies. Flexion-extension lateral views should be obtained only after a three-view series has been cleared and only upon recommendation by a spine consultant. Flexion-extension radiographs may not detect ligamentous instability if paraspinal spasm is present. Therefore, in the acute situation, other studies (eg, CT, MRI) may be preferable to rule out a fracture or significant ligamentous injury.

## DIFFERENTIAL DIAGNOSIS

Acute disk herniation (normal radiographs with or without neurologic deficit)

Cervical sprain (normal radiographs with muscle pain/ tenderness)

High thoracic fracture (evident on swimmer's view or thoracic radiographs)

## ADVERSE OUTCOMES OF THE DISEASE

Severe injury may result in complete or incomplete quadriplegia. Nerve compression with radiculopathy may also occur. Chronic neck pain and fatigue may result from deformity or associated muscle injury.

## TREATMENT

The cervical spine must be immobilized at the time of extrication of the patient from the accident scene. In addition, bracing of the cervical spine and the use of a spine board should be used during transport of patients who sustain high-energy trauma or who have suspected neck injuries. Immediate IV steroids (methylprednisolone 30 mg/kg bolus followed by a continuous drip of 5.4 mg/kg/hr for 23 hours) should be initiated for patients who have sustained a spinal cord injury.

Patients whose initial radiographs and neurologic examination are normal but who have persistent pain should wear a cervical collar for 7 to 10 days. The clinical examination and radiographs should be repeated if symptoms persist. If these radiographs are normal, flexion-extension lateral radiographs and an MRI scan should be obtained. If these studies are normal, the patient may start a neck stretching and strengthening physical therapy program with scapular stabilization.

## ADVERSE OUTCOMES OF TREATMENT
Neurologic deficits may develop or worsen during treatment.

## REFERRAL DECISIONS/RED FLAGS
Patients with instability or with a fracture, dislocation, subluxation, or neurologic deficit require further evaluation. A high index of suspicion for occult injury should be maintained in patients who are intoxicated, uncooperative, or unconscious.

SECTION 8 ■ SPINE

# FRACTURES OF THE THORACIC OR LUMBAR SPINE

## DEFINITION

Fractures of the thoracic or lumbar spine generally occur as a result of high-energy trauma such as motor vehicle accidents or falls from a height. They may also occur following minimal trauma in patients who have diminished bone strength from osteoporosis, tumors, infections, or long-term steroid use.

The fracture pattern usually determines fracture stability and likelihood of neural injury. Simple compression fractures involving only the anterior half of the vertebral body are generally stable, as are some burst fractures (compression fractures extending to the posterior third of the vertebral body). Flexion-distraction injuries that disrupt the posterior ligamentous complex are highly unstable. These injuries are often associated with abdominal injuries such as bowel lacerations.

## CLINICAL SYMPTOMS

Moderate to severe back pain related to a traumatic event is the most common presenting symptom. The pain is exacerbated by motion. Numbness, tingling, weakness, or bowel and bladder dysfunction suggest nerve root or spinal cord injury. In addition, decreased bowel motility may occur secondary to an ileus in patients with lumbar spine fractures.

## TESTS

### Physical Examination

Inspect the trunk, chest, and abdomen for swelling and ecchymosis. Patients with lap belt (flexion/distraction) injuries often demonstrate ecchymosis or contusions over the anterior iliac spines. Tenderness to palpation or light percussion occurs at the level of injury. Hematoma formation and a step-off (forward shift) or gap between spinous processes with swelling are the hallmarks of an unstable flexion-distraction or burst fracture. Evaluate motor and sensory function of all nerve roots distal to the injury. Diffuse numbness, weakness, loss of reflexes, ankle clonus, or a positive Babinski sign indicates spinal cord injury. Examination of perianal sensation, sphincter function, and the bulbocavernosus reflex are particularly important with an associated spinal cord injury. Evaluate the abdomen and chest for possible associated injuries.

## Diagnostic Tests

AP and lateral radiographs of the thoracic and lumbar spine are indicated. When a spine fracture is identified, the radiograph should be scrutinized for adjacent or nonadjacent fractures as well. CT scans with reconstructions offer the best information with respect to the need for surgical stabilization.

In the lateral view, compression and burst fractures show loss of height of the anterior wall of the vertebral body and resultant kyphotic deformity (**Figure 1**). Burst fractures by definition evidence an injury to the middle column, which can be best seen on a CT scan. Unstable flexion-distraction injuries show widening of the space between adjacent spinous processes on the AP and/or lateral view. The AP view may reveal transverse process fractures or widening of the interpedicular distance that also confirms an unstable burst fracture (**Figure 2**). Rotation of one vertebral body in relation to the one below also indicates instability. Any injury other than a simple compression fracture requires additional imaging studies.

# DIFFERENTIAL DIAGNOSIS

Herniated lumbar disk (no fracture, patient able to walk, single nerve root involvement)

Thoracic or lumbar muscle strain (no neurologic findings or fractures)

Visceral injuries (abnormal abdominal examination and radiographs, ultrasound, or CT scan)

# ADVERSE OUTCOMES OF THE DISEASE

Loss of nerve or spinal cord function, persistent painful instability or deformity, and impaired function are serious sequelae of certain injuries to the spine.

# TREATMENT

Preventing neurologic injury, restoring stability, and restoring normal function are the goals of treatment. Initial extrication, transportation, and evaluation in the emergency department require the use of spinal precautions, including a spine board and log rolling. If radiographs reveal no fracture or instability and no neurologic deficits are present, these precautions may be lifted after confirmation by a specialist.

Isolated transverse process fractures do not affect stability of the spine but do indicate significant injury to adjacent muscles and possible injury to the kidneys. A thoracolumbar corset may be used to decrease symptoms.

Simple compression fractures with wedging of less than 20° and no posterior vertebral or posterior element involvement can

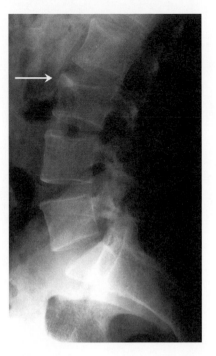

**Figure 1**
Lateral radiograph showing a minimal compression fracture of the lumbar spine.

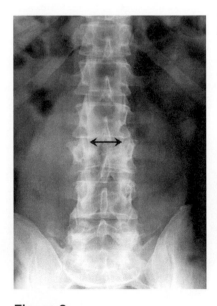

**Figure 2**
AP radiograph showing a burst fracture of the lumbar spine with widening of the interpedicular distance (double-headed arrow).

SECTION 8 ■ SPINE

be managed with a thoracolumbosacral orthosis (TLSO) for 8 to 12 weeks, to be worn during sitting and standing activities. Pain management may require short-term oral narcotics. Walking may be encouraged, but bending, stooping, twisting, and lifting more than 20 lb should be discouraged. The patient should return to work as quickly as possible, with job modifications as needed. Exercises to strengthen trunk flexor and extensor muscles can supplement walking after the brace is removed.

Other injuries usually require more aggressive treatment. Patients with a spinal cord injury should be started on a steroid protocol as soon as possible. Patients with unstable burst fractures, flexion-distraction injuries, or fracture-dislocations are usually treated by internal fixation and spinal fusion.

## ADVERSE OUTCOMES OF TREATMENT

Progressive collapse with kyphotic deformity may occur, resulting in chronic pain and/or neurologic compromise. Chronic muscle pain may also develop if the trunk muscles are not adequately strengthened after immobilization is discontinued.

## REFERRAL DECISIONS/RED FLAGS

Any neurologic deficit is a sign of significant injury and requires further evaluation. Burst fractures, flexion-distraction injuries (or any injury to the posterior column of the spine), fractures with vertebral rotation, and fracture-dislocations all require further evaluation and treatment.

SECTION 8 ■ SPINE

# LOW BACK PAIN: ACUTE

## SYNONYMS

Low back strain
Lumbar sprain
Pulled low back

## DEFINITION

Although the term low back pain (LBP) more properly
describes a symptom rather than a diagnosis, it can be
appropriately used as a diagnostic category. For more than 80%
of patients with LBP, a more specific diagnosis is not possible.

LBP is the most frequent cause of lost work time and
disability in adults younger than 45 years. Most symptoms,
however, are of limited duration, with 80% of patients
demonstrating significant improvement and returning to work
within 1 month. The 4% of patients whose symptoms persist
longer than 6 months generate 80% to 90% of the costs to
society for treating LBP.

A low back strain is an injury to the paravertebral spinal
muscles. The term sprain is used to describe ligamentous
injuries that may include the facet joints or anulus fibrosus. In
the latter condition, the disk does not herniate into the spinal
canal, but substances may leak from the nucleus pulposus that
induce inflammation and cause irritation of the lumbosacral
nerve roots. Because of the deep location of the lumbar soft
tissues, however, localizing an injury to a specific structure is
difficult, if not impossible. Furthermore, in this area, regardless
of which muscle or ligamentous structures have been injured,
the treatment protocols are identical.

A history of repeated lifting and twisting or operating
vibrating equipment may be associated with LBP. However,
individuals who engage in little physical exertion may also
report similar symptoms. Factors associated with reports of
LBP include poor fitness, job dissatisfaction, smoking, and
various psychosocial issues.

## CLINICAL SYMPTOMS

Patients report the acute onset of LBP, often following a lifting
episode. The lifting may be a trivial event, such as leaning over
to pick up a piece of paper. The pain often radiates into the
buttocks and posterior thighs (**Figure 1**). Patients may have
difficulty standing erect and may need to change position
frequently for comfort. This condition may first be experienced
in the early adult years.

**ICD-9 Codes**

**847.1**
Sprains and strains of other and
unspecified parts of back, thoracic

**847.2**
Sprains and strains of other and
unspecified parts of back, lumbar

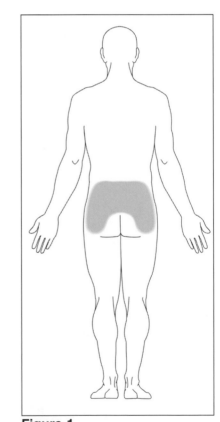

**Figure 1**

Typical pain diagram for a patient
with LBP.

SECTION 8 ■ SPINE

## TESTS

### Physical Examination

Examination reveals diffuse tenderness in the low back or sacroiliac region. Range of motion of the lumbar spine, particularly flexion, is typically reduced and painful. The degree of lumbar flexion and the ease with which the patient can extend the spine are good parameters by which to evaluate progress. Lower extremity reflexes and the motor and sensory function of the lumbosacral nerve roots are normal.

### Diagnostic Tests

Plain radiographs usually are not helpful to diagnose acute LBP. In adolescents and young adults, there is little or no disk space narrowing, whereas in adults older than 30 years, there is variable disk space narrowing and/or spurs. These changes are widely prevalent and are not considered pathologic but rather physiologic signs of aging.

For patients with atypical symptoms, such as pain at rest or at night or a history of significant trauma, AP and lateral radiographs should be obtained. These views help to identify pathologic processes such as infection, neoplasms (visualize up to T10), fracture, or spondylolisthesis.

## DIFFERENTIAL DIAGNOSIS

Ankylosing spondylitis (family history, morning stiffness, limited mobility of the lumbar spine)

Drug-seeking behavior (symptom amplification, inconsistent and nonphysiologic examination)

Extraspinal causes (ovarian cyst, nephrolithiasis, pancreatitis, ulcer disease, aortic aneurysm, retroperitoneal tumors)

Fracture of the vertebral body (major trauma or minimal trauma with osteoporosis)

Herniated disk (unilateral radicular pain symptoms that extend below the knee and are equal to or greater than the back pain)

Infection (fever, chills, sweats, elevated erythrocyte sedimentation rate)

Multiple myeloma (night sweats, men older than 50 years)

## ADVERSE OUTCOMES OF THE DISEASE

Functional impairment is the primary disability. This can be of great significance for any patient whose normal activities are strenuous and whose general health is otherwise excellent, but young adults in particular have difficulty accepting a condition that may impair function for several weeks.

# Treatment

Before any treatment is begun, a complete history should be taken and the patient should be thoroughly evaluated to rule out any significant neurologic findings. If signs of neurologic deficits such as dorsiflexion weakness, plantar flexion weakness, or urinary frequency are found, a referral to a specialist is indicated.

For the patient with LBP with or without sciatic symptoms and with no significant neurologic deficits, treatment has two phases. The initial phase deals with symptomatic relief; the second phase focuses on return to activity.

Phase one, or symptomatic treatment, should include avoidance of intense physical activity. Pain management can be initiated with aspirin, acetaminophen, or NSAIDs. Steroid dose packs, narcotic medication, or muscle relaxants are not recommended as primary pain management tools for most patients who present with acute LBP. It is important to inform the patient that in most cases the symptoms of acute LBP resolve quickly, with the patient able to return to work and other activities within a few days.

As the acute pain improves, phase two treatment can begin. A variety of approaches may be used, all of which focus on helping the patient return to full activity. Initially, the patient may need lighter duty or shorter hours at work. Flexibility in allowing such arrangements benefits both the employee, in increased self-esteem, and the employer, in decreased costs. As pain diminishes and activity increases, the patient should be referred to a physical therapist for an exercise program focusing on an aerobic activity (walking, running, bicycling, swimming, using an elliptical machine) plus strengthening of trunk flexors and extensors. Once the patient is established in this program, he or she may transition to a health club or a home exercise program such as the one described below. Patients who continue to exercise and remain fit have fewer recurrences of LBP.

A patient who is unable to return to work within 4 weeks should be referred to a specialist for further evaluation and treatment.

# Physical Therapy Prescription

The formal physical therapy prescription should include an evaluation to determine specific segmental restrictions and muscle dysfunction. Before developing a rehabilitation program, it is important to determine whether lumbar spine muscle asymmetry, especially of the multifidus, is present. Formal physical therapy may include a combination of mobilization of the restricted segments and stabilization exercises emphasizing endurance. A home exercise program for LBP (see p 761) includes a combination of stretching and stabilization exercises. The cobra stretch and knee to chest exercises are good general stretching exercises for the low back. Side bridges and hip bridges are excellent exercises to improve stability of the low back muscles.

## ADVERSE OUTCOMES OF TREATMENT

NSAIDs may cause gastric, renal, or hepatic complications. Although uncommon, spinal manipulation may result in a lumbar disk herniation.

## REFERRAL DECISIONS/RED FLAGS

Neurologic abnormalities, unresponsive pain syndromes, or an unusual clinical presentation indicates the need for further evaluation.

SECTION 8 ■ SPINE

# HOME EXERCISE PROGRAM FOR ACUTE LOW BACK PAIN

Perform the exercises in the order listed. Apply heat to the low back for 20 minutes before performing the exercises. If the pain worsens or if it does not improve after performing the exercises for 3 to 4 weeks, call your doctor.

| Exercise Type | Muscle Group/ Area Targeted | Number of Repetitions/Sets | Number of Days per Week | Number of Weeks |
|---|---|---|---|---|
| Cobra stretch | Low back | 10 repetitions | Daily | 3 to 4 |
| Knee to chest | Low back | 10 repetitions/3 sets | Daily | 3 to 4 |
| Side bridges | Quadratus lumborum | 5 repetitions | Daily | 3 to 4 |
| Hip bridges | Hip extensors Low back extensors | 5 repetitions | Daily | 3 to 4 |

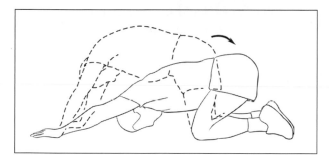

## Cobra Stretch

Crouch on your hands and knees. First rock forward onto your extended arms, allowing your back to sag. Hold for 5 seconds. Then rock back and sit on your bent knees with your arms extended and your head tucked in. Hold for 5 seconds. Repeat 10 times.

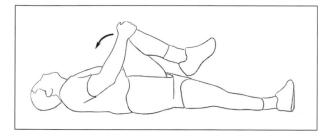

## Knee to Chest

Lie on your back on the floor with your knees bent and your feet flat on the floor. Grasp one knee and bring it up to your chest as far as it will go. Then lower the leg back to the floor. Repeat with the other leg. Then do both legs together. Repeat this sequence 10 times.

SECTION 8 ■ SPINE

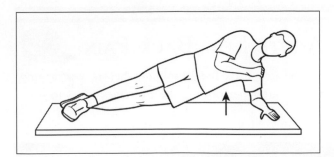

## Side Bridges

Lie on your side on the floor. With your elbow bent at 90°, lift your body off the floor as shown, keeping your body straight. Hold the position for 15 seconds and then repeat on the other side. Perform 5 repetitions daily.

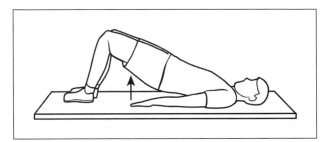

## Hip Bridges

Lie on your back on the floor with your arms at your sides, your knees bent, and your feet flat on the floor. Lift your pelvis so that your body is in a straight line from your shoulders to your knees. Hold this position for 15 seconds. Perform 5 repetitions daily.

# Low Back Pain: Chronic

## Definition

Chronic low back pain (LBP) is used to describe LBP of more than 3 months' duration. These symptoms usually present between 30 and 60 years of age. Symptoms are typically recurrent and episodic, but in some patients the pain is unremitting. Although the diagnosis of degenerative disk disease (DDD) is sometimes used in such cases, this term is being abandoned because it implies that DDD is a specific disorder of the spine that requires specific treatment. This suggests to patients that they are "ill" with a "disease," whereas often the symptoms are the result of physiologic changes of aging. Once chronic LBP has been identified, however, a thorough evaluation is required to exclude causes such as cancer, stenosis, deformity, osteoporosis, infection, and abdominal conditions such as aneurysm, ulcer, or retroperitoneal tumor. All patients with chronic LBP should be evaluated not only by a spine specialist but also by their internist, family practitioner, or, for women, their gynecologist.

Degeneration of the intervertebral disk is a physiologic event of aging and may be modified by factors such as injury, repetitive trauma, infection, heredity, and tobacco use. As the hydrophilic properties of the nucleus pulposus degrade, the disk loses height and the segmental ligaments develop laxity. Motions such as translation and twisting may create tears within the anulus fibrosus. Chronic LBP may develop.

## Clinical Symptoms

Low back pain that radiates to one or both buttocks is the hallmark symptom (**Figure 1**). The pain is often described as "mechanical" in that it is aggravated by activities such as bending, lifting, stooping, or twisting. Patients may report stiffness or have a history of intermittent sciatica (pain radiating down the back of the leg), but discomfort in the back is the predominant symptom. The pain is typically relieved with lying down or a night's rest. Some patients, however, have difficulty sleeping because of the symptoms.

Depression is not the cause of chronic LBP, but it can complicate treatment. Therefore, early recognition will greatly assist with symptom resolution.

**ICD-9 Codes**

**722.52**
Degeneration of lumbar intervertebral disk, lumbar, or lumbosacral disk

**724.2**
Low back pain, chronic

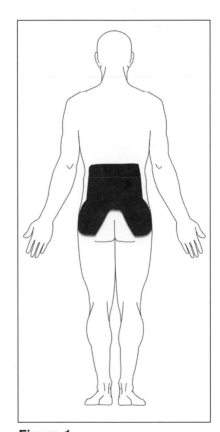

**Figure 1**

Typical pain diagram for a patient with chronic LBP.

SECTION 8 ■ SPINE

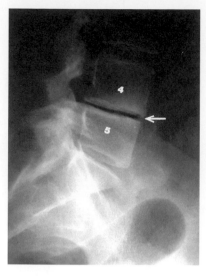

**Figure 2**

Lateral radiograph showing marked degenerative changes affecting the disk between L4 and L5 (arrow). Note the extreme disk space narrowing.

# TESTS

## *Physical Examination*

Lumbar and sacroiliac tenderness is a common finding. Patients may also exhibit a side or forward list from muscle spasm. Motor and sensory function of the lower extremity nerve roots as well as the lower extremity reflexes are normal. Straight-leg raising and spinal motion may be mildly restricted. Although not characteristic, nonorganic findings such as widespread sensitivity to light touch, nonanatomic localization of symptoms, inappropriate pain behaviors, and inconsistent actions may be seen with this condition. (See Physical Examination—Spine: Special Tests, p 731.)

## *Diagnostic Tests*

AP and lateral radiographs often show age-appropriate changes, such as anterior osteophytes and reduced height of the intervertebral disks. Often there is a "vacuum sign," with apparent air (nitrogen) in the disk space (**Figure 2**).

# DIFFERENTIAL DIAGNOSIS (PARTIAL LIST)

Degenerative disorders (imaging abnormalities)

Developmental defects (abnormal radiographs)

Infection (elevated erythrocyte sedimentation rate, C-reactive protein, temperature)

Inflammation (other joint involvement, elevated erythrocyte sedimentation rate)

Metabolic disease (abnormal laboratory studies)

Neoplasms (weight loss, night pain, fatigue)

Neurologic disorders (long tract signs)

Psychosocial issues (depression, worker's compensation issues, positive Waddell signs)

Referred pain (aortic aneurysm, pelvic tumor, renal disorders)

Trauma (history of injury)

# ADVERSE OUTCOMES OF THE DISEASE

In patients with more severe symptoms, vocational and recreational activities may be limited. Sleep disturbances, mood swings, and sexual dysfunction may occur, and concentration may be adversely affected. Deconditioning, which may be the result of reduced activity, is frequently associated with the condition and may aggravate the symptoms as well as increase any occupational dysfunction.

# Treatment

Before treatment is initiated, the patient should have undergone a thorough clinical evaluation with appropriate laboratory tests and multiple imaging studies to exclude pathologic processes other than normal physiologic aging. Thus, once these conditions have been ruled out, a more appropriate term for the condition might be chronic benign LBP.

Narcotic abuse is a cause for concern in this population. By definition, the patient with chronic LBP has experienced pain for a lengthy period and frequently has received a variety of medications, including addictive muscle relaxants and narcotics. In addition, many of these patients are deconditioned, depressed, unemployed, angry, and demanding, so management of the condition is often challenging. Referral to a comprehensive pain management program is warranted. These programs employ a wide range of strategies, including comprehensive evaluations with thorough psychological testing, injections, biofeedback, cognitive/behavior conditioning programs, spinal cord stimulation, psychotherapy, and detoxification programs.

In addition, a return-to-activity program is also essential to overcome the deconditioning that is typical in the patient with chronic LBP. This can be initiated on an individual or group (class) basis and is typically overseen by a physical therapist. Once a comprehensive management program has been developed, the primary care physician can follow the patient, emphasizing the need to maintain "well behavior." Pain relapses are common, and referral back to the pain management center may be necessary. Because of the difficulty of assessing and managing these patients, a comprehensive team approach is often necessary for a successful outcome.

# Physical Therapy Prescription

Chronic LBP is difficult to treat using any single approach. Often the trunk muscles are weak and unable to stabilize the spine during daily activities. Therefore, a home exercise program should consist of stabilization exercises including modified side bridges, hip bridges, bird dog exercises, and abdominal bracing (see pp 767-768). Aerobic or cardiovascular conditioning consistent with the patient's general health is also helpful. If the patient's symptoms do not improve after adhering to the home program for 3 to 4 weeks, formal physical therapy may be ordered. The physical therapist must conduct an extensive evaluation of the mobility and strength of the lumbar spine to determine a treatment approach. Use of pain modalities is limited with chronic LBP.

Section 8 ■ Spine

## ADVERSE OUTCOMES OF TREATMENT

NSAIDs may cause gastric, renal, or hepatic complications. Avoid labeling patients as "disabled" because this may negatively affect the patient's motivation. Narcotic dependency or abuse can become a problem for these patients.

## REFERRAL DECISIONS/RED FLAGS

Further evaluation is needed for patients who have fever, chills, unexplained weight loss, a history of cancer, significant night pain, or a history of pain for more than 6 to 12 months. Other indications for additional evaluation include the presence of pathologic fractures, obvious deformity, saddle anesthesia, loss of major motor function, bowel or bladder dysfunction, abdominal pain, or visceral dysfunction.

## REFERENCE

1. Beck AT, Beamesderfer A: Assessment of depression: The depression inventory. *Mod Probl Pharmacopsychiatry* 1974;7:151-169.

# HOME EXERCISE PROGRAM FOR CHRONIC LOW BACK PAIN

Perform the exercises in the order listed. Apply heat to the low back for 20 minutes before performing the exercises. You should not experience pain with the exercises. If the pain worsens or if it does not improve after performing the exercises for 3 to 4 weeks, call your doctor.

| Exercise Type | Muscle Group | Number of Repetitions/Sets | Number of Days per Week | Number of Weeks |
|---|---|---|---|---|
| Modified side bridges | Quadratus lumborum | 5 repetitions | Daily | 3 to 4 |
| Hip bridges | Back and hip extensors | 5 repetitions | Daily | 3 to 4 |
| Bird dog | Back extensors | 5 repetitions | Daily | 3 to 4 |
| Abdominal bracing | Abdominals | 5 repetitions | Daily | 3 to 4 |

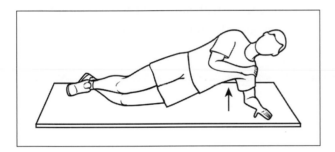

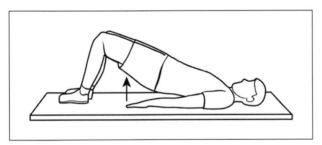

## Modified Side Bridges

Lie on your side on the floor with your knees bent. With your elbow bent at 90°, lift your body off the floor as shown, keeping your body straight. Hold the position for 15 seconds and then repeat on the other side. Perform 5 repetitions daily.

## Hip Bridges

Lie on your back on the floor with your arms at your sides, your knees bent, and your feet flat on the floor. Lift your pelvis so that your body is in a straight line from your shoulders to your knees. Hold this position for 15 seconds. Perform 5 repetitions daily.

SECTION 8 ■ SPINE

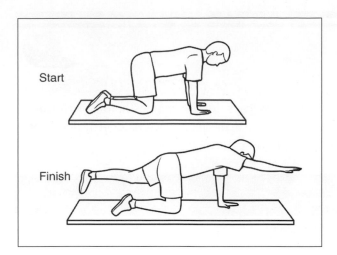

## Bird Dog

Kneel on the floor on your hands and knees. Lift your right arm straight out from the shoulder, level with your body, at the same time you lift your left leg straight out from the hip. Hold this position for 15 seconds. Repeat with the opposite arm and leg. Perform 5 repetitions daily.

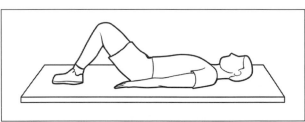

## Abdominal Bracing

Lie on your back on the floor with your arms at your sides, your knees bent, and your feet flat on the floor. Contract your abdominal muscles so that your stomach is pulled away from your waistband. Hold this position for 15 seconds. Perform 5 repetitions daily.

SECTION 8 ■ SPINE

# LUMBAR HERNIATED DISK

## SYNONYMS
Lumbar radiculopathy
Neurogenic leg pain
Sciatica

## DEFINITION
The intervertebral disk is composed of the nucleus pulposus, a gel-like material that cushions axial compression; the anulus fibrosus, a specialized ligamentous structure surrounding the nucleus pulposus that helps to stabilize the spine; and the superior and inferior cartilaginous end plates. Activities such as lifting and twisting increase pressure on the nucleus pulposus. Lumbar disk herniations usually develop over time as the weaker posterolateral portion of the anulus fibrosus develops fissures that permit the egress of other disk components that herniate into the lumbar canal adjacent to the exiting lumbar nerve root. The resultant herniated disk syndrome (commonly called sciatica) causes pain, numbness, and/or weakness in one or both lower extremities, depending on the anatomic location of the herniation. The pain results in part from direct mechanical compression of the nerve root and in part from chemical irritation of the nerve root by substances within the nucleus pulposus.

Lumbar disk herniation most commonly occurs at the L4-5 or L5-S1 levels, with subsequent irritation of the L5 or S1 nerve root. Herniations at more proximal intervertebral levels constitute only 5% of all lumbar disk herniations.

Lumbar disk herniations affect approximately 2% of the population. Even though only 10% of these patients have symptoms that persist longer than 3 months, the numbers are so great that this represents approximately 600,000 patients. Most of these patients improve with nonsurgical care, but those who continue to remain symptomatic generally consider surgical management to improve their quality of life.

## CLINICAL SYMPTOMS
The onset of symptoms is often abrupt, but it may be insidious. Unilateral radicular leg pain frequently follows the onset of acute low back pain. The theory is that the initial posterolateral disk bulge results in low back pain that then becomes sciatic pain as the herniation emerges past the anulus to the spinal canal.

**ICD-9 Codes**
**722.10**
Displacement of thoracic or lumbar intervertebral disk without myelopathy

**724.4**
Thoracic or lumbosacral neuritis or radiculitis, unspecified (Radicular syndrome of lower limb)

SECTION 8 ■ SPINE

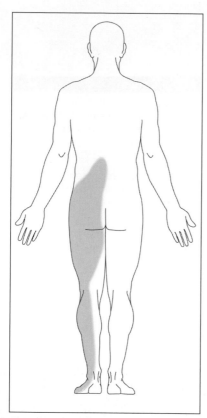

**Figure 1**
Pain diagram of patient with lumbar radiculopathy.

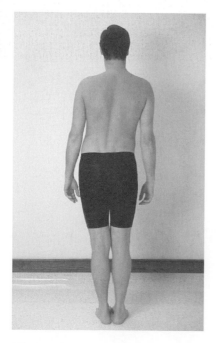

**Figure 2**
Trunk shift, or "list," to right.

The pain is often severe and is exaggerated by sitting, walking, standing, coughing, and sneezing. Typically, the pain radiates from the buttock down the posterior or posterolateral leg to the ankle or foot (**Figure 1**). Patients have a difficult time finding a position of comfort. Usually, lying on the back with a pillow under the knees or lying on the side in a fetal position provides some relief.

Upper or midlumbar radiculopathy (L1 to L4 nerve root compression) refers pain to the anterior aspect of the thigh and often does not radiate below the knee.

# TESTS

## Physical Examination

As the patient stands, look for the presence of a trunk list to one side (**Figure 2**). The patient may also evidence limited forward flexion with dysrhythmia of the paraspinous muscles (ie, they contract asymmetrically). With the patient sitting, perform the seated straight-leg raising test (see Physical Examination—Spine: Special Tests, p 728). As the knee is extended on the symptomatic side, a patient with true sciatic tension will lean back to relieve the pressure on the exiting nerve root. This sign has a high correlation with a herniated lumbar disk. Even more specific is the crossed straight-leg raising sign: when the nonsymptomatic extremity is elevated, the patient reports buttock or sciatic pain on the symptomatic side. Evaluate motor and sensory function of the lumbosacral nerve roots as well as the deep tendon reflexes.

With the patient supine, perform supine straight-leg raising on the involved and uninvolved limbs. This test places the L5 and S1 nerve roots on stretch. Ipsilateral restriction of straight-leg raising is common with a variety of lumbar spine problems, but a positive crossed straight-leg raising test (pain that occurs in the involved leg or buttock when the uninvolved leg is lifted) is highly specific for lumbar nerve root entrapment. To put the upper lumbar nerve roots on stretch, perform the reverse straight-leg raising test (see Physical Examination—Spine: Special Tests, p 730). Classic findings include the following (**Figure 3**):

- The L3-4 disk (L4 nerve root) may produce weakness in the anterior tibialis, numbness in the shin, pain in the thigh, and an asymmetric knee reflex. About 5% of disk ruptures occur at this level.

- The L4-5 disk (L5 nerve root) may produce weakness in the great toe extensor, numbness on the top of the foot and first web space, and pain in the posterolateral thigh and calf. There is no predictable reflex test for a herniated

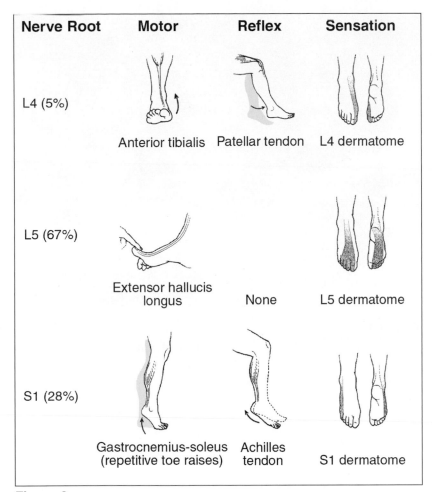

| Nerve Root | Motor | Reflex | Sensation |
|---|---|---|---|
| L4 (5%) | Anterior tibialis | Patellar tendon | L4 dermatome |
| L5 (67%) | Extensor hallucis longus | None | L5 dermatome |
| S1 (28%) | Gastrocnemius-soleus (repetitive toe raises) | Achilles tendon | S1 dermatome |

**Figure 3**

Typical motor, sensory, and reflex findings with common lumbar radiculopathies.

Adapted from Kasser JR (ed): *Orthopaedic Knowledge Update* 5. Rosemont, IL, American Academy of Orthopaedic Surgeons, 1996, pp 609–624.

lumbar disk at the L4/L5 level. Thus, checking the extensor hallucis longus is especially important as this may be the only sign to confirm an L5 radiculopathy.

- The L5-S1 disk (S1 nerve root) may produce weakness in the great toe flexor as well as in the gastrocnemius-soleus complex, with inability to sustain tiptoe walking, numbness in the lateral foot, pain and ache in the posterior calf, and an asymmetric ankle reflex.

## Diagnostic Tests

Plain radiographs usually demonstrate age-appropriate changes with no specific findings. MRI should be ordered to confirm the diagnosis if symptoms persist longer than 4 weeks, if a significant neurologic deficit is identified, or as a part of the preoperative evaluation (**Figure 4**). MRI is otherwise not necessary unless there are progressive neurologic changes or intolerable pain.

SECTION 8 ■ SPINE

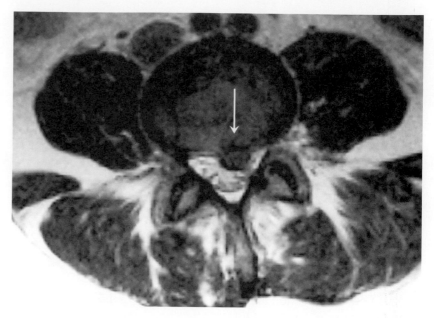

**Figure 4**
Preoperative axial MRI scan showing herniated lumbar disk (arrow).

## DIFFERENTIAL DIAGNOSIS

Cauda equina syndrome (perianal numbness, urinary overflow incontinence or retention, reduced anal sphincter tone, bilateral involvement)

Demyelinating conditions (clonus)

Extraspinal nerve entrapment (abdominal or pelvic mass)

Hip or knee arthritis (decreased internal rotation of hip, knee deformity or effusion)

Lateral femoral cutaneous nerve entrapment (sensory only, lateral thigh)

Spinal stenosis (older population)

Thoracic cord compression (clonus, spasticity, high sensory pattern, abdominal reflexes)

Trochanteric bursitis (no tension signs, pain down lateral thigh and leg, exquisite tenderness over the trochanter)

Vascular insufficiency (absent posterior tibial pulse, claudication, trophic changes)

## ADVERSE OUTCOMES OF THE DISEASE

Cauda equina syndrome with permanent motor loss, urinary incontinence, and sensory numbness may develop. Specific root deficit, with permanent dysesthesia, pain, or weakness, may occur.

## TREATMENT

NSAIDs should be used in the acute phase, along with 1 to 2 days of minimal activity. Narcotic medication may be helpful in the acute phase for selected patients but typically should not be prescribed for longer than 7 days. Patients should limit sitting, prolonged standing, or walking. Patients should be reassured that most disk herniations resolve without residual problems.

Most patients who have a lumbar disk herniation will improve within 3 to 4 weeks. If they do not, an evaluation by a specialist should be obtained.

Physical therapy as described for acute low back pain (see pp 761-762) is also appropriate for patients with a lumbar herniated disk. Patients with true radiculopathy with a lumbar herniated disk take longer to recover, however, and usually require activity modification for at least 4 to 8 weeks. Both aerobic conditioning and trunk strengthening are essential for the best outcome. Patients whose symptoms do not improve and who experience a clear decrease in their quality of life are candidates for surgical diskectomy. Profound or progressive neurologic disorders, including cauda equina syndrome, require urgent surgery.

Epidural steroid injections (up to three in a 6-month period), which are usually administered under radiologic guidance, may be considered. These injections should be avoided in any patient who presents with a significant neurologic deficit. Although the risk of significant complications is low, epidural steroid injections should not be recommended without consideration of these risks. Also, if the patient experiences no relief of symptoms, repeating the injections later is not warranted.

The effectiveness of manipulative therapy, traction, or acupuncture for patients with a confirmed lumbar herniated disk remains unproved in randomized controlled trials despite many anecdotal reports of the efficacy of these therapies.

## ADVERSE OUTCOMES OF TREATMENT

NSAIDs may cause gastric, renal, or hepatic complications. Progression of neurologic deficit or persistent numbness and weakness may occur despite treatment.

## REFERRAL DECISIONS/RED FLAGS

Patients with any of the following conditions need further evaluation: cauda equina syndrome, urinary retention, perianal numbness, motor loss, severe single nerve root paralysis, progressive neurologic deficit, radicular symptoms that persist for more than 6 weeks, intractable leg pain, or recurrent episodes of sciatica that interfere with the patient's life activities.

SECTION 8 ■ SPINE

# LUMBAR SPINAL STENOSIS

## SYNONYM
Neurogenic claudication

## DEFINITION

Lumbar spinal stenosis is the narrowing of one or more levels of the lumbar spinal canal with subsequent compression of the nerve roots. Anatomically, lumbar stenosis affects as many as 30% of the population older than 60 years, yet only a portion of these individuals will have symptoms. In elderly patients, spinal stenosis is typically degenerative in origin. Younger patients with achondroplasia or other disorders that cause a small spinal canal may experience clinical symptoms in their 20s or 30s.

Degenerative lumbar spinal stenosis occurs most commonly at the L3-4, L4-5, and L2-3 levels. Although central lumbar stenosis is uncommon at L5-S1, lateral degenerative changes at this level may cause compression of the L5 (higher) nerve root.

## CLINICAL SYMPTOMS

The stenosis may be quite advanced before symptoms occur. Onset of symptoms may be insidious, or develop quickly without any history of injury. A common pattern of presentation is neurogenic claudication that causes radicular symptoms (with or without associated back pain) in one or both legs (**Figure 1**). Neurogenic claudication differs from vascular claudication, but these conditions may coexist in elderly patients (**Table 1**). With neurogenic claudication, symptoms progress from a proximal to a distal direction. Walking or prolonged standing causes fatigue and weakness in the legs. Sitting or lying generally relieves the pain. Vascular insufficiency may be difficult to differentiate from lumbar spinal stenosis.

Extension of the spine narrows the lumbar spinal canal, flexion increases the canal diameter. Therefore, patients may obtain short-term relief by leaning forward (stooping). For example, these patients often lean on the cart while grocery shopping. The length of time that symptomatic relief lasts after sitting will vary. Patients may also awaken at night with back and/or leg pain after a few hours of sleep.

Lumbosacral pain occurs less commonly and is associated with walking or standing. A vague aching in the legs associated with leg weakness may also be reported.

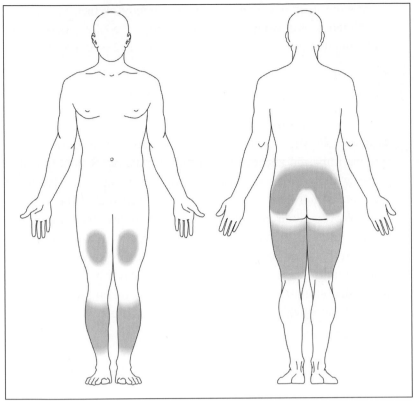

**Figure 1**

Typical pain diagram for a patient with spinal stenosis. Some patients may have severe stenosis but little thigh or leg pain.

**Table 1 Comparison of Vascular and Neurogenic Claudication**

| Evaluation | Vascular | Neurogenic |
| --- | --- | --- |
| Claudication distance | Fixed | Variable |
| Relief of pain | Standing | Sitting-flexed |
| Walk uphill | Pain | No pain |
| Bicycle ride | Pain | No pain |
| Type of pain | Cramp, tightness | Numbness, ache, sharp |
| Pulses | Absent | Present |
| Bruit | Present | Absent |
| Skin | Loss of hair, shiny | Normal |
| Atrophy | Rare | Occasional |
| Weakness | Rare | Occasional |
| Back pain | Uncommon | Common |
| Limitations of spinal movement | Uncommon | Common |

Reproduced from Herkowitz HN: Spinal stenosis: Clinical evaluation. *Instr Course Lect* 1992;41:184.

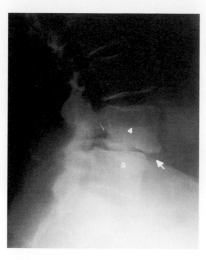

**Figure 2**
Lateral radiograph of a patient with degenerative spondylolisthesis at L4 on L5 (arrow).

Spondylolisthesis (degenerative or spondylolytic), vascular insufficiency, and osteoarthritis of the hips are often associated with spinal stenosis. Obesity may also be an associated factor.

# TESTS

## Physical Examination
True muscle weakness in the legs is uncommon. Proprioception may be impaired and result in a mildly positive Romberg test. Sensory changes are segmental if present but may involve more than one spinal level. Reflexes may be diminished. The anterior and posterior tibial pulses will be normal unless the patient has concomitant vascular disease. Some patients will have a lumbar deformity. Bowel or bladder symptoms may be reported, but anal sphincter tone is rarely decreased. Because many patients have concomitant prostate disease or stress incontinence, genitourinary evaluation is necessary to differentiate these processes.

## Diagnostic Tests
AP and lateral radiographs (including up to T10 in the lateral view) may show spondylolisthesis or significant narrowing of the intervertebral disk (**Figure 2**). Osteopenia may be present.

# DIFFERENTIAL DIAGNOSIS
Abdominal aortic aneurysm (palpable pulsatile mass)

Arterial insufficiency (distance to claudication constant, recovery after rest, absent or diminished pulses)

Diabetes mellitus (abnormal glucose metabolism, nonsegmental numbness, skin changes)

Folic acid or vitamin $B_{12}$ deficiency (confirmed by laboratory tests, anemia)

Infection (mild temperature elevation, elevated erythrocyte sedimentation rate, elevated C-reactive protein, intervertebral disk narrowing with reactive changes in the adjacent vertebral end plates)

Tumor (patchy neurologic deficit, bone destruction, night pain)

# ADVERSE OUTCOMES OF THE DISEASE
The rate of progression varies widely. Many patients tolerate this condition well and never develop any neurologic deficit. However, pain and limited function may become significant and lead to an adverse quality of life with secondary depression. Standing erect may become impossible, forcing the patient to adopt a stooped posture. Claudication may develop after walking only a few feet. Although cauda equina syndrome must be considered, this syndrome is rare.

# Treatment

Many patients with lumbar spinal stenosis are elderly and have comorbidities that require consideration when weighing treatment options. Initial treatment generally includes NSAIDs and physical activity. Water therapy is a good initial activity for the elderly, deconditioned patient with mild symptoms. Narcotic medication is rarely required. Epidural steroid injections (up to three in a 6-month period), which are usually administered under radiologic guidance, may be considered. Epidural steroid injections improve symptoms in about 50% of patients, but the improvement usually lasts only 4 to 6 months.

Patients who are becoming nonambulatory and report a decreased quality of life are candidates for surgical management. The age of the patient is less important than comorbidities in predicting surgical outcomes. Patients with degenerative spondylolisthesis and/or scoliosis in addition to lumbar spinal stenosis may require spinal fusion in addition to decompression of the stenotic segments.

# Adverse Outcomes of Treatment

Neural damage during decompression is possible but unlikely with improved techniques. Prolonged use of NSAIDs may cause renal failure, hepatotoxicity, and gastrointestinal ulcer disease. The chronic use of narcotics is associated with its own set of problems when these drugs are used inappropriately.

# Referral Decisions/Red Flags

Any neurologic deficit, gait disturbance, or bowel and bladder dysfunction should be evaluated further. Because these changes may not improve following surgery, the goal of treatment is to prevent progression. If nonsurgical treatment is ineffective, specialty consultation is indicated. Night pain that disturbs sleep usually indicates advanced disease for which further evaluation is indicated.

Section 8 ■ Spine

# METASTATIC DISEASE

## DEFINITION

Malignant tumors involving the spine may be either primary (rare) or metastatic (common). Metastatic disease to the vertebrae occurs at some time in the clinical course of the disease in approximately 50% of all patients who have solid tumors. The highest incidence occurs with carcinoma of the breast, lung, prostate, colon, thyroid, and kidney.

Osseous involvement of the vertebrae is much more common than involvement of the spinal cord or dura. The most likely etiology is hematogenous spread, whereby neoplastic cells in the vertebral body are deposited through the Batson plexus, a unique venous plexus of the spine characterized by collateral connections to the inferior vena cava and a general lack of valves.

Metastatic disease may become clinically evident through one of several different presentations: (1) as an incidental finding in asymptomatic patients; (2) in patients with known primary tumors who are being evaluated for possible metastatic disease by bone scan, MRI, or CT; (3) as neurologic findings in patients with or without previous history of a primary tumor; or (4) as the primary presenting symptom of cancer in patients who were not aware they had a primary tumor.

## CLINICAL SYMPTOMS

Pain is the most common presenting symptom. The pain may be first noted following trivial trauma, is typically constant, and worsens progressively as the days or weeks pass. This pain is usually due to minor vertebral fractures secondary to the weakness created by the metastatic process. Weight-bearing activities (standing, sitting) aggravate the pain, whereas lying down typically results in relief. Pain that prevents sleep and persists through the night is highly suspicious for a neoplasm.

With compression of the nerve roots, the pain associated with cervical or lumbar tumors also radiates to the extremities. Similar nerve root entrapment by tumors in the thoracic spine causes a band-like distribution of pain around the chest. When the compression involves a nerve root, radicular symptoms and associated sensory loss and/or motor weakness are restricted to a single extremity. If more generalized sensory and motor dysfunction occurs, and especially if the patient reports bowel or bladder dysfunction or difficulty walking, cervical or thoracic cord compression or cauda equina syndrome may be present.

The rate of disease progression and neurologic dysfunction may be slow, evolving over weeks or months, or rapid in more aggressive tumors. Progression may be more difficult to identify in patients taking high dosages of pain medication for metastatic disease elsewhere. Acute onset of quadriplegia or paraplegia may occur (infrequently) with rapid enlargement of a soft-tissue tumor mass or following a pathologic fracture that compresses the spinal cord.

# TESTS

## Physical Examination

An area of tenderness to palpation and/or percussion along the spinous processes is common. Tumors in the posterior elements (lamina, spinous process) may be palpable. A patient with a vertebral body collapse may develop increased kyphosis at the level of fracture. Assess motor and sensory function of all nerve roots distal to the lesion. Check deep tendon and other appropriate spinal cord reflexes. If the primary tumor has not been previously diagnosed, the patient will need a complete evaluation for staging purposes with particular emphasis on the thyroid, breasts, chest, kidney, and prostate. Consultation with an oncologist is warranted.

## Diagnostic Tests

Initial radiographic evaluation requires high-quality AP and lateral radiographs. Cervical spine radiographs should also include odontoid views and show all vertebrae from the occiput to T1. Lumbar spine radiographs should include the bodies of T10 to the tip of the coccyx, with a spot lateral view of the lumbosacral junction if needed for clarity. A radiopaque marker placed next to an area of percussion tenderness helps identify the area of concern. The lateral view may show collapse with loss of height of the vertebral body or areas of bony destruction with lytic or blastic lesions in the vertebral body. Often the first radiologic sign of tumor involvement is loss of integrity of a pedicle, as seen on the AP view and often described as the "winking owl" sign because of the asymmetry of the involved and uninvolved pedicles (**Figure 1**).

A technetium Tc 99m bone scan is the best screening study to identify widespread metastatic disease because it evaluates the spine as well as other axial (pelvis) and appendicular (extremity) bones. This study will generally be negative in patients with multiple myeloma.

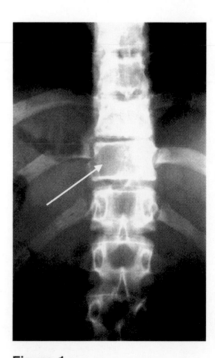

**Figure 1**

AP radiograph of the spine demonstrates a missing pedicle (arrow), indicative of a metastatic or a primary tumor (the "winking owl" sign).

SECTION 8 ■ SPINE

# DIFFERENTIAL DIAGNOSIS

Degenerative arthritis (fracture rare, bone dense)

Infection (loss of disk space, sclerosis)

Multiple myeloma (men older than 50 years, fracture from trivial trauma)

Osteoporotic fracture (generalized osteopenia, pedicles intact)

Traumatic fracture (normal bone, widening of bone in AP and lateral views)

# ADVERSE OUTCOMES OF THE DISEASE

Involvement of one area of the spine with metastatic disease does not usually change the overall survival rate, but spinal deformity and/or intractable pain poses considerable problems in patient care. Spinal involvement with neurologic deficit compromises quality of life and may shorten lifespan with complications of paraplegia. Quadriplegia and paraplegia are the most serious sequelae of pathologic fractures.

# TREATMENT

Treatment of spinal tumors is based on the type of tumor, the degree of bony involvement, the type of symptoms, and physician/patient preference. Chemotherapy, hormone therapy, or radiation is appropriate for asymptomatic tumors detected during evaluation for metastatic disease. Radiation therapy is appropriate for painful metastases without serious deformity or neural compression. Alternative methods are considered in tumors that are insensitive to radiation (renal cell carcinoma). With pain and neurologic deficit, the most effective way to improve neural function and overall function is surgical decompression and stabilization, generally with adjunctive postoperative radiation therapy. Surgical intervention results in improved neurologic function in approximately 85% of patients.

# ADVERSE OUTCOMES OF TREATMENT

Neurologic deterioration persists in some patients, despite adequate decompression, because of recurrent tumor or tumor involvement in the vascular supply to the spinal cord. Surgical wound complications are more common when the surgery follows radiation therapy or the patient is taking oral steroids.

# REFERRAL DECISIONS/RED FLAGS

Patients with known prior malignancies and spinal symptoms or patients with intractable pain require specialty evaluation, as do patients in whom trivial trauma produces a spinal fracture, even in the presence of osteoporosis.

# Scoliosis in Adults

## Definition

Scoliosis is a lateral curvature of the spine. In adults, the condition is classified as either a deformity that developed during childhood or a deformity that developed after skeletal maturity, usually secondary to degenerative spondylosis and/or degenerative spondylolisthesis. Changes that occur with aging, including osteoporosis, degenerative disk disease, spinal stenosis, and degenerative spondylolisthesis, may contribute to and/or confound the symptoms and progression of either condition.

**ICD-9 Codes**

**737.30**
Scoliosis (and kyphoscoliosis), idiopathic

**737.43**
Curvature of spine associated with other conditions, scoliosis

## Clinical Symptoms

The most common presenting symptom is pain localized to the region of the deformity. The most common overlapping syndrome is degenerative spondylosis, which may also cause lower lumbar pain. Because age-related changes in the spine are present in nearly everyone, a thorough evaluation is required to identify the most likely source of pain. Radicular pain is most commonly associated with compression of the L4 or L5 nerve root due to asymmetric hypertrophy of the facet joints, asymmetric disk degeneration, and mild rotatory subluxation. Neurologic changes are infrequent but most commonly involve the extensor hallucis longus muscle.

In some patients, the chief presenting symptom is a progressive spinal deformity. Some report that they are "getting shorter." These patients may also report that the "hump" on their back is getting bigger, or that they are leaning to the side more.

Cardiopulmonary decompensation rarely is evident in adult-onset scoliosis. Symptoms related to pulmonary compromise are associated with more severe thoracic curves, including both idiopathic and neuromuscular curves.

## Tests

### Physical Examination

The entire spine should be inspected and palpated with the patient standing. The relative height of the shoulders and iliac wings should be noted, as should any asymmetry at the waist. Decompensation is evaluated by measuring the distance a plumb line from C7 deviates to the right or left of the gluteal cleft. Forward bending also exaggerates the asymmetry of the posterior rib cage and thoracolumbar junction. Neurologic

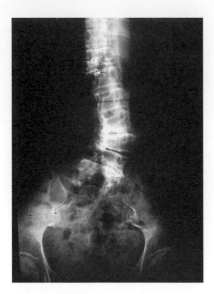

**Figure 1**
PA radiograph of the spine demonstrating advanced thoracolumbar kyphoscoliosis.

examination should include evaluation of reflexes as well as motor and sensory function of the lumbosacral nerve roots. In addition, pathologic reflexes should be assessed as well as a gait analysis looking for ataxia or evidence of spinal cord compression (myelopathy).

### Diagnostic Tests

Weight-bearing full-length PA and lateral radiographs should be obtained on a 36″ cassette (**Figure 1**). Electromyography is rarely indicated but occasionally may be helpful to distinguish radiculopathy from neuropathy.

## DIFFERENTIAL DIAGNOSIS

Congenital scoliosis (vertebral body abnormality, childhood or adolescent presentation)

Degenerative disk disease with asymmetric disk space collapse (normal vertebral shape, sharp curve over few segments)

Degenerative spondylolisthesis with accompanying lateral listhesis and disk degeneration (forward or backward slip of vertebral body)

Neuromuscular scoliosis (neurologic abnormalities and weakness)

Severe disk herniation with sciatic scoliosis and radiculopathy (unilateral neurologic signs, normal vertebral contour)

Traumatic or pathologic vertebral fracture (wedge-shaped vertebral body, history of trauma)

Vertebral osteomyelitis (fever, severe local pain, lysis of bone in vertebral body, narrowing of disk)

## ADVERSE OUTCOMES OF THE DISEASE

Increased pain and deformity with diminished functional activity are possible. With increased cosmetic deformity, patients may become more introverted.

## TREATMENT

Most cases of scoliosis in adults can be managed with NSAIDs and exercise. Exercise programs should begin with water therapy and progress to trunk strengthening as the symptoms decrease and the patient's tolerance increases. Aerobic activity is also recommended. Swimming is a particularly good exercise because it accomplishes trunk strengthening as well as aerobic conditioning.

## ADVERSE OUTCOMES OF TREATMENT

NSAIDs may cause gastric, renal, or hepatic complications. Complications of surgical management may include increased pain, increased deformity, infection, pseudarthrosis, instrumentation failure, and/or paralysis. The postoperative complication rate is much higher in adults than in adolescents. Patients must clearly understand the risks and benefits of this major surgery before undergoing the procedure. Elderly patients especially should be informed of the risks inherent in these surgeries in older patients. The physician should discuss the risks of both mortality and neurologic deficits.

# REFERRAL DECISIONS/RED FLAGS

Progressive neurologic deterioration requires emergency management. Patients who experience progressive pain and in whom the deformity progresses may be considered for major spinal fusion surgery. Patients who report that they cannot walk more than two blocks because of pain, respiratory dysfunction, or weakness require specialty evaluation. Any change in the deformity requires specialty evaluation as well.

SECTION 8 ■ SPINE

# SPINAL ORTHOSES

## CERVICAL

### Soft Cervical Collar

This foam-covered orthosis is appropriate for short-term use in cervical sprains or intermittent use to alleviate pain in patients with cervical spondylosis. The most common error is selecting a soft cervical collar that is too wide, thus thrusting the neck into extension. A collar that positions the neck in approximately 10° of flexion maximizes the space for the nerve roots as they pass through the vertebral foramen. Patients should be on an isometric exercise program to avoid loss of intrinsic muscle support. Soft cervical collars worn at night are also helpful.

### Philadelphia Collar

This molded polystyrene brace provides better control of cervical rotation and is preferred for transport and initial immobilization of patients with suspected cervical fractures. Some physicians prefer this support to the cervical collar in the treatment of acute sprains. Unless rotational control is necessary (C1-2 injury), most patients prefer the greater comfort of a soft cervical collar.

### Rigid Cervical Orthoses

A hard cervical collar limits flexion and extension better than a soft cervical collar. Greater restriction of neck motion is obtained by a brace that extends from the neck to the midthoracic spine. For example, the Miami J orthosis (Jerome Medical, Moorestown, NJ) is basically a Philadelphia collar that has a rigid plastic component extending to the middle of the chest. As such, it greatly restricts rotation that primarily occurs in the upper cervical spine as well as the flexion and extension and lateral bending that occur to a greater degree in the lower cervical spine.

### Halo Brace

This brace provides superior immobilization of the cervical spine. The halo portion is rigidly secured to the head by four screws inserted into the outer table of the skull. Bars connect the halo to a plastic vest that surrounds the chest. Minimal cervical spinal motion occurs in a patient wearing this brace.

## THORACIC

### Thoracolumbosacral Corset

A standard lumbosacral corset with a proximal extension provides adequate support for patients with osteoporosis or acute thoracic sprains involving the lower thoracic spine. Some corsets are equipped with metal stays or plastic inserts that are bent to conform to the patient's spine. Women may not comply with this brace because breast irritation may occur. The orthotist may need to modify the brace to ensure patient compliance.

## Jewett-type Three-point Orthosis
The basic principle of this type of orthosis is three-point fixation, with pressure over the sternum and pubis anteriorly and over the midspine posteriorly. Most are aluminum and bendable to fit the patient. These braces limit flexion and extension of the thoracic spine but provide limited rotational control. Because of their limited contact areas and light weight, these orthoses are well tolerated by patients. This type of orthosis is useful for patients with thoracic sprains or minimal compression fractures.

## Total-contact Thoracolumbosacral Orthosis (TLSO)
These braces are either prefabricated modules that are fitted based on measurements of the torso or are made from a plaster mold of the patient's torso. The latter type provides better total contact and rotational control but is quite expensive. These braces usually are constructed of hard plastic anterior and posterior clamshells that are lined with a soft material and attach together on the sides. These braces are used primarily as definitive treatment in patients with stable fractures of the thoracolumbar spine or as a postoperative aid following spinal fusion.

# LUMBAR

## Elastic Belts
These braces do not limit lumbar spine motion and probably do not prevent injury. With a mild lumbar strain, they do provide some abdominal support and can certainly remind the patient to be careful during various activities.

## Lumbosacral Corset
The standard lumbosacral corset can be worn with or without internal stays of metal or plastic. These devices provide very little restriction of motion and are most useful as an adjunct to pain control following a lumbar sprain or acute disk herniation. The time period of bracing should be short and accompanied by an exercise program once the acute pain has subsided.

## Rigid Orthoses
See the descriptions for the three-point and total-contact orthoses.

SECTION 8 ■ SPINE

# SPONDYLOLISTHESIS: DEGENERATIVE

**ICD-9 Code**

**738.4**
Acquired spondylolisthesis

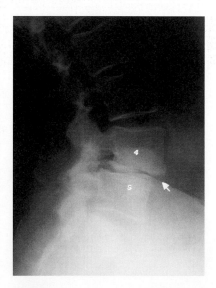

**Figure 1**
Lateral radiograph of a patient
with degenerative
spondylolisthesis at L4 on L5
(arrow).

## SYNONYM
Pseudospondylolisthesis

## DEFINITION
Degenerative spondylolisthesis is forward slippage of a lumbar vertebral body that is caused by degeneration and alterations in the facet joints in conjunction with degenerative changes in the intervertebral disk. By definition, the lamina and pars interarticularis are intact. This condition occurs most frequently between the fourth and fifth vertebral bodies. Degenerative spondylolisthesis is more common in women older than 40 years. These patients also tend to be mildly to moderately overweight.

Retrolisthesis is posterior slippage of a lumbar vertebral body on the vertebrae below. This condition also develops secondary to degenerative changes.

## CLINICAL SYMPTOMS
Back pain that is aggravated by bending, lifting, or twisting activities is common. Narrowing of the lateral recesses may cause a radiculopathy. Narrowing of the central canal may cause neurogenic claudication or other symptoms of spinal stenosis.

## TESTS

### Physical Examination
Inspect and palpate the spine for any curvature, loss of lordosis, or step-off of the spinous processes. Evaluate motor and sensory function of the L1-S4 nerve roots. Diminished knee and/or ankle reflexes are often present; however, these findings are common in elderly patients. Motor examination is usually normal, but strength testing after walking may reveal weakness in toe or heel walking or in great toe dorsiflexion strength.

### Diagnostic Tests
AP and lateral radiographs are important. The lateral view will show slippage of one vertebra onto another, usually with the superior vertebra displaced several millimeters relative to the one below (**Figure 1**). The involved disk space frequently shows degeneration and narrowing.

## DIFFERENTIAL DIAGNOSIS

Iatrogenic instability (following diskectomy or decompression)

Isthmic spondylolisthesis (pars defect) (findings on radiographs and single-photon emission CT [SPECT] scans)

Pathologic fracture (from tumor)

Posttraumatic instability (history of fracture)

## ADVERSE OUTCOMES OF THE DISEASE

Disabling back pain or functional neurologic impairment associated with spinal canal stenosis or radiculopathy is possible.

## TREATMENT

Initial management should include NSAIDs and exercise. Many patients with degenerative spondylolisthesis are overweight, and they should be advised of the benefits of weight loss. Weight loss alone is unlikely to eliminate the patient's symptoms, however, because the forces generated by the trunk and spinal muscles will not be influenced by weight reduction. Patients may find an abdominal binder to be helpful occasionally, but more rigid braces are typically poorly tolerated and are seldom worn. Patients may engage in activities as tolerated because activity will not cause injury, although it may be uncomfortable. Nonsurgical management is often successful for several years in these patients, but they usually consider surgical management eventually.

## ADVERSE OUTCOMES OF TREATMENT

NSAIDs may cause gastric, renal, or hepatic complications and may interact with other medications.

## REFERRAL DECISIONS/RED FLAGS

Patients with symptoms of spinal stenosis (neurogenic claudication) after walking two blocks or less require further evaluation. Patients with cauda equina syndrome (perianal numbness and/or bowel or bladder impairment) require immediate evaluation.

SECTION 8 ■ SPINE

# SPONDYLOLISTHESIS: ISTHMIC

**ICD-9 Code**

**738.4**
Acquired spondylolisthesis

## DEFINITION

Spondylolisthesis occurs when one vertebral body slips in relation to the one below. In children this usually occurs between L5 and S1. A defect develops at the junction of the lamina with the pedicle (pars interarticularis), leaving the posterior element without a bony connection to the anterior element. Most likely this condition represents a cyclic loading event (fatigue fracture) that evolves over time in the adolescent years and fails to heal. If only the defects are present, the patient has spondylolysis. When the vertebral body slides forward, producing the "slip" or "listhesis," the condition is called spondylolisthesis and classified as isthmic. Patients who participate in activities that place stress on this area, such as gymnastics and football, have a higher incidence of this condition. For example, the incidence of spondylolysis in female gymnasts is nearly sixfold the incidence in less active age-matched females.

## CLINICAL SYMPTOMS

Spondylolisthesis may be asymptomatic or minimally symptomatic. However, adolescent and adult patients may also develop significant back pain that radiates posteriorly to or below the knees and worsens with standing (**Figure 1**). Frequently, patients report spasms in the hamstring muscles manifested by the inability to bend forward. In addition, markedly limited straight-leg raising is demonstrated on examination (see Physical Examination—Spine: Special Tests, p 728). True nerve compression symptoms are rare, although the fibrocartilaginous tissue in the region of the pars interarticularis does compress the L5 nerve roots in patients with isthmic spondylolisthesis.

## TESTS

### Physical Examination

Examination may reveal diminished lumbar lordosis and flattening of the buttocks. With significant spondylolisthesis, a step-off is noted, with the spinous process of the slipped vertebra that is "left behind" being more prominent than the one above.

Hamstring spasm markedly limits the patient's ability to bend forward or the height to which the examiner can raise the patient's straight leg with the patient supine (straight-leg raising test). Neurologic deficits are uncommon.

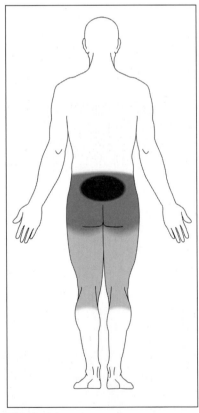

**Figure 1**

Typical pain diagram for a patient with isthmic spondylolisthesis. Distribution of leg symptoms will generally follow the L5 dermatome on one or both sides.

## Diagnostic Tests

With forward slippage (spondylolisthesis), lateral radiographs demonstrate forward translation of L5 relative to S1 (expressed as a percentage of the AP width of the vertebral body) (**Figure 2**). A defect in the pars interarticularis (a "collar" on the "Scotty dog") is evident on the oblique views (**Figure 3**). This is the only radiographic abnormality if the condition is limited to spondylolysis.

Increasing slippage can be evaluated with radiographs taken at 6-month intervals (or sooner if symptoms increase) until skeletal maturity is achieved.

# DIFFERENTIAL DIAGNOSIS

Intervertebral disk injury (no step-off or slip, no defect seen on plain radiograph)

Intervertebral diskitis (elevated erythrocyte sedimentation rate, fever)

Osteoid osteoma (night pain, abnormal bone scan, pain relieved with aspirin)

Spinal cord tumor (sensory findings, upper motor neuron signs)

Tethered spinal cord (pain, hamstring tightness, upper motor neuron signs)

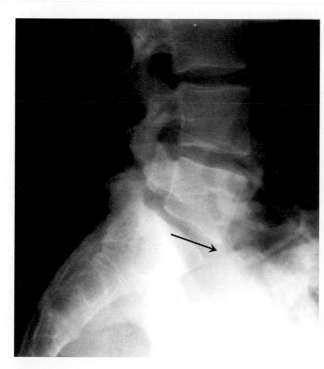

**Figure 2**
Lateral radiograph of a grade 2 to 3 spondylolisthesis at the lumbosacral junction (arrow).

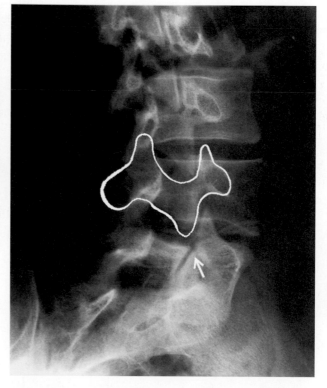

**Figure 3**
Oblique radiograph shows a normal "Scotty dog" appearance to the lamina (outlined area). In the vertebra below, the Scotty dog has a "collar" (arrow), which is the site of the pars interarticularis defect of spondylolisthesis.

SECTION 8 ■ SPINE

## ADVERSE OUTCOMES OF THE DISEASE

Progressive or complete slip of the vertebral body, chronic back pain and disability, paralysis of the lower lumbar nerve roots (usually L5), or bowel and bladder involvement (cauda equina syndrome) are possible.

## TREATMENT

Isthmic spondylolisthesis differs from degenerative spondylolisthesis in that these patients are often skeletally immature at the outset of the condition, so a single-photon emission CT (SPECT) scan should be performed in the young patient to assess metabolic activity in the area of the defect in the pars interarticularis. If the area of the defect is active and the patient is skeletally immature, some surgeons recommend surgical stabilization or fixation of the defect. Once the patient reaches skeletal maturity, fixation of the defect is not warranted.

Skeletally mature patients need not be restricted from any activity. Progression of this condition in an adult is rare. Most cases of progression in adults occur in patients with spondylolisthesis following decompression surgery without spinal fusion.

In adults, nonsurgical treatment with NSAIDs and exercise is recommended. Surgery is recommended only in patients with a decreased quality of life whose symptoms have not responded to a well-planned and faithfully followed nonsurgical regimen.

## ADVERSE OUTCOMES OF TREATMENT

Despite treatment, progression of the forward slip may continue.

## REFERRAL DECISIONS/RED FLAGS

Patients with significant pain and/or obvious slippage need further evaluation.

# PEDIATRIC ORTHOPAEDICS

**Section Editor**
Peter D. Pizzutillo, MD
Director, Orthopaedic Surgery
St. Christopher's Hospital for Children
Philadelphia, Pennsylvania

Joseph B. Chandler, MD
Director of Medical Services, Atlanta Braves
Resurgens Orthopaedics
Atlanta, Georgia

Tanya Maxwell, MS, L/ATC
Peachtree Orthopaedic Clinic
Atlanta, Georgia

# PEDIATRIC ORTHOPAEDICS—OVERVIEW

The often-quoted statement "Children are not just small adults" is particularly germane to pediatric disorders of the musculoskeletal system. Fractures, soft-tissue injuries, neurologic disorders, and infections have unique features and different considerations in children. Furthermore, the effect of growth must always be considered because it may be a positive or negative factor in the treatment of these disorders. For these reasons, this book includes this separate section on pediatric orthopaedics.

## COMMON PRESENTING SYMPTOMS IN CHILDREN

When a child presents with persistent pain and local swelling and/or refuses to use a limb or bear weight on a lower extremity, a detailed physical examination is indicated to identify a specific cause and recommend effective treatment.

## AGE AND SEX

Because degenerative joint disease takes years to develop, pain from a skeletal deformity is uncommon during childhood. Therefore, understanding the natural history of these conditions is critical to knowing whether treatment is needed. Some "deformities" in children are normal for the age. For example, genu varum, or bowlegs, is normal at birth, but by the time a child reaches age 3 years, a "knock-knee" alignment, or relatively large amount of genu valgum, is normal.

Considering age and sex can be helpful when evaluating children. For example, a boy between the ages of 4 and 8 years who has proximal thigh pain and a limp most likely has Legg-Calvé-Perthes disease. Similar symptoms in adolescent boys suggest a slipped capital femoral epiphysis. Female infants are more likely than male infants to have hip dysplasia, whereas clubfoot is more common in male infants. Adolescent girls are more likely to have scoliosis, but kyphosis of the spine is more common in adolescent boys.

## GROWTH

Growth, with its associated remodeling potential, may be a tremendous ally in treatment. This is particularly true in the newborn period, when simply bracing a very dysplastic hip for a few months will result in a normal joint that functions well for a lifetime. Certain angular deformities in pediatric fractures also may remodel completely. This allows greater latitude in closed management of fractures in children.

Growth may exacerbate some pediatric disorders, however. Fractures that damage the physis, or growth plate, may cause progressive angulation or shortening of the limb. Progressive angulation also may occur from asymmetric compression on one side of the physis. As a result, growth from that side of the physis is inhibited and an angular deformity develops. Examples include progressive bowleg deformity in infantile tibia vara (occurring in obese children who start walking at an early age) and rickets (weakening of the bony structure at the growth plate).

## NEUROMUSCULAR DISORDERS

Many pediatric neuromuscular disorders such as cerebral palsy, myelomeningocele, and muscular dystrophy cause muscle weakness and muscle imbalance (greater weakness on one side of the joint). Muscle imbalance plus growth results in contracture of the muscle and possible bony deformity. For example, in a child with cerebral palsy, the hip adductor and flexor muscles are often more spastic and therefore stronger than the opposing hip abductors and extensors. With growth, this muscle imbalance may cause progressive contracture of the adductors and flexors, as well as dysplasia of the femur and acetabulum, and subluxation or dislocation of the hip.

## VARIABLES IN SOFT-TISSUE INJURIES

As children grow, their coordination and strength also are developing. As a result, competitive sports require adaptation of the game to the age and size of the child. Overuse injuries in the adult primarily manifest themselves as either microscopic tears or complete rupture of the musculotendinous junction or within the substance of the tendon. In children, the bone-tendon junction is the weak link. The result is different types of overuse syndromes. For example, Osgood-Schlatter disease results from microscopic avulsion fractures at the insertion of the patellar tendon during adolescence when the child is relatively big and active and when the relatively weak secondary ossification center of the proximal tibia is developing.

SECTION 9 ■ PEDIATRIC ORTHOPAEDICS

# VARIABLES IN INFECTION AND ARTHRITIS

The higher incidence of hematogenous osteomyelitis in children is related to the unique anatomy of metaphyseal circulation in children. Likewise, a child's spine is more susceptible to hematogenous diskitis and osteomyelitis for similar reasons. Hematogenous septic arthritis also is more common in children. Chronic arthritides such as juvenile rheumatoid arthritis also are different in children. The etiology of this difference is less clear but may be related to a developing immune system causing a different response to triggering agents.

# PEDIATRIC ORTHOPAEDICS PRINCIPLES OF EVALUATION AND EXAMINATION

## INSPECTION/PALPATION

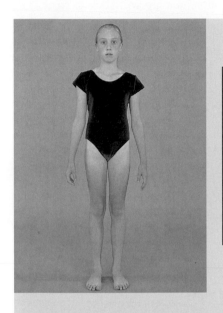

### Anterior view

With the patient standing, inspect alignment of the legs for knock-knee (genu valgum), bowleg (genu varum), internal femoral torsion (patellae point toward one another), external femoral torsion (patellae face away from each other and not straight ahead), and limb-length inequality (pelvis not level). Also, look for increased angulation at the elbow or extreme shoulder height asymmetry. Look for asymmetry in the angle formed by the humerus and forearm (elbow carrying angle). It is normal for the elbow to be in slight varus alignment. Unilateral deformity may indicate an acute injury or deformity from a congenital or traumatic growth disturbance.

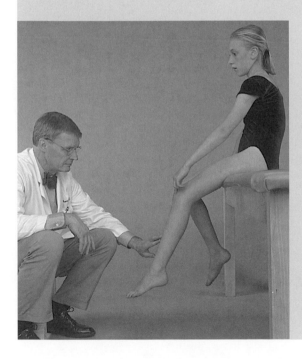

### Palpation

A young child may not be able to verbalize the site of his or her pain. Initiate palpation by touching an area that is probably not involved. Palpate from this area to the region of suspected involvement. Even though the child may be apprehensive and crying, a change in discomfort can be identified as the tender area is palpated.

# RANGE OF MOTION

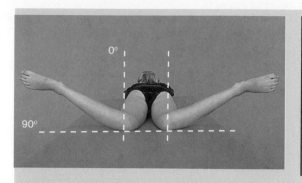

## Hip internal rotation

Measure internal rotation with the hip in extension for a more accurate reflection of femoral torsion. With the patient prone, flex the knees to 90° (the Zero Starting Position) and rotate the legs outward. This maneuver positions the hip into internal rotation. With restricted unilateral motion, one hip will allow a greater arc of motion than the other. With increased femoral anteversion, internal rotation will exceed external rotation by 30° or more.

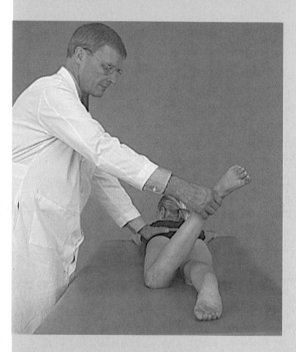

## Hip external rotation

With the child prone and knees together, rotate the legs inward while stabilizing the pelvis. This maneuver positions the hip in external rotation. Compare the two sides. Rotation of the hips is typically symmetric.

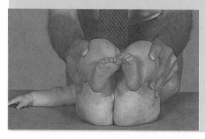

## Hip abduction–infants

Assess hip abduction in neonates and infants with the hips flexed, as some degree of hip flexion contracture is normal in children this age. Thigh lengths should be equal. Abduct the child's legs. Abduction in children this age should be symmetric and should exceed 50°. Limited abduction suggests developmental dislocation of the hip.

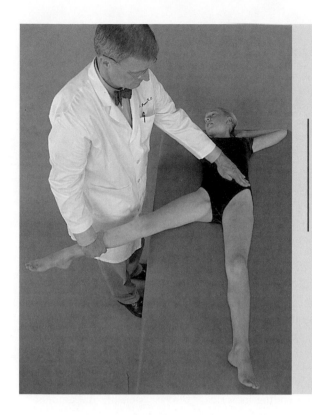

### *Hip abduction–older children*

Assess hip abduction with the hip in extension and the pelvis level. Place one finger on the contralateral anterior superior iliac spine. This hand will sense when the pelvis starts to tilt (limit of hip abduction). Abduct the hip until the pelvis starts to tilt and estimate the degree of movement.

# SPECIAL TESTS

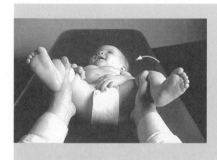

### *Barlow test*

The Barlow test dislocates an unstable neonatal hip. Stabilize the pelvis by placing one hand on the pelvis (symphysis pubis). Place your other hand with the long finger over the greater trochanter and the thumb on the medial thigh. Flex and then adduct the hip, using very little force. If the hip is located but unstable, the femoral head will dislocate with a clunk or with a sensation of slippage as the thigh is adducted.

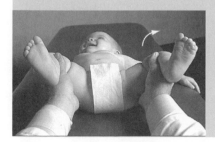

### *Ortolani maneuver*

The Ortolani maneuver reduces a dislocated hip in a neonate or young infant. Flex the hips to 90°. Place your long finger over the greater trochanter and your thumb over the inner thigh. Abduct both hips, one hip at a time, pushing the femoral head into the acetabulum with your long finger. This test is positive if there is a clunk or sensation of reduction, which occurs as the femoral head slips over the rim of the acetabulum and relocates.

SECTION 9 ■ PEDIATRIC ORTHOPAEDICS

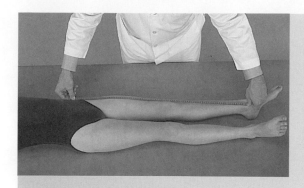

## Limb-length discrepancy

Measure with a tape measure from the anterior superior iliac spine to the prominence of the medial malleolus. Alternatively, different-sized wooden blocks can be placed under the short leg while the patient is standing. The thickness of the blocks under the leg when the iliac crests are level indicates the amount of limb-length discrepancy.

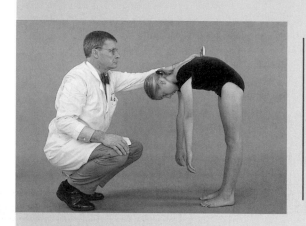

## Scoliosis, forward bending

The vertebral body rotates with scoliosis, pulling the transverse process and ribs posteriorly on the convex side. The resulting posterior prominence is more apparent with the forward bending test. Ask the patient to bend forward with the knees straight and with both arms hanging free. Examine the back from behind, in front, and from the side of the patient. A prominence on forward bending indicates scoliosis. Measure the amount of trunk asymmetry with a scoliometer.

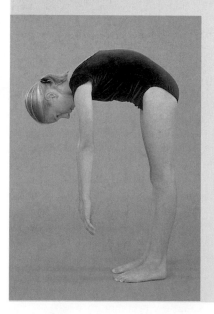

## Kyphosis

Examine the thoracic spine from the side. Look for excessive roundback deformity in the thoracic spine. Ask the patient to bend forward with arms hanging free. If the patient is not able to touch the toes, the reason may be tight hamstrings secondary to Scheuermann kyphosis or spondylolisthesis in the lower lumbar spine.

# ANTERIOR KNEE PAIN

## DEFINITION

Pain about the anterior aspect of the knee is a common problem in active adolescents and is primarily the result of repetitive stress. The most common causes are patellar maltracking, a pathologic plica, or a symptomatic bipartite patella.

Anterior knee pain caused by altered patellofemoral forces secondary to abnormal patellar tracking in the trochlear groove of the femur is common and has many different names, including patellofemoral stress syndrome (PFSS), miserable malalignment syndrome, and anterior knee syndrome.

A plica is a normal fold of the synovium that may become thickened and/or fibrotic secondary to a direct blow or repetitive stress.

A bipartite patella is a failure of an ossification center of the patella to fuse, most commonly the superior lateral corner (**Figure 1**). A bipartite patella is typically seen as an incidental finding on radiographs; however, it may become symptomatic as a result of a direct blow or following repetitive stress from flexion-extension exercises.

## CLINICAL SYMPTOMS

Patients with anterior knee pain typically report a history of vague parapatellar pain, frequently activity related. With PFSS or symptomatic plica, the pain frequently increases with flexion-extension activities such as running, kicking, and jumping, as well as with squatting, walking downhill or down stairs, or prolonged sitting. Giving way with these activities is occasionally reported. Infrequently, a patient will report that the knee locks, defined as a temporary inability to bend or extend the knee following an activity that places a high stress load on the patellofemoral joint (eg, squatting or kneeling). Swelling is rarely reported.

A bipartite patella may be asymptomatic until the patient falls on the knee, presumably altering the fibrous union between the unfused ossicle and the remainder of the patella. In the acute setting, tenderness and swelling are localized to the superolateral corner of the patella. In chronic cases, patients report pain after running and jumping activities.

| ICD-9 Codes |
| --- |
| **717.9** |
| Pathologic plica |
| **719.46** |
| Patellofemoral pain |
| **736.6** |
| Bipartite patella |

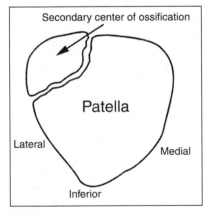

**Figure 1**

The separate ossification center seen in bipartite patella.

**SECTION 9 ■ PEDIATRIC ORTHOPAEDICS**

## TESTS

### Physical Examination

If asked to place one finger on the spot that hurts the most, adolescents with PFSS often will report that they cannot identify an exact spot but will state that their knee "hurts all over" and make a sweeping gesture over the front of the knee. In contrast, a patient with symptomatic plica or bipartite patella typically can localize his or her symptoms. Plica pain typically is localized to the medial border of the patella, whereas pain associated with bipartite patella will occur over the junctional area, typically the upper outer border. Hip rotation should be assessed to exclude the possibility of slipped capital femoral epiphysis, which can masquerade as anterior knee pain. Assess the overall alignment of the extremity. Patients with PFSS often have hip varus, knee valgus, and foot pronation, which can result in lateral tracking of the patella in the femoral groove.

Strength of the abdominal and paravertebral muscles, as well as the muscles of the hip, should be evaluated, as should flexibility of the muscles of the lower leg. Tight, weak muscles of the core and leg can result in greater stress to the patellofemoral joint (**Figure 2**). A positive apprehension sign (see Physical Examination—Knee and Lower Leg: Special Tests, p 480) implies true patellar instability rather than PFSS. Patellar compression may cause pain but is often nonspecific. A thorough knee examination is needed to rule out other causes of pain.

In patients with a symptomatic patella plica, examination may reveal a clicking sensation with knee flexion and extension. The tender plica occasionally may be palpated along the medial border of the patella.

### Diagnostic Tests

Screening radiographs include AP, lateral, and skyline views of the knee. The skyline view is beneficial because it shows both the location of the patella in the femoral groove and the thickness of the cartilage. Adolescents with PFSS have a normal patellofemoral joint space. Special imaging studies such as CT or MRI may be required for patients who have persistent pain.

## DIFFERENTIAL DIAGNOSIS

Articular cartilage defects (swelling, abnormal MRI)

Infection (rare) (erythema, effusion, severe pain, elevated C-reactive protein)

Neoplasm (rare) (severe pain, night pain, abnormal bone scan)

**Hamstrings**

Semitendinosus

Biceps femoris

Semimembranosus

**Dorsiflexors**

Tibialis anterior

Extensor digitorum longus

Extensor hallucis longus

Peroneus tertius

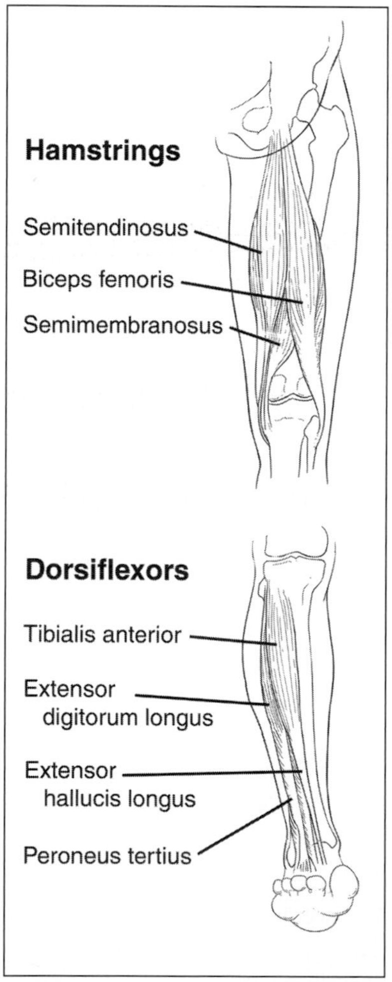

**Figure 2**

Muscle groups that tend to lose flexibility during the adolescent growth spurt.

Osteochondritis dissecans (swelling, abnormal radiographs and MRI)

Patellar subluxation or dislocation (marked positive apprehension sign, marked hypermobility of the patella)

## ADVERSE OUTCOMES OF THE DISEASE

The long-term prognosis is good in patients treated nonsurgically for symptomatic bipartite patella, symptomatic plica, or PFSS. The natural history of PFSS, which is commonly seen in adolescents, is not well defined. Most patients recover uneventfully. In the absence of true patellar subluxation or dislocation, progression to chondromalacia is rare.

## TREATMENT

Symptoms associated with PFSS are often improved by rest from aggravating activities, strengthening of the medial head of the quadriceps, and stretching of the muscles of the lower extremity. Core strengthening exercises also are beneficial. Strengthening the hip, abdominal, and trunk muscles will help better position the body and therefore diminishes the forces across the patellofemoral joint. A brace to help elevate the patella in the trochlear groove (infrapatellar strap) or guide the patella more centrally in the groove (sleeve/pad or doughnut) may be beneficial. Orthotics can be used to decrease foot pronation because the latter can enhance apparent knee valgus. Surgical management of PFSS is rarely recommended.

Treatment of symptomatic plica includes rest for 7 to 10 days with the knee in an extended position, or if symptoms are mild, activity modification. Occasionally, oral NSAIDs may be helpful in diminishing symptoms. Icing the area often provides relief. Arthroscopic excision of a symptomatic plica is rarely required in adolescents but may be considered if a prolonged trial (3 to 6 months) of nonsurgical measures fail.

Treatment of a bipartite patella is similar to that of symptomatic plica. Patients often recover after several days (5 to 7) of rest or immobilization, or use of a brace with a lateral pad combined with a decrease in flexion-extension activities followed by quadriceps strengthening. In the unusual case of persistent pain over the fibrous junction of the ossicle with the patella, surgery to remove the unfused ossicle may be required.

## ADVERSE OUTCOMES OF TREATMENT

Persistent effusion of the knee may indicate inflammatory disease (eg, juvenile rheumatoid arthritis) or infection (eg,

SECTION 9 ■ PEDIATRIC ORTHOPAEDICS

Lyme disease). Pain, hypersensitivity to touch, and limited knee motion suggests the presence of complex regional pain syndrome.

## REFERRAL DECISIONS/RED FLAGS

Pain at rest or that increases at night requires further evaluation to rule out neoplastic processes. A joint effusion, increased generalized joint laxity, or joint line pain should raise concern for internal derangement. Marked apprehension with lateral deviation of the patella suggests patellar instability, and specialty evaluation may be warranted.

# BACK PAIN

## SYNONYM
Backache

## DEFINITION
Pain in the thoracic or lumbar spine is not as common in children as in adults, but when it does occur and is present for more than a few weeks, it is more often due to organic causes (sometimes serious).

## CLINICAL SYMPTOMS
The nature of onset, as well as the location, character, and radiation of the pain should be determined. Back pain accompanied by neurologic signs and symptoms (eg, radicular pain, muscle weakness, gait abnormalities, sensory changes, bowel and bladder dysfunction) or systemic symptoms (eg, fever, malaise, and weight loss) suggest an organic cause. Night pain often signals a more serious problem such as neoplasm.

## TESTS

### Physical Examination
Examine the spine with special emphasis on identifying deformities, loss of motion, muscle spasm, and areas of tenderness. Assess gait, motor and sensory function of all appropriate nerve roots, straight leg and reverse straight leg raising tests, deep tendon reflexes, and pathologic reflexes (Babinski sign). Test superficial abdominal reflexes by lightly stroking the skin in a diagonal direction toward the umbilicus. Perform the test in all four quadrants. A normal reflex is deviation of the umbilicus toward the side of the test in all four quadrants. Asymmetric abdominal reflexes may be the only finding in a child with syringomyelia or other spinal cord pathology; however, this reflex may be absent or asymmetric in healthy children.

Neurologic deficits may develop as a late manifestation of a tumor; therefore, a normal neurologic examination does not rule out serious problems in the early stages of disease.

### Diagnostic Tests
The extent of the evaluation depends on the duration and degree of symptoms as well as the results of the physical examination. No laboratory or radiographic studies are necessary if the examination is normal and symptoms are mild and of limited duration.

**ICD-9 Codes**

**724.1**
Pain in thoracic spine

**724.2**
Low back pain

SECTION 9 ■ PEDIATRIC ORTHOPAEDICS

For symptoms in the thoracic and lumbar regions, weight-bearing AP and lateral radiographs of the entire spine provide important information because these views permit good visualization of vertebral elements and surrounding soft tissues. Oblique views may be helpful for patients who have symptoms in the lumbar spine.

AP, lateral, oblique, and open-mouth odontoid views of the cervical spine are indicated for patients with neck pain. Flexion-extension lateral views of the cervical spine are indicated to rule out instability.

The need for additional imaging studies (eg, bone scan, MRI, CT) depends on the suspected etiology. The need for and sequencing of these tests depends on the differential diagnosis.

## DIFFERENTIAL DIAGNOSIS

Differential diagnosis of pediatric back pain is shown in **Table 1**. Muscle strain is the most common cause of thoracic and lumbar pain in children. Scheuermann disease may present with pain in the thoracic and thoracolumbar regions, while spondylolysis and spondylolisthesis are common causes of pain in the lumbar and lumbosacral regions. Idiopathic scoliosis rarely causes pain in children, but scoliosis associated with syringomyelia, tethered spinal cord, or neoplasms may present as back pain.

## ADVERSE OUTCOMES OF THE DISEASE

When back pain has an organic cause, failure to diagnose may result in progression of the condition. In certain conditions, such as instability of the upper cervical spine, tumors, or infections, failure to diagnose may ultimately result in spinal cord or peripheral nerve injury.

## TREATMENT

Treatment of back pain in children is diagnosis specific. Because of the extensive differential diagnoses, it is not possible to discuss all aspects of treatment here.

If there are no ominous symptoms or neurologic abnormalities, then observation with activity modifications and mild analgesics is appropriate initially. More extensive studies will be necessary if the pain does not improve within 1 to 2 months, if the pain becomes worse, or if new symptoms and abnormal physical findings develop.

## ADVERSE OUTCOMES OF TREATMENT

Adverse outcomes of treatment are also diagnosis specific. The principal adverse outcome is lack of improvement or worsening of symptoms despite treatment. This indicates failure to recognize an underlying organic cause for the pain.

## Table 1 Differential Diagnosis of Back Pain in Children

| Etiology | Condition |
|---|---|
| *Congenital* | Congenital spine anomalies |
| | Diastematomyelia |
| *Developmental* | Scoliosis |
| | Kyphosis (Scheuermann disease) |
| *Traumatic* | Upper cervical spine instability |
| | Occult fractures |
| | Pathologic fractures |
| | Muscle strain |
| | Spondylolysis and spondylolisthesis |
| | Herniated disk |
| | Slipped vertebral apophysis |
| *Infectious* | Diskitis |
| | Vertebral osteomyelitis |
| | Tuberculosis |
| *Systemic* | Chronic infection |
| | Storage diseases |
| | Juvenile osteoporosis |
| *Juvenile arthritis* | Ankylosing spondylitis |
| | Juvenile rheumatoid arthritis |
| *Neoplastic* | |
| Benign | Osteoid osteoma |
| | Osteoblastoma |
| | Aneurysmal bone cyst |
| | Langerhan cell histiocytosis |
| Malignant | Spinal cord tumor |
| | Neuroblastoma |
| | Leukemia |
| | Osteogenic sarcoma |
| | Metastatic disease |
| *Psychogenic* | |

# REFERRAL DECISIONS/RED FLAGS

The following factors suggest a serious underlying etiology: (1) persistent or increasing pain; (2) night pain; (3) pain accompanied by systemic symptoms such as fever, malaise, or weight loss; (4) neurologic symptoms or findings; (5) bowel or bladder dysfunction; (6) onset of symptoms at a young age, especially 4 years of age or younger (possible tumor); and (7) a painful thoracic scoliosis. If these findings occur, further evaluation is necessary.

SECTION 9 ■ PEDIATRIC ORTHOPAEDICS

# ELBOW PAIN

**ICD-9 Code**

**719.42**
Pain in joint, upper arm

## DEFINITION

Elbow pain in children is most often caused by an acute or chronic injury to bone or soft tissues. Excessive throwing and the subsequent valgus stress cause most chronic elbow pain in children. The principal focus of this chapter is soft-tissue injuries. Fractures are discussed in separate chapters.

## CLINICAL SYMPTOMS

Patients with acute conditions report pain, tenderness, swelling, and most often a history of falling on an outstretched arm. For those with chronic pain, activity-related aching pain at the involved area is common.

## TESTS

### Physical Examination

For patients with acute conditions, evaluate the status of the median, ulnar, and radial nerves distal to the injury. Assess radial and ulnar pulses as well. With obvious deformity, position or splint for comfort and proceed with radiographs. In other children, attempt to find the site of maximum tenderness and perform a gentle evaluation of elbow motion.

For children with chronic pain, assess the point of maximum tenderness. Mild swelling and limited motion may be present. Palpate for a mass to exclude an atypical tumor. Palpate the ulnar nerve while moving the elbow to rule out a subluxating ulnar nerve.

### Diagnostic Tests

AP and lateral radiographs of the elbow should be obtained for all acute injuries. A fracture or dislocation may be obvious or subtle. The radial head should be directed toward the capitellum on all views. Comparison views are helpful with subtle injuries.

With chronic pain, AP and lateral radiographs may be normal or may show an avulsion fracture, fragmentation and heterotopic ossification of the medial epicondyle (Little Leaguer elbow), or fragmentation and irregularity of the capitellum.

**Table 1  Differential Diagnosis of Elbow Pain in Children**

| Etiology | Condition |
| --- | --- |
| *Acute Pain* | |
| Trauma | Dislocation |
| | Lateral condyle fracture |
| | Hemarthrosis |
| | Medial condyle fracture |
| | Medial epicondyle fracture |
| | Radial head fracture |
| | Occult fracture |
| | Olecranon fracture |
| | Sprain |
| | Subluxation of the radial head (nursemaid's elbow) |
| | Supracondylar humerus fracture |
| Infection | |
| *Chronic Pain* | |
| Overuse | Osteochondritis of the capitellum |
| | Panner disease |
| | Little Leaguer elbow |
| | Traction apophysitis |
| Neoplasm | |

# DIFFERENTIAL DIAGNOSIS

**Table 1** lists the differential diagnoses. Selected conditions are described thereafter.

## Occult Fractures

A posterior fat pad sign is associated with occult fractures in children. Overlying the distal humerus are anterior and posterior fat pads. These structures are within the elbow joint capsule. In a normal elbow, the anterior fat pad can be seen on a lateral radiograph, but the posterior fat pad usually is not seen. Any process that causes an elbow effusion will elevate the anterior and posterior fat pads and make both structures visible (**Figure 1**). In children who have a positive posterior fat pad sign and no evidence of fracture on initial radiographs, the incidence of a subsequent bony injury ranges from 6% to 76%. The greater incidence is noted in studies that include repeat AP, lateral, and oblique radiographs obtained 2 to 3 weeks after the injury.

A child with a posterior fat pad sign and no apparent fracture on initial radiographs or signs of septic arthritis should be assumed to have an occult, nondisplaced fracture. A posterior long arm splint or a long arm cast should be used for 2 to 3 weeks. Bony injuries

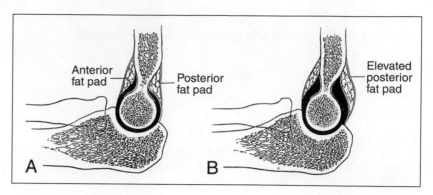

**Figure 1**

Normal anterior and posterior fat pads (**A**) and anterior and posterior fat pads elevated from an effusion (**B**).

Reproduced with permission from Skaggs DL, Mirzayan R: The posterior fat pad sign in association with occult fracture of the elbow in children. *J Bone Joint Surg Am* 1999;81:1429-1433.

that demonstrate only a posterior fat pad sign at initial evaluation are usually mild, nondisplaced fractures. If no tenderness is noted at the 2- to 3-week evaluation, immobilization can be discontinued. In this situation, there is no evidence that repeat radiographs alter treatment.

## Dislocation

Dislocation of the elbow is typically posterior. Associated injuries such as fracture of the medial epicondyle or other fractures can occur. The medial epicondyle fracture can be displaced and incarcerated in the joint. Closed reduction usually is successful.

## Hemarthrosis

An elbow hemarthrosis is a diagnosis of exclusion. Examination demonstrates swelling of the joint, and radiographs typically show a posterior fat pad sign. Aspiration of the joint is diagnostic and will decrease discomfort.

## Sprains

Elbow sprains are uncommon in children because the bone is the weak link. Short-term immobilization is appropriate.

## Subluxation of the Radial Head

This condition, also called a pulled elbow or nursemaid's elbow, is the most common elbow injury in children younger than age 5 years. This injury is associated with increased ligamentous laxity. The mechanism of injury is a pull on the forearm when the elbow is extended and the forearm pronated. The annular ligament, which wraps around the neck of the radius, slips proximally and becomes interposed between the radius and ulna.

Immediately after the injury, the child will cry, but the initial pain quickly subsides. Thereafter, the child is reluctant to use the arm but otherwise does not appear to be in great distress. The extremity is held by the side with the elbow slightly flexed and the forearm pronated. Tenderness over the radial head and resistance on attempted supination of the forearm are the only consistent findings. Radiographs are normal.

To reduce the subluxation, place your thumb over the radial head and supinate the forearm. If this maneuver fails to produce the snap of reduction, then flex the elbow. Resistance may be perceived just before reaching full flexion. As the elbow is pushed through that resistance, the annular ligament will slip back into normal position and a snap will be perceived as the radial head reduces. If the reduction is successful, the child will begin to use the extremity normally in a few minutes. The exception is the child who presents 1 to 2 days after injury. At this time, swelling of the annular ligament may both obscure the snap that signals a successful reduction and also prevent immediate resumption of normal function. However, if the elbow has full flexion and supination, the radial head has been reduced. Immobilization is probably not necessary, as parents report that slings are quickly discarded.

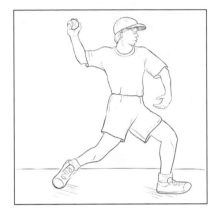

**Figure 2**
The throwing motion imposes valgus stress on the elbow.

## Infection

Infection as a cause of acute elbow pain is relatively uncommon. For example, in one study of pediatric infections, the elbow accounted for only 12% of septic arthritis. These conditions, however, should be considered when evaluating a child with elbow pain. The possibility of infection is more likely with an acute onset of pain, no history of injury, and an elevated temperature.

## Chronic Pain

These injuries may affect either the medial (tension) or lateral (compression) side of the humerus. Medial injuries can be acute (avulsion fracture of the medial epicondyle) or gradual in onset (traction apophysitis of the medial epicondyle, better known as Little Leaguer elbow) (**Figure 2**). Lateral involvement is secondary to osteonecrosis of the capitellum. When children younger than age 10 years are affected, the condition typically is called Panner disease and has a good prognosis.

Chronic injuries generally are self-limited. Resting the arm, with no throwing for 3 to 6 weeks, is indicated followed by rehabilitation to restore elbow motion and upper extremity strength. Osteonecrosis of the capitellum in adolescents, called osteochondritis dissecans or OCD, has a more guarded prognosis (**Figure 3**). This condition can result in an

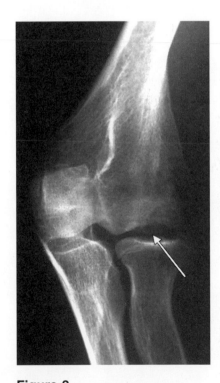

**Figure 3**
AP radiograph demonstrating radiolucency typical of osteochondritis dissecans of the capitellum (arrow).
Reproduced from Peterson RK, Savoie FH III, Field LD: Osteochondritis dissecans of the elbow. *Instr Course Lect* 1999;48:393-398.

osteochondral loose body, which causes a locking or catching sensation, and is more likely to cause residual symptoms and consideration of surgical treatment. Intra-articular loose bodies secondary to osteochondritis dissecans should be removed surgically if they are causing pain and/or intermittent locking of the joint.

Tumors, although very uncommon about the elbow in children, are more likely with chronic pain, no history of injury, pain at rest, night pain, and pain that is getting worse.

# FOOT AND ANKLE PAIN

## DEFINITION

Foot and ankle pain in a child generally is caused by specific clinical conditions; however, trauma, infection, and tumors are potential causes as well.

## CLINICAL SYMPTOMS

A history of a significant injury combined with localized findings generally suggests some type of trauma. However, children have numerous minor injuries to the lower extremities, and parents might attribute symptoms to a particular injury or episode when, in fact, the actual condition has nothing to do with trauma. Furthermore, injuries in younger children may occur away from the parents or others, and young children are typically unable to give an exact account of how the injury occurred.

Determining whether the problem is acute or chronic also provides information about its etiology. A recent onset of symptoms generally is associated with traumatic or infectious conditions.

Questions about systemic symptoms such as malaise, swelling, and fever are important with either acute-onset conditions or chronic symptoms. Fever and swelling are more likely to suggest infectious or possibly malignant conditions.

## TESTS

### Physical Examination

Infections in the foot usually have a history of direct penetrating injuries such as a nail puncture wound. If the incident occurred within the preceding 24 to 72 hours, the diagnosis is most likely a soft-tissue cellulitis or abscess.

Physical examination often can localize the area of tenderness to a specific anatomic site. This step is extremely helpful in arriving at the correct diagnosis. Older children can often point with one finger to the spot that hurts the most, which helps localize the anatomic site and greatly narrows the differential diagnosis.

The foot should be examined for areas of swelling, erythema, or ecchymosis. Ecchymosis is generally a sign of traumatic injury, whereas erythema suggests an inflammatory or infectious process. The ankle and subtalar joints should be evaluated for range of motion and tenderness on range of motion. Decreased inversion and eversion of the subtalar joint can suggest a tarsal coalition, whereas painful range of motion of the joint can indicate an inflammatory or infectious process.

**ICD-9 Codes**

**682.7**
Abscess, foot

**732.5**
Juvenile osteochondrosis of foot

**733.44**
Aseptic necrosis of bone, talus

**733.49**
Osteonecrosis of navicular

**754.61**
Tarsal coalition

**755.66**
Hallux valgus

**E920.9**
Nail puncture wound

SECTION 9 ■ PEDIATRIC ORTHOPAEDICS

## Diagnostic Tests

Radiographs are needed when a fracture or chronic process is suspected. Physical examination should be used to determine whether the problem is in the foot or ankle. If the problem is localized to the foot, AP, lateral, and oblique views of the foot are taken. AP and lateral views of the ankle can be ordered if the ankle is the area of concern. If findings on the radiographs could be a normal variant, comparison views of the opposite foot can be taken.

More sophisticated imaging studies are sometimes necessary. A bone scan can be helpful if a stress fracture or infectious process is suspected. CT is generally best for benign bony lesions, whereas MRI provides better information on soft-tissue lesions and malignant processes.

# DIFFERENTIAL DIAGNOSIS

## Hindfoot

### Calcaneal apophysitis

Calcaneal apophysitis is characterized by pain in the posterior aspect of the heel that occurs after play and sports activities and most commonly affects active, prepubertal children. Tenderness at the posterior aspect of the calcaneus is common. Radiographs typically are not needed. Short-term activity modifications or restriction is indicated. Detailed information about calcaneal apophysitis is provided on pp 819-820.

### Os trigonum

The os trigonum is an accessory ossicle of the posterior talus that usually is a normal anatomic variant. However, this secondary center of ossification may become symptomatic in older adolescents and adults, particularly those who participate in ballet or soccer. Patients commonly report posterior ankle pain that is activity related. Pain also develops secondary to posterior impingement of the os trigonum between the talus and tibia during plantar flexion. Surgical excision may be required.

### Osteochondral lesion of the talus

This lesion typically affects adolescents, particularly athletes. The pain is exacerbated by activity and is localized to the ankle region. Radiographs of the ankle usually confirm the diagnosis, although MRI may be necessary in some cases. Osteochondritis dissecans of the talus may result in ankle pain with activity, swelling, and locking of the ankle joint. Treatment includes immobilization or sometimes surgery depending on the size, location, and degree of displacement. Detailed information about osteochondral lesions of the talus is provided on pp 915-916.

### Tarsal coalition

Tarsal coalition is the most common cause of rigid flatfeet in children. Symptoms typically develop during the second decade. The onset of pain generally is insidious but can be associated with an injury or change in activity or perceived as recurrent ankle sprains. Hindfoot motion is markedly restricted, and spasm of the peroneal muscles can be elicited by quickly inverting the foot. Talocalcaneal bars are difficult to see on routine radiographs; therefore, CT is necessary to confirm the diagnosis. Treatment depends on the presentation of symptoms. Detailed information about tarsal coalition is provided on pp 947-949.

## Midfoot

### Osteonecrosis of the navicular

This condition, sometimes called Köhler disease, primarily affects children (usually boys) ages 4 to 8 years. Patients limp, turn out their foot while walking, and may report pain in the medial arch. Radiographs show a dense, fragmented, thin navicular (**Figure 1**). A short leg walking cast for 4 to 8 weeks relieves pain, improves walking (less pain), and may speed resolution of the osteonecrosis. However, the eventual outcome is good whether casting or activity modifications are chosen.

### Accessory navicular

Accessory navicular is an anatomic variant in which a secondary center of ossification forms at the medial aspect of the navicular and may become symptomatic during adolescence. Patients report pain and swelling on the medial side of the foot. Activity or shoe wear may exacerbate the pain. Radiographs may be necessary, depending on the presentation and history of symptoms. Treatment generally is limited to short-term activity restrictions or shoe modifications. However, a walking cast or even surgical treatment may be necessary, depending on the symptoms and history. Detailed information about accessory navicular is provided on pp 817-818.

## Forefoot

### Freiberg infraction

Freiberg infraction is osteonecrosis that most commonly involves the head of the second metatarsal, most likely a result of trauma, and typically affects adolescents. The pain is exacerbated by activity. Examination reveals tenderness under the involved metatarsal head, sometimes swelling on the dorsal aspect of the metatarsal head and pain at the extremes of dorsiflexion and plantar flexion. Radiographs usually show evidence of the condition within 2 to 3 weeks of the onset of symptoms (**Figure 2**). Treatment options include activity

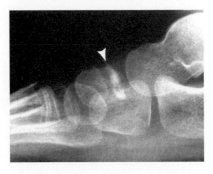

**Figure 1**
Lateral radiograph of the foot showing a shattered, fragmented navicular (arrowhead).

Reproduced from Kasser JR (ed): *Orthopaedic Knowledge Update* 5. Rosemont, IL, American Academy of Orthopaedic Surgeons, 1996, pp 503-514.

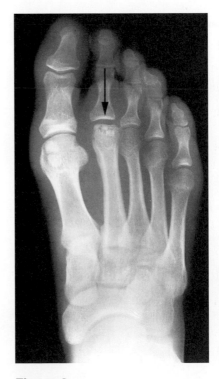

**Figure 2**
Radiograph showing Freiberg infraction. Note flattening and fragmentation at the head of the second metatarsal (arrow).

SECTION 9 ■ PEDIATRIC ORTHOPAEDICS

modifications, a metatarsal pad, or short-term casting. Occasionally, surgical treatment is required to remove loose bodies or to realign the metatarsal head.

### Hallux valgus

Hallux valgus may develop during adolescence. At this age, most patients are asymptomatic, but some may report pain. Treatment principles are similar to those for adults. Detailed information about hallux valgus is presented on pp 648-650.

## Other Foot Problems

### Enthesitis

Enthesitis is characterized by pain and inflammation at a bone-tendon insertion but is uncommon in children. Disorders such as Achilles tendinitis or plantar fasciitis may be the presenting symptoms of a seronegative spondyloarthropathy.

### Infection

Infection in the foot usually is secondary to a direct penetrating injury, such as a nail puncture wound. If symptoms develop within 24 to 72 hours after the injury, the cellulitis or abscess usually is secondary to a *Staphylococcus aureus* infection. If swelling and erythema develop several days after the injury, the infection usually is a septic arthritis or osteomyelitis secondary to *Pseudomonas aeruginosa* that requires surgical débridement.

### Sprains, strains, and fractures

Sprains, strains, and fractures of the foot and ankle occur but are relatively uncommon until late adolescence. Most of these injuries in children can be managed by nonsurgical modalities. In a child who has a history of an inversion injury and tenderness over the distal fibular physis, the most likely diagnosis is a nondisplaced fracture of the physis. This injury is best treated with a cast.

### Tumors

Tumors in the foot and ankle are uncommon at all ages. The most common benign bony tumor in children is a unicameral or aneurysmal bone cyst involving the calcaneus. Osteoid osteoma affecting the tarsal bones also occurs in children. Ewing sarcoma affecting the tarsal bones or diaphysis of metatarsals is the most common malignant bony lesion involving the foot. The pain, swelling, and radiographic findings in this tumor may mimic osteomyelitis. Of the malignant soft-tissue lesions, synovial cell sarcoma is most common in the foot. Typical symptoms include onset during the second decade of a slowly enlarging mass.

# GROWING PAIN

## DEFINITION

Growing pain is a condition for which there is no uniform diagnostic consensus. Typically, it is a diagnosis made after more specific pathologic conditions are excluded. Although its true etiology is unknown, growing pain or leg aches are often thought to be the result of overactivity (muscular strain or fatigues). The condition typically occurs in an otherwise healthy, active child. Growing pain is more common in boys, in children with ligamentous laxity, and in 2- to 5-year-old children. Older children, however, also may be affected. The pain or discomfort is commonly localized to the calf but may be perceived in the foot, ankle, knee, or thigh. The problem is often bilateral, but parents may report that one leg seems to hurt more than the other or that one leg hurts some nights while the other leg hurts different nights.

**ICD-9 Code**
**729.5**
Pain in limb

## CLINICAL SYMPTOMS

Leg pain is often described as mild to moderate, intermittent in character, and more noticeable in the evening or at night or following a day of increased activity or sport. In fact, most children do not limp during the day. Parents generally report using warm or cold compresses, massage, or simple analgesics to relieve the symptoms. Constitutional symptoms such as fever, weight loss, loss of appetite, or malaise are rarely reported.

## TESTS

### Physical Examination

Examination of the affected extremity should focus on identifying any masses, inflammation, lymphadenopathy, abnormal joint movement, instability, muscle group atrophy, and any neurologic deficits. With growing pain, the examination is normal in all aspects, although the affected extremity can be tender to deep pressure. Flexible flatfeet may be noted, but the gait and pattern of shoe wear is normal.

### Diagnostic Tests

Plain radiographs should be considered in children who have a higher intensity of pain or more prolonged symptoms, a history of pain at rest that is not relieved by simple analgesics, or an associated mass. Bone scan, CT, or MRI should be considered if a specific lesion, such as bone or soft-tissue tumor, stress fracture, bone or joint infection, or tarsal coalition, is suspected.

Metabolic work-up may be needed if the history and review of systems suggest certain conditions such as leukemia or an endocrinopathy.

## DIFFERENTIAL DIAGNOSIS

Calcaneal apophysitis (heel pain with activity)

Köhler disease (unilateral, pain with activity, foot turned out with walking)

Metabolic/systemic disease (history and review of systems suggestive of leukemia, endocrine disorder, renal osteodystrophy, juvenile chronic arthritis, rheumatic disease)

Subacute osteomyelitis (unilateral, activity-related symptoms)

Trauma (unilateral, toddler's or stress fracture)

Tumor (unilateral, pain more persistent and severe)

## ADVERSE OUTCOMES OF THE DISEASE

Growing pain has a benign and self-limiting course, although the leg aches may occur intermittently for several months. Permanent long-term impairment has not been noted.

## TREATMENT

An explanation of the natural history and expected outcome and perhaps a recommendation about use of simple analgesics usually are sufficient to allay parental fears and to avoid overtreatment. Short-term use of NSAIDs and/or a short period of rest or immobilization before resuming activities, as the level of pain allows, also can be recommended. Surgical treatment is not indicated.

## ADVERSE OUTCOMES OF TREATMENT

Overuse of pain medication with subsequent psychological aspects and unnecessary testing are possible.

## REFERRAL DECISIONS/RED FLAGS

Patients with a history of severe, persistent pain along with constitutional symptoms (eg, fever, night sweats, malaise, poor appetite, weight loss) need further evaluation. Findings on physical examination that indicate masses, significant inflammation, lymphadenopathy, circulatory compromise, neuropathy, or myopathy also are a concern. A serious error is to diagnose growing pain or leg aches while overlooking the more specific underlying conditions listed in the differential diagnosis.

SECTION 9 ■ PEDIATRIC ORTHOPAEDICS

# ACCESSORY NAVICULAR

## DEFINITION

Accessory navicular is an anatomic variant in which a secondary center of ossification forms in the medial portion of the tarsal navicular bone at the attachment of the posterior tibialis tendon. During adolescence, this may become prominent and symptomatic by virtue of its size, or from repetitive sprains and microfractures at the attachment of the ossicle to the navicular. Symptoms are more common in girls. The disorder is fairly common, with one study observing a 14% incidence of symptoms during adolescence.

**ICD-9 Code**
**732.5**
Juvenile osteochondrosis of foot

## CLINICAL SYMPTOMS

Patients typically report pain and swelling on the medial side of the foot. The pain is exacerbated with activity or with pressure from the overlying shoes. Severe pain is uncommon.

## TESTS

### Physical Examination

Tenderness and mild swelling over the medial aspect of the navicular (insertion of the posterior tibialis tendon) is typical. Inversion of the foot against resistance may be painful. A flexible pes planus may be present.

### Diagnostic Tests

Radiographs are not necessary with a typical examination and mild symptoms. With persistent or severe symptoms, AP, lateral, and oblique radiographs of the foot will document the disorder and exclude other possibilities. The AP and lateral views should be weight bearing to best demonstrate pes planus or other alignment problems. The oblique view, obtained with the patient supine, often provides the best profile of the accessory ossicle (**Figure 1**). Some patients have a cornuated navicular (shaped like a horn of plenty), resulting from fusion of the accessory ossicle to the navicular.

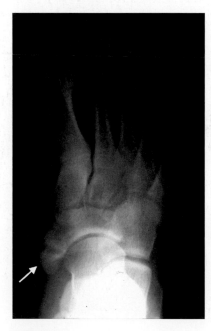

**Figure 1**
AP radiograph of the foot demonstrating accessory navicular (arrow).

## DIFFERENTIAL DIAGNOSIS

Flexible pes planovalgus (developmental or acquired)

Posterior tibial tendinitis (swelling in the region of the posterior tibial tendon)

Tarsal coalition (restricted inversion, eversion of the heel)

# Adverse Outcomes of the Disease

Patients may experience persistent pain or a limp.

# Treatment

Most patients can be treated with short-term restriction of activities and/or shoe modifications to relieve pressure over the prominent navicular (soft material medial to the bump and/or stretching of the shoe). A short period of time in a walking cast may permit healing of the repetitive microfractures and resolution of symptoms. In most cases, the bump is not large and symptoms resolve with cessation of growth. Excision of the prominent portion of the navicular is the treatment of choice for patients with persistent, disabling symptoms.

# Adverse Outcomes of Treatment

Postoperative infection and a tender medial scar that is irritated by shoe wear are both possible.

# Referral Decisions/Red Flags

Persistent pain signals the need for further evaluation.

# CALCANEAL APOPHYSITIS

## SYNONYM
Sever disease

**ICD-9 Code**
**732.5**
Juvenile osteochondrosis of foot

## DEFINITION
Calcaneal apophysitis most commonly affects active, prepubertal children and is characterized by pain in the posterior aspect of the heel that occurs after play and sports activities. This condition is caused by repetitive stress and microtrauma on the calcaneal apophysis. This weak link is obliterated when the apophysis fuses to the main body of the calcaneus, a process that occurs around age 9 years in girls and age 11 years in boys.

## CLINICAL SYMPTOMS
Patients have posterior heel pain and a limp that is activity related.

## TESTS

### Physical Examination
Examination reveals tenderness at the posterior aspect of the calcaneus.

### Diagnostic Tests
Radiographs are not diagnostic, and sclerosis at the secondary ossification center is normal (**Figure 1**). With bilateral

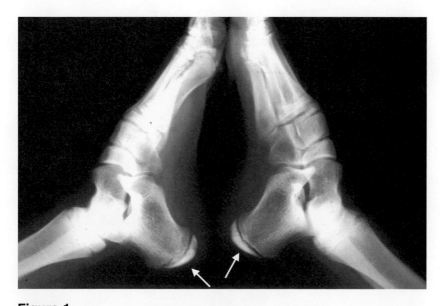

**Figure 1**
Radiograph of the feet reveals irregular calcaneal apophyses (arrows) that are normal. There are no radiographic findings consistent with calcaneal apophysitis (Sever disease).

SECTION 9 ■ PEDIATRIC ORTHOPAEDICS

involvement and a typical history, radiographs probably are not necessary. With unilateral involvement, a lateral view of the heel is necessary to rule out a unicameral bone cyst.

## Differential Diagnosis

Achilles tendinitis (can be associated with Reiter syndrome or other seronegative spondyloarthropathies)

Infection (unilateral, elevated erythrocyte sedimentation rate, swelling)

Tumor (unilateral, swelling, night pain)

## Adverse Outcomes of the Disease

Pain, a limp, and activity modifications are possible, but there are no long-term sequelae.

## Treatment

Treatment includes short-term modification or restriction of the precipitating activity. Shoe modifications using a ¼" heel lift or heel cushion and Achilles tendon stretching can be helpful. Casting is rarely needed but can be used for 4 to 6 weeks if the pain and limp are recalcitrant. Neither surgery nor steroid injection is indicated.

## Adverse Outcomes of Treatment

There are no long-term sequelae.

## Referral Decisions/Red Flags

Suspicion of tumor or osteomyelitis indicates the need for further evaluation. When treatment does not relieve discomfort, additional diagnostic studies are indicated to rule out infection or neoplastic disease.

# Cavus Foot Deformity

## Synonyms
High-arched foot
Pes cavus

## Definition
Pes cavus is a foot with an abnormally high arch. The forefoot
is fixed in equinus relative to the hindfoot. Other terms, such as
cavovarus and equinocavovarus, describe additional changes in
the hindfoot or ankle.

Children with a cavus foot frequently have an underlying
neuromuscular disorder with associated muscle weakness or
spasticity. Unless there is a known cause for the cavus foot,
children who present with this condition should undergo a
thorough diagnostic evaluation. Patients with systemic
neuromuscular diseases or idiopathic cavus feet usually have
bilateral involvement. Unilateral deformity is associated with
localized disorders of the lumbosacral spinal cord.

## Clinical Symptoms
Parents often note changes in the arch and toes, difficulty in
fitting shoes, or difficulty with repeated ankle sprains. Pain is
infrequent during childhood, but with time, painful callosities
develop underneath the prominent metatarsal heads. A family
history should be obtained because some causes of cavus feet
are genetic disorders. Inquire about bowel or bladder symptoms
that may be present with spinal cord lesions.

## Tests

### Physical Examination
Inspect the lower extremity to evaluate the alignment of the
ankle, heel, midfoot, and toes, and check the plantar aspect of
the foot for callosities. A careful neurologic examination of the
lower extremities also is necessary. Examine the spine for
curvatures, paraspinal spasm, and midline defects such as
dimpling or abnormal hairy patches. Examine the upper
extremity for weakness of the intrinsic muscles of the hand.

### Diagnostic Tests
Weight-bearing AP and lateral radiographs of the foot and the
entire spine should be obtained. On the spinal radiographs, look
for congenital malformations, diastematomyelia, widening of

| ICD-9 Codes | |
|---|---|
| **736.75** | Cavovarus deformity of foot, acquired |
| **754.59** | Varus deformities of feet, other (Talipes cavovarus) |

SECTION 9 ■ PEDIATRIC ORTHOPAEDICS

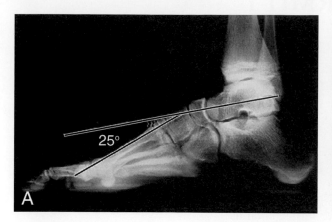 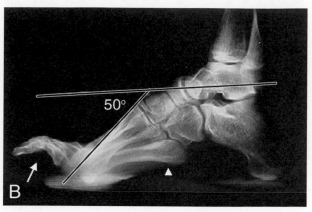

**Figure 1**

Radiographs demonstrating cavus foot. **A,** Radiograph demonstrates a positive (22°) (Meary's angle caused by cavus foot and associated forefoot equinus. In a normal foot, a line drawn through the long axis of the talus would go through the first metatarsal. **B,** Radiograph of the foot of a patient with a more severe deformity (Meary's angle = 53°). Note the claw toes (arrow) and the hypertrophy of the cortices of the fifth metatarsal (arrowhead) resulting from excessive lateral forefoot weight bearing.

the interpedicular distance, and atypical curve patterns. On the lateral view of a normal foot, a line typically passes through the axis of the talus and first metatarsal. With a cavus foot, dorsal angulation is noted on lines drawn through the axis of the talus and the first metatarsal (Meary's angle) (**Figure 1**).

Nerve conduction velocity studies and MRI of the spine may be indicated. Electromyography may distinguish myopathic from neuropathic conditions.

# DIFFERENTIAL DIAGNOSIS

Charcot-Marie-Tooth disease (peripheral neuropathy with abnormal nerve conduction velocity studies, autosomal dominant most common)

Clubfoot (incomplete correction)

Diastematomyelia (hairy patch on the spine, abnormal spinal radiographs and MRI)

Friedreich ataxia (gait abnormalities, autosomal recessive)

Idiopathic (may be familial, very uncommon, diagnosis of exclusion)

Lipomyelomeningocele (soft-tissue prominence on the lower spine, may be noted only on MRI)

Muscular dystrophy (previous diagnosis)

Myelomeningocele (previous diagnosis)

Poliomyelitis (previous diagnosis)

Spinal cord tether (possible unilateral foot deformity)

Spinal cord tumor (commonly unilateral deformity)

Trauma (residuum of tendon laceration or fracture)

# ADVERSE OUTCOMES OF THE DISEASE

Outcome and progression depend on the disease process.

# TREATMENT

Underlying spinal cord pathology requires surgical treatment. Foot deformities may be accommodated in the early stage of the disorder by shoe modifications and arch supports. In children, cavus feet tend to progress, and progressive deformities require surgical treatment to correct the deformity and balance muscle forces to maintain the correction. Arthrodesis should not be used primarily but may be helpful as a salvage procedure.

# ADVERSE OUTCOMES OF TREATMENT

With patients who have progressive loss of sensation and proprioception, skin ulcers are more common if the foot remains in an unbalanced position, and Charcot arthropathy of the ankle is more likely to occur after a previous triple arthrodesis. In patients who remain ambulatory, degenerative changes develop in the ankle joint in those who have undergone triple arthrodesis of the foot.

# REFERRAL DECISIONS/RED FLAGS

Further evaluation is recommended upon diagnosis.

SECTION 9 ■ PEDIATRIC ORTHOPAEDICS

# CHILD ABUSE

**ICD-9 Code**

**995.50**
Child abuse, unspecified

## SYNONYMS
Munchausen syndrome by proxy
Nonaccidental trauma
Shaken baby syndrome

## DEFINITION
Approximately 2.4 million reports of child abuse are filed annually in the United States, and 4,000 children die every year as a result of abuse or neglect. Most cases of abuse involve children younger than age 3 years. Firstborn children, premature infants, stepchildren, and handicapped children are at a greater risk. Failure to recognize injuries of child abuse results in a child being returned to the same environment and a 25% risk of serious reinjury and a 5% risk of death.

The critical issue in identifying child abuse is whether the history given by the family adequately explains the child's injuries. Soft-tissue injuries such as bruising, burns, or scars are seen in most patients. Toddlers typically have normal bruises over the chin, the brow, elbows, knees, and shins, but bruises on the back of the head, buttocks, abdomen, legs, arms, cheeks, or genitalia are suspicious for abuse. Fractures also are common in child abuse cases, and these children are more likely to have an additional abdominal injury as a result of blunt trauma.

## THE INVESTIGATIVE INTERVIEW
The guiding principle for the conduct of the interview is to remain objective while calmly and methodically questioning the family. Seldom is a single physical finding conclusive for a diagnosis of child abuse; additional injuries and risk factors in the home must be identified. Other guidelines of the investigative interview include the following:

- interview individual family members in private;
- be attentive, nonjudgmental, and avoid leading questions during the history;
- carefully document the given history of injury verbatim, as well as its source;
- establish a scenario for the injury from each witness, noting carefully any inconsistencies;
- identify who primarily is responsible for feeding and disciplining the child;
- identify all family members and other individuals who have access to the child;

- identify individuals outside the family who have been with the child without family supervision;
- assess for risk factors: boyfriends, stepparents, baby-sitters, and even larger siblings, as these individuals are often abusers;
- note any delay in seeking medical attention for injuries.

When obtaining the social history, inquire about unusual stresses on the family, such as recent loss of a job, separation or divorce, death in the family, housing problems, or inadequate funds for food. Alcohol abuse in the home is a risk factor for child abuse, and maternal cocaine use increases the risk of abuse fivefold.

If family members later change their account of how the injury occurred or any other aspect of the history, do not alter the original account, but date and record the revision as an addendum to the record.

# TESTS

## Physical Examination
Carefully conduct a head-to-toe examination to evaluate the child for any suspicious soft-tissue injuries. A thorough examination is important because in most cases of confirmed abuse, there is evidence of prior abuse. Note, in detail, any suspicious soft-tissue injuries. Palpate the face, spine, and upper and lower extremities for tenderness suggestive of fracture. Examine the abdomen for swelling and tenderness. Inspect for physical signs of sexual assault such as bruising or chafing of the genitalia. Physical findings of sexual abuse can be subtle. A physician specializing in sexual abuse may be required to examine the child.

## Diagnostic Tests
If the child's mental status is abnormal, evaluate for subdural hematoma and retinal hemorrhage secondary to violent shaking. Check bleeding studies when there is bruising, and order a toxicology screening if there is a history of substance abuse in the family or if there is abnormal mental status. CT of the abdomen is indicated if the head-to-toe examination shows abdominal tenderness or if the results of liver function tests are elevated.

AP and lateral radiographs of all long bones, the hands, feet, spine, and the chest, as well as a skull series, are standard. Do not order a single radiograph or so-called "baby gram." This study does not provide adequate detail and may miss subtle fractures. While there is no predominant fracture pattern seen in child abuse, certain fractures are more suspicious for child

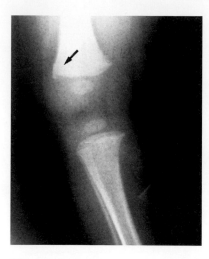

**Figure 1**
AP radiograph of the distal femur with a "corner" or "chip" fracture (arrow).

abuse than others. Fractures considered highly specific for child abuse include posterior rib fractures, scapula fractures, fractures of the posterior process of the spine, and fractures of the sternum. One type of fracture unique to child abuse is the "corner" or "chip" fracture of the metaphysis that avulses the edge of the metaphysis from the epiphysis because of downward traction or pull on the extremity (**Figure 1**). Spiral fractures are caused by rotational injury, and transverse or oblique fractures are caused by a direct blow. Rib fractures also are common and, when healed, may appear only as fusiform thickening of the ribs. A bone scan may be helpful in detecting rib fractures, but it may not show skull fractures or long bone fractures near the epiphyseal growth plates.

Fractures considered to be of moderate specificity for abuse include multiple, especially bilateral, fractures, fractures of different ages, epiphyseal separations, vertebral body fractures, fractures of the fingers, and complex skull fractures. Multiple fractures at various stages of healing without explanation strongly suggest a history of child abuse (**Figure 2**).

The age of fractures can be estimated by their appearance. Seven to 14 days after the injury, new periosteal bone and callus formation can be seen; by 14 to 21 days after the initial injury, there is loss of the definition of the fracture line and maturation of the callus with trabecular formation. More dense callus is seen 21 to 42 days after injury. As the bone remodels to a more normal configuration, fractures older than 6 weeks are distinguished by subtle fusiform sclerotic thickening that is best seen when compared with a normal contralateral bone.

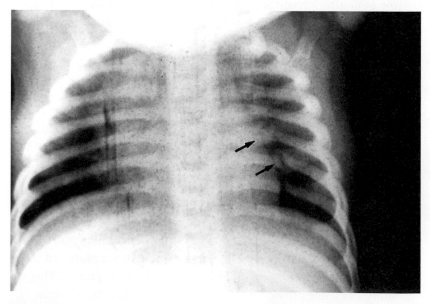

**Figure 2**
Radiograph demonstrating rib fractures at various stages of healing (arrows).

Fractures of low specificity for abuse include clavicle fractures and linear skull fractures. Of note, a vague history of injury or other risk factors for child abuse outweigh fracture specificity in determining child abuse.

It is important to avoid overdiagnosing child abuse. Spiral fractures of the tibia, the so-called "toddler's fracture," can occur in 1- to 3-year-old children as a result of a relatively trivial fall. Spontaneous fractures can occur in diseases such as osteogenesis imperfecta. The presence of osteopenia, a family history of osteogenesis imperfecta, as well as the presence of blue sclera would suggest this disease. Pathologic fractures also are seen in osteomyelitis, tumor, rickets, neuromuscular disease, and other metabolic diseases.

## THE FINAL DIAGNOSIS OF CHILD ABUSE

Once pathologic fractures are excluded, determine whether the child's fracture has been caused by either accidental trauma or inflicted trauma. A diagnosis of accidental trauma can be made when an acute injury is brought promptly to medical attention, has a plausible mechanism of injury, and lacks other risk factors for child abuse. Suspicious injuries must be reported as child abuse.

## REPORTING CHILD ABUSE

In the United States, any physician who reports suspected child abuse in good faith is protected from both civil and criminal liability, but failure to report suspected child abuse exposes the physician to liability. Sexual abuse is a criminal offense and must always be reported. Eliciting help from the hospital's child protection committee is helpful and appropriate. In addition to making notes in the medical record, the physician may be asked to complete a notarized affidavit summarizing findings in the abuse case and stating that the child may be at risk for injury or loss of life if returned to the home environment. The child may then be placed in a foster home until an investigation is completed. The physician must be prepared to defend his or her findings in custodial hearings if the family challenges the actions of child protective services.

SECTION 9 ■ PEDIATRIC ORTHOPAEDICS

# CLUBFOOT

**ICD-9 Code**

**754.51**
Talipes equinovarus

## SYNONYMS
Congenital clubfoot
Talipes equinovarus

## DEFINITION
Clubfoot, sometimes called talipes equinovarus, is a congenital deformity characterized by four distinct components: plantar flexion (equinus) of the ankle, adduction (varus) of the heel (hindfoot), high arch (cavus) at the midfoot, and adduction of the forefoot (**Figure 1**).

While there are many theories about the causes of clubfoot, none has been proved. Most cases are idiopathic and occur in an otherwise normal infant. Neuromuscular clubfoot is secondary to disorders such as myelomeningocele, arthrogryposis, and congenital constriction band syndrome. Only idiopathic clubfoot is discussed here.

The incidence of clubfoot in boys is twice that in girls. If a family has one child with a clubfoot, the risk in subsequent siblings is 3% to 4%. If one parent and one child in a family have clubfoot, the risk in subsequent children is 25%.

## CLINICAL SYMPTOMS
Infants with clubfoot typically appear as if they could walk on the top or dorsolateral aspect of the foot. In most patients, all four components of a clubfoot are present to some degree, but different aspects of the deformity may be more striking. Plantar flexion (equinus) usually is most severe and is characterized by the foot pointing down, a drawn-up position of the heel, and the inability to pull the calcaneus down when dorsiflexing the foot. The high arch (cavus) may be difficult to see, but with a severe clubfoot, it is indicated by a transverse crease across the sole of the foot. Occasionally, forefoot adduction is relatively severe while the other components appear less severe.

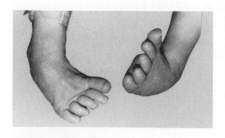
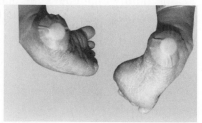

**Figure 1**
Bilateral congenital clubfoot, seen in a newborn.

# TESTS

## Physical Examination

Examination should rule out neuromuscular disorders and determine whether muscle function and sensation are intact. In rare instances, congenital absence of the anterior compartment muscles will occur in association with rigid clubfoot. Absence of muscle function and altered sensation can indicate a spinal cord disorder such as lipomyelomeningocele.

A true idiopathic clubfoot is not fully correctable by passive manipulation. Therefore, a foot that can be placed in a normal position by manipulation is talipes equinovarus caused by intrauterine molding rather than a true clubfoot. This problem typically resolves without therapy.

## Diagnostic Tests

Radiographs usually are not necessary to confirm the diagnosis or to begin treatment. However, they should be obtained if the diagnosis is unclear or if nonsurgical treatment is failing. Standardized stress views provide the most information about the rigidity of deformity and differential diagnosis.

# DIFFERENTIAL DIAGNOSIS

Arthrogryposis (stiffness and weakness of multiple joints of the upper and/or lower extremities)

Congenital constriction band syndrome (partial or circumferential bands of indented skin and underlying tissue, variable distal amputations and deformities including clubfoot)

Distal arthrogryposis (autosomal dominant condition, stiffness of the hands and feet)

# ADVERSE OUTCOMES OF THE DISEASE

When left untreated, children with clubfoot will have a severe disability. Not only are walking and shoe wear severely impaired, but there is the psychological trauma of living with what many perceive as a grotesque deformity.

Even with successful treatment, the affected foot will be smaller and less mobile than a normal foot. The difference is not as obvious with bilateral involvement but is readily apparent with unilateral involvement. The shoe of the affected foot is typically 1 to 1½ sizes smaller than the normal foot. In addition, the calf muscles are smaller in the affected leg and may present a cosmetic problem for which there is no good solution.

# TREATMENT

Manipulation and casting should commence immediately upon diagnosis; untreated, the deformity will only become stiffer and more resistant to nonsurgical treatment. Two to 4 months of manipulation and casting are required to correct a clubfoot. The success rate of casting depends on many variables, including the rigidity of the deformity and the experience and skill of the physician. Correction by manipulation usually requires prolonged splinting to minimize the potential for recurrence. Recurrence after casting is most common within the first 2 to 3 years of life, but can happen up to age 5 to 7 years.

Surgery is required when nonsurgical treatment fails, usually after 3 to 4 months of treatment. Initial reconstructive procedures range from heel cord lengthening to a complete posterior, medial, and lateral release of the foot. The purpose of surgery is to lengthen or release contracted tendons and ligaments so that the bones can be positioned in normal alignment. Casting is done after surgery to allow healing of the tendon and remodeling of the tarsal bones. Although less common, recurrence also is possible after surgical treatment.

Treatment is successful if the foot is in a good weight-bearing position and the child can run and play without pain.

# ADVERSE OUTCOMES OF TREATMENT

Recurrent deformity is more likely to occur if the treatment program did not completely correct the deformity. Overcorrection is possible after surgical release and results in a severe flatfoot with lateral translation of the heel. Flatfoot can also result from casting if the hindfoot varus is not fully corrected before the foot is manipulated into dorsiflexion.

# REFERRAL DECISIONS/RED FLAGS

Immediate diagnosis and specialty evaluation in the first week of life provide the best chance for successful correction by casting and manipulation. Neurologic abnormalities or stiff joints suggest an underlying disorder associated with the clubfoot deformity.

# Complex Regional Pain Syndrome

## Synonyms

Causalgia
CRPS
Reflex sympathetic dystrophy
RSD

**ICD-9 Codes**

**337.21**
Reflex sympathetic dystrophy of the upper limb

**337.22**
Reflex sympathetic dystrophy of the lower limb

## Definition

Complex regional pain syndrome (CRPS) describes a constellation of signs and symptoms characterized by dysfunctional, debilitating pain that is not anatomic in distribution and is disproportionate to the inciting injury. CRPS is classified as either type I (reflex sympathetic dystrophy [RSD]) or type II (causalgia). Type I CRPS is a pain syndrome that principally involves the extremities and is associated with varying degrees of autonomic dysfunction. Type I CRPS is more common in children and adolescents, particularly in children between the ages of 9 and 15 years. The diagnosis is often delayed because of the confusing clinical presentation of musculoskeletal, neurologic, and inflammatory symptoms.

## Clinical Symptoms

An older child or adolescent with type I CRPS commonly presents after a minor twisting injury or contusion. Signs and symptoms typically include excessive pain and hypersensitivity to light touch, cold intolerance, transient swelling, and skin discoloration in the extremity (most commonly the foot and ankle). Weight bearing, joint range of motion, and limb mobility may be severely restricted by pain, weakness, and joint stiffness.

## Tests

### Physical Examination

Type I CRPS is a diagnosis of exclusion. Early in the disease the physical examination can be confusing and may delay the diagnosis. The patient may be unable to bear weight on an affected lower extremity or may refuse to move an affected upper extremity. Localized soft-tissue edema and skin hyperemia are visible. Active range of motion is limited, and attempts at passive range of motion elicit severe pain. Minor sensory stimuli, such as brushing against bed sheets, cause severe burning pain in a localized but nonanatomic distribution.

SECTION 9 ■ PEDIATRIC ORTHOPAEDICS

### Diagnostic Tests

Plain radiographs, three-phase bone scan, and MRI, along with laboratory studies such as erythrocyte sedimentation rate, C-reactive protein, and other hematologic tests are most useful to eliminate the common differential diagnoses.

In the early stages of type I CRPS, routine studies are within normal limits. Tests specific for type I CRPS such as thermography, cold testing, and sympathetic blockade (the gold standard) may help confirm the diagnosis in equivocal cases. In patients with long-standing symptoms, radiographs reveal limb osteopenia, and MRI shows edema of soft tissues and bones.

## DIFFERENTIAL DIAGNOSIS

Contusion
Inflammatory synovitis
Ligament sprain
Musculoskeletal infection
Neoplasm
Occult fracture
Spinal pathology
Tendinitis

## ADVERSE OUTCOMES OF THE DISEASE

Long-term symptoms are associated with dystrophic changes such as muscle wasting, joint contracture, thickening of the nails, and the appearance of coarse hair on the extremities. The most feared complications are chronic pain, limb dystrophy, and permanent limb dysfunction. Most patients, however, fully recover if diagnosed early and appropriately treated.

## TREATMENT

Physical therapy is the mainstay of treatment. Frequent sessions focusing on desensitization, joint mobility, and weight bearing help to restore function within 4 to 6 weeks. Low doses of antidepressants (commonly amitriptyline) or anticonvulsants (commonly gabapentin) are effective in diminishing symptoms and facilitating rehabilitation in patients who initially are unresponsive to physical therapy. Narcotics and other pain medications are best used under careful supervision in the earliest stages of type I CRPS and have a limited long-term role in children.

Paravertebral sympathetic chain blockade by selective injection or epidural infusion is necessary only if other treatment regimens fail. A team approach to management enhances outcomes.

## ADVERSE OUTCOMES OF TREATMENT

Inability to resolve the pain ultimately may result in severe disability, including loss of limb function.

## REFERRAL DECISIONS/RED FLAGS

Early diagnosis and referral are most likely to result in complete resolution of the pain complex.

SECTION 9 ■ PEDIATRIC ORTHOPAEDICS

# Congenital Deficiencies of the Lower Extremity

## Conditions

Fibular deficiency (fibular hemimelia)
Tibial deficiency (tibial hemimelia)
Longitudinal deficiency of the femur, partial (proximal femoral focal deficiency)

## Definition

Congenital deficiencies of the lower extremity are obvious at birth, and their appearance can be alarming to parents. Support and counseling by the physician can be critical while the parents are attempting to understand their child's condition. Limb-length discrepancy is the primary functional disability. The discrepancy remains proportional, but the absolute amount increases as the child grows. Many patients will function best with an appropriate amputation. It should be emphasized to the parents that these patients can be quite functional with a prosthesis. Furthermore, many of these patients are otherwise healthy and this also can be emphasized to the parents.

Even though surgical treatment usually is not done until the child is 1 year of age or older, early referral to a specialist is helpful. This allows the surgeon time to gain the parents' trust, as the concept of amputation is not easy to accept in a small infant when the absolute discrepancy is small. Providing the parents with an opportunity to meet other affected children at a more advanced stage of growth and development also will be reassuring.

## Fibular Deficiency

Fibular deficiency, sometimes called fibular hemimelia or congenital absence of the fibula, is a sporadic disorder of unknown etiology. It is the most common long bone deficiency (**Figure 1**). Limb-length discrepancy is universal, ranging from 2 to 16 cm by skeletal maturity.

The deficiency often extends to the lateral border of the foot with associated defects, including absence of the lateral ray(s) of the foot, anomalous bony fusions of the tarsal bones, valgus alignment of the hindfoot, and equinus positioning of the ankle with a ball-and-socket-like ankle joint. Associated milder deformities may occur in the thigh with genu valgum secondary to hypoplasia of the lateral femoral condyle along with mild shortening of the femur.

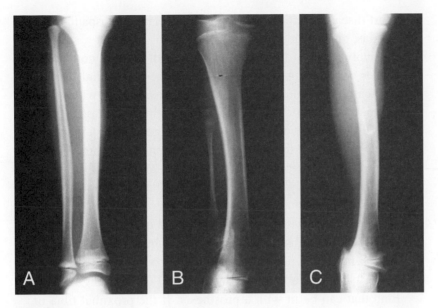

**Figure 1**

Radiographs demonstrate three types of fibular deficiency according to the Kalamchi classification. **A,** Type IA: minimal shortening of the fibula with a ball-and-socket ankle. **B,** Type IB: only partial fibula present. **C,** Type II: complete absence of the fibula.

Reproduced from Kasser JR (ed): *Orthopaedic Knowledge Update* 5. Rosemont, IL, American Academy of Orthopaedic Surgeons, 1996, pp 437-451.

The goal of treatment is a functional limb. The limb-length discrepancy will increase as the child grows, and the degree of anticipated final discrepancy, in combination with the stability of the hindfoot, will determine the surgical treatment. If the anticipated discrepancy is large (8 to 16 cm) and/or the hindfoot is unstable, disarticulation at the ankle and prosthetic fitting is recommended during the first 2 years of life. If the anticipated discrepancy is small and the hindfoot is stable, other modalities to equalize the leg lengths may be considered.

A situation to be avoided is when a patient undergoes multiple procedures to maintain a nonfunctional foot and equalize large limb-length discrepancies, only to find the leg must be amputated during adolescence. A careful assessment of hindfoot function and anticipated limb-length discrepancy at maturity can help avoid this scenario.

## TIBIAL DEFICIENCY

Tibial deficiency, also called tibial hemimelia or congenital absence of the tibia, is characterized by partial or complete absence of the tibia (**Figure 2**). This disorder may be sporadic or familial, with most inherited cases secondary to autosomal dominant transmission. Familial cases usually have bilateral involvement and upper extremity deficiencies. Other disorders that may be associated with tibial deficiency include congenital

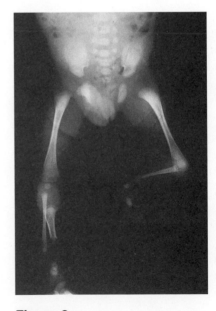

**Figure 2**

Radiograph of an infant with bilateral tibial deficiency. The patient's right lower limb has incomplete absence of the tibia; the left tibia is completely absent.

heart disease, cleft palate, imperforate anus, hypospadias, hernias, and gonadal malformations.

Involvement of the medial aspect of the foot is common with talipes equinovarus (clubfoot) and absence of medial ray(s). Ironically, tibial deficiency also can be associated with polydactyly. Shortening of the involved limb is present and, with unilateral involvement, the anticipated discrepancy is typically large (8 to 16 cm). Knee flexion contracture is found when the tibia is totally absent or if the quadriceps is deficient, and the fibula may appear as a bony projection lateral to the lateral femoral condyle.

Treatment is based on function of the quadriceps muscle and the presence or absence of a proximal tibia. If a proximal tibia is present and the quadriceps is functional, disarticulation at the ankle will provide the child with a good end-bearing residual limb that can be fit with a prosthesis. If the proximal tibia or quadriceps muscle is absent, knee disarticulation and fitting with an appropriate prosthesis will provide the best function. In both situations, the limb-length discrepancy can be made up by the length of the prosthesis. Of course the best function occurs when knee function can be salvaged, but even with the knee disarticulation, function is very satisfactory.

# Longitudinal Deficiency of the Femur, Partial

Longitudinal deficiency of the femur, partial (LDFP), also called proximal femoral focal deficiency (PFFD), is an uncommon, sporadic condition of unknown etiology characterized by dysgenesis of the proximal femur with coxa vara and/or pseudarthrosis of the femoral neck. Shortening of the femur is marked, and limb-length discrepancy at maturity ranges from 7 to 25 cm. Associated abnormalities are common and include hip dysplasia, hypoplasia of the lateral femoral condyle, knee instability with absent anterior cruciate ligament, and partial or complete fibular deficiency. Associated deficiencies in other organ systems are uncommon.

While several classification systems exist, the most simple (and perhaps useful) classification is that by Torode and Gillespie (**Figure 3**). Type A is a congenital short femur, in which the foot lies opposite the midpoint of the contralateral tibia when the limb is gently extended. Overall length discrepancy is less than 20%. In type B, the thigh is very short, with external rotation of the hip and flexion contractures of both the hip and knee, and the foot lies approximately at the level of the contralateral knee. The overall length discrepancy is about 40%. Type C is characterized by an extremely short

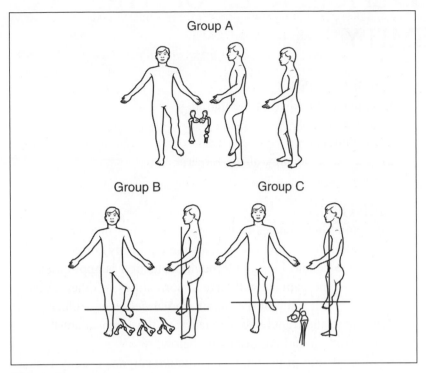

**Figure 3**

Classification of LDFP, or PFFD.

Adapted from Gillespie R: Classification of congenital abnormalities of the femur, in Herring JA, Birch JG (eds): *The Child with a Limb Deficiency*. Rosemont, IL, American Academy of Orthopaedic Surgeons, 1998, p 69.

femur with pistoning and instability of the hip joint. The foot lies well proximal to the opposite knee.

Patients with type A deficiency can be treated with a limb equalization procedure (limb lengthening, contralateral epiphysiodesis, or both). Types B and C usually require some form of amputation and prosthetic fitting because of the expected severe limb-length discrepancy at maturity. Depending on the severity of the hip abnormality, some form of reconstruction also may be necessary. However, in almost all cases, the child will be able to walk, even if the femoral head and acetabulum are completely absent.

SECTION 9 ■ PEDIATRIC ORTHOPAEDICS

# Congenital Deficiencies of the Upper Extremity

## Conditions

Hypoplasia/Absence of the thumb
Radial deficiency
Ulnar deficiency
Transverse deficiency of the forearm

## Definition

Congential deficiencies of the upper extremity may be either longitudinal (affecting one side of the extremity) or complete transverse deficiencies. A thorough evaluation is appropriate because some patients will have abnormalities in other organ systems. Deficiency of the thumb, radial deficiency, ulnar deficiency, and transverse deficiency of the forearm are the most common and are discussed below.

As a general principle, reconstructive surgery usually is not performed before the infant is 6 to 18 months of age; however, early specialty evaluation is helpful to allay anxiety of the parents and grandparents. Furthermore, early consultation allows time for parents to gain an understanding and realistic expectations of the expected function and appearance after surgical treatment. Finally, some of these disorders will not benefit from surgical treatment, but early discussion concerning principles of prosthetic management will be helpful.

## Hypoplasia/Absence of the Thumb

The extent of the deficiency is variable. A hypoplastic thumb may be small, unstable, or thin due to deficient development of the thenar musculature. Other disorders are common, including congenital heart disease (Holt-Oram syndrome), craniofacial abnormalities, and vertebral anomalies (VATER association). Fanconi anemia also can develop in later childhood.

If untreated, patients adapt by using the pinch function between the index and long fingers to substitute for the deficient thumb. Patients with unilateral involvement (eg, a normal opposite upper extremity) generally have excellent overall function with minimal impairment.

Surgical management is based on the magnitude of the deficiency. Reconstruction is indicated when the hypoplastic thumb is of adequate size and the carpometacarpal joint is stable. Index pollicization (transfer of the index finger to the thumb position, leaving the hand with three fingers) is recommended for more severe deformities.

# RADIAL DEFICIENCY

Radial deficiency, sometimes called radial hemimelia or radial clubhand, is characterized by radial deviation of the hand; variable presence and stiffness of the thumb, index, and long fingers; variable shortening and bowing of the forearm segment; and variable range of motion at the elbow. Associated disorders include congenital heart disease (Holt-Oram syndrome), craniofacial abnormalities, and vertebral anomalies (VATER association). TAR syndrome (thrombocytopenia with absent radius) also is possible. The unique aspect of TAR syndrome is the presence of an essentially normal thumb. In other syndromes, if the radius is deficient, then the thumb also is hypoplastic or absent.

Surgical management is designed to improve the alignment and appearance of the hand relative to the forearm. A centralization procedure ideally is performed between 6 and 18 months of age. Untreated patients can still function surprisingly well. Therefore, surgical treatment is contraindicated in patients with short forearms and/or limited elbow motion. These patients do better if the hand remains closer to the midline (eg, radially deviated).

# ULNAR DEFICIENCY

Ulnar deficiencies include a variety of disorders involving either a partial or complete absence of skeletal and soft-tissue elements on the ulnar (postaxial) border of the forearm and hand. Conditions range from hypoplasia of the ulna, in which the ulna is completely present but short, to total aplasia of the ulna, which may be associated with congenital fusion of the radius to the humerus (radiohumeral synostosis). Digital deficiencies are common and variable.

Compared with radial and thumb deficiencies, ulnar deficiencies are not associated with anomalies of other organ systems. However, patients with ulnar deficiencies are more likely to have disorders elsewhere in the skeletal system, including tibial deficiency and longitudinal deficiency of the femur, partial (also called proximal femoral focal deficiency).

Surgical treatment is not commonly indicated for ulnar deficiency, except for associated digital deformities. Syndactyly release, web space reconstruction, and other procedures, when indicated, can improve hand function.

SECTION 9 ■ PEDIATRIC ORTHOPAEDICS

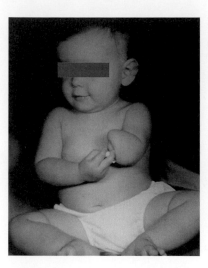

**Figure 1**

Infant with unilateral transverse deficiency of the forearm already using affected limb to assist the uninvolved extremity.

# Transverse Deficiency of the Forearm

Transverse deficiency of the forearm, sometimes called congenital below-elbow amputation, is characterized by complete absence of the hand and wrist and a hypoplastic or partially absent forearm. Elbow function is good, even if the radial head is dislocated. This disorder is sporadic, typically unilateral, and generally is not associated with abnormalities in other organ systems, although patients may have congenital constriction band syndrome and other musculoskeletal anomalies.

Children with unilateral transverse deficiency of the forearm have minimal functional limitations. Bimanual activities are often performed using the medial aspect of the affected forearm to assist the opposite, uninvolved extremity (**Figure 1**). The principal deficit is cosmetic, which is particularly troublesome during the teenage years.

Surgical treatment is rarely necessary. Primitive digital remnants, if present, occasionally are removed for cosmetic reasons.

Prosthetic management is of great interest to families of infants with this condition. The best time to introduce the prosthesis is controversial, though many centers favor an aggressive "fit when they sit" protocol. This approach is based on the developmental principle that normal bimanual activities begin when an infant is able to sit independently, at about age 6 to 8 months. Others recognize that a prosthesis often impedes an infant's ability to crawl and favor the first fitting after an infant is able to stand and walk independently.

Prosthetic options include the standard body-powered design, consisting of a shoulder harness and a hook terminal device; a myoelectric design, consisting of a mechanical hand that is opened and closed by voluntary forearm muscle activity; and a passive design, consisting of a lightweight, durable, cosmetically appealing, nonmovable hand. The optimal design is based on a number of factors and is best determined on an individual basis.

The principal benefit of prosthetic management is cosmetic, which may be more significant to the parents than the child prior to the teenage years. Function is not consistently improved by any of the prosthetic designs, leading to a high rate of prosthetic rejection.

# CONGENITAL DEFORMITIES OF THE LOWER EXTREMITY

## CONDITIONS

Coxa vara
Congenital dislocation of the knee
Congenital dislocation of the patella
Posteromedial bowing of the tibia
Anterolateral bowing of the tibia
Calcaneovalgus foot
Congenital vertical talus
Congenital short first metatarsal
Congenital curly toe
Polydactyly

## DEFINITION

These conditions are, by definition, present at birth; however, some disorders, such as congenital dislocation of the patella, may not be apparent until the child is older.

## CLINICAL SYMPTOMS

For most of these conditions, pain is not present during infancy and early childhood.

## TESTS

### Physical Examination

Deviations from normal evoke suspicion, although there is a range of normal. The lower extremities of a newborn have been compressed in the uterus. Therefore, a hip flexion contracture of 40° to 60° and a knee flexion contracture of 20° to 30° are normal in newborns. Likewise, in utero, the ankles and feet are pressed into a dorsiflexed position; therefore, calcaneovalgus posture of the foot is normal.

Disproportionate shortening of the upper and lower extremities or spine suggests a generalized skeletal dysplasia. Other organ systems should be evaluated to rule out other genetic and chromosomal disorders.

### Diagnostic Tests

AP and lateral radiographs of the affected extremity are standard.

## COXA VARA

This condition is a relatively uncommon hip disorder characterized by a decrease in the normal neck-shaft angle of

| ICD-9 Codes | |
|---|---|
| **754.41** | Congenital dislocation of the knee |
| **754.43** | Anterolateral bowing of the tibia |
| **754.43** | Posteromedial bowing of the tibia |
| **754.44** | Congenital dislocation of the patella |
| **754.61** | Congenital vertical talus |
| **754.62** | Calcaneovalgus foot |
| **755.02** | Polydactyly of toes |
| **755.38** | Congenital short first metatarsal |
| **755.60** | Congenital deformities of the lower extremity |
| **755.62** | Coxa vara |

SECTION 9 ■ PEDIATRIC ORTHOPAEDICS

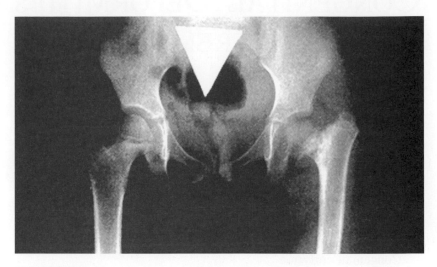

**Figure 1**

Pelvic radiograph demonstrating congenital coxa vara in a 5-year-old child.

Reproduced from Kasser JR (ed): *Orthopaedic Knowledge Update* 5. Rosemont, IL, American Academy of Orthopaedic Surgeons, 1996, p 353.

the femur (**Figure 1**). The types of coxa vara are congenital, acquired, and developmental. Congenital coxa vara is associated with congenital short femur and proximal femoral focal deficiency. Acquired coxa vara is secondary to metabolic or traumatic conditions. Developmental coxa vara is an idiopathic condition that develops in early childhood.

The bony deformity alters the mechanics of the hip and causes abductor muscle weakness, a Trendelenburg gait abnormality, and, if unilateral, a limb-length discrepancy. Untreated, the deformity and gait abnormality progress. A realignment osteotomy can improve hip function.

# CONGENITAL DISLOCATION OF THE KNEE

This condition presents as hyperextension of the knee at birth, which ranges from a mild positional deformity that readily responds to short-term splinting to a frank dislocation of the tibia on the femur that is complicated and difficult to treat (**Figure 2**). Associated abnormalities such as hip dislocation or clubfoot are common in patients with true subluxation or dislocation of the knee.

# CONGENITAL DISLOCATION OF THE PATELLA

Congenital dislocation of the patella may not be apparent for several months after birth. Persistent flexion contracture of the knee and external rotation of the leg are suggestive of the diagnosis. The patella may not be palpable in its dislocated

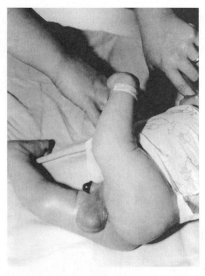

**Figure 2**

Clinical photograph of a newborn with bilateral congenital dislocation of the knees. The patient also had associated bilateral dislocated hips and a left clubfoot.

lateral position. Ultrasound is helpful in confirming the diagnosis in a younger child whose patella has not started to ossify. Surgical treatment is necessary and is more complicated than what is required for adolescents and adults with recurrent dislocation of the patella.

# POSTEROMEDIAL BOWING OF THE TIBIA

This idiopathic deformity is most obvious and rather striking at birth (**Figure 3**). Posteromedial bowing of the tibia causes the neonate's foot to be in apparent dorsiflexion and valgus, and the deformity initially can be misclassified as a calcaneovalgus foot. The affected limb also is short. The bowing improves with growth, and realignment osteotomy is rarely necessary. A variable degree of limb-length discrepancy persists and typically requires a shoe lift and possibly contralateral epiphysiodesis.

# ANTEROLATERAL BOWING OF THE TIBIA

This condition might or might not be apparent at birth and is often associated with neurofibromatosis (**Figure 4**). Anterolateral bowing of the tibia often progresses to congenital pseudarthrosis of the tibia, a condition that results in an unstable extremity, requires complicated operations and even then has a high failure rate. Infants with anterolateral bowing of the tibia need bracing to prevent, if possible, progression to pseudarthrosis.

SECTION 9 ■ PEDIATRIC ORTHOPAEDICS

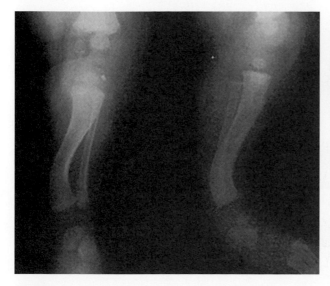

**Figure 3**

Radiograph of infant with congenital posteromedial bow of the tibia.

Reproduced from Kasser JR (ed): *Orthopaedic Knowledge Update* 5. Rosemont, IL, American Academy of Orthopaedic Surgeons, 1996, p 441.

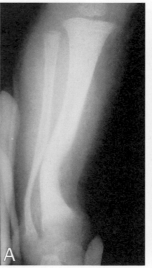
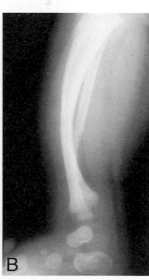

**Figure 4**

AP (**A**) and lateral (**B**) radiographs showing anterolateral bowing of the tibia.

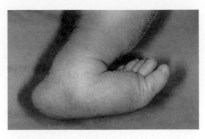

**Figure 5**

Clinical photograph of a calcaneovalgus foot in a neonate.

# CALCANEOVALGUS FOOT

This condition is common in neonates and is characterized by marked dorsiflexion of the ankle such that the foot may be pressed against the tibia (**Figure 5**). Examination should include an evaluation for deficient activity of the plantar flexors from lipomyelomeningocele or some other neurologic condition. If the child has no neuromuscular disorder, spontaneous correction without sequelae is expected.

# CONGENITAL VERTICAL TALUS

This rigid flatfoot deformity might or might not be recognized at birth (**Figure 6**). The condition may be idiopathic, familial, or associated with a neuromuscular or chromosomal abnormality. Most patients do not respond to serial casting and require surgical treatment.

# CONGENITAL SHORT FIRST METATARSAL

Shortening of the great toe is obvious and is often associated with hallux varus. If the great toe is deviated, problems with shoe wear develop. Strapping is ineffective, and surgical treatment is required.

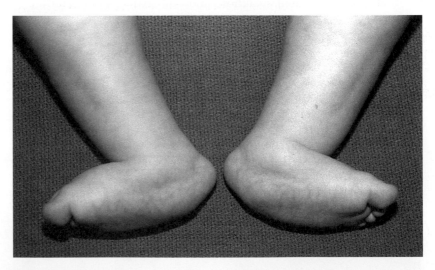

**Figure 6**

Clinical photograph of the feet of a 9-month-old infant with bilateral congenital vertical talus.

Reproduced from Kasser JR (ed): *Orthopaedic Knowledge Update* 5. Rosemont, IL, American Academy of Orthopaedic Surgeons, 1996, p 507.

## CONGENITAL CURLY TOE

This idiopathic condition is characterized by flexion and medial rotation of the toe. Most children are asymptomatic. Strapping is ineffective. If problems develop with shoe wear, surgical treatment of the toe flexors is often successful.

## POLYDACTYLY

The presence of accessory toes often causes trouble with shoe wear (**Figure 7**). Deletion is best performed around 10 months of age, a time when anesthetic problems are less but before the child begins to walk. An earlier consultation often helps the parents understand the treatment and the rationale for timing of surgery.

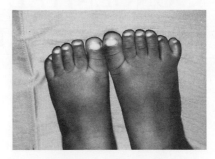

**Figure 7**
Clinical photograph of the feet of a child with postaxial polydactyly of the right foot.

SECTION 9 ■ PEDIATRIC ORTHOPAEDICS

# CONGENITAL DEFORMITIES OF THE UPPER EXTREMITY

**ICD-9 Codes**

**755.01**
Polydactyly of fingers

**755.11**
Syndactyly of fingers without fusion of bone

**755.50**
Congenital dislocation of the radial head

**755.53**
Congenital radial-ulnar synostosis

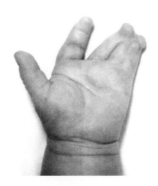

**Figure 1**
Clinical photograph of the hand of a child with complex syndactyly of the ulnar three fingers. Note how the long finger is pulled toward the shorter ring and little fingers.

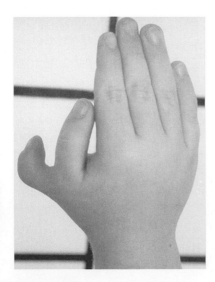

**Figure 2**
Clinical photograph of the hand of a child with polydactyly expressed as a duplicated thumb.

## CONDITIONS

Syndactyly
Polydactyly
Congenital radioulnar synostosis
Congenital dislocation of the radial head

## DEFINITION

Congenital deformities are, by definition, present at birth. Syndactyly and polydactyly are obvious; however, congenital dislocation of the radial head and congenital radioulnar synostosis usually are not identified until the child is 3 to 10 years of age.

## SYNDACTYLY

Syndactyly is a condition characterized by the lack of normal separation between fingers or toes (**Figure 1**). It can vary from a thin web of skin to a bony fusion (synostosis) between the phalanges. In complete syndactyly, the digits are joined to the tips. In partial syndactyly, there can be increased webbing at the base of the digits or webbing to just short of the tips. Other malformations occur in about 5% of patients.

Because the fingers differ in length, growth may cause progressive deviation of the conjoined fingers. Use of the digits is limited, and cosmesis is an issue for patients. Therefore, children with hand syndactyly should be assessed for surgical treatment. In most cases, a skin graft will be needed. The growth differential of syndactyly of the toes is less significant, and function is rarely limited. Therefore, correction of syndactyly of the toes often is not required.

## POLYDACTYLY

Polydactyly is the presence of extra digits in the hand or foot, usually adjacent to the thumb or great toe (preaxial) or lateral to the little finger (postaxial) (**Figure 2**). Extra digits can vary in appearance from a vestigial digit attached by a narrow bridge of skin to a normal-appearing digit with its own metacarpal/metatarsal. Radiographs usually are not needed for diagnostic purposes, only for prognosis and planning surgical treatment.

Polydactyly of the hand may not cause functional difficulties, but it is a significant cosmetic deformity. Accessory digits of the foot frequently cause difficulty in shoe wear. Vestigial digits can be ablated by application of a circumferential suture at the base of the skin bridge. Otherwise, removal of extra digits should be delayed until the child is 9 to 10 months of age, a time when anesthesia problems are less but before the child will be psychologically affected by the operation. Early consultation often helps the parents understand the treatment. Surgical deletion may be performed earlier if the extra digit interferes with function or if the parents have significant concerns.

# CONGENITAL RADIOULNAR SYNOSTOSIS

In congenital radioulnar synostosis, the proximal ends of the radius and ulna fail to separate, resulting in an inability to pronate and supinate the forearm. Children substitute shoulder motion to place the hand in a pronated or supinated position. When the condition is unilateral, there are fewer symptoms because the normal opposite extremity can be used for many activities. This abnormality often is not detected until children are old enough to start using their hands in a purposeful manner.

Limited pronation and supination of the forearm can be readily detected, even during examination of the newborn. Because many young children have lax wrist ligaments, the distal end of the radius and ulna, not the hand, should be grasped and gently pronated and supinated to assess forearm rotation.

After ossification occurs, radiographs demonstrate bony union of the proximal radius and ulna (**Figure 3**).

No treatment is needed if the forearm is in a satisfactory position. Patients with bilateral involvement are more likely to have functional limitations. Surgery to divide the synostosis and restore motion has not been successful in most series. Surgical treatment usually is reserved for patients with disability secondary to a forearm positioned in either extreme pronation

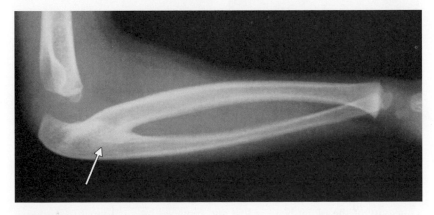

**Figure 3**
Radiograph demonstrating radioulnar synostosis. Fusion of the proximal radius and ulna is apparent (arrow).

or supination. Osteotomy to realign the forearm can improve function. This procedure usually is not done until the child is at least age 4 years and may be delayed until the adolescent or adult years if the degree of disability is questionable.

# CONGENITAL DISLOCATION OF THE RADIAL HEAD

Congenital dislocation of the radial head can occur in several directions but most commonly develops posteriorly and typically is bilateral. Elbow deformity and limited motion are the presenting symptoms, but these may not be noticed by the parents for several years. Occasionally, children report pain.

Examination reveals that elbow motion is limited. Rotation is often more limited than flexion and extension. The dislocated radial head often presents as a palpable prominence on the lateral side of the elbow.

Radiographs of the elbow demonstrate the dislocation. The radial head is dome shaped (convex) instead of its normal concave appearance (**Figure 4**).

The deformity and limited elbow motion associated with this condition are often well tolerated. Attempts at open reduction in young children have met with little success. Excision of the radial head after growth is completed can be considered for pain relief but usually does not improve motion.

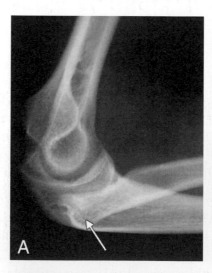
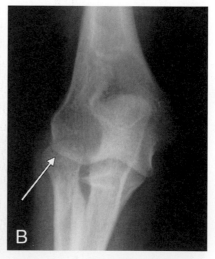

**Figure 4**
Radiographs demonstrating congenital dislocation of the radial head.
**A,** On the lateral view, the radial head is dislocated posteriorly and does not articulate with the humerus (arrow). **B,** On the AP view, the normal concavity of the radial head is lost and replaced by a convexity (arrow).

# Developmental Dysplasia of the Hip

## Synonyms

Congenital dysplasia of the hip
Congenital dislocation of the hip
Congenital subluxation of the hip

### ICD-9 Codes

**754.30**
Congenital dislocation of the hip, unilateral

**754.31**
Congenital dislocation of the hip, bilateral

## Definition

Developmental dysplasia of the hip (DDH) encompasses all dysplastic hip disorders, ranging from an in utero rigid dislocation to a typical perinatal hip dislocation to a hip dysplasia that develops during childhood from either extreme ligamentous laxity or from neuromuscular disorders such as cerebral palsy or myelomeningocele. The various nomenclatures previously used (eg, congenital dislocation of the hip, congenital dysplasia of the hip, congenital disease of the hip) were imprecise and confusing because some patients had a hip problem that was neither congenital nor dislocated.

Typical DDH is associated with ligamentous laxity and usually is detectable at birth. Common characteristics include prevalence in the left hip (3:1 ratio), female gender (5:1 ratio), and breech presentation (20% for frank breech presentation). DDH is rarely seen in blacks but is more common in whites of northern European ancestry, American Indians, and families with a history of DDH. Development of torticollis also is associated with DDH.

## Clinical Symptoms

Neonates are asymptomatic. Parents often notice a limp, a waddling gait pattern, or a limb-length discrepancy when the infant begins to walk.

## Tests

### Physical Examination

The physical examination is key to the early diagnosis. The examination should be done on a firm surface with the infant relaxed. Hip instability may not be detected if the infant is crying or upset.

Two maneuvers are helpful in detecting hip instability during the neonatal examination (**Figure 1**). The Barlow test should be performed first and is a "sign of exit" as the femoral head dislocates from the socket. To perform this test, flex the infant's hips and knees to 90°, then place your thumb along the medial

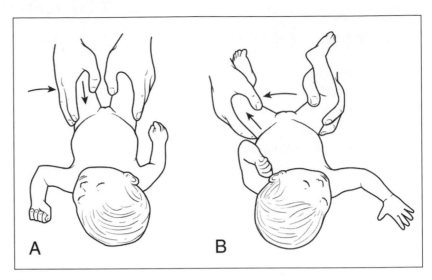

**Figure 1**
Barlow (**A**) and Ortolani (**B**) maneuvers.

thigh and the long finger along the lateral axis of the femur. Apply gentle pressure to the knee in a posterior direction while adducting the femur. A positive Barlow test is a "clunk," as the femoral head dislocates from the socket and slides over the posterior lip of the acetabulum.

The Ortolani maneuver is a "sign of relocation" as the femoral head is manipulated back into the acetabulum. To perform this maneuver, flex the hips and knees to 90° and position your hands similar to the Barlow maneuver. Abduct the hip while applying gentle pressure from your long finger over the greater trochanter and then pushing the femoral head anteriorly. A positive Ortolani sign is a "clunk" as the femoral head slides over the posterior lip of the acetabulum and into the socket.

In a neonate who has a dislocated hip, the adductors become contracted. As a result, in patients 1 to 3 months of age or older, the hip cannot be relocated by the Ortolani maneuver. The key to diagnosing DDH at this age is recognizing limited hip abduction. In infants, this is most easily detected by flexing the hips and knees to 90° and maximally abducting both hips. Asymmetric abduction suggests unilateral DDH. A unilateral dislocation also is indicated by shortening of the thigh, or a positive Galeazzi sign (unequal knee heights with the hips and knees flexed to 90°). Bilateral DDH is not as obvious. Thigh lengths are equal, and abduction is symmetric. Bilateral DDH is suggested by hip abduction limited to less than 45°.

## Diagnostic Tests
Because a neonate's femoral head is cartilaginous, radiographs of the hip can be difficult to interpret at this time. Radiographs are more accurate in detecting bony changes in the femoral

head and acetabulum in infants who are 4 to 8 months old. In most neonates, the physical examination is sufficient to make the diagnosis and initiate treatment.

Ultrasound can provide information concerning whether the hip joint is unstable or dislocated and is particularly useful before the femoral head has ossified (**Figure 2**). There is a debate about whether ultrasound screening of newborns should be selective or universal. Currently, most physicians are selectively screening infants and recommend an ultrasound only if the infant is at increased risk for DDH or has an equivocal examination.

## DIFFERENTIAL DIAGNOSIS

Cerebral palsy (mild spastic diplegia with tightness of adductors)

Congenital coxa vara (decreased abduction associated with decreased femoral neck-shaft angle)

Congenital short femur (limb-length discrepancy)

Fracture of the femur (limited motion associated with pain and swelling)

## ADVERSE OUTCOMES OF THE DISEASE

The longer the hip is dislocated, the less likely that closed reduction will be successful. If left untreated, DDH can lead to premature degenerative joint disease (osteoarthritis), causing pain and limited function.

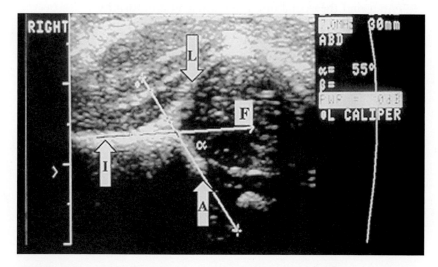

**Figure 2**
Ultrasound of neonatal hip and measurements used to determine unstable hip. I = ilium; L = labrum; A = acetabulum; F = femoral head.

SECTION 9 ■ PEDIATRIC ORTHOPAEDICS

# Treatment

Treatment depends on the magnitude of the problem and the age of the patient. The goal of treatment is to concentrically reduce the femoral head into the socket and maintain the reduction while the acetabulum develops and the hip stabilizes. If DDH is detected within the first 3 months, most hips will reduce and stabilize with a dynamic positioning device, such as a Pavlik harness. The harness holds the hips in flexion and abduction, allowing the femoral head to reduce concentrically into the acetabulum. Consistent, full-time wearing of the brace is necessary for the child with an unstable joint to develop a stable hip joint.

The Pavlik harness is less successful if the DDH is detected in an infant between 3 and 9 months of age. At this age, an orthosis may be tried for 2 to 3 weeks to see if the femoral head will reduce into the acetabulum. If it does not, the harness should be abandoned because the brace will aggravate the deformity if the femoral head remains dislocated. For older infants, an examination under anesthesia, arthrogram, and either closed or open reduction with application of a spica cast are necessary.

# Adverse Outcomes of Treatment

Failure of reduction of the femoral head into the socket, persistent hip instability, and osteonecrosis of the femoral head are serious complications associated with treatment. Osteonecrosis can interfere with the growth of the proximal femur and the acetabulum, resulting in a deformity.

# Referral Decisions/Red Flags

An infant who has suspected instability or dislocation requires specialty evaluation.

# DISKITIS

**ICD-9 Codes**

**722.92**
Thoracic diskitis

**722.93**
Lumbar diskitis

## DEFINITION

Diskitis is an infection that occurs in or around the intervertebral disk and, in children, is most often a bacterial infection of hematogenous origin. MRI consistently shows inflammation at the anterior corner of one or both adjacent vertebrae (**Figure 1**). These findings, together with the results of microvascular studies, support the concept that diskitis begins as a foci of osteomyelitis in the anterior metaphyseal corner of one vertebra and subsequently spreads to the adjacent disk. Diskitis can occur anywhere in the spine, but it most commonly affects the low thoracic and lumbar regions. Children between ages 2 and 7 years are most commonly affected, and in this age group, diskitis often can be treated with oral antibiotics. Diskitis can develop in young adolescents as well, and in this age group the causative organisms and treatment requirements are similar to those of adults.

## CLINICAL SYMPTOMS

Onset of symptoms is insidious, and delay in diagnosis is usual. Children who are able to communicate may be able to localize the pain to the back, but they also may perceive their pain as abdominal or thigh discomfort. Toddlers are frequently first seen when they refuse to walk. Therefore, the differential diagnosis must include not only spinal disorders, but abdominal, pelvic, and lower extremity processes as well.

## TESTS

### Physical Examination

Children rarely appear systemically ill. Fever, if present, may be low grade. Toddlers may refuse to walk or even sit unsupported. Those who will walk often lean forward and place their hands on their thighs for support (psoas sign). Percussion of the spinous processes may help localize the pain. Passive spinal motion is resisted. If both lower extremities are elevated simultaneously, the back and hips are held rigid. The single straight-leg raising test also may be positive.

### Diagnostic Tests

White blood cell count is often within normal limits, but the erythrocyte sedimentation rate and C-reactive protein usually are elevated. Blood cultures may be positive.

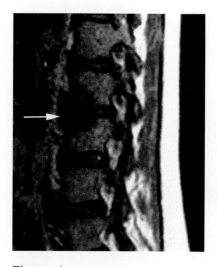

**Figure 1**
T1-weighted MRI scan showing the characteristic signal changes of diskitis at L2-3.

SECTION 9 ■ PEDIATRIC ORTHOPAEDICS

AP and lateral radiographs of the spine should be obtained as part of the initial assessment. However, irregularity of the vertebral end plates and narrowing of the disk usually are not apparent until 2 or 3 weeks after onset of symptoms.

MRI will confirm the diagnosis and clearly define the extent of the process. A bone scan is usually, but not always, positive early in the disease and may be of value when localization is unclear.

Because of the low yield and necessity for general anesthesia, aspiration of the disk usually is not recommended in young children who have a typical clinical picture.

A tuberculin skin test should be performed, unless done recently.

## Differential Diagnosis

Epidural abscess (rare, neurologic symptoms)

Herniated disk (teenagers, radicular symptoms)

Pyelonephritis (flank pain, pyuria)

Retrocecal appendicitis (systemic symptoms, pain with hip extension)

Retroperitoneal mass (may require MRI to differentiate)

Septic arthritis of the hip (marked pain on movement of the hip)

Spinal tuberculosis (spares the disk, involves bone, usually thoracolumbar area)

Spine tumor (neurologic abnormalities, may require MRI to differentiate)

## Adverse Outcomes of the Disease

Even though persistent disk space narrowing is common and may progress to spontaneous fusion of the adjacent vertebrae, residual problems are rare unless chronic osteomyelitis occurs.

## Treatment

Because *Staphylococcus aureus* is the most common organism identified, a penicillinase-resistant antibiotic or cephalosporin usually is used. A common regimen consists of 2 to 4 days of intravenous administration, followed by 4 to 6 weeks of oral antibiotics.

Initial bed rest should be followed by a gradual return to activities, as symptoms permit. With the routine use of antibiotics, immobilization in a body cast or brace is required less frequently but can be quite successful in reducing severe or recalcitrant pain. Physical therapy programs are not recommended.

Surgical débridement is almost never necessary.

## Adverse Outcomes of Treatment

Antibiotic allergies or secondary gastrointestinal problems can develop.

## Referral Decisions/Red Flags

Persistent fever, vertebral osteomyelitis and/or collapse, diagnostic dilemma, presence of a psoas abscess, and any neurologic deficit or suspicion of epidural abscess indicate the need for further evaluation.

Section 9 ■ Pediatric Orthopaedics

# EVALUATION OF THE LIMPING CHILD

## DEFINITION

Many conditions cause a child to limp. Establishing the correct diagnosis can be challenging because the possibilities are extensive and include various diseases and injuries, as well as various anatomic sites, ranging from the spine to the foot (**Table 1**). In addition, the history is often vague, the complaints nonfocal, and the examination unremarkable despite diagnostic possibilities that carry significant implications.

## CLINICAL SYMPTOMS

### *Is the problem acute or chronic?*

A recent onset of limping makes infectious or traumatic conditions more likely, although trauma is not as common as might be expected. Young children often fall, and parents tend to attribute one of these episodes as the cause of the limp. Therefore, the history should begin by asking the parents how long they have noticed the limp rather than what caused the child to limp. Unless an infection or other serious process is suspected, problems of short duration may be observed, but chronic problems need further evaluation with laboratory and radiographic studies.

### *What time of the day is the limp worst?*

Most musculoskeletal conditions are exacerbated by activity and relieved by rest. Therefore, parents often report that the pain or limp is worst in the afternoon. However, with transient synovitis of the hip or juvenile rheumatoid arthritis, the limp is more pronounced in the morning. Pain at night suggests leukemia or other neoplasms.

### *Are there systemic symptoms?*

Questions about malaise, swelling, fever, and loss of endurance are important, even with an acute onset. With chronic symptoms, the review of systems should be more extensive.

## TESTS

### *Physical Examination*

Ask older children to place one finger on "the one spot that hurts the most" to localize the anatomic site and narrow the differential diagnosis. Palpate the spine and lower extremities of younger children to identify areas of tenderness. Inspect the spine and lower extremities for swelling or skin changes.

**Table 1  Causes of Limping in Children**

| | With Trauma | With Fever or Systemic Illness | Without Trauma, Fever, or Systemic Illness |
|---|---|---|---|
| **Bones** | Fracture | Osteomyelitis | Benign bone tumor |
| | Child abuse fracture | Hemoglobinopathy | Aneurysmal bone cyst |
| | Stress fracture | Hand-foot syndrome | Unicameral bone cyst |
| | Periostitis | Sickle cell crises | Osteoid osteoma |
| | | Gaucher crises | Fibrous dysplasia |
| | | Neuroblastoma | Langerhans cell histiocytosis |
| | | Leukemia | Ewing sarcoma |
| | | Ewing sarcoma | Limb-length discrepancy |
| | | | Malignant bone tumor |
| | | | Osteogenic sarcoma |
| | | | Unicameral bone cyst |
| **Joints** | Sprain | Septic arthritis | Juvenile rheumatoid arthritis |
| | Dislocation | Lyme arthritis | Pauciarticular |
| | Hemarthrosis | Systemic juvenile rheumatoid arthritis | Polyarticular |
| | | Systemic lupus erythematosus | Hemophilic arthropathy |
| | | Other collagen vascular disease | Pigmented villonodular synovitis |
| | | Reactive arthritis/arthralgia | |
| | | Acute rheumatic fever | |
| | | Sarcoidosis | |
| | | Sickle cell disease | |
| | | Leukemia | |
| **Soft tissue** | Bursitis | Abscess | Charcot-Marie-Tooth disease |
| | Contusion | Cellulitis | Diastematomyelia |
| | Enthesitis | Dermatomyositis/polymyositis | Muscular dystrophy |
| | Muscle strain | | Overuse syndrome |
| | Nerve injury | Spider/insect bite | Rhabdomyosarcoma |
| | | Trichinosis | Spinal cord tumor |
| | | Viral myositis | |

## Table 1  Causes of Limping in Children (Continued)

| | With Trauma | With Fever or Systemic Illness | Without Trauma, Fever, or Systemic Illness |
|---|---|---|---|
| **Spine and pelvis** | Avulsion fracture vertebra | Diskitis | Spondylolysis/spondylolisthesis |
| | Disk herniation | Osteomyelitis–pelvis | Disk herniation |
| | | Sacroiliac septic arthritis | |
| | | Ankylosing spondylitis | |
| **Hip** | Avulsion fracture | Septic arthritis–hip | Developmental dysplasia of the hip |
| | Anterior superior iliac spine–sartorius | Osteomyelitis–proximal femur | Transient synovitis |
| | Anterior inferior iliac spine–rectus femoris | | Legg-Calvé-Perthes disease |
| | Slipped capital femoral epiphysis, acute | | Slipped capital femoral epiphysis, chronic |
| **Knee** | Avulsion fracture–patella | Septic arthritis–knee | Popliteal cyst |
| | Toddler's fracture of the tibia | Osteomyelitis adjacent bone | Discoid meniscus |
| | Referred hip pain | | Meniscal tear |
| | | | Osgood-Schlatter disease |
| | | | Sinding-Larsen-Johansson disease |
| | | | Osteochondritis dissecans |
| | | | Patella instability |
| **Foot and ankle** | Toddler's fracture of the tibia | Septic arthritis–ankle | Accessory navicular |
| | Stress fracture–foot | Puncture wound | Freiberg infraction |
| | Puncture wound–foot | Osteomyelitis | Köhler disease |
| | | Foreign body | Sever apophysitis |
| | | | Tarsal coalition |

Muscle weakness or atrophy is a sentinel sign of a significant process. In a young child, these findings are best determined by measuring and comparing limb girths at symmetric locations. For example, asymmetry in thigh girth of 1 cm or more measured 6 to 8 cm above the patella indicates a significant knee problem that requires additional laboratory and radiographic studies.

## Diagnostic Tests

A temperature of 100.4°F (38°C) or higher suggests an inflammatory or neoplastic process and the need for additional studies, such as a CBC, erythrocyte sedimentation rate, and appropriate radiographs. AP and lateral radiographs are indicated when a fracture or a chronic process is suspected. Different diagnostic possibilities dictate special views. For example, a tunnel view is indicated to rule out osteochondritis dissecans in an older child who has been limping and had knee pain for several weeks after sports activity. A bone scan often localizes the site of disease in patients with a limp that cannot be diagnosed by routine studies. However, this test is not always positive, even with a chronic process. For example, leukemia may cause increased, decreased, or even normal uptake on bone scans. CT is generally best for benign bony lesions. MRI provides better information on soft-tissue lesions and sarcomas; however, before proceeding to these tests, consult with an appropriate specialist to avoid ordering expensive studies that provide limited information.

SECTION 9 ■ PEDIATRIC ORTHOPAEDICS

# FLATFOOT

**ICD-9 Codes**
**734.0**
Pes planus (acquired)
**754.61**
Congenital pes planus

## SYNONYMS

Flexible flatfoot
Peroneal spastic flatfoot
Pes planus
Pronated foot
Valgus foot

## DEFINITION

Flatfoot is defined as an abnormally low or absent longitudinal arch. Flexible flatfoot is more common and is considered a normal foot shape in infants and in up to 20% of adults. Rigid flatfoot is an uncommon condition that is discussed in greater detail in the chapter on tarsal coalition.

Flexible flatfoot in children is always bilateral. These patients have a visible arch when they are not standing and have normal mobility of the subtalar joint (inversion and eversion of the hindfoot). Rigid flatfoot may be unilateral or bilateral. These patients have persistent flattening of the longitudinal arch in non–weight-bearing positions and have restricted subtalar motion.

Patients with neuromuscular conditions and underlying hypotonia and patients with pathologic ligamentous laxity (Marfan syndrome, Ehlers-Danlos syndrome, Down syndrome) may have a flatfoot that initially is flexible but with time may progress to a rigid deformity.

## CLINICAL SYMPTOMS

Flexible flatfoot usually is asymptomatic. Occasionally, however, children with flexible flatfeet report activity-related generalized pain and fatigue in the feet, ankles, and legs, as well as aching pain at night. Adolescents with flexible flatfeet often have an associated contracture of the Achilles tendon and may report focal pain and have redness and callosities under the bony prominence beneath the sagging arches.

## TESTS

### Physical Examination

The heel is in valgus alignment, which gives the medial malleolus a prominent appearance, and the foot is rotated outward in relation to the leg (**Figure 1**). With severe pes planovalgus, the medial border of the foot is convex, and the

# FRACTURES IN CHILDREN

Fractures are more common in children than in adults, due in part to their boisterous play and in part to the different characteristics of their bone. The strength of bone gradually increases as a child grows, but it is not until late adolescence that a child's bone is as strong as that of most adults. As a result, bone is the weak link in children, and ligamentous injuries are uncommon until late adolescence.

Fractures are uncommon in children younger than 3 years of age. Infants and young children usually are protected by their restrained activity, even though their bones are weaker. However, intentional abuse as a cause of fracture is significantly higher in young children, as described in the chapter on child abuse. After age 3 years, the incidence of fractures gradually increases until it peaks during adolescence. The incidence is also higher in boys and during the summer months.

Plasticity of bone, or the modulus of elasticity, is greater in children. Therefore, a child's bone can bend or deform without completely breaking. As a result, torus and greenstick fractures are common fracture patterns in children, but these injuries are rarely seen in adults.

Bone healing also is more rapid in children. For example, a fracture of the femur in an adult requires 16 to 20 weeks of immobilization if treated by closed means. By comparison, the same fracture requires only 2 weeks of immobilization in an infant and 4 to 6 weeks of casting in young children. Because of more rapid healing, nonunion is very uncommon in children.

Fractures involving the growth plate or physis are unique to children, accounting for 15% to 20% of all pediatric fractures. These injuries are described in a separate chapter.

Bone remodeling is greater in children, and some deformities will spontaneously correct. The potential for remodeling is greater in younger children, in fractures close to the physis, and in fractures angulated in the plane of motion. For example, a fracture of the distal radius with 35° of volar or dorsal angulation in a 5-year-old child will completely remodel in 1 to 2 years, even if no reduction is performed. In this instance, the primary reason for reduction is to relieve the pressure on adjacent soft tissues. Angular correction in other planes is less predictable, and rotational deformities typically do not correct.

Pediatric fractures present special problems in diagnosis and management. A fracture might not be visible on routine radiographs when it involves only the physis and when the secondary ossification center has not ossified. Young children are also less tolerant of major blood loss, and a child with a displaced femur fracture or multiple trauma needs to be monitored carefully.

The most common management of displaced fractures in children is closed reduction and casting, whereas displaced fractures in adults often require internal or external fixation devices. The thick periosteum in children helps in maintaining the reduction. Pediatric fractures also heal more rapidly, which reduces the duration of and complications associated with immobilization. Furthermore, unlike adults, complications of prolonged bed rest such as pneumonia and thrombophlebitis are very uncommon in children. Thus, body casts can be used to treat complex pediatric fractures involving the spine, pelvis, and lower extremities.

# FRACTURES OF THE GROWTH PLATE

## DEFINITION

Any fracture that involves the epiphyseal growth plate (the physis) is called a physeal fracture. The five-part Salter-Harris classification has been the system most commonly used to describe these injuries. However, there is concern that a Salter-Harris type V fracture does not occur and that this system does not describe all fracture patterns. Recently, a new classification system, the Peterson classification, was proposed that delineates six types and has sound anatomic, epidemiologic, and outcome associations (**Figure 1**). Fracture types progress from lesser to greater seriousness of injury, frequency of occurrence, and level of surgical intervention required.

## CLINICAL SYMPTOMS

Patients have acute pain, localized tenderness and swelling, and may have deformity and restricted motion of the involved site. There is always a history of trauma.

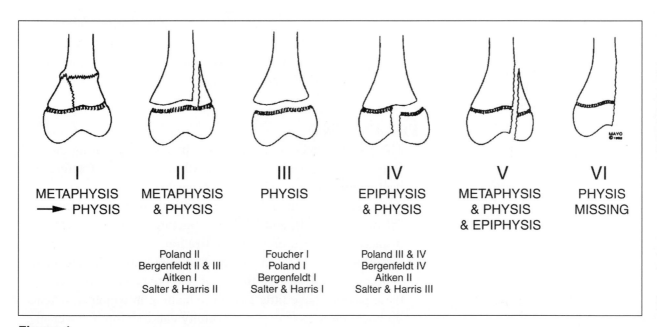

| I | II | III | IV | V | VI |
|---|---|---|---|---|---|
| METAPHYSIS → PHYSIS | METAPHYSIS & PHYSIS | PHYSIS | EPIPHYSIS & PHYSIS | METAPHYSIS & PHYSIS & EPIPHYSIS | PHYSIS MISSING |
| | Poland II Bergenfeldt II & III Aitken I Salter & Harris II | Foucher I Poland I Bergenfeldt I Salter & Harris I | Poland III & IV Bergenfeldt IV Aitken II Salter & Harris III | | |

**Figure 1**

Peterson classification of physeal injuries.

Reproduced with permission from Peterson HA: Physeal Fractures: Part 3. Classification. *J Pediatric Orthop* 1994:14:439-448.

# TESTS

## Physical Examination

Tenderness and swelling are localized and always present with maximum tenderness over the growth plate. Vascular and neurologic compromise are rare, as the fracture does not involve muscle compartments.

## Diagnostic Tests

AP and lateral radiographs usually identify the fracture. If not, oblique views will nearly always identify the fracture. Nondisplaced type III fractures show only soft-tissue swelling.

# DIFFERENTIAL DIAGNOSIS

Contusion (swelling and ecchymosis near a joint, negative radiographs)

Dislocation (evident on radiographs)

Fracture of the metaphysis of a long bone (radiographs show no involvement of the physis)

Osteochondral fracture (involves articular surface but not the physis)

Sprain (swelling, maximum tenderness over the ligament, and negative radiographs)

# ADVERSE OUTCOMES OF THE DISEASE

Premature growth arrest (partial or complete) will result in diminished bone length and angulation deformity. Nonunion and overgrowth are rare.

# TREATMENT

The goal is reduction, maintaining the reduction during the healing process, and avoiding growth arrest. These fractures heal rapidly, usually within 4 to 6 weeks.

Closed reduction and cast immobilization are indicated in fracture types I, II, and III. Some fractures will be minimally displaced and need only immobilization. In adolescents (over age 14 years in boys and 12 years in girls), mild displacement is acceptable because in the event that premature arrest occurs, these patients have little growth remaining in which significant limb-length discrepancy or deformity can develop. Conversely, in these same patients, less angular deformity can be accepted because there is less time for the fracture to remodel before the patient reaches skeletal maturity.

Fracture types IV and V involve the cartilage of both the growth plate and the articular surface. Therefore, anatomic reduction is required to ensure a congruous joint surface and to prevent development of a bone bridge (usually called a physeal bar) between the epiphysis and metaphysis. In most instances, open reduction and internal fixation is necessary to obtain and maintain reduction.

Fracture type VI is by definition always an open fracture; therefore, immediate surgical attention is necessary. Physeal bars always develop after this injury and, if the patient has significant growth remaining, reconstructive surgery will be required.

## ADVERSE OUTCOMES OF TREATMENT

Failure to recognize the fracture and its potential for growth arrest and failure to maintain anatomic reduction are the most common causes of a poor outcome. Physeal bars do not become evident for at least 3 months after fracture, and some not for many months. Follow-up of at least 1 year (unless the patient reaches skeletal maturity earlier) is mandatory. Longer follow-up is needed for physeal fractures of the femur, tibia, and the more complex injuries (types IV, V, and VI).

## REFERRAL DECISIONS/RED FLAGS

Displaced physeal fractures require reduction and maintenance of reduction. All type VI fractures, and many type IV and V fractures, require immediate surgery. All patients require long-term follow-up.

SECTION 9 ■ PEDIATRIC ORTHOPAEDICS

# FRACTURES ABOUT THE ELBOW

## ICD-9 Codes

**812.40**
Fractures of distal humeral physis

**812.41**
Supracondylar fracture, distal humerus

**812.42**
Lateral condyle fracture; lateral epicondyle fracture, distal humerus

**812.43**
Medial condyle fracture; medial epicondyle fracture, distal humerus

**813.01**
Olecranon fracture, proximal forearm

**813.06**
Radial neck fracture, proximal forearm

## DEFINITION

Fractures about the elbow are common in children. Injuries involving the distal humerus account for more than 80% of these fractures (**Table 1**).

Supracondylar fractures of the distal humerus are the most common elbow fractures in children, typically affecting children between the ages of 2 and 12 years. This fracture is above the physis. Most are extension fractures with the distal fragment displaced posteriorly (**Figure 1**).

The next most common injury is a fracture of the lateral condyle of the distal humerus. Fracture of the medial condyle is uncommon; however, whether on the lateral or medial side, condylar fractures are serious because the fracture typically involves the growth plate of the distal humerus and the articular surface of the elbow (**Figure 2**).

Fracture of the lateral epicondyle is uncommon. Fracture of the medial epicondyle is the third most common elbow fracture (**Figure 3**). The epicondyles are secondary ossification centers at sites of muscle origin. Fractures of the medial or lateral epicondyle do not involve the articular surface and do not adversely affect growth. Therefore, epicondyle fractures of the distal humerus, even when displaced, have limited consequences unless the elbow joint is concomitantly dislocated and the fragment is incarcerated into the joint.

Fractures across the entire physis of the distal humerus are uncommon. These injuries occur most frequently in infants and small children as a result of child abuse.

In children, the metaphyseal portion of the radial neck is the weak link. Therefore, the valgus force that causes a fracture of the radial head in adults will result in a fracture of the radial neck in children.

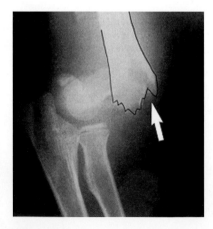

**Figure 1**

Radiograph of a displaced supracondylar fracture (humerus is outlined).

Reproduced from Sullivan JA, Anderson SJ (eds): *Care of the Young Athlete*, Rosemont, IL, American Academy of Orthopaedic Surgeons, 2000, p 317.

### Table 1   Types of Elbow Fractures in Children

| Distal Humerus | Proximal Forearm |
| --- | --- |
| Supracondylar | Radial neck |
| Lateral condyle | Olecranon |
| Medial condyle | |
| Lateral epicondyle | |
| Medial epicondyle | |
| Distal humeral physis | |

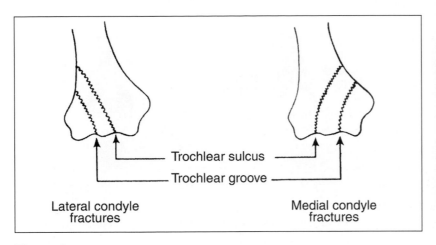

**Figure 2**

Typical fracture patterns of lateral and medial condyles of distal humerus in children.

Reproduced with permission from Milch H: Fractures and fracture-dislocations of the humeral condyles. *J Trauma* 1963;3:592–607.

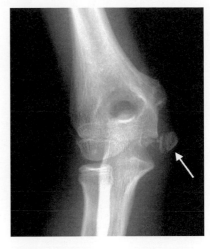

**Figure 3**

Radiograph demonstrating a displaced fracture of the medial epicondyle (arrow).

Olecranon fractures are uncommon in children. These injuries usually involve the articular surface and, when displaced, require an open or closed reduction.

# CLINICAL SYMPTOMS

Patients have acute pain, tenderness, swelling, and most often a history of falling on an outstretched arm. The child often refuses to use the limb and holds it at the side with the elbow flexed. Swelling can be severe, but with nondisplaced or minimally displaced fractures, swelling may be mild.

# TESTS

## Physical Examination

Evaluate the status of the median, ulnar, and radial nerves distal to the injury. Assess distal pulses and capillary filling. With obvious deformity, position or splint the limb in a position of comfort and order radiographs. In other children, attempt to find the site of maximum tenderness and gently evaluate elbow motion.

## Diagnostic Tests

AP and lateral radiographs of the elbow are necessary. The fracture may be obvious or subtle. Oblique views and comparison radiographs of the opposite elbow are helpful with subtle injuries. The radial head should be directed toward the distal humerus (capitellum) on both AP and lateral views.

An abnormal posterior fat pad sign is associated with fractures about the elbow, and the presence of this sign is

SECTION 9 ■ PEDIATRIC ORTHOPAEDICS

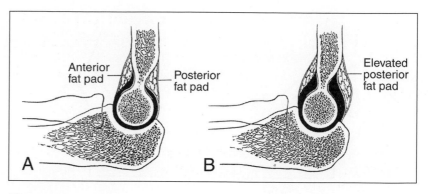

**Figure 4**

Normal anterior and posterior fat pads (**A**) and anterior and posterior fat pads elevated from an effusion (**B**).

Reproduced with permission from Skaggs DL, Mirzayan R: The posterior fat pad sign in association with occult fracture of the elbow in children. *J Bone Joint Surg Am* 1999;81:1429-1433.

particularly helpful with subtle or occult fractures. In a normal elbow, the anterior fat pad can be seen on a lateral radiograph, but the posterior fat pad is not visualized. Any process that causes an elbow effusion will elevate both anterior and posterior fat pads (**Figure 4**). The posterior fat pad is, therefore, often visible with elbow fractures in children, even when these injuries are not obvious on initial radiographs.

# DIFFERENTIAL DIAGNOSIS

Dislocation of the elbow (typically posterior, evident on radiographs)

Hemarthrosis of the elbow (swelling, limited motion, no other positive findings)

Monteggia fracture-dislocation (fracture of proximal ulna and dislocation of the radial head)

Sprain (swelling, tenderness over the involved ligament, no evidence of fracture)

Subluxation of the radial head (typical history and age, tenderness over radial head, negative radiographs)

# ADVERSE OUTCOMES OF THE DISEASE

Supracondylar fractures have the highest incidence of neurovascular problems. Median, ulnar, and radial nerve injuries are associated with this fracture. The brachial artery may be injured, and compartment syndrome involving the volar forearm muscles may develop. Failure to recognize this problem in a timely fashion will result in necrosis of forearm muscles and subsequent contractures (Volkmann ischemic contracture). Malunion with loss of the normal carrying angle (cubitus varus) may occur.

Condyle fractures may be missed, particularly in very young children who have limited ossification of the distal humerus. In these children, only a thin wafer of metaphyseal fragment will be apparent, with the rest of the fracture involving the cartilaginous physis and trochlea and, therefore, not visible on plain radiographs. Fractures displaced 2 mm or more often are associated with delayed union, nonunion, or malunion (rotational and/or cubitus valgus). Condyle fractures of the humerus that are initially nondisplaced may become displaced, even when immobilized, by contraction of the forearm muscles attaching at the condyle. These injuries require close follow-up and repeat radiographs.

Medial epicondyle fractures of the distal humerus do not commonly cause residual problems, even when markedly displaced, unless associated with dislocation of the elbow and a fracture fragment that is not recognized as being entrapped in the joint.

Fractures across the entire distal physis of the humerus have complications that are similar but typically less severe than supracondylar fractures. In addition, the potential for child abuse should be recognized and appropriately investigated.

Fractures of the radial neck that are angulated more than 30° may be associated with loss of forearm rotation, premature closure of the growth plate, and osteonecrosis of the radial head.

Fractures of the olecranon that have 2 mm or more disruption of the articular surface need reduction to prevent progressive arthritic changes.

# TREATMENT

Nondisplaced fractures can be treated with splint or cast immobilization. Condyle fractures, in particular, need repeat radiographs in 3 to 5 days. Displaced fractures need reduction and, in most cases, pinning. The exception is medial or lateral epicondyle fractures of the humerus and radial neck fractures with less than 30° of angulation.

# ADVERSE OUTCOMES OF TREATMENT

These are the same as the adverse outcomes of the disease. In addition, postoperative infection can develop.

# REFERRAL DECISIONS/RED FLAGS

Any displacement or angulation, inability to extend all fingers of the affected hand, failure of over-the-counter medications to provide pain relief, and absent or diminished radial pulse are signs that further evaluation is necessary.

SECTION 9 ■ PEDIATRIC ORTHOPAEDICS

# FRACTURES OF THE CLAVICLE AND PROXIMAL HUMERUS

## DEFINITION

The clavicle is a common site of fracture in children, with most occurring in the middle third. However, fractures can occur at either end as well. Those close to the sternoclavicular joint can be serious because the great vessels are located just posterior to the joint. Those at the distal third of the clavicle generally heal rapidly in children and typically do not require surgery.

Fractures of the proximal humerus account for about 5% of fractures in children. These fractures can occur in neonates during delivery or in older children as a result of a fall. Metaphyseal fractures typically occur in children between ages 5 and 12 years, whereas physeal fractures (those involving the growth plate) most commonly occur in children between ages 13 and 16 years. Peterson type III (Salter type II) is the most common pattern of physeal fracture.

## CLINICAL SYMPTOMS

Newborns with a fracture of the clavicle or proximal humerus may refuse to move the arm, a condition called pseudoparalysis. Clavicle fractures in children are characterized by acute pain, tenderness, swelling, and a palpable deformity. Fractures of the proximal humerus are less obvious because of the overlying deltoid muscle.

## TESTS

### Physical Examination
Identify the point of maximum tenderness, and check the overlying skin for any tenting or blanching. Assess motor and sensory functions of the axillary, musculocutaneous, median, ulnar, and radial nerves. Radial and ulnar pulses should be checked as well.

### Diagnostic Tests
For suspected injury to the clavicle, obtain an AP radiograph of the clavicle. AP and axillary views of the shoulder are necessary for suspected injury of the proximal humerus (**Figure 1**).

## DIFFERENTIAL DIAGNOSIS

Cleidocranial dysostosis (absence of some or all of the clavicle, frontal bossing)

Congenital muscular torticollis (asymmetric neck motion, plagiocephaly)

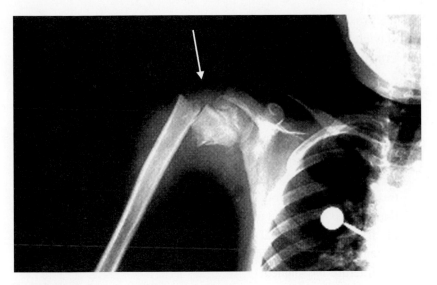

**Figure 1**
AP radiograph demonstrating a proximal humerus fracture (arrow) in a 5-year-old boy who fell from a tree.

Congenital pseudarthrosis of the clavicle (atrophic ends of bone at "fracture")

Obstetric brachial plexus palsy (inability to spontaneously move fingers/wrist/elbow)

Pathologic fracture (injury through a bone cyst or underlying bone disorder)

Septic arthritis/osteomyelitis of the shoulder (no visible fracture, fever, pain with range of motion)

Shoulder dislocation (evident on radiographs)

Soft-tissue injury to shoulder (contusion)

## ADVERSE OUTCOMES OF THE DISEASE

Malunion, physeal bar and growth arrest, neurologic or vascular compromise of the involved extremity, and/or osteomyelitis in an open fracture can occur.

## TREATMENT

### Newborns

These fractures heal without incident and fully remodel. No treatment is needed for fractures of the clavicle. For fractures of the proximal humerus, immobilize the arm for comfort.

### Young Children

Middle-third clavicle fractures do not require realignment, as they will remodel and straighten with time. Observation and immobilization in a sling or a figure-of-8 strap is satisfactory. Unless posterior displacement with involvement of the great vessels and/or respiratory difficulties are present, fractures of

SECTION 9 ■ PEDIATRIC ORTHOPAEDICS

the proximal third also can be treated with a sling. Distal-third clavicle fractures generally heal without reduction or surgery. Fractures of the proximal humerus usually are best treated with a sling. Reduction usually is not needed unless there is more than 40° of angulation.

### Adolescents

Clavicle fractures in this age group usually require only a sling or figure-of-8 strap unless the fracture is tenting or blanching the overlying skin. Fractures of the proximal humerus can be treated with a sling but may require reduction if there is more than 30° to 40° of angulation or less than 50% apposition of the fragments. Physical therapy rarely is required unless the patient has poor range of motion or atrophy several weeks after the fracture has healed.

## ADVERSE OUTCOMES OF TREATMENT

Recurrence, malunion, growth arrest of the physis, and resulting deformity are possible.

## REFERRAL DECISIONS/RED FLAGS

Neurovascular compromise, difficulty in breathing, skin tenting or blanching over the fracture site, open fractures, displacement of more than 50%, and/or angulation of more than 40° indicate the need for further evaluation.

# FRACTURES OF THE DISTAL FOREARM

## DEFINITION

The distal third of the forearm is the most common location for fractures in children, accounting for 20% to 40% of all pediatric fractures. The different types of fractures, in order of relative severity, are listed in **Table 1**. Fractures of the distal forearm are uncommon before age 4 years, but torus and greenstick fractures may occur in this younger age group. After age 10, fractures involving the growth plate of the distal radial physis are more common.

A torus fracture is characterized by buckling of the cortex on only one side of the bone and is the least complicated injury. The most common torus fracture involves the dorsal surface of the distal radius. A metaphyseal fracture isolated to the distal radius typically is nondisplaced. In a greenstick fracture, the cortex is disrupted on the tension side but is intact or only buckled on the compression side. A Galeazzi fracture is a displaced fracture of the distal radius with a dislocation of the distal ulna or a fracture of the distal ulnar physis (**Figure 1**).

## CLINICAL SYMPTOMS

Patients typically report a fall on an outstretched extremity. Acute pain, tenderness, and swelling are noted. With displaced fractures, the deformity is obvious. Symptoms following a torus fracture may not be immediately obvious.

### Table 1   Types of Distal Radius Fractures in Children

Torus fracture*

Metaphyseal fracture, complete

Greenstick fracture

Greenstick fractures of the distal radius and ulna

Complete fracture of the distal radius and greenstick fracture of the distal ulna

Complete fracture of the distal radius and ulna

Physeal fracture

Galeazzi fracture

* Typically nondisplaced or minimally displaced

**ICD-9 Codes**

**813.42**
Galeazzi fracture
Greenstick fracture of the distal radius
Metaphyseal fracture of the distal radius, complete
Physeal fracture of the distal radius
Torus fracture of the distal radius

**813.44**
Complete fracture of the distal radius and ulna
Greenstick fractures of the distal radius and ulna

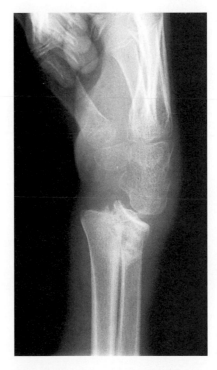

**Figure 1**

Lateral radiograph demonstrating a significantly displaced fracture of the distal radial physis in an 11-year-old boy who presented late.

Reproduced from Waters PM: Forearm and foot fractures, in Richards BS (ed): *Orthopaedic Knowledge Update: Pediatrics.* Rosemont, IL, American Academy of Orthopaedic Surgeons, 1996, pp 251-257.

SECTION 9 ■ PEDIATRIC ORTHOPAEDICS

## TESTS

### Physical Examination

Evaluate the status of the median, ulnar, and radial nerves distal to the fracture. Assess circulation at the fingertips. Examine the skin carefully, as puncture wounds are indicative of a grade I open fracture.

### Diagnostic Tests

AP and lateral radiographs of the forearm should show both the wrist and elbow joints. Comparison views are rarely needed with these injuries.

## DIFFERENTIAL DIAGNOSIS

Child abuse (multiple injuries)

Osteomyelitis of the distal radius or ulna (no history of injury, fever, marked tenderness)

Pathologic fracture through a bone cyst or other tumor (evident on radiographs)

Septic arthritis of the wrist (subacute onset, no history of injury, fever, marked swelling)

Wrist sprain (acute symptoms, but uncommon in children)

## ADVERSE OUTCOMES OF THE DISEASE

Malunion or crossunion (synostosis) with loss of forearm rotation, compartment syndrome (uncommon), and osteomyelitis in open fractures are possible.

## TREATMENT

Most of these fractures heal without incident and can be treated by closed means. Residual angulation typically will remodel completely if 1 to 2 years of growth remain. The considerable remodeling potential of distal forearm fractures is related to the large amount of growth from the distal radial and ulnar physis, which contributes approximately 80% of forearm length.

Torus fractures and nondisplaced fractures of the distal radius are stable but should be immobilized in a short arm cast or splint for comfort and to protect the bone from a second fall that could cause exacerbation of the injury. To ensure compliance and prevent further injury, most children are better treated in a short arm cast. Displaced fractures are treated initially by immobilization in a long arm cast to prevent forearm rotation. The duration of immobilization depends on the age of the child and extent of injury.

For displaced fractures of the distal forearm, the degree of angulation that can be accepted depends on the plane of angulation and the amount of growth remaining. Loss of rotational alignment is the only absolute indication for both reduction and remanipulation. Distal forearm fractures that are angulated in the volar or dorsal plane often remodel in children, even if a reduction was not performed. The principal reason for reduction is to relieve the pressure on adjacent soft tissues; therefore, closed reduction generally is indicated for angulation of 10° to 15° or more.

Unlike adults, most children with Galeazzi injuries can be treated by closed reduction.

Exploration of the fracture under general anesthesia with irrigation and débridement is critical for any open fracture, even if the wound is only a small puncture.

## ADVERSE OUTCOMES OF TREATMENT

Reangulation is fairly common in completely displaced fractures, particularly when reduction is incomplete. The decision to remanipulate the fracture depends on the age of the child, the degree of healing, and the plane of angulation. Significant malunion with loss of functional wrist and forearm motion can occur but is relatively uncommon. Synostosis with loss of forearm pronation and supination is more common with open fractures. Physeal fractures may be complicated by an arrest of growth and resulting deformity at the wrist.

## REFERRAL DECISIONS/RED FLAGS

Inability to extend all fingers, pain not relieved by over-the-counter medications, neurologic dysfunction, dislocation of the distal ulna, and/or angulation of greater than 10° to 15° require further evaluation.

SECTION 9 ■ PEDIATRIC ORTHOPAEDICS

# FRACTURES OF THE PROXIMAL AND MIDDLE FOREARM

**ICD-9 Codes**

**813.00**
Fracture, closed, upper end of forearm, unspecified

**813.20**
Fracture, middle forearm, closed, unspecified part

## DEFINITION

In children, fractures of the proximal or midportion of the forearm typically cause disruption of both the radius and the ulna (**Figure 1**). Other injury patterns include a Monteggia fracture-dislocation (radial head dislocation associated with a fracture of the ulna), a both-bone fracture, or isolated fracture of the ulna. An isolated ulna fracture usually occurs secondary to a direct blow as the child places the forearm in front of the face to deflect an oncoming blow.

## CLINICAL SYMPTOMS

Patients have acute pain, tenderness, and swelling, usually in association with a fall on the outstretched arm.

## TESTS

### Physical Examination

Assess median, ulnar, and radial nerve function distal to the fracture site. Severe or inordinate pain on passive extension of the fingers should raise concern for possible compartment syndrome.

### Diagnostic Tests

Full-length AP and lateral radiographs of the forearm that include the wrist and elbow are indicated. The radial head should align with the capitellum on both views. A Monteggia injury should be excluded if a fracture of the ulna is present. In a Monteggia injury, dislocation of the radial head is usually anterior but could be posterior or lateral.

## DIFFERENTIAL DIAGNOSIS

Child abuse (multiple injuries)

Osteogenesis imperfecta (previous history, thin bony cortices)

Osteomyelitis of the proximal radius or ulna (fever, swelling)

Pathologic fracture through a bone cyst or tumor (evident on radiographs)

Septic arthritis of the elbow (fever, swelling, markedly restricted motion)

## ADVERSE OUTCOMES OF THE DISEASE

If recognized early, a Monteggia fracture-dislocation in children can be treated by closed reduction. However, failure to diagnose

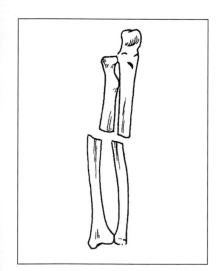

**Figure 1**

Drawing of a fracture of the middle third of the forearm.

Adapted with permission from Müller ME, Nazarian S, Koch P, et al (eds): *The Comprehensive Classification of Fractures of Long Bones.* Berlin, Germany, Springer-Verlag, 1990, pp 96-105.

the injury in a timely fashion will necessitate open reduction, reconstructive surgery, or acceptance of the deformity. Proximal forearm fractures are more likely to cause complications such as malunion, compartment syndrome, or loss of forearm rotation.

## TREATMENT

Irrigation and débridement of open fractures are indicated. Both-bone forearm fractures that are angulated more than 15° and all Monteggia fracture-dislocations require closed reduction and immobilization in a long arm cast for 6 to 10 weeks. In adolescents, internal fixation may be required.

## ADVERSE OUTCOMES OF TREATMENT

Recurrence of the deformity, malunion, loss of forearm rotation, and compartment syndrome are possible. Both-bone fractures can develop a synostosis or bony bar connecting the radius and ulna.

## REFERRAL DECISIONS/RED FLAGS

Inability to extend all fingers, pain not relieved by over-the-counter pain medications, and angulation greater than 15° indicate the need for further evaluation.

# FRACTURES OF THE FEMUR

## ICD-9 Codes

**820.00**
Femoral neck fracture, closed, unspecified type

**820.21**
Intertrochanteric femur fracture, closed

**821.00**
Femoral shaft fracture, closed, unspecified part

**821.22**
Distal femoral physeal fracture, closed

**821.23**
Supracondylar femur fracture, closed

## DEFINITION

Fractures of the femur in children are usually the result of significant trauma, although they can occur after simple falls. Fractures can occur anywhere in the femur (eg, femoral neck, intertrochanteric region, femoral shaft, supracondylar region, distal femoral physis) and can be transverse, oblique, spiral, or comminuted. Most involve the femoral shaft and heal without incident in 6 to 12 weeks. Traditional closed treatment, such as traction or spica casting, is giving way to surgical fixation in older children and adolescents to enable early mobility and improve outcome.

## CLINICAL SYMPTOMS

Patients have acute pain, swelling, inability to bear weight, deformity, and a history of trauma.

## TESTS

### Physical Examination

Pain and disability will be immediate. Tenderness, deformity, or swelling may localize the fracture. Tibial and peroneal nerve function distal to the knee should be evaluated, as should circulation at the ankle.

### Diagnostic Tests

AP and lateral radiographs of the femur, including the hip and knee joints, should be obtained. Stress views may be necessary to identify physeal fractures of the distal femur.

## DIFFERENTIAL DIAGNOSIS

Child abuse (metaphyseal corner fractures or multiple fractures in various stages of healing)

Knee injury (especially collateral ligament tears)

Osteogenesis imperfecta (multiple fractures after trivial trauma)

Pathologic fracture through a cyst or bony tumor (evident on radiographs)

Slipped capital femoral epiphysis (common in overweight adolescents)

## ADVERSE OUTCOMES OF THE DISEASE

Malunion, either angular or rotational, along with growth derangement and limb-length discrepancy are possible.

Osteonecrosis of the femoral head may occur with a displaced or nondisplaced fracture of the femoral neck. Fractures of the distal femoral physis may be misdiagnosed as a knee sprain.

# TREATMENT

The type of treatment depends on the location of the fracture in the femur, the fracture pattern, and the age of the patient. Immobilization by a spica cast or initial treatment by traction followed by casting are time-honored and effective modalities, especially well suited to young children who tolerate recumbency and heal rapidly.

Nondisplaced femoral neck and intertrochanteric fractures may be treated with cast immobilization. These injuries should be monitored closely with radiographs for evidence of displacement. Displaced fractures should be treated by immediate reduction and fixation to minimize the risk of complications.

Femoral shaft fractures can be treated with immediate spica casting or traction until early callus formation provides enough stability for the fracture to maintain alignment in a spica cast. This treatment is routine for young children up to age 6 years and for children 6 to 10 years of age who do not meet the indications for other types of treatment. Minor angulation will remodel.

Older children may be candidates for fixation of femoral shaft fractures that enables them to get out of bed and return to school earlier. Supracondylar fractures and fractures of the distal femoral physis are difficult to reduce and hold in casts and often will require surgical fixation to maintain the reduction.

# ADVERSE OUTCOMES OF TREATMENT

These are similar to the adverse outcomes of the disease.

# REFERRAL DECISIONS/RED FLAGS

Virtually all femoral fractures require at least a short hospitalization. Open fractures and fractures with vascular compromise require urgent treatment.

SECTION 9 ■ PEDIATRIC ORTHOPAEDICS

# FRACTURES OF THE TIBIA

**ICD-9 Code**
**823.80**
Fracture of tibia, unspecified part,
closed

## DEFINITION

Diaphyseal and proximal metaphyseal fractures occur more commonly in younger children, but growth plate and intra-articular fractures are more prevalent in older children. The tibia is a common site of fracture in children who are victims of child abuse. A list of various fracture types, age of peak incidence, and potential complications is provided in **Table 1**.

## CLINICAL SYMPTOMS

Most patients present with a history of injury causing the acute onset of pain and inability to walk. Toddler's fractures (minimally displaced spiral fractures of the diaphysis and/or metaphysis of the tibia), minimally displaced or incomplete metaphyseal fractures in older children, and stress fractures are characterized by a vague history of injury or insidious onset with minimal swelling or localizing signs and a limp.

**Table 1    Tibial Fractures and Potential Complications**

| Fracture Type | Age of Peak Incidence | Pitfalls/Complications |
| --- | --- | --- |
| *Proximal* | | |
| Tibial spine fracture | Older child | Chronic laxity of knee |
| Tibial tubercle avulsion | Older child, adolescent | Growth arrest Compartment syndrome |
| Metaphyseal fracture | Younger child | Genu valgum |
| *Diaphyseal* | | |
| Toddler's fracture | 1 to 3 years | Failure to recognize Overdiagnosis |
| Stress fracture | Older child, adolescent | Failure to recognize Overdiagnosis |
| Complete fracture | | Varus malunion Compartment syndrome |
| *Distal* | | |
| Physeal fracture | Older child, adolescent | Malunion Growth arrest |
| Triplane/Tilleaux fractures* | Adolescent | Failure to recognize Degenerative arthritis |

*Complex fracture of distal tibia occurring near end of growth

# TESTS

## Physical Examination

Assess superficial peroneal, deep peroneal, and posterior tibial nerve function. Evaluate dorsalis pedis and posterior tibialis pulses, as well as capillary refill. Assess for possible compartment syndrome, particularly in proximal physeal and midshaft fractures with muscle contusion. Look carefully for any puncture wounds or abrasions that would signify an open fracture.

## Diagnostic Tests

AP and lateral radiographs of the tibia that show the knee and ankle are necessary. For injuries thought to involve the knee or ankle, center the radiographs in these areas. Oblique radiographs and CT can be helpful in visualizing complex fractures of the distal tibia, such as triplane or Tilleaux fractures. A bone scan can be helpful in identifying a stress fracture or other occult injuries.

# DIFFERENTIAL DIAGNOSIS

Child abuse (multiple injuries, metaphyseal beak or corner fractures)

Ligament injuries (unusual in prepubertal children)

Osteogenesis imperfecta (previous history, thin bony cortices)

Pathologic fracture through a bone cyst or tumor (evident on radiographs)

Stress fracture (indolent onset)

# ADVERSE OUTCOMES OF THE DISEASE

Early potential problems include compartment syndrome and vascular injuries. These complications are less common but may be more difficult to diagnose in children. Remodeling is unpredictable in deformities of greater than 10°, and malunion with subsequent degenerative arthritis may occur. Growth arrest is common with distal tibial physeal injuries but less likely with proximal injuries.

# TREATMENT

Treatment focuses on minimizing angular deformity, restoring joint congruity, and avoiding or identifying compartment syndrome or vascular injuries. Toddler's fractures, stress fractures, and certain nondisplaced fractures can be managed with immobilization in a short leg walking cast. Displaced shaft fractures often require manipulative reduction and long leg casting. These patients are best managed with hospital admission overnight for observation and elevation. Early splitting of the cast to accommodate swelling may be necessary. The duration of casting depends upon the age of the child and the extent of the fracture.

Displaced intra-articular or physeal fractures need closed or open reduction and limited internal fixation supplemented by cast immobilization. All open fractures require surgical exploration and débridement.

## ADVERSE OUTCOMES OF TREATMENT

These are the same as adverse outcomes of the disease. In addition, infection may develop after open treatment.

## REFERRAL DECISIONS/RED FLAGS

Patients who report pain after immobilization that is not relieved by mild analgesics or over-the-counter medications need further evaluation. Patients who have lacerations or deep abrasions overlying the fracture site should be treated as if they have an open fracture. Inability to correct angular deformities to less than 10° is considered a problem. Proximal or distal tibial fractures that involve the physis or articular surface need further evaluation.

# Genu Valgum

## Definition

Genu valgum (knock-knees) is alignment of the knee with the tibia laterally deviated (valgus) in relation to the femur. At birth, the child is bowlegged, with a genu varum of 10° to 15°. The bowing gradually straightens to 0° by 12 to 18 months of age. Continued growth produces maximum genu valgum at age 3 to 4 years that averages 10° to 15° (**Figure 1**). With subsequent growth, the genu valgum decreases, and normal adult alignment of 5° to 10° genu valgum occurs by early adolescence. Young children have a fairly wide range of normal knee alignment (two standard deviations typically is ± 10°).

**ICD-9 Code**
**736.41**
Genu valgum, acquired

## Clinical Symptoms

Parental concern is the usual reason for the visit.

## Tests

### Physical Examination

Measure the child's height and then plot it on a height nomogram. Measure the tibiofemoral angle using a goniometer or by measuring the intermalleolar (IM) distance. The IM distance is the distance between the medial malleoli with the medial femoral condyles touching. The IM distance has the disadvantage of being a relative rather than an absolute measurement and is not reproducible.

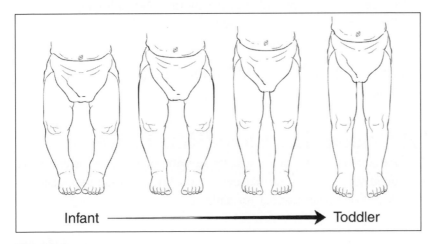

Infant ⟶ Toddler

**Figure 1**

Normal progression from bowlegs of infancy through slow evolution to a physiologic valgus angle of about 12° at age 3.

Reproduced from Gomez JE: Growth and Maturation, in Sullivan JA, Anderson SJ (eds): *Care of the Young Athlete*. Rosemont, IL, American Academy of Orthopaedic Surgeons 25-32.

## Diagnostic Tests

Radiographs usually are not necessary, but should be considered when the valgus is more than 15° to 20°, or if the child is short statured. A weight-bearing AP radiograph on a 36- x 43-cm cassette with the film centered at the knees and the feet pointing straight ahead provides screening for a possible skeletal dysplasia, as well as accurate measurement of the tibiofemoral angle (genu valgum).

# Differential Diagnosis

Hypophosphatemic rickets (short stature, wide physis, low serum phosphorus)

Multiple epiphyseal dysplasia (short stature, multiple joint involvement)

Pseudoachondroplasia (short stature, early arthritic change)

# Adverse Outcomes of the Disease

None

# Treatment

Observation is the treatment of choice for an otherwise normal 3- to 4-year-old child with marked genu valgum. Shoe modifications are ineffective, and long leg braces are not indicated because this condition spontaneously corrects more than 99% of the time. The child shown in **Figure 2** is a 3-year, 6-month-old boy referred for evaluation of knock-knees. His height is in the 70th percentile, and his development is normal. Genu valgum measured 18° by clinical examination. The patient was considered to be within normal limits, and an explanation was provided to the mother. No radiographs or further follow-up was required.

# Adverse Outcomes of Treatment

None

# Referral Decisions/Red Flags

Patients of short stature and those with asymmetric or excessive genu valgum need further evaluation (greater than two standard deviations from normal for age).

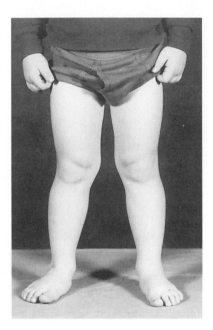

**Figure 2**

Clinical photograph of boy referred for evaluation of "knock-knees." The patient was considered to be within normal limits.

Reproduced from Greene WB: Genu varum and genu valgum in children. *Instr Course Lect* 1994;43:151-159.

# Genu Varum

## Synonym
Bowlegs

ICD-9 Code
**736.42**
Genu varum, acquired

## Definition
Genu varum (bowlegs) is an angular deformity at the knee with the tibia medially deviated (varus) in relation to the femur. At birth, genu varum of 10° to 15° is normal. The bowing gradually straightens to 0° by age 12 to 18 months. Continued growth then results in progressive valgus with maximum genu valgum of 10° to 15° occurring at age 3 to 4 years. Young children have a fairly wide range of normal knee alignment (two standard deviations is ± 10°).

The most common cause of bowlegs in children 18 to 36 months of age is physiologic genu varum, a condition that resolves without treatment (normal variation of growth).

## Clinical Symptoms
Parental concern is the usual reason for the visit.

## Tests

### Physical Examination
Measure the child's height and then plot it on a height nomogram. Quantify the genu varum either by using a goniometer to measure the degree of varus deformity. It is also important to assess tibial torsion.

### Diagnostic Tests
Radiographs are appropriate if the child is under the 25th percentile for height, the varus is relatively severe for the child's age, there is excessive internal tibial torsion, the varus is increasing after age 16 months, or there is significant asymmetry of the two sides. Obtain weight-bearing AP radiographs of the lower extremities on a 36- x 43-cm cassette with the film centered at the knees and the feet pointing straight ahead (**Figure 1**). Assess radiographs for the tibiofemoral angle, the width of the growth plate (widened in rickets and certain skeletal dysplasias), and the slope of the proximal tibia (medial aspect depressed in infantile tibia vara). Infantile tibia vara and physiologic genu varum can be difficult to differentiate in children under age 3 years, but radiographic measurement can help. The right limb shown in Figure 1 has medial depression of the tibial physis and an increased tibial metaphyseal-diaphyseal angle of 20°. This radiographic picture suggests a

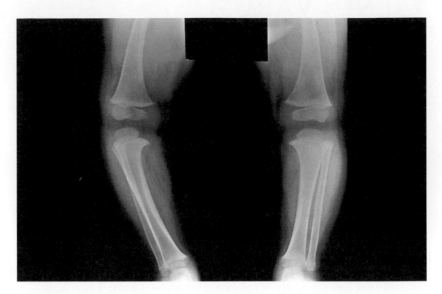

**Figure 1**

Radiograph demonstrating genu varum in a 1-year, 6-month-old girl.

Reproduced from Greene WB: Infantile tibia vara. *Instr Course Lect* 1993;42:525-538.

high probability of infantile tibia vara (which is also referred to as Blount's disease), and a long leg brace was prescribed.

## DIFFERENTIAL DIAGNOSIS

Hypophosphatemic rickets (short stature, widened physis, and low serum phosphorus level)

Infantile tibia vara (obese children who begin walking at an early age; associated internal tibial torsion, depression of the medial aspect of the proximal tibial physis)

Metaphyseal chondrodysplasia (short stature, widened physis, normal serum phosphorus level)

Physiologic genu varum (spontaneous correction by age 2½ to 3 years, normal tibial metaphyseal-diaphyseal angle)

## ADVERSE OUTCOMES OF THE DISEASE

The principal adverse outcome is persistent varus deformity.

## TREATMENT

For young children with infantile tibia vara, bracing can be successful. After age 30 to 36 months, tibial osteotomy may be required.

## ADVERSE OUTCOMES OF TREATMENT

The deformity can recur.

## REFERRAL DECISIONS/RED FLAGS

The presence of disorders other than physiologic genu varum indicates the need for further evaluation.

# INTOEING AND OUTTOEING

## SYNONYMS

*Intoeing*
Pigeon-toed

*Outtoeing*
External rotation contracture of infancy
External tibial torsion
Femoral retroversion

**ICD-9 Codes**
**736.89**
Acquired deformity of lower limb
**781.2**
Abnormality of gait

## DEFINITION

Intoeing means that the foot turns in more than expected during walking and running activities. With outtoeing, the child's foot turns out more than expected.

By age 2 years, children typically walk with the foot turned out relative to the line of progression, a phenomenon that is obvious when observing a child's footprints in the snow or sand. When walking on level ground, the foot typically is turned out at an angle of 10° to 20° to the line of progression.

Intoeing may be secondary to foot deformities or may be due to inward rotation of the femur or tibia, or a combination of the two. Increased internal torsion of the femur (femoral anteversion) is the most common finding. Excessive outtoeing, although not as frequent a concern as intoeing, is similar in that excessive rotation may occur in the femur (femoral retroversion), the tibia (external tibial torsion), or both. In many cases, intoeing and outtoeing are variations of normal development.

Understanding normal development of femoral and tibial torsion, as well as the changes that occur in hip rotation, is critical in evaluating these children. Inward femoral rotation (anteversion) is greatest at birth (approximately 40°) and gradually declines to adult values of 10° to 15° by age 8 years. The tibia normally twists outward between the knee and ankle. Tibial torsion is typically neutral or 0° at birth and gradually increases to 20° to 40° by age 3 to 4 years. Tibial torsion is often asymmetric, with the left side commonly less severe.

Although not an absolute measurement, the easiest way to assess femoral anteversion is by measuring hip rotation. It is important to realize that clinical measurement of hip rotation does not profile the degree of bony femoral torsion until neonatal tightness of the hip joint capsule resolves. Due to intrauterine positioning, a neonate is born with tightness of the hip joint capsule. This creates an external contracture and increased external rotation of the hip even though femoral torsion is maximum at birth. The effect of this capsular contraction on measurement of hip rotation does not completely resolve until the infant is at least age 1 year and sometimes even up to age 2 years.

# Clinical Symptoms

Typically, medical attention is sought because parents or grandparents are concerned about how the child is walking. In children, intoeing and outtoeing usually do not cause pain or interfere with development or stability in gait. With severe intoeing, children may stumble or trip more frequently as they catch their toes on the back of the trailing leg.

# Tests

## Physical Examination

The physical examination should include the following steps:

- Measurement of foot progression angle (angle that the foot makes relative to the line of progression as the child walks)
- Measurement of hip rotation (femoral torsion)
- Measurement of tibial torsion (thigh-foot angle)
- Observation of the posture of the foot
- Evaluation for possible neuromuscular disorders

Observe the child walking and estimate the foot progression angle. The foot progression angle does not identify the site of the problem; however, it quantifies the severity of the problem and distinguishes whether there is an intoeing or outtoeing disorder.

Hip rotation approximates femoral torsion. Hip rotation should be measured with the hip in extension. Placing the child in the prone position is the most reliable method to measure hip rotation. Flex the knee to 90° and position the leg in the Zero Starting Position (**Figure 1**). Rotate both legs simultaneously to measure internal rotation. The degree of internal rotation is the angle of the leg from the Zero Starting Position (**Figure 2**). To assess external rotation, place one hand on the buttocks and move the leg into external rotation. The degree of external rotation is the angle of the leg when the pelvis starts to tilt.

The average range of hip rotation for a child older than age 2 years is approximately 50° of internal rotation and 40° of external rotation. An excessive amount of internal rotation (greater than 65°) coupled with a limited degree of external rotation indicates increased femoral anteversion. Likewise, after 2 years of age, an excessive amount of external rotation

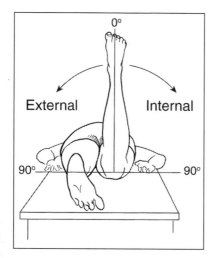

**Figure 1**

Hip rotation: Zero Starting Position.

Reproduced from Greene WB, Heckman JD (eds): *The Clinical Measurement of Joint Motion.* Rosemont, IL, American Academy of Orthopaedic Surgeons, 1994, pp 106-107.

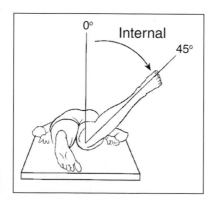

**Figure 2**

Measuring internal rotation of the hip.

Reproduced from Greene WB, Heckman JD (eds): *The Clinical Measurement of Joint Motion.* Rosemont, IL, American Academy of Orthopaedic Surgeons, 1994, pp 106-107.

coupled with limited internal rotation indicates reduced femoral torsion (femoral retroversion).

Tibial torsion is most easily assessed by measuring the thigh-foot angle (the axis of the foot relative to the axis of the thigh with the knee flexed to 90° and the hip and foot in a neutral or Zero Starting Position alignment) (**Figure 3**). A neutral or internal thigh-foot angle indicates internal tibial torsion (**Figure 4**).

Foot posture is assessed for metatarsus adductus, a possible cause of intoeing, as well as hindfoot alignment. Increased heel valgus or pes planovalgus may be perceived by the parents as the leg turning out.

Neuromuscular disorders may cause intoeing or outtoeing. Furthermore, these children may be brought to a physician with the parents concerned about intoeing or outtoeing before the underlying disorder has been diagnosed. This is particularly common in patients with mild cerebral palsy. Therefore, assess for appropriate motor milestones (**Table 1**) and examine for spasticity, muscle contractures, clonus, and a stiff or imbalanced gait.

External rotation contracture of infancy may persist and cause concern. These children are typically brought to a physician between the ages of 6 to 12 months, a time when they are starting to pull to a stand or are in walkers. The parents are concerned about the posture of the lower extremities. Boys and black children are more commonly affected. The right leg typically is affected more often. Examination reveals 60° to 70° of external rotation and only 20° to 30° of internal rotation. The hip rotation is usually symmetric, but the right leg typically is more externally rotated because the tibial torsion has advanced to a greater degree on that side. In the absence of neuromuscular disease and muscle imbalance, normal growth will correct this condition without the need for special shoes, braces, or exercise therapy.

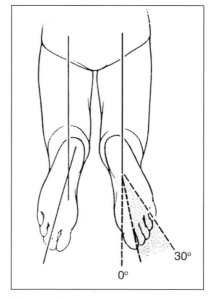

**Figure 3**

Normal range of thigh-foot angle.

Adapted with permission from Alexander IJ: *The Foot: Examination and Diagnosis*, New York, NY, Churchill Livingstone, 1990, p 115.

| Table 1 | Gross Motor Developmental Screens During Early Childhood | |
| --- | --- |
| **Age** | **Activity** |
| 2 years | Stairs, one step at a time |
| 2 ½ years | Jumps |
| 3 years | Stairs, alternating feet |
| 4 years | Hops on one foot |
| 5 years | Skips |

Adapted with permission from Paine RS, Oppe TE: Neurological examination of children, in *Clinics in Developmental Medicine, Nos 20/21*. London, England, William Heinemann Medical Books.

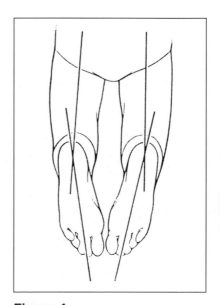

**Figure 4**

Bilateral internal tibial torsion.

Adapted with permission from Alexander IJ: *The Foot: Examination and Diagnosis*, New York, NY, Churchill Livingstone, 1990, p 115.

Section 9 ■ Pediatric Orthopaedics

## Diagnostic Tests

Radiographs are rarely needed unless the child has evidence of short stature.

# DIFFERENTIAL DIAGNOSIS

Cerebral palsy or other neuromuscular disorders (developmental delay, spasticity, muscle weakness)

Femoral anteversion (increased internal rotation of the hip)

Femoral retroversion (increased external rotation of the hip)

Metatarsus adductus (forefoot adducted)

Skeletal dysplasia (short stature)

Tibial torsion (increased internal or external rotation of the tibia)

# ADVERSE OUTCOMES OF THE DISEASE

If intoeing persists, the child may have a cosmetically unpleasant gait pattern and may trip more frequently, but this condition has not been linked to degenerative arthritis in adulthood. Most children, however, function quite well. If intoeing caused by increased femoral anteversion persists, the tibia may compensate and external tibial torsion may develop. This condition is rarely associated with knee problems and has been associated with the ability to run quickly.

Outtoeing, except in neuromuscular disorders, often improves with age and rarely requires treatment.

# TREATMENT

Shoe modifications, braces, and exercises do not alter developmental changes in femoral or tibial torsion. Casting occasionally is necessary in metatarsus adductus.

Slow correction of femoral anteversion to an acceptable degree is typical. An associated increase in external tibial torsion will diminish the degree of intoeing. In rare cases, children may have persistent tripping or an unsightly gait and surgical correction by rotational osteotomy of the femur may be indicated. The procedure generally is done after age 7 to 8 years to allow for spontaneous resolution.

In children with cerebral palsy and other neuromuscular disorders, both abnormal femoral and tibial torsion persist in a much higher percentage of patients and are more likely to require surgical correction due to their impact on gait.

## ADVERSE OUTCOMES OF TREATMENT

Risks of surgery include failure to heal, infection, over- or undercorrection of the deformity, or postoperative angular deformity. Risks of casting for metatarsus adductus are minimal.

## REFERRAL DECISIONS/RED FLAGS

Physicians who are familiar with the evaluation and examination of this problem can adequately reassure parents regarding the frequent resolution of these deformities. When metatarsus adductus persists in an infant older than age 6 months, or internal tibial torsion or abnormal femoral anteversion persists past age 4 years and the deformity is significant, further evaluation is warranted. Specialty evaluation is sometimes necessary to allay parents' or grandparents' concern.

# JUVENILE RHEUMATOID ARTHRITIS

**ICD-9 Codes**

**714.30**
Polyarticular juvenile rheumatoid arthritis, chronic or unspecified

**714.32**
Pauciarticular juvenile rheumatoid arthritis

## SYNONYMS

JRA

Still's disease

## DEFINITION

The American Rheumatic Association lists four criteria for diagnosing juvenile rheumatoid arthritis (JRA): (1) chronic synovial inflammation of unknown cause; (2) onset in children younger than age 16 years; (3) objective evidence of arthritis in one or more joints for 6 consecutive weeks; and (4) exclusion of other diseases. Pauciarticular JRA involves four or fewer joints after 6 months of symptoms, whereas polyarticular JRA involves five or more joints. Systemic JRA is the subgroup characterized by an illness beginning with high spiking fevers—temperatures above 102.7°F (39.3°C). The number of joints involved is not included in the definition of systemic-onset JRA, but most patients in this group have several affected joints.

## CLINICAL SYMPTOMS

Pain, swelling, and stiffness are less severe in JRA than in the adult form.

Pauciarticular JRA is the most common pattern. Age at onset typically is younger than age 4 years, and girls are affected four times more often than boys. The parents will comment that the child is irritable, lethargic, or shows a reluctance to play. The disease commonly begins in a single joint, most frequently the knee, ankle, wrist, or finger joints. Uveitis is most likely to develop in children with this type of JRA and a positive antinuclear antibody (ANA) test.

The polyarticular form is characterized by symmetric involvement of the knees, wrists, fingers, and ankles and is more common in girls. The onset of the seronegative form typically occurs in children between ages 1 and 3 years, and the seropositive form usually begins in adolescence and is virtually indistinguishable from adult rheumatoid arthritis.

Systemic onset commonly occurs in children between the ages of 4 and 9 years and at onset is associated with spiking fevers, polyarthralgias, myalgias, an evanescent maculopapular rash with central clearing, and a high erythrocyte sedimentation rate.

# Tests

## Physical Examination
Evaluate the joints for swelling effusion, warmth, decreased range of motion, and adjacent muscle atrophy.

## Diagnostic Tests
The erythrocyte sedimentation rate is often normal. A positive ANA test indicates a tendency for uveitis.

# Differential Diagnosis
Leukemia (night pain, bone pain more than joint pain or effusion)

Osteomyelitis (fever, more severe pain)

Septic arthritis (fever, single joint involvement, more severe pain and effusion)

# Adverse Outcomes of the Disease
Spontaneous remission is common, but end-stage arthritis may occur. Blindness may develop with untreated uveitis.

# Treatment
NSAIDs are the mainstay of treatment. Other medications, such as methotrexate, are used if synovitis is persistent. Etanercept is approved for use in children and is effective in treating refractory polyarticular JRA. Anti-interleukin 6 currently is used for systemic JRA. Intra-articular injection of corticsteroids is effective in the treatment of pauciarticular JRA.

Splinting and orthotics help maintain functional joint alignment. Physical therapy is helpful in maintaining joint motion and strength when the pain has diminished. Regular ophthalmologic slit lamp examinations for uveitis are necessary, with the frequency of this examination dependent on the type of JRA, results on ANA test, and age of the child.

# Adverse Outcomes of Treatment
NSAIDs can cause gastric, renal, or hepatic complications. The use of methotrexate requires monitoring of hepatic function every 3 months and symptomatic relief of centrally induced nausea. Prior to the use of etanercept, reactive purified protein derivative skin evaluation is indicated because susceptibility to infection is of concern.

# Referral Decisions/Red Flags

Failure of NSAIDs, splinting, and physical therapy to relieve symptoms indicates the need for further evaluation. Persistent active synovitis also is an indication that the patient needs additional evaluation.

# KYPHOSIS

## SYNONYMS
Juvenile kyphosis
Postural round back
Scheuermann disease

**ICD-9 Codes**

**732.0**
Scheuermann disease

**737.0**
Postural kyphosis

## DEFINITION
Kyphosis is a curvature of the sagittal plane of the spinal column. It originates from the Greek word *kyphos*, meaning "hump backed," and refers to a curve pointing backward (the apex of the curve is posterior). The normal thoracic spine has a kyphosis of 20° to 40° (Cobb angle measured from T5 to T12). Kyphosis measuring between 40° and 50° is considered borderline normal. Any kyphosis greater than 50° is considered hyperkyphosis. Conditions associated with kyphosis in children are listed in the differential diagnosis.

Postural kyphosis and Scheuermann disease are the most common causes of hyperkyphosis in children. Both conditions present during adolescence. Postural kyphosis is more common in girls, and Scheuermann disease is more common in boys. The kyphosis usually is more severe in Scheuermann disease, but radiographs are necessary to differentiate these disorders. By definition, Scheuermann disease has irregularities of the vertebral end plates, and more than 5° of anterior wedging must be observed in at least three successive vertebra.

## CLINICAL SYMPTOMS
Most patients are seen because of either poor posture or poor posture with back pain. When present, the pain usually is activity related and relieved by rest.

## TESTS

### Physical Examination
The Adams forward bend test is the best way to profile the kyphosis. This test is done by viewing the child from the side. Children with Scheuermann disease and other pathologic causes of kyphosis usually have sharp angulation in the spine, whereas patients with postural kyphosis have a more normal spinal profile (**Figure 1**). Patients with postural kyphosis have normal flexibility (ie, the spine flattens in the supine position).

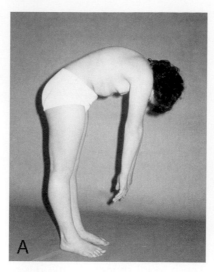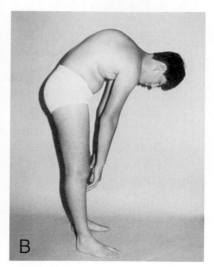

**Figure 1**

Adams forward bend test. **A,** Normal spine profile. **B,** Angulated spine profile seen in a patient with Scheuermann disease.

Reproduced with permission from Staheli L (ed): *Pediatric Orthopaedic Secrets.* Philadelphia, PA, Hanley & Belfus, Inc, 1998, p 286.

## Diagnostic Tests

Weight-bearing AP and lateral radiographs of the spine should be obtained. The x-ray tube should be positioned 6' from the patient, preferably with a 14″ x 36″ film and a grid. The patient's breasts and gonads should be shielded when possible. Look for bony abnormalities, including congenital abnormalities.

Measure curve magnitude on the lateral radiograph using the Cobb method. The upper thoracic vertebrae may not be well visualized; therefore, by definition, kyphosis is measured from T5 to T12. The angle is a line drawn along the superior end plate of T5 and a line drawn on the inferior end plate of T12. Any curvature exceeding 50° is considered abnormal.

## DIFFERENTIAL DIAGNOSIS

Congenital (hemivertebra or anterior failure of segmentation)

Iatrogenic (eg, after laminectomy)

Juvenile rheumatoid arthritis (severe systemic juvenile rheumatoid arthritis requiring prolonged steroids)

Neurofibromatosis (café au lait spots, subcutaneous neurofibromas, inguinal and/or axillary freckling)

Neuromuscular (cerebral palsy, poliomyelitis)

Pathologic fracture (leukemia, Gaucher disease, thalassemia, osteogenesis imperfecta, juvenile osteoporosis, and any condition requiring prolonged use of steroids)

Tuberculosis (Pott disease)

## ADVERSE OUTCOMES OF THE DISEASE

Scheuermann kyphosis can progress to significant deformities. Respiratory function, however, is not affected until the curve is well over 100°. Congenital kyphosis may cause stretch and dysfunction of the spinal cord.

## TREATMENT

Postural kyphosis can be observed or treated with an exercise program. Scheuermann kyphosis in a skeletally immature patient requires brace treatment and possibly spinal fusion, if the condition is severe. Bracing is not effective in patients with congenital deformities, and progressive deformities often require surgical management.

## ADVERSE OUTCOMES OF TREATMENT

Bracing may fail to prevent progression. Surgical treatment may be complicated by pseudarthrosis, wound infection, pneumonia, and/or spinal cord injury.

## REFERRAL DECISIONS/RED FLAGS

Patients with Scheuermann kyphosis or any type of congenital kyphotic deformity require further evaluation.

# LEGG-CALVÉ-PERTHES DISEASE

**ICD-9 Code**

**732.1**
Juvenile osteochondrosis of hip and pelvis

## SYNONYMS

Aseptic necrosis of the femoral head
Avascular necrosis of the femoral head
Idiopathic osteonecrosis of the femoral head

## DEFINITION

Legg-Calvé-Perthes disease (LCPD) is idiopathic osteonecrosis of the femoral head in children. LCPD typically affects children between the ages of 4 and 8 years, but the range of onset is 2 to 12 years of age. It is unilateral in 90% of patients, four times more common in boys, and uncommon in blacks. The prognosis is worse in older children and in those who have more severe involvement (ie, greater degree of osteonecrosis).

After the bone dies and loses structural integrity, the articular surface of the femoral head may collapse, leading to deformity and arthritis. However, because bone repair is relatively rapid in children, the prognosis in LCPD is significantly better when compared with adults who develop osteonecrosis of the femoral head.

## CLINICAL SYMPTOMS

Typically, the child has been limping for 3 to 6 weeks at the initial visit. Activity worsens the limp, making symptoms more noticeable at the end of the day. If the child reports pain, it is typically an aching in the groin or proximal thigh.

## TESTS

### Physical Examination

Examination reveals mild to moderate restriction of hip motion. Abduction, in particular, is limited and typically measures 20° to 30° compared with 60° to 70° on the uninvolved side. However, limited abduction may not be apparent unless movement of the pelvis is recognized. Examine abduction by placing one hand on the opposite pelvis and using the other hand to abduct the hip. The degree of abduction is recorded when the pelvis starts to move or tilt. Another technique is to align the pelvis in neutral and abduct (spread) both extremities.

### Diagnostic Tests

AP and frog-lateral radiographs of the pelvis should be obtained. Increased density of the femoral head is an early sign of LCPD. The crescent sign indicates that a shear fracture has occurred in the subchondral bone (**Figure 1**). In the early stage of LCPD, plain radiographs may be normal, and MRI may be necessary to demonstrate the osteonecrosis. In a child with bilateral involvement, screening AP radiographs of the hand and knee are needed to rule out epiphyseal dysplasia or thyroid disease.

## Differential Diagnosis

Atypical septic arthritis (increasing pain and constitutional symptoms)

Gaucher disease (osteonecrosis secondary to cerebroside and infarcts)

Hypothyroidism (delayed development)

Multiple epiphyseal dysplasia (bilateral, mild short stature, autosomal dominant)

Sickle cell anemia (osteonecrosis secondary to vascular infarcts)

Spondyloepiphyseal dysplasia (bilateral, marked short stature)

Stickler syndrome (bilateral, short stature)

Transient synovitis (pain more noticeable in the morning)

## Adverse Outcomes of the Disease

Residual deformity of the femoral head may progress to osteoarthritis of the hip; however, the onset of severe arthritic symptoms varies ranging from adolescence to the geriatric years. The latter is obviously more common and preferred.

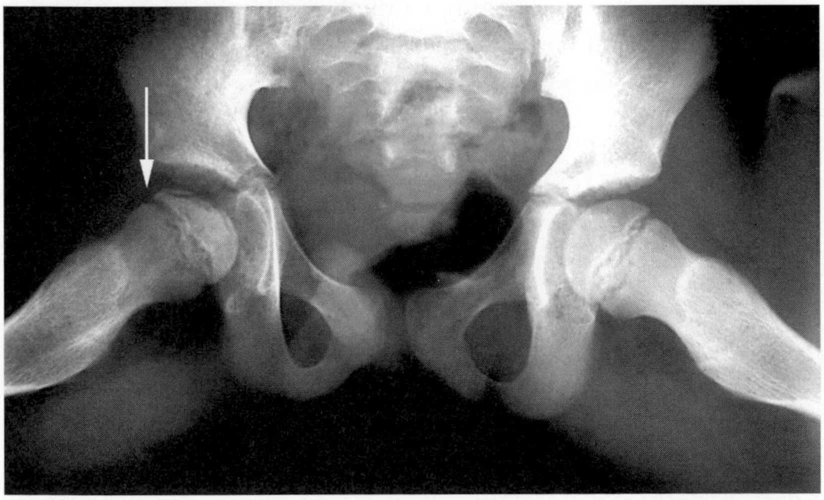

**Figure 1**
Radiograph of a 7-year-old boy with a 2-month history of right hip pain. The subchondral fracture (arrow) is through 75% of the femoral head.
Reproduced from Beaty JH: Legg-Calvé-Perthes disease: Diagnostic and prognostic techniques. *Instr Course Lect* 1989;38:291-296.

# TREATMENT

The physiology of the healing process in LCPD involves revascularization of the femoral head, removal of necrotic bone, and replacement with viable bone that is initially relatively weak (woven bone) and remodeling of woven bone to the normal lamellar bone. While this process occurs more rapidly and with greater consistency in children, it is still a biologic phenomenon that requires many months. Unfortunately, no current interventions accelerate this process. Furthermore, no treatment modality consistently produces good outcomes or prevents deformity of the femoral head.

Observation may be acceptable for children who are unlikely to develop significant deformity. Therefore, observation is commonly indicated for children younger than age 6 years who do not exhibit significant subluxation and who maintain at least 40° to 45° of abduction. Older children who have no involvement of the lateral portion of the femoral head also may be observed.

The principal reason for treatment with an abduction brace is to contain the femoral head within the acetabulum, thus maintaining the femoral head in as much of a spherical state as possible. An abduction brace that extends only to the distal thigh does not alter the natural history of severe LCPD in children who are 6 years of age or younger. As a general rule, osteotomy is reserved for older children. Note that none of these treatment modalities completely contains the femoral head during all phases of gait.

Before any treatment is initiated, motion must be regained. A short period of bed rest and traction is commonly required. The abduction brace is generally worn all day and is discontinued when the lateral portion of the femoral head has regenerated, a process that generally takes 12 to 18 months.

# ADVERSE OUTCOMES OF TREATMENT

No improvement in natural history, postoperative infection, and limb-length discrepancy are all possible.

# REFERRAL DECISIONS/RED FLAGS

Children younger than age 6 years who have significant involvement of the femoral head or less than 40° of abduction require further evaluation. Children age 6 years or older require further evaluation.

# LITTLE LEAGUER ELBOW

## SYNONYMS

Medial epicondylar fracture or avulsion
Olecranon stress fracture
Osteochondritis dissecans of the elbow
Panner disease
Traction apophysitis of the elbow
Valgus-extension overload syndrome

## DEFINITION

Little Leaguer elbow is the name given to several pathologic entities that share a common etiology (overuse in the overhead throwing athlete) and a common age group (range, 8 to 16 years old). This term, however, is too general; it is preferable and more accurate to use the name of specific pathologic entities when possible. These include (1) injuries resulting from traction or tension (eg, traction apophysitis of the medial epicondyle or olecranon, medial epicondylar fragmentation or avulsion, olecranon avulsion, and ulnar collateral ligament sprains or tears) and (2) injuries resulting from compression (eg, osteochondritis dissecans [OCD] of the capitellum and Panner disease) (**Figure 1**).

Traction apophysitis of the medial epicondyle is inflammation or injury to the unfused medial epicondyle that occurs as a result of overuse in the skeletally immature overhead throwing athlete. Fragmentation of the medial epicondyle may occur in the young athlete (age 8 to 12 years), whereas avulsion of the medial epicondyle typically occurs in patients closer to physeal closure (age 12 to 14 years). Traction apophysitis of the olecranon, likewise, is an injury to the unfused olecranon physis in the young throwing athlete. Fragmentation of the olecranon epiphysis is rare, and avulsion is less common than with the medial epicondyle. Delayed or failed closure of the olecranon physis more commonly occurs as a result of overuse and may result in chronic pain.

Injuries of the ulnar collateral ligament are now recognized with alarming frequency in the adolescent overhead throwing athlete. This injury is more completely described in the chapter on ulnar collateral ligament injuries.

OCD occurs in the adolescent age group (typically older than age 12 years) after the capitellum has ossified. This condition is characterized by focal osteonecrosis of the capitellum (but rarely the radial head) with varying degrees of subchondral separation and is frequently associated with overuse in the

SECTION 9 ■ PEDIATRIC ORTHOPAEDICS

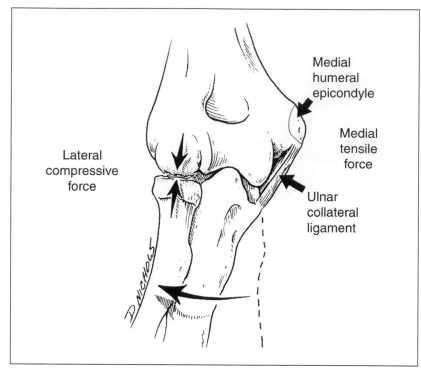

**Figure 1**

Drawing illustrating forces at the elbow: compression on the lateral side and tension on the medial side. Medial forces cause a medial humeral epicondyle stress fracture in the skeletally immature patient rather than an ulnar collateral ligament sprain, as seen in adults.

Reproduced with permission from Andrews JR, Zarins B, Wilk KE (eds): *Injuries in Baseball*. Philadelphia, PA, Lippincott-Raven, 1998.

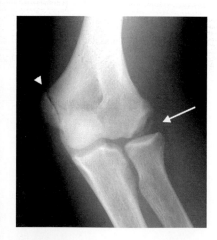

**Figure 2**

AP radiograph of a left-handed baseball pitcher reveals osteochondritis dissecans lesion of the capitellum (arrow) with an open medial humerus epiphysis (arrowhead).

Reproduced from Hutchinson MR, Ireland ML: Overuse and throwing injuries in the skeletally immature patient. *Instr Course Lect* 2003;52:25-36.

thrower (**Figure 2**). Loose body formation is common, leading to mechanical symptoms.

Panner disease, which is often confused with OCD, is seen in children younger than age 12 years and consists of a focal avascular lesion of the capitellum that typically is self-limited with a good prognosis.

# CLINICAL SYMPTOMS

These conditions occur in the young overhead throwing athlete with a history of overuse. There is often a history of an excessive number of pitches per game, excessive number of innings pitched per week (or year), year-round participation in the throwing sport, and the premature use of the breaking ball (curveball or slider) before adequate skeletal maturity. Pain, either chronic or acute, is the most common symptom.

# TESTS

## *Physical Examination*

Tenderness to palpation is the most common physical finding and may be medial (medial epicondylar traction apophysitis, medial epicondylar fragmentation/avulsion, ulnar collateral ligament injuries), lateral (OCD, Panner disease), or posterior (olecranon traction apophysitis/avulsion). Flexion contractures are common, and instability may be seen in ulnar collateral ligament injuries or severe OCD with loss of capitellar lateral bony support.

### Diagnostic Tests

Radiographs of the elbow help to establish most of these diagnoses. In these patients, obtaining a comparison view of the contralateral side is essential to better visualize subtle changes. MRI often is necessary to confirm OCD, Panner disease, and ulnar collateral ligament injuries.

## DIFFERENTIAL DIAGNOSIS

Cubital tunnel syndrome/ulnar neuritis (rarely seen in this age group)

Fractures of the radial head, olecranon, or supracondylar humerus (radiographs differentiate)

Lateral epicondylitis/tendinosis (rarely seen in this age group)

Medial epicondylitis/tendinosis (rarely seen in this age group)

## ADVERSE OUTCOMES OF THE DISEASE

Persistent pain, inability to participate in sports, chronic instability, and loss of motion are possible. Medial epicondylar avulsion may lead to late ulnar palsy. OCD may lead to loose body formation and, in more severe cases, osteoarthritis.

## TREATMENT

Because these conditions technically are overuse injuries, the most critical component of treatment is rest. A period of at least 3 to 6 months of rest from throwing is appropriate for these problems. In OCD, abstaining from pitching for 1 year may be necessary. Physical therapy is helpful during this time to help maintain strength and restore motion. Immobilization should be avoided, except for possible brief periods in the acute phase, given the likelihood of significant and perhaps permanent loss of motion. Unfortunately, even with appropriate rest, the athlete may not be able to resume pitching, and a change in position or sport may be recommended. While nonsurgical care usually is appropriate, surgical intervention is occasionally necessary.

SECTION 9 ■ PEDIATRIC ORTHOPAEDICS

## ADVERSE OUTCOMES OF TREATMENT

Surgery carries a small risk of infection, hardware failure, or neurovascular injury. Despite appropriate treatment, persistent pain and disability may occur.

## REFERRAL DECISIONS/RED FLAGS

Further evaluation is needed if nonsurgical treatment fails.

## PREVENTION

Given the increasing incidence of overuse injuries and the likelihood that results will be suboptimal despite appropriate care, prevention must be emphasized. Education of athletes, parents, and coaches is critical, and governing bodies of youth baseball organizations must be willing to make rule changes for the long-term benefit of these athletes. Year-round pitching should be avoided, and participation in baseball showcases should be restricted. Participation in other sports should be encouraged. General physical conditioning and proper pitching mechanics should be emphasized. Current recommendations for pitchers are given in **Tables 1** and **2**.

| Table 1 | Recommended Ages for Learning Various Pitches |
|---|---|
| **Pitch** | **Recommended Age (Years)** |
| Changeup | 11 to 12, or when sufficient velocity and control have been developed with the fastball |
| Curveball | 14.5 |
| Slider | 18 |

| Table 2 | Recommended Pitching Limits | |
|---|---|---|
| **Age (Years)** | **Maximum Number of Pitches Thrown per Game** | **Maximum Number of Innings Pitched per Week** |
| 8 to 10 | 50 | 6 |
| 11 to 14 | 75 | 6 |
| 15 to 18 | 90 to 100 | 10 |

# METATARSUS ADDUCTUS

## SYNONYM

Metatarsus varus

**ICD-9 Code**
**754.53**
Metatarsus varus

## DEFINITION

Metatarsus adductus is a common congenital deformity characterized by medial deviation (adduction) of the forefoot (**Figure 1**). In one prospective study, the deformity was observed in 13% of full-term infants. Metatarsus adductus often resolves spontaneously, but it may persist.

## CLINICAL SYMPTOMS

Symptoms are absent during infancy. Parental concern typically initiates evaluation.

## TESTS

### Physical Examination

The most striking feature is convexity of the lateral border of the foot. The hindfoot is in neutral or increased valgus and never demonstrates a varus posture. Normal ankle dorsiflexion is also present. These latter two findings are important because

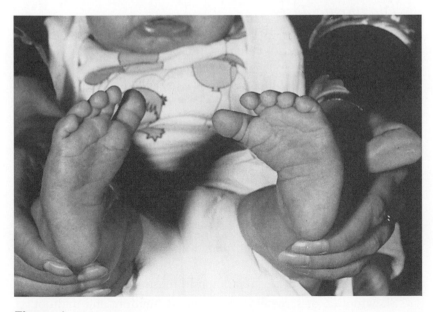

**Figure 1**

Three-month-old infant with obvious metatarsus adductus. The foot appears to be supinated; however, when the foot was placed in a weight-bearing position, the hindfoot alignment was normal.

Reproduced from Greene WB: Metatarsus adductus and skewfoot. *Instr Course Lect* 1994;43:161-177.

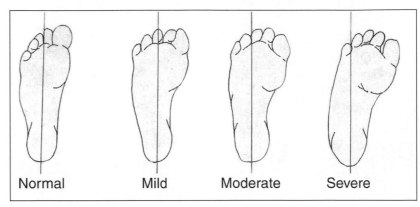

**Figure 2**

Classification of metatarsus adductus as described by Bleck.

Reproduced with permission from Bleck EE: Metatarsus adductus: Classification and relationship to all kinds of treatment. *J Pediatr Orthop* 1983;3:2-9.

some children with severe metatarsus adductus may, at first inspection, appear to have a clubfoot deformity.

The severity of metatarsus adductus can be assessed using the heel bisector line (**Figure 2**). Normally, a line bisecting the heel crosses the forefoot between the second and third toes. Metatarsus adductus is considered mild when the heel bisector crosses the third toe, moderate when the heel bisector goes between the third and fourth toes, and severe when the heel bisector crosses between the fourth and fifth toes. Flexibility of the forefoot should be assessed, and perhaps the simplest criteria is to define a flexible foot as one in which the second toe can easily be brought in line with the heel bisector.

## Diagnostic Tests

Radiographs are rarely needed, but stress views can be useful in differentiating this condition from an atypical clubfoot. Obtaining serial photocopies of the foot is a low-cost, no-risk method of charting the progression of metatarsus adductus (**Figure 3**).

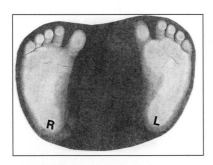

**Figure 3**

Photocopy of feet of a 9-month-old infant with bilateral metatarsus adductus.

Reproduced from Greene WB: Metatarsus adductus and skewfoot. *Instr Course Lect* 1994;43:161-177.

# DIFFERENTIAL DIAGNOSIS

Cavus foot (high arch, heel in varus)

Clubfoot (heel in varus, ankle in equinus)

Hyperactive abductor hallucis ("monkey toe," lateral border of the foot straight)

Internal tibial torsion (foot rotated in; lateral border of the foot straight)

Skeletal dysplasia (most common in diastrophic dwarfism)

Skewfoot (Z or serpentine foot; valgus hindfoot and midfoot, severe forefoot adduction)

# ADVERSE OUTCOMES OF THE DISEASE

Abnormal shoe wear and subsequent discomfort with prolonged standing are possible. Some children are emotionally stressed when teased about their foot alignment.

# TREATMENT

Most newborns are not treated, although parents are advised to avoid positioning the infant prone with the feet turned in, a position that accentuates metatarsus adductus. Because metatarsus adductus corrects spontaneously in most children, the decision to begin treatment may be delayed until the infant is 6 months old; however, it is reasonable to initiate treatment earlier if the deformity is severe and inflexible.

Stretching exercises done by the parents, and the use of nighttime splints or outflare shoes, have not been proved effective. The reports advocating these modalities have included younger patients whose metatarsus adductus may have resolved spontaneously.

Serial casting is the gold standard of nonsurgical management, and if started at age 6 to 9 months, has a high degree of success. Casts are applied for 2-week periods, and usually three or four casts will suffice. Casting can be successful in children ages 1 to 3 years, but at these ages, casting is more difficult and is associated with a higher rate of failure. The cast should be applied in a manner that molds the forefoot into abduction without accentuating heel valgus. A long leg cast is probably more effective.

Surgical treatment has limited indications.

# ADVERSE OUTCOMES OF TREATMENT

Recurrent deformity may occur despite serial casting. Exacerbating heel valgus while casting may result in development of a severe flatfoot or skewfoot deformity. Degenerative changes at the tarsometatarsal joints have been noted after a complete tarsometatarsal surgical release. Damage to the physis of the first metatarsal and subsequent shortening of that bone is the unique complication of correcting metatarsus adductus by metatarsal osteotomies.

# REFERRAL DECISIONS/RED FLAGS

Residual metatarsus adductus in an infant age 6 months or a rigid metatarsus adductus in an infant older than age 3 months signals the need for further evaluation.

SECTION 9 ■ PEDIATRIC ORTHOPAEDICS

# Neonatal Brachial Plexus Palsy

## Synonym
Obstetrical palsy

## Definition
Neonatal brachial plexus palsy, sometimes called obstetrical palsy, is a motor and sensory deficit of the upper extremity that results from a stretch injury to the brachial plexus during labor and delivery. Three patterns of palsy may occur: Erb palsy, Klumpke palsy, and pan plexus palsy. Erb palsy is most common and is defined as a lesion involving the upper portion of the brachial plexus. An Erb palsy primarily affecting C5 and C6 results in weakness of elbow flexion and weakness of shoulder abduction, flexion, and external rotation. If the Erb palsy includes C7, then wrist flexion and elbow extension also are affected. Klumpke palsy is a lesion of the lower plexus that affects primarily the hand and wrist. Pan plexus palsy is involvement of the entire plexus.

The injury can range from a minor stretch of the nerves to a partial or complete rupture of the nerve substance or to an avulsion of the nerve root from the spinal cord. Prognosis for neurologic recovery depends on the severity of the injury. With a mild injury, nerve signal transmission is interrupted temporarily, but the nerve structure itself is not disrupted. Recovery is complete with this type of injury.

The prognosis is poorer with disruption of nerve substance (ie, axon, sheath, or supporting connective tissue), and these infants are likely to have some degree of permanent impairment. Most patients have a "mixed" lesion, with different nerve branches having different degrees of neural disruption.

## Clinical Symptoms
Irritability in the supraclavicular triangle may be present during the first few weeks after birth.

## Tests

### Physical Examination
Examination findings vary depending on the pattern of nerve injury and include diminished movement and sensation in the upper extremity. Initially, the upper extremity appears to be flail. The classic appearance of a neonate with Erb palsy is the "waiter's tip" position (ie, shoulder adducted and internally rotated, elbow extended, forearm pronated, and wrist flexed) (**Figure 1**). A Horner sign can appear in lower plexus lesions. Phrenic nerve paralysis occurs in approximately 5% of patients.

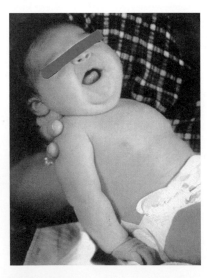

**Figure 1**
Typical posture ("waiter's tip" position) of child with Erb palsy.

Repeated examinations of muscle and sensory function are needed to correlate the physical findings with an anatomic location of injury and to assess the degree and rate of neurologic recovery. Failure to recover muscle balance results in contractures and limited motion, particularly at the shoulder and elbow.

*Diagnostic Tests*
Radiographs should be ordered if results of physical examination suggest a fracture of the clavicle or humerus. If the infant does not recover full function, electromyography and nerve conduction velocity studies may help guide decision making for surgical options. These studies are best obtained by the surgeon who can direct specific questions to the electromyographer.

# DIFFERENTIAL DIAGNOSIS

Clavicle fracture (tenderness and deformity on palpation, pain on passive range of motion, possible pseudoparalysis)

Humerus fracture (swelling, deformity, and pain with range of motion of the arm, possible pseudoparalysis)

Proximal humeral osteomyelitis (cessation of normal motion, but infant may not appear toxic)

Septic shoulder joint (cessation of normal motion, but infant may not appear toxic)

# ADVERSE OUTCOMES OF THE DISEASE

The prognosis varies depending on the severity of the neurologic injury. A good prognosis correlates with early spontaneous recovery of function. Joint contractures and limited motion develop if the patient has significant muscle weakness. In children with Erb palsy, muscle imbalance also can result in posterior dislocation of the shoulder and/or radial head instability.

# TREATMENT

Initial treatment consists of a 3-month program designed to rest and then stretch the muscles while awaiting spontaneous recovery. During the first month, management focuses on protecting the injured extremity. Careful examination and documentation of the initial functional deficit allow for an accurate assessment of the amount and timing of later recovery. After the first month, gentle passive range of motion is needed several times a day to stretch the strong muscles and to move the joints through a full range of motion. Special attention to external rotation of the shoulder with the flexed elbow at the side will help prevent posterior subluxation of the shoulder.

During the third month, the infant should be reexamined to document recovery of muscle function. Additional evaluation is appropriate at this time for those infants who do not recover palpable function in all muscle groups.

No single treatment predictably restores full function. Therefore, accurate assessment of the level and severity of injury, prevention of secondary deformity, and a plan to optimize recovery and ultimately the functional outcome for the child are the cornerstones of treatment.

Recent advances in intraoperative electrodiagnostic testing and microsurgical techniques have led to a greater interest in early surgical treatment. The dilemma is that some spontaneous recovery will be sacrificed if surgery is done too early, but a longer period of observation may compromise potential results. Furthermore, there is no true repair of these lesions, and the neural reconstruction is a complex process of nerve grafts and nerve transfers. Determining whether an early operation alters the natural history of recovery, and which procedure is best, is difficult to measure and is still being assessed.

Early plexus surgery is an option for certain carefully evaluated infants because it may improve the level of ultimate recovery. An infant who has plateaued in recovery without regaining palpable elbow flexion, shoulder abduction, or external rotation by age 4 to 6 months should be considered for plexus exploration. An infant who has a pan plexus palsy has a poor prognosis for recovery of hand function and should be considered for plexus exploration even earlier than 4 to 6 months.

Children ages 2 to 4 years with significant muscle imbalance about the shoulder, elbow, and hand should undergo appropriate muscle releases and tendon transfers to provide a balanced upper extremity. Earlier procedures may be indicated if shoulder dislocation or significant contracture occurs.

## ADVERSE OUTCOMES OF TREATMENT

Neurologic deficit may not improve after surgical treatment. Bony deformities can develop and progress despite tendon transfers. Diminished overall growth potential of the extremity may occur.

## REFERRAL DECISIONS/RED FLAGS

If full recovery does not occur within 3 to 4 months, further evaluation is recommended. Sepsis or skeletal trauma (child abuse) must be suspected if there is sudden loss of function in an extremity that moved well at birth.

# OSGOOD-SCHLATTER DISEASE

## SYNONYMS

Osteochondritis of the inferior patella
Osteochondritis of the tibial tuberosity
Tibial tubercle traction apophysitis

**ICD-9 Code**
**732.4**
Osgood-Schlatter disease

## DEFINITION

Osgood-Schlatter disease (or condition) is an overuse injury that
occurs in the growing child. It results from repetitive stress
where a too-tight quadriceps "pulls" on the apophysis
(secondary ossification center) of the tibial tubercle during a
time of rapid growth (approximately age 11 to 13 years).
Overuse explains the fivefold greater incidence in patients who
are active in sports and the two to three times greater incidence
in boys. Sinding-Larsen-Johansson disease is a similar disorder
that occurs at the junction of the patellar tendon and the distal
pole of the patella.

## CLINICAL SYMPTOMS

Patients report pain that is exacerbated by running, jumping,
and kneeling activities. Pain also can occur after prolonged
sitting with the knees flexed.

## TESTS

### Physical Examination

Examination reveals tenderness and swelling at the insertion of the
patellar tendon into the tibial tubercle in Osgood-Schlatter disease
and at the inferior pole of the patella in Sinding-Larsen-Johansson
disease. These conditions may occur in both knees simultaneously,
but one side may be more symptomatic. Although knee motion
usually is not restricted, kneeling is painful during the acute phase.
The knee and patellofemoral joints are stable.

### Diagnostic Tests

AP and lateral radiographs of the knee may be normal or show
soft-tissue swelling. In Osgood-Schlatter disease, small spicules of
heterotopic ossification may be seen anterior to the tibial
tuberosity (**Figure 1**). In Sinding-Larsen-Johansson disease,
elongation of the inferior pole of the patella may be apparent,
along with "fragmentation" in the area, caused by repetitive stress
on the growth center. When a patient has bilateral symptoms,
radiographs are rarely needed, but they should be obtained with
unilateral involvement to rule out tumors.

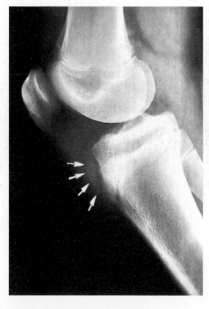

**Figure 1**
Radiograph showing symptomatic
tibial tubercle ossicle (arrows)
in a 13-year-old boy with Osgood-
Schlatter disease.

Reproduced from Stanitski CL: Knee overuse
disorders in the pediatric and adolescent athlete.
*Instr Course Lect* 1993;42:483-495.

SECTION 9 ■ PEDIATRIC ORTHOPAEDICS

## DIFFERENTIAL DIAGNOSIS

Infection (rare, elevated erythrocyte sedimentation rate)
Neoplasm (rare, unilateral)

## ADVERSE OUTCOMES OF THE DISEASE

The long-term prognosis for patients who undergo nonsurgical treatment is good, with minimal adult disability. Some residual prominence of the tibial tubercle is common, particularly in patients who have fragmentation of the epiphysis and heterotopic ossification during the active phase of the disease. These patients occasionally report discomfort when walking.

Rarely, an avulsion fracture through the tibial apophysis can occur with activity in symptomatic patients; therefore, these patients require rest from activity.

## TREATMENT

Symptoms are often controlled adequately with intermittent use of ice after sports, coupled with occasional use of NSAIDs, use of a protective knee pad, and stretching exercises. Decreasing exercise for the muscles of the lower extremity to permit healing of the microscopic avulsion fractures is the key to treating severe symptoms.

Occasionally, immobilization is needed for severe or recalcitrant symptoms. This usually can be accomplished with a prefabricated knee immobilizer that is removed once a day for bathing and range-of-motion exercises.

Another important aspect in management is helping the parents and patient understand the anticipated duration that sports activities may be restricted. In patients with Osgood-Schlatter disease, activity may need to be discontinued or modified for an average of 2 to 3 months or more or until symptoms subside.

Surgical treatment is not commonly needed except in the rare case of an avulsion of the ossification center or for excising a heterotopic ossification over the tibial tubercle.

## ADVERSE OUTCOMES OF TREATMENT

These are the same as the adverse outcomes of the disease. Rarely, avulsion fracture of the tibial tubercle can occur if children continue to participate in activity, despite significant pain.

## REFERRAL DECISIONS/RED FLAGS

Unilateral pain at rest or pain not directly over the tibial tubercle should raise concerns of a neoplastic or another disorder.

# OSTEOCHONDRAL LESIONS OF THE TALUS

## SYNONYMS

Osteochondral fracture
Osteochondritis dissecans

ICD-9 Code

**733.44**
Aseptic necrosis of bone, talus

## DEFINITION

Osteochondral lesions of the hyaline cartilage and underlying subchondral bone of the weight-bearing surface of the talus may occur acutely after trauma (osteochondral fracture) or may develop secondary to idiopathic subchondral avascularity (osteochondritis dissecans [OCD] of the talus), appearing similarly to OCD of the knee. These abnormalities may cause fissuring and collapse of the joint surface of the talus, delamination of joint cartilage from the underlying bone, loose fragment formation, and hyaline cartilage defects within the ankle joint.

## CLINICAL SYMPTOMS

Patients present with ankle pain, swelling or recurrent effusion, a sensation of catching or popping, or occasional giving way. The symptoms may occur acutely after an injury or intermittently with vigorous activities over a period of weeks to months. A history of frequent ankle swelling, often misdiagnosed as a chronic ankle sprain, is not uncommon.

## TESTS

### Physical Examination

Examination of the ankle reveals limited, painful active and passive range of motion, a palpable effusion, and tenderness along the anterior joint line. Ligamentous stress testing and subtalar joint mobility are normal.

### Diagnostic Tests

Mortise views of the ankle reveal an articular surface defect surrounded by a halo of lucent bone on the weight-bearing surface of the talus. Acute osteochondral lesions are often smaller and wafer-shaped on the lateral talus, whereas more chronic OCD lesions are deeper and cup-shaped on the posteromedial talus. CT is useful for staging of medial lesions (**Figure 1**). MRI best defines the extent of the cartilage surface disruption and its adjacent subchondral avascularity. Synovial fluid visualized between the OCD lesion and the adjacent bone of the talar body suggests an unstable lesion with little healing potential.

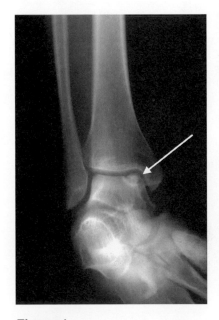

**Figure 1**
AP mortise radiograph of the ankle shows nondisplaced osteochondritis of the talus (arrow).

# DIFFERENTIAL DIAGNOSIS

Acute osteochondral fracture (acute onset, hemarthrosis, pain)

Erosive osteomyelitis (rare) (subacute, joint effusion, pain with motion)

Neoplasm (rare) (insidious onset, night pain, joint swelling)

Osteochondral dissecans lesion of the talus (indolent onset, pain, swelling, locking of the ankle joint)

Osteonecrosis of the talus (joint surface collapse from previous trauma, steroid use, sickle cell disease, delayed onset, decreased ankle motion)

Septic arthritis of the ankle with resultant chondrolysis (rare) (pain, postinfection progressive decrease in ankle motion)

# ADVERSE OUTCOMES OF THE DISEASE

Long-term complications include ankle pain, stiffness, synovitis of the ankle joint, and premature osteoarthritis.

# TREATMENT

Patients who have not reached skeletal maturity have the capacity to heal and should be evaluated for healing potential with immobilization. Adolescents approaching skeletal maturity have a limited capacity for healing.

# ADVERSE OUTCOMES OF TREATMENT

When large lesions fail to heal, loose body formation and osteoarthritis of the ankle joint may develop.

# REFERRAL DECISIONS/RED FLAGS

Osteochondral lesions are best treated with early intervention and thus require early referral.

# OSTEOMYELITIS

## DEFINITION

Osteomyelitis is an infection in bone that is usually bacterial in origin. In children, osteomyelitis usually develops as a result of hematogenous seeding but can be secondary to direct contamination (eg, open fracture, nail puncture wound).

The metaphysis of long bones is the most common location of osteomyelitis in children because the circulation is sluggish at the metaphyseal-physeal barrier, where small vessels are required to make a "U-turn." Untreated, the infection spreads through the medullary canal and penetrates the metaphyseal cortex causing a subperiosteal abscess. The growth plate usually is not penetrated. Acute osteomyelitis presents within 2 weeks of disease onset and is the main focus of this chapter.

Subacute osteomyelitis is a more balanced response between host and organism that results in a quasicontained lesion in the bone and typically presents after 1 month to several months. The diagnosis is often delayed because symptoms are often vague and other findings such as fever and abnormal laboratory studies are not remarkable. There are two types of subacute osteomyelitis. Cavitary subacute osteomyelitis occurs in the epiphysis or metaphysis and is characterized by a small, localized area of radiolucency surrounded by reactive bone. In cavitary osteomyelitis, cultures are often negative and similar to diskitis. Initial treatment may be a 6-week trial of oral antibiotics. The second type of subacute osteomyelitis simulates a neoplastic process and, therefore, mandates a biopsy with or without débridement. These lesions typically are in the diaphysis but also may be metaphyseal. Periosteal elevation and cortical thickening are the early radiographic signs.

Chronic osteomyelitis is characterized by necrotic bone harboring bacteria (sequestrum).

## CLINICAL SYMPTOMS

Pain, swelling, tenderness, erythema, increased localized warmth, and generalized malaise are associated with acute osteomyelitis. When the lower extremity, pelvis, or spine is involved, refusal to walk or limping is an early symptom, particularly in a young child. Pseudoparalysis (failure to use a limb despite normal neuromuscular structures) is observed when the upper extremity is affected.

---

**ICD-9 Codes**

**730.00**
Acute osteomyelitis, site unspecified

**731.00**
Chronic osteomyelitis, site unspecified

SECTION 9 ■ PEDIATRIC ORTHOPAEDICS

# Tests

## Physical Examination

An elevated temperature of 100.4°F (38°C) or higher is typical but not always present. Tenderness is common in the involved region. Motion of the adjacent joint may be limited, but not to the degree observed in septic arthritis. Other sites of infection such as cellulitis and septic arthritis should be investigated.

## Diagnostic Tests

Laboratory studies should include a CBC with differential and erythrocyte sedimentation rate, as these tests confirm an inflammatory process and are parameters in monitoring response to treatment. A C-reactive protein is a better test for monitoring early response to treatment, but whether this study is helpful at diagnosis is unclear. Neonates and children who are seen early in the disease process may not have an abnormal WBC, elevated erythrocyte sedimentation rate, or significant fever. A blood culture should be obtained, as it will identify the infecting organism in 40% to 50% of patients.

AP and lateral radiographs of the suspected area are necessary. Early in the disease process, radiographs are normal or show only soft-tissue swelling, but negative radiographs help in ruling out a fracture or neoplastic process. Seven to 10 days after the onset of symptoms, osseous changes are apparent and include periosteal elevation and/or destruction of bone with areas of radiolucency and no surrounding reactive bone.

Although not often needed in acute osteomyelitis, MRI or a bone scan should be considered in unclear situations. MRI is more definitive but more expensive. Ultrasound may show an area of periosteal elevation and provide direction for aspiration.

Aspiration should be done if the area of potential bone involvement is identified, the site is accessible, and a neoplastic process has been ruled out. A 20-gauge or larger bore needle and syringe should be used to obtain the specimen. Positive results can confirm the diagnosis, and the specimen can help guide antibiotic therapy through evaluation of a Gram stain and the subsequent results of culture.

# Differential Diagnosis

Acute leukemia (indolent onset, diffuse tenderness, night pain)
Acute rheumatic fever (migratory arthralgia)
Cellulitis (erythema and swelling of subcutaneous tissues)
Langerhans cell histiocytosis (pain, "hole in a bone" appearance)
Malignant bone tumors (Ewing sarcoma most often simulates osteomyelitis)
Septic arthritis (joint swelling and severe restriction of motion)

# ADVERSE OUTCOMES OF THE DISEASE

Growth disturbance and limb-length discrepancy, chronic osteomyelitis, destruction of adjacent joints, pathologic fracture, and bone defects leading to limb dysfunction are possible.

# TREATMENT

Intravenous antibiotic should be started immediately after obtaining initial diagnostic tests and cultures. *Staphylococcus aureus* is the most common pathogen, and antibiotic selection should cover this organism in all age groups. Antibiotic selection should also cover Group B streptococci and enteric rod organisms in neonates. In children ages 6 months to 4 years, *Haemophilus influenzae* is also covered if vaccination is incomplete.

Frequently, when the patient is seen approximately 4 to 7 days after onset, or the abscess or symptoms persist despite antibiotic therapy, surgical drainage is needed. Surgery for acute osteomyelitis consists primarily of drainage of the subperiosteal abscess. In chronic osteomyelitis, resection of necrotic and avascular tissue is required.

The typical course of antibiotics is 6 weeks but may be longer depending on clinical response and laboratory values. The indication and time to switch from intravenous to oral antibiotics is controversial at present, but an early change to oral medication (after up to 7 days of intravenous therapy) is feasible in many patients, particularly those who present early.

Immobilization of the affected bone decreases pain and should continue for 3 weeks or more to assist the healing process and protect against pathologic fracture. The bone is weaker not only from osseous destruction, but the woven bone that is initially formed in the healing process does not have the same strength as lamellar bone.

Osteomyelitis secondary to nail puncture wounds usually is caused by *Pseudomonas aeruginosa*. This infection requires surgical débridement and antibiotic therapy for 2 to 3 weeks. Failure to débride this infection adequately can lead to chronic osteomyelitis that is difficult to eradicate. A shorter course of antibiotics may be acceptable if the contaminated area is small and can be aggressively débrided.

# ADVERSE OUTCOMES OF TREATMENT

These are the same as the adverse outcomes of the disease.

# REFERRAL DECISIONS/RED FLAGS

A team approach provides the best management of osteomyelitis.

SECTION 9 ■ PEDIATRIC ORTHOPAEDICS

# PEDIATRIC SPORT PARTICIPATION

Sports participation during childhood offers a number of potential benefits that lead to lifelong habits of fitness. Children develop specific skills, learn the importance of teamwork, acquire leadership skills, and develop confidence. All of these attributes result in improved self-esteem. Physical activity also provides an appropriate outlet for releasing stress.

It is important to help children choose an activity routine that is fun, developmentally appropriate, and realistic given individual, family, and community resources. One way to create exercise prescriptions for adults is to use the mnemonic FITT, which stands for frequency, intensity, time (duration), and type of activity. This can be useful for creating a physical activity prescription for children as well.

Suggestions for increasing physical activity can include walking or bicycling for transportation and planning physical activity rather than sedentary activities with friends. Many adolescents, especially girls, may not be active because they think organized sports are the only type of exercise that "counts." Therefore, it is important to help adolescents identify the physical activity they may already be getting (eg, walking), as well as to reinforce the benefits of other lifetime activities such as bicycling, dancing, skating, and swimming.

Potential disadvantages of organized sports include burnout, injuries, and an overemphasis on winning. Adults who lead children's sports activities sometimes forget that sports should be for the child and should be fun (**Table 1**).

Children are not merely small adults. They have unique needs that must be considered. For example, children are more heat sensitive than adults and tend not to drink enough. They rarely will admit that they are tired. Therefore, practices should be scheduled during the cooler hours of the day and include adequate breaks. Adults in charge should ensure that adequate amounts of fluids that children like to drink are readily available and encouraged.

### Table 1  Reasons Children Want to Play Sports

| | |
|---|---|
| To have fun | To make new friends |
| To improve their skills | To succeed or win |
| To learn new skills | To become physically fit |
| To be with their friends | |

Reproduced from Landry GL: Benefits of sports participation, in Sullivan JA, Anderson SJ (eds): *Care of the Young Athlete*. Rosemont, IL, American Academy of Orthopaedic Surgeons, pp 1-8.

# Readiness for Sports Participation

Overall readiness must be based on the individual child and his or her eagerness to participate, not the parents' desire. A variety of sport activities should be offered, and the child should be allowed to choose.

The attrition rate for youth sport participation is 35% annually. Many athletes drop out because of burnout, not being able to participate, or because they are not matched to their level of skill. **Table 2** lists the developmental skills for sports and sports recommendations during childhood.

Motor development in infants and toddlers is limited, but aquatic programs for infants and toddlers are popular. A recent policy statement developed by the American Academy of Pediatrics noted that children generally are not developmentally ready for swimming lessons until after their fourth birthday and that aquatic programs for infants and toddlers have not been shown to decrease the risk of drowning.

Children 3 to 5 years of age have developed the fundamental skills of crawling, walking, jumping, and running. Vision, however, is relatively imprecise. Children at this age have difficulty tracking moving objects. Therefore, "keeping their eye on the ball" will be difficult. Furthermore, children in this age group have very short attention spans and are egocentric in their learning. Appropriate activities for this age include running, tumbling and throwing, but team and competitive sports are inappropriate.

Children between the ages of 6 and 10 years begin transitional skill development. Prior to this age they could throw, but now they are ready to work on accuracy. Some children at this age are very proficient; others are not. At about age 7 to 8 years, children begin to communicate and cooperate as a group effort; however, their attention span is still limited. Team sports in this group should be modified to ensure that practices are short and fun and that skills instruction is limited to 10 to 20 minutes. Include egocentric activities to practice the material taught. Modify the rules to stress high scoring and full participation.

Adolescents can develop complex sport skills that require rapid decision making. Certainly for some children, waiting until adolescence to become involved in competitive sports that require complex skills and interactions, such as football, wrestling, hockey, and basketball, prevents the burnout that occurs when these sports are pushed on the child at an earlier age. Adolescents also have fairly good attention spans, so chalk talks and the like can be used with this group.

SECTION 9 ■ PEDIATRIC ORTHOPAEDICS

## Table 2   Developmental Skills and Sports Recommendations During Childhood

**Early Childhood (2 to 5 years)**

Motor skills

  Limited fundamental skills

  Limited balance skills

Learning

  Extremely short attention span

  Poor selective attention

  Egocentric learning (trial and error)

  Visual and auditory cues are important

Vision

  Not fully mature before ages 6 to 7 (farsighted)

  Difficulty tracking and judging velocity of moving objects

Sports recommendations

  Emphasize fundamental skills with minimal variation and limited instruction

  Emphasize fun, playfulness, exploration, and experimentation rather than competition

  Activities: Running, swimming, tumbling, throwing, catching

**Middle Childhood (6 to 9 years)**

Motor skills

  Continued improvement in fundamental skills

  Posture and balance become more automatic

  Improved reaction times

  Beginning transitional skills

Learning

  Short attention span

  Limited development of memory and rapid decision making

Vision

  Improved tracking

  Limited directionality

Sports recommendations

  Emphasize fundamental skills and beginning transitional skills

  Flexible rules of sports

  Allow free time in practices

  Short instruction time

  Minimal competition

  Activities: Entry-level soccer and baseball

**Table 2 Developmental Skills and Sports Recommendations During Childhood (Continued)**

**Late Childhood (10 to 12 years)**

Motor skills

  Improved transitional skills

  Ability to master complex motor skills

  Temporary decline in balance control at puberty

Learning

  Selective attention

  Able to use memory strategies for sports such as football and basketball

Vision

  Adult patterns

Sports recommendations

  Emphasis on skill development

  Increasing emphasis on tactics and strategy

  Emphasize factors promoting continued participation

  Activities: Entry-level for complex skill sports (eg, football, basketball)

(Adapted with permission from Nelson MA: Developmental skills and children's sports. *Physician Sportsmed* 1991;19:67-97.)

SECTION 9 ■ PEDIATRIC ORTHOPAEDICS

# PREPARTICIPATION PHYSICAL EVALUATION

## DEFINITION

Although it is not intended to substitute for a routine annual physical examination, the preparticipation physical evaluation (PPE) is often the only contact an older child or adolescent has with a physician. Therefore, this examination should be as comprehensive as possible.

The PPE has a number of goals, as listed below:

1. Identify conditions that would predispose children to serious injury or death.
2. Identify current medical or psychological conditions that could be worsened by exercise.
3. Diagnose previously undetected conditions.
4. Assess general health and risk-taking behaviors.
5. Satisfy school, state, and insurance requirements.
6. Assess fitness level and performance parameters (optional).

## TYPES OF EVALUATIONS

One of two types of PPE is appropriate. The first is an examination by the athlete's personal physician. This is perhaps the preferred method; however, it is not always feasible because of lack of access, cost considerations, or time constraints. The second is the "station" method in which athletes move through several stations for different parts of the evaluation. This approach allows for large numbers of athletes to be evaluated in a short time at relatively little cost. Specialists are often available to expedite consultations, and coaches and athletic trainers usually are involved to help maintain order and facilitate communication.

A standard form can be used with either of these methods.

## COMPONENTS OF THE PPE

### Timing and Interval

Optimal timing for the PPE is 6 weeks prior to the beginning of the athletic season. This allows adequate time for further consultation, diagnostic testing, or rehabilitation of identified problems. Comprehensive evaluations should be performed at every new level of school (elementary school, middle school, high school), with either interval or comprehensive evaluations repeated annually.

## History

Most clinically relevant conditions should be uncovered during the medical history. Often the history given by adolescents is inaccurate or incomplete; therefore, parental input is desirable. Questions should emphasize symptoms related to the cardiovascular system, such as dizziness or syncope with exercise, chest pain, shortness of breath, palpitations, and fatigability. Use of a questionnaire often helps to ensure completeness and reminds athletes or parents of previous injuries and illnesses. Because many important cardiovascular conditions have a hereditary component, obtaining a family history also is critical. The family history should include details about any sudden death in a close relative prior to the age of 50 years, Marfan syndrome, long QT syndrome, or other significant cardiovascular conditions.

## Physical Examination

The examination component begins with a thorough general examination, including cardiovascular and musculoskeletal examinations.

### Cardiovascular examination

The cardiovascular examination should include evaluation of peripheral pulses, murmurs, and blood pressure. **Table 1** summarizes important aspects of the screening cardiovascular examination. Note that all diastolic murmurs and grade 3/6 systolic murmurs warrant further evaluation. Hypertrophic cardiomyopathy (HCM) may produce a systolic murmur that cannot be distinguished from an innocent murmur. The murmur of HCM increases in intensity with a Valsalva maneuver

**Table 1  Cardiovascular Screening in Athletes**

| Condition | Cardiovascular Examination | Abnormality |
|---|---|---|
| Hypertension | Blood pressure | Varies with age—general guideline is > 135/85 mm Hg in adolescents |
| Coarctation of aorta | Femoral pulses | Decreased intensity of pulse |
| Hypertrophic cardiomyopathy | Auscultation with provocative maneuvers (standing, supine, Valsalva) | Systolic ejection murmur that intensifies with standing or Valsalva maneuver |
| Marfan syndrome | Auscultation | Aortic (decrescendo diastolic murmur) or mitral (holosystolic murmur) insufficiency |

Adapted with permission from Maron BJ, Thompson PO, Puffer JC, et al: Cardiovascular preparticipation screening of competitive athletes: A statement for health professionals from the Sudden Death Committee (clinical cardiology) and Congenital Cardiac Defects Committee (cardiovascular disease in the young), American Heart Association. *Circulation* 1996;94:850-856.

SECTION 9 ■ PEDIATRIC ORTHOPAEDICS

(decreased ventricular filling, increased obstruction) and decreases with squatting (increased ventricular filling, decreased obstruction). Note that it will also increase in intensity when the athlete moves from a squatting to a standing position.

Blood pressures obtained during the PPE often are elevated; sometimes this is due to the use of a blood pressure cuff that is too small, particularly in large adolescents, or that a table of age-based norms was not used. However, at times the athlete's blood pressure is truly elevated. Hypertension is rarely severe enough to disqualify an athlete from participation, but it needs to be identified and followed by the athlete's regular physician.

### Musculoskeletal examination

The musculoskeletal examination is of particular importance because it typically accounts for 50% of the abnormal physical findings identified on the PPE. The examination should focus on areas previously injured or on areas that are symptomatic. Most musculoskeletal injuries are detected on the basis of the history alone. A 2-minute musculoskeletal screening examination is a quick examination for detecting musculoskeletal problems in asymptomatic individuals.

Some authorities recommend a sport-specific approach to the physical examination. This method emphasizes those areas that are most commonly injured or diseased in each specific sport. For example, a swimmer's examination would focus on the shoulders and ears (otitis externa), whereas a wrestler's examination would emphasize the skin, body fat composition, and the shoulders.

### Diagnostic Tests

Routine screening radiographs and laboratory tests are not indicated. These tests should be ordered based on information solicited during the history and physical examination.

## REFERRAL DECISIONS/RED FLAGS

Any history of the following physical findings indicates the need for further evaluation and possible specialty consultation.

1. Early fatigue, dizziness, syncope, chest pain, shortness of breath, or palpitations with exercise
2. Family history of sudden death or significant cardiovascular condition
3. Physical signs of Marfan syndrome
4. Significant head or spinal injury
5. Best-corrected vision of less than 20/40 in either eye
6. Previous heat illness
7. Significant musculoskeletal problem or injury

Once the PPE has been completed, recommendations for unrestricted clearance, clearance after further evaluation or treatment, limited participation, or total restriction can be made. Often these decisions will be made together with the athlete, parents, and consultants. Guidelines for conditions referable to the cardiovascular system can be found in the 26th Bethesda Conference published in the *Journal of the American College of Cardiology*. Guidelines for most other conditions are presented in the *Preparticipation Physical Evaluation* monograph published by the Physician and Sports Medicine, 4530 W. 77th Street, Minneapolis, MN 55435. To obtain a copy of this monograph, contact AAP Publications, 1-800-433-9016.

SECTION 9 ■ PEDIATRIC ORTHOPAEDICS

# SCOLIOSIS

## DEFINITION

Scoliosis is a lateral curvature of the spine of greater than 10°. The curve(s) can occur in the thoracic or lumbar spine (occasionally in both) and are associated with rotation of the vertebrae and sometimes with excessive kyphosis or lordosis. Idiopathic scoliosis is most common, but it can develop secondary to other problems (**Table 1**).

Idiopathic scoliosis usually develops in early adolescence. The male-to-female ratio is nearly equal in patients with curves of less than 20°. However, girls are seven times more likely than boys to have a significant, progressive curvature that requires treatment. Progression typically occurs in girls between the ages of 10 and 16 years.

## CLINICAL SYMPTOMS

Parents may notice that the child's clothes do not hang correctly. More commonly, the curvature is identified during a school screening program or routine examination. Pain is not characteristic in adolescents with idiopathic scoliosis.

**Table 1   Etiologic Classification of Structural Scoliosis**

| Type | Possible Cause |
| --- | --- |
| Idiopathic | |
| Congenital | Failure of formation—hemivertebra<br>Failure of segmentation—bony bar joining one side of two or more adjacent vertebrae |
| Neuromuscular | Cerebral palsy<br>Muscular dystrophy<br>Myelomeningocele<br>Spinal muscular atrophy<br>Friedreich ataxia (spinocerebellar degeneration) |
| Vertebral disease | Tumor<br>Infection<br>Metabolic bone disease |
| Spinal cord disease or anomaly | Tumor<br>Syringomyelia |
| Disease associated | Neurofibromatosis<br>Marfan syndrome<br>Connective tissue disorders |

SECTION 9 ■ PEDIATRIC ORTHOPAEDICS

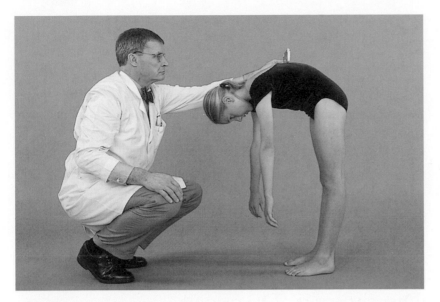

**Figure 1**
Physician using a scoliometer to quantify degree of scoliotic deformity. This patient demonstrates no deformity.

The presence of significant pain suggests another condition and requires further evaluation.

# Tests

## *Physical Examination*

Mild degrees of scoliosis may not be apparent when the patient is standing. Findings such as uneven shoulder height or pelvic asymmetry are inaccurate in detecting mild degrees of scoliosis; such findings are often present in the absence of spinal curvature.

The forward bending test is the most sensitive clinical method of documenting the problem; this test accentuates the vertebral and rib rotational deformities that are part of the abnormality. Observe the back from behind as the patient bends forward with the feet together, knees straight, and the arms hanging free. Elevation of the rib cage and/or prominence of the lumbar paravertebral muscle mass on one side is a positive finding. The deformity can be quantified in degrees using an inclinometer such as the scoliometer (**Figure 1**). Inclinations of greater than 5° to 7° should be evaluated further.

The examination should include evaluation for other conditions associated with scoliosis. Assess the trunk and lower extremities for skin lesions, cavus feet, limb-length discrepancy, abnormal joint laxity, and, most importantly, neuromuscular abnormalities. Left-sided thoracic curvatures have a significant association with spinal cord abnormalities, necessitating detailed evaluation and further diagnostic testing.

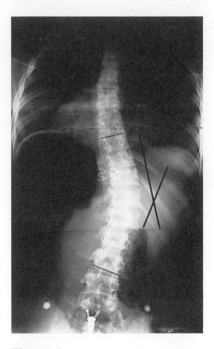

**Figure 2**

PA radiograph of the entire spine on a long cassette demonstrating a scoliotic deformity and the Cobb method of measuring its magnitude.

## Diagnostic Tests

Posteroanterior and lateral full-length radiographs with the patient standing and the knees straight should be obtained. The x-ray tube should be positioned 6' from the cassette, a 14" x 36" grid. Positioning patients with their backs to the x-ray source and using modern image-enhancing equipment minimizes exposure of the breasts and gonads.

The Cobb angle is the standard method of quantifying the degree of curvature and is determined by measuring the intersecting angle of perpendiculars (congruent angle) to the upper end plate of the most superior and the lower end plate of the most inferior vertebrae in the curve (**Figure 2**). By convention, radiographs of the spine are viewed, measured, and described as if the patient were being examined from behind.

## DIFFERENTIAL DIAGNOSIS

See Table 1 for a list of differential diagnoses.

## ADVERSE OUTCOMES OF THE DISEASE

Patients with hypokyphosis of the thoracic spine are at increased risk for restrictive pulmonary disorders. Therefore, serial pulmonary function tests are indicated until skeletal maturity and the curve has stabilized.

Progression of the curve is possible. If the curve is less than 50° at skeletal maturity, progression usually ceases. When an idiopathic thoracic curve is greater than 60°, progression in adulthood is common and can compromise respiratory function, although significant reduction in pulmonary function is unusual with a curve of less than 90° in an otherwise healthy individual. Back pain can occur in adulthood. In most patients, the back pain is not a major disability, but disabling pain is more likely to develop in patients who have decompensated lumbar or thoracolumbar curvatures.

## TREATMENT

Many idiopathic curves never progress to a degree that requires brace or surgical treatment. Regular observation during adolescence is appropriate. The frequency of observation depends on the degree of curve and the amount of growth remaining (**Table 2**).

Exercise therapy does not influence progression of scoliosis.

Brace treatment is reserved for patients with progressive curves in the range of 20° to 45°. It is not always effective, however, even with a well-made orthosis and good patient compliance. The goal of bracing is to arrest progression;

## Table 2   Guidelines for Observation

| Scoliometer Reading | Stage of maturity | |
| --- | --- | --- |
| | *Premenarche* | *Postmenarche* |
| < 5° | Recheck 3 months | Recheck 5 to 6 months |
| > 5° | Radiographs | Radiographs |
| | | |
| Curve magnitude | *Risser 0-2** | *Risser 3-5** |
| < 20° | Recheck 3 months | Recheck 6 to 12 months |
| 20°–30° | Brace or recheck 3 months | Repeat radiograph 3 months |
| 30°–45° | Brace | Brace or repeat radiograph 3 months |

*Risser sign is progression of ossification of the iliac apophysis

therefore, bracing is not necessary for curves that are unlikely to progress or when limited growth remains. Bracing also is ineffective for large curves even when several years of growth remain.

Surgery consisting of a spinal fusion is appropriate for idiopathic curves of greater than 50° or for curves of 40° to 50° that are likely to progress. Scoliosis of other etiologies is more likely to progress, and bracing and/or surgery may be advisable prior to reaching the guidelines for adolescent idiopathic scoliosis.

## ADVERSE OUTCOMES OF TREATMENT

The spinal curve may progress despite brace treatment, requiring surgical intervention. Surgical results can be adversely affected by infection, neurologic injury, or failure of the fusion mass to become solid. Regardless of the technique or instrumentation used, a solid bony fusion is the goal of any surgical procedure.

## REFERRAL DECISIONS/RED FLAGS

Patients with an obvious curvature or mild scoliosis with more than 5° of inclination should be evaluated radiographically to document the degree of scoliosis and estimate the likelihood of progression. Patients with unusual findings—convex left thoracic curves, pain, abnormal neurologic findings, bowel or bladder dysfunction, or deformities of the feet—require further evaluation for other than an idiopathic etiology.

SECTION 9 ■ PEDIATRIC ORTHOPAEDICS

# SEPTIC ARTHRITIS

## SYNONYMS
Infected joint
Pyarthrosis

## DEFINITION
Joint infections are more common in children and develop as a result of either hematogenous seeding from sources such as respiratory infection or impetigo or by direct extension from penetrating wounds or an adjacent osteomyelitis. The latter occurs mostly in the hip. Septic arthritis typically affects the large joints of the lower extremities and occasionally the sacroiliac joint. As a result of the release of proteolytic enzymes from the bacteria, neutrophils, and other inflammatory cells, microscopic articular cartilage damage can be detected within 48 to 72 hours of inoculation.

## CLINICAL SYMPTOMS
Patients typically have an acute onset of guarding of the involved joint. The pain is often poorly localized initially. Children will frequently limp or stop walking or refuse to move the upper extremity (pseudoparalysis). Malaise, elevated temperature, and loss of appetite soon develop.

## TESTS

### Physical Examination
The patient typically appears ill at presentation. For comfort, the joint is held in a position that accommodates distention. An affected hip will be positioned in flexion, abduction, and external rotation, while an involved knee or elbow is positioned in slight flexion. The child is apprehensive and resists attempts to examine the affected extremity.

### Diagnostic Tests
Any suspicion of joint infection requires immediate aspiration and analysis of the joint fluid. The results are corroborated with the findings on physical examination and results of other laboratory tests (**Table 1**).

Plain radiographs typically are not helpful in confirming an early diagnosis but are useful in excluding other disorders. Initial radiographs appear normal. Joint space widening, fat pad signs, and soft-tissue swelling develop later. Ultrasound can be useful, particularly in the hip, in the early screening for a joint effusion; however, this imaging study has a variety of technical

**Table 1    Typical Laboratory Results Associated With Septic Arthritis**

| Condition | Erythrocyte Sedimentation Rate | Blood Culture | Joint Culture | Blood WBC | Joint WBC |
|---|---|---|---|---|---|
| Septic joint | 30 mm/hr in most patients; gradual decrease unpredictable in neonates | Positive 30% to 40% | Positive 60% to 70% | 15,000/mm$^3$ (variable) often not elevated early | 20 to 250,000/ mm$^3$ |
| Transient synovitis | < 20 mm/hr (average 18) | Negative | Negative | Normal | Normal |
| Juvenile rheumatoid arthritis | Normal to 40 mm/hr (average 25) | Negative | Negative | Normal | Variable |

limitations. Furthermore, the absence of joint effusion on ultrasound does not rule out a septic process.

# DIFFERENTIAL DIAGNOSIS

Acute leukemia (bone pain more common, less swelling of the joint)

Acute osteomyelitis (no significant joint effusion)

Juvenile rheumatoid arthritis (more gradual onset, less "sick" appearance)

Lyme disease (indolent onset)

Reactive arthritis (less severe pain and effusion)

Rheumatic fever (arthralgia, less effusion)

Transient synovitis (hip only, less "sick" appearance)

Traumatic hemarthrosis (history of trauma)

# ADVERSE OUTCOMES OF THE DISEASE

If untreated, septic arthritis invariably causes articular cartilage erosions, capsular scarring, and subsequent painful arthritis. Delay in treatment may result in secondary joint arthrosis developing later in life with associated joint stiffness and pain. Delay in treating septic arthritis of the hip joint in a young child can result in subluxation, dislocation, and/or osteonecrosis of the femoral head.

# TREATMENT

Prompt intravenous antibiotic administration and joint drainage is the treatment of choice. The selection of the initial antibiotic is based on the most likely infecting organism(s) (**Table 2**). Changes in treatment are based on results of culture studies (**Table 3**). If the

### Table 2 Causative Organisms and Preferred Antibiotics for Septic Arthritis

| Organism | Typical Age | Antibiotic |
| --- | --- | --- |
| *Staphylococcus aureus* | All ages | Oxacillin |
| Group B streptococci | Neonate to 3 months | Ampicillin |
| Group A streptococci | 3 months to adolescence | Oxacillin |
| *Kingella kingae* | Neonate to 6 years | Cefotaxime |
| *Haemophilus influenzae* | Neonate to 3 months | Cefotaxime |
| Gram-negative coliforms | Neonate to 3 months | Ceftriaxone |
| Gonococcus | Adolescence | Ceftriaxone |

### Table 3 Preferred Antibiotics Pending Culture Results

| Patient Age | Antibiotic |
| --- | --- |
| Neonate | Oxacillin plus cefotaxime or gentamicin |
| Younger than 6 years old | Oxacillin plus cefotaxime |
| 6 years to adolescence | Oxacillin |
| Adolescence | Oxacillin plus ceftriaxone |

infection is diagnosed early and is not severe, and if the joint can be decompressed by aspiration, then treatment by antibiotics alone may be satisfactory. Otherwise, surgical decompression is indicated. To minimize the risk of osteonecrosis, a septic hip joint requires prompt surgical drainage.

## ADVERSE OUTCOMES OF TREATMENT

The adverse outcomes of treatment have more to do with failure to diagnose and/or properly treat a septic joint. Surgical decompression must be done promptly and thoroughly. Failure to adequately débride the joint may prolong the duration of infection and/or increase the risk for recurrence. To be predictably effective, antibiotics must be selected based on culture reports or historic guidelines. Antibiotics must be delivered in therapeutic doses for an appropriate period of time (usually 2 to 3 weeks).

## REFERRAL DECISIONS/RED FLAGS

A team approach provides the best management of septic arthritis in children. Joint aspiration and fluid analysis are essential in confirming the diagnosis.

# Seronegative Spondyloarthropathies

## Synonyms

Ankylosing spondylitis
Psoriatic arthritis
Reiter syndrome

## Definition

The seronegative spondyloarthropathies have the following characteristics in common: (1) inflammation of tendon, fascia, or joint capsule insertions (enthesitis); (2) pauciarticular arthritis, usually involving the lower extremity; (3) extra-articular inflammation involving the eye, skin, mucous membranes, heart, and bowel; and (4) association with the HLA-B27 antigen.

## Clinical Symptoms

Unlike that in adults, the onset of ankylosing spondylitis in children is more likely to affect the joints of the lower extremities. Asymmetric pauciarticular arthritis involving the lower extremity in children age 9 years or older, particularly in boys, should suggest the possibility of ankylosing spondylitis. The family history is often positive.

Reiter syndrome, with its triad of conjunctivitis, enthesitis, and urethritis, may be triggered in young children by infectious diarrhea caused by *Yersinia*, *Campylobacter*, *Salmonella*, or *Shigella*. In adolescents, nongonococcal urethritis secondary to *Chlamydia* or trachoma may cause Reiter syndrome. All three components of the disorder are not necessarily present in every patient, nor are they always present at the same time. The Achilles tendinitis or plantar fasciitis associated with Reiter syndrome can be extremely painful.

Psoriatic arthritis is considered uncommon in children, but approximately one third have the onset of this disorder before age 15 years, especially girls. Arthritis frequently antedates skin problems when this disorder occurs in childhood. A family history of psoriasis is a helpful clue when joint symptoms occur first.

Arthritis of inflammatory bowel disease, either ulcerative colitis or Crohn disease, typically causes symptoms before age 21 years, but only 15% of patients are diagnosed before age 15 years. Arthralgia without joint effusion is twice as common as arthritis with joint effusion.

SECTION 9 ■ PEDIATRIC ORTHOPAEDICS

## TESTS

### Physical Examination

A purplish discoloration may occur around the joint and is one of the distinguishing features of a juvenile spondyloarthropathy. Likewise, a child with ankylosing spondylitis may have an enthesitis, such as patellar tendinitis, Achilles tendinitis, or plantar fasciitis. Although children with ankylosing spondylitis may not have back pain, limited mobility of the spine can be present.

Mild conjunctivitis or an acute anterior uveitis causing painful red eyes and photophobia also are associated with Reiter syndrome.

In psoriatic arthritis, monoarticular involvement of the knee is the most common presentation. Progression to other joints proceeds in an asymmetric fashion. Compared with other spondyloarthropathies, upper extremity involvement and tenosynovitis involving the digits and nail pits is more common in psoriatic arthritis.

Pauciarticular arthritis of the lower extremity in inflammatory bowel disease typically is of short duration and either resolves spontaneously or with treatment of the bowel lesion. However, progressive ankylosing spondylitis may develop in some patients.

### Diagnostic Tests

The presence of the HLA-B27 antigen and a positive family history for spondyloarthropathy support the diagnosis of ankylosing spondylitis. Sterile pyuria supports the diagnosis of Reiter syndrome.

## DIFFERENTIAL DIAGNOSIS

Juvenile rheumatoid arthritis (often younger age at onset, upper extremity joint commonly affected, synovitis more impressive)

Various overuse syndromes (localized and more often unilateral)

## ADVERSE OUTCOMES OF THE DISEASE

Many lower extremity problems associated with the childhood spondyloarthropathies resolve spontaneously, but persistent erosive arthritis may develop. Ultimately, changes in the sacroiliac joint develop in children with ankylosing spondylitis.

## TREATMENT

NSAIDs, muscle strengthening, orthotics for the painful joint, and counseling about activity modifications are indicated.

## Adverse Outcomes of Treatment

NSAIDs can cause gastric, renal, or hepatic complications.

## Referral Decisions/Red Flags

Loss of function or inability to control pain indicates the need for further evaluation.

# SHOES FOR CHILDREN

A child's shoes were once considered an indicator of the family's economic status. A barefooted child suggested poverty and deprivation. Later the child's shoe became a focus of medical treatment. Many physicians thought that by modifying the child's shoes, lower limb deformity could be corrected and disability in later life prevented. During the past several decades, clinical studies have clarified the role shoes play in a child's life. The accumulated data are now sufficiently large to establish recommendations for children's footwear.

## NORMAL FOOT DEVELOPMENT

Clinical studies have consistently shown that the bare human foot has the following attributes: (1) excellent mobility; (2) thickening of the plantar skin to as much as 1 cm; (3) alignment of the phalanges with the metatarsals, causing the toes to spread; (4) variable arch height; and (5) an absence of most common foot deformities. These findings show that satisfactory foot development occurs in the barefoot environment.

Arch development has been documented in several studies. The arch develops spontaneously during a child's first 6 to 8 years, and the range of normal is very broad. About 15% of adults have flexible flatfeet, which are considered a variation of normal and typically are not associated with disability.

## EFFECTS OF SHOES ON THE FOOT

The primary role of shoes is to protect the foot. Indeed, if shoes are not fitted properly, toe deformities are likely to develop.

Wearing shoes does not affect how soon a child will begin to walk. Infants do well in stockings around the house. At this age, soft shoes may be used for appearance or to protect the foot when outside. Soft, flexible shoes are best for the toddler. If the toddler's foot is chubby, a high-top shoe can be helpful to keep the shoe on the foot, but this type of shoe does not affect the growth or development of the foot. High-top shoes also may be necessary in children with conditions that cause ligamentous laxity or hypotonia.

## CHARACTERISTICS OF A GOOD SHOE

For children, the features of a good shoe include the following five "F's":

- *Flexible*. The shoe should allow as much free motion as possible. As a test, make certain that the shoe can be easily flexed in your hand.
- *Flat*. Avoid high heels that force the foot forward, cramping the toes.
- *Foot-shaped*. Avoid pointed toes or other shapes that are different from the normal foot.
- *Fitted generously*. Better too large than too short. Allow about a fingerbreadth of room for growth.
- *Friction like skin*. The sole should have about the same friction as skin. Soles that are slippery or adherent can cause the child to fall.

# THE "CORRECTIVE" SHOE

The concept that shoes could be therapeutic appears to be based on the once widely accepted assumption that the growing foot needs support and could be molded by a corrective shoe. The assumption that external forces could correct deformity led to the development of various orthotic inserts and heel modifications. Although uncontrolled studies reported improvements with such devices, two controlled prospective studies on the effect of shoe modifications and arch development published in 1989 showed no difference between treated and untreated feet. In essence, shoe inserts do not modify or alter intoeing, outtoeing, or flexible flatfeet. In fact, shoe inserts can be harmful. Adults who wore shoe modifications as children often remember the experience as negative and, in one study, were shown to have lower self-esteem than control subjects.

Some shoe modifications are useful. These are not corrective but produce some immediately desirable effect: Shoe lifts for the short leg equalize limb length and improve walking. Shoe inserts for older children or adolescents with rigid foot deformities can redistribute weight-bearing forces and reduce discomfort or skin breakdown if sensation is impaired. Shock-absorbing footwear with cushioned soles can help in the management of overuse syndromes.

# CURRENT PROBLEMS

The design of shoes has improved over the past decade. Currently, the major problems in shoes affect girls. The prevalence of constrictive and deforming shoes for girls, including heel elevations, pointed toes, and tight fit, causes deformity (bunions) and instability, both of which increase the risk of ankle injuries.

SECTION 9 ■ PEDIATRIC ORTHOPAEDICS

# RECOMMENDATIONS

1. Shoes should be regarded as a form of clothing, designed to simulate the barefoot state.

2. Walking and playing barefooted in a safe environment is an acceptable alternative to wearing shoes for infants and children.

3. For most children, shoes should be flexible, flat, shaped like the foot, and have soles that provide friction similar to skin.

4. Cushioning of the sole can reduce the risk of overuse conditions around the foot.

5. Shoe modifications are not "corrective." Inserts are useful only for load redistribution and do not change the shape of the foot.

6. Physicians should promote public education about healthy footwear for children.

7. Prescribing unnecessary shoe inserts and modifications is expensive for the family and society. More importantly, these can be uncomfortable and embarrassing for the child.

SECTION 9 ■ PEDIATRIC ORTHOPAEDICS

# SLIPPED CAPITAL FEMORAL EPIPHYSIS

## SYNONYM
Slipped epiphysis

## DEFINITION
Slipped capital femoral epiphysis (SCFE) is displacement of the femoral head through the physis that typically occurs during the adolescent growth spurt.

During adolescence, the orientation of the physis of the proximal femur changes from horizontal to oblique. That, coupled with the patient's increased body size, may cause intolerable shear at the relatively weak physis. The result is microscopic fractures and gradual slippage of the femoral head posteriorly and usually also medially. Occasionally, an acute event causes sudden displacement of the femoral head—in essence, a fracture or unstable slip.

Obesity, male gender, and greater involvement with sports activities are predisposing factors. Increased femoral retroversion also is a risk factor and probably explains the greater incidence of SCFE among blacks.

A small percentage of patients with SCFE have an endocrine disorder that alters the strength or growth of the physis. Hypothyroidism and growth hormone deficiency are most common, but SCFE also has been observed in panhypopituitarism, hyperthyroidism, and multiple endocrine neoplasia. Growth hormone deficiency usually is diagnosed before SCFE develops, but in children with hypothyroidism, SCFE often occurs before the endocrine disorder has been diagnosed.

The mean age at presentation is 12 years for girls (typical range: 10 to 14 years) and 13 years for boys (typical range: 11 to 16 years). Onset before or after the typical age range is associated with some type of endocrinopathy.

Bilateral involvement is more common than originally understood and is seen in 40% to 50% of patients who are followed to closure of the growth plate.

## CLINICAL SYMPTOMS
Pain exacerbated by activity is the most common presenting symptom. Pain usually is localized to the anterior proximal thigh, but in one third of patients it is referred to the distal thigh and, on rare occasions, at the ankle. The clinical examination is easy and almost pathognomonic. Therefore, it is worthwhile to perform a screening examination for SCFE on all adolescents who present with lower extremity pain.

**ICD-9 Code**

**732.2**
Nontraumatic slipped upper femoral epiphysis

SECTION 9 ■ PEDIATRIC ORTHOPAEDICS

# Tests

## Physical Examination

Loss of hip internal rotation is the most sensitive and specific finding and is readily apparent, even with minimal displacement of the femoral head. SCFE is the only pediatric disorder that causes greater loss of internal rotation when the hip is moved into a flexed position. Assessing internal rotation with the hip flexed to 90° is an effective screening maneuver and is easily done on all adolescents who have lower extremity pain.

Abduction and extension also are decreased. The affected extremity may be between 1 and 3 cm shorter than the unaffected extremity, depending on the severity of the slip. In addition, patients typically walk with the affected extremity externally rotated.

## Diagnostic Tests

AP and frog-lateral radiographs of the pelvis confirm the diagnosis (**Figure 1**). On rare occasions, the femoral head is displaced only in a posterior direction. In these situations, the AP radiograph will appear normal or will show slight valgus malalignment of the femoral head. No displacement is evident in a few patients, but in this preslip phase, the physis is widened.

The severity of displacement is classified as mild, moderate, or severe as measured by the degree of posterior displacement. Most authors rate a mild SCFE as less than 30°, moderate as 30° to 50°, and severe as greater than 50°.

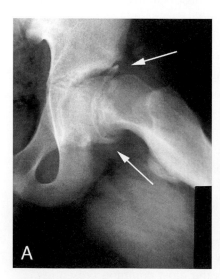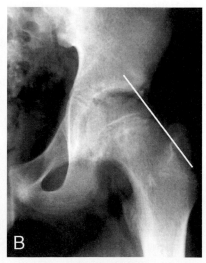

**Figure 1**
Radiographs of the pelvis showing mild SCFE of the right hip.
**A,** Posterior displacement of the femoral head (arrows) is profiled on the frog-lateral radiograph. **B,** On the AP view, mild degrees of medial displacement can be recognized by drawing a line along the lateral aspect of the femoral neck. When SCFE is present, the line on the involved hip will either miss the femoral head or transect less of it than on the uninvolved hip.

# DIFFERENTIAL DIAGNOSIS

Endocrinopathy (atypical age, constitutional symptoms)

Legg-Calvé-Perthes disease (in younger age range)

Meralgia paresthetica (lateral femoral cutaneous nerve entrapment)

Neoplasm (night pain, no restriction of hip internal rotation in flexion)

# ADVERSE OUTCOMES OF THE DISEASE

Progressive arthritis, chondrolysis, and osteonecrosis may occur. Individuals vary, but on average, the degree of displacement correlates with the duration of symptoms. Severe SCFE predisposes the hip to symptomatic degenerative changes by the time the patient is a young or middle-aged adult, but stabilization of a mild or moderately displaced SCFE provides good long-term function, with symptomatic arthritis either not occurring or not developing until the older adult years. Therefore, making the diagnosis as early as possible is important.

# TREATMENT

The goals of treatment for adolescents with SCFE are to prevent further slippage of the femoral head, promote closure of the physis, and avoid osteonecrosis and chondrolysis. Treatment is based on the duration of symptoms and the degree of displacement. Most patients are treated by in situ stabilization. Patients with severe deformity may require a realignment osteotomy. With an unstable SCFE, patients have severe pain after a fall, are unable to walk, and have radiographic evidence of severe displacement. These patients require emergent reduction and stabilization.

# ADVERSE OUTCOMES OF TREATMENT

Patients are at risk for recurrent slippage until the physis closes. After stabilization, this problem is not common because the typical patient with SCFE is nearing completion of growth. Furthermore, insertion of the screw promotes closure of the growth plate. Chondrolysis and osteonecrosis also may occur.

# REFERRAL DECISIONS/RED FLAGS

Further evaluation for surgical treatment should occur immediately upon diagnosis.

SECTION 9 ■ PEDIATRIC ORTHOPAEDICS

# SPONDYLOLISTHESIS

## DEFINITION

Spondylolisthesis occurs when one vertebral body slips forward in relation to the vertebral body below. In children, spondylolisthesis occurs most frequently between L5 and S1 when a defect develops at the junction of the lamina with the pedicle (pars interarticularis) (**Figure 1**). The resultant spondylolysis means that the posterior elements (lamina and spinous process) have only a fibrous tissue connection to the anterior elements (pedicle and vertebral body). As a consequence, the vertebral body may slide forward, producing the "slip" or spondylolisthesis. Most likely this condition is a fatigue or stress fracture that occurred in the preadolescent years and failed to heal. Children who participate at a high level in activities that place hyperextension stresses on this area, such as gymnastics and football, have a higher incidence of this condition.

## CLINICAL SYMPTOMS

Back pain may develop that is worse with standing and that radiates to or below the knees (**Figure 2**). Symptoms are more common with more than 50% slippage. Spasms in the hamstring muscles, manifested by the inability to bend forward, accompanied by limited straight-leg raising test are frequently found in symptomatic patients. True nerve root compression symptoms (radiculopathy), however, are infrequent in children.

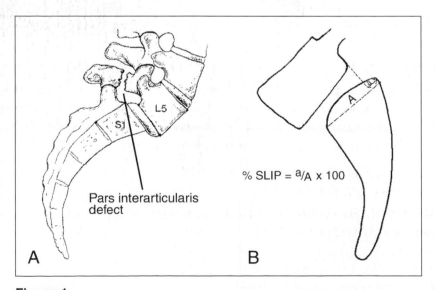

$$\% \text{ SLIP} = a/A \times 100$$

**Figure 1**
**A,** Drawing of a grade I L5-S1 spondylolisthesis (lateral view).
**B,** Determination of slip percentage.

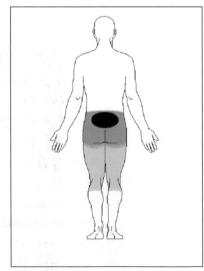

**Figure 2**
Typical pain diagram for a patient with adolescent spondylolisthesis.

# TESTS

## Physical Examination

Typical posture includes flexion of the hips and knees, backward tilting of the pelvis, and flattening of the normal lumbar lordosis. With marked slippage, a step-off can be palpated, with the spinous process of the slipped vertebra more prominent than the one above.

Hamstring spasm is manifested by marked limitation in forward bending and a limited passive straight-leg raising test. Motor and sensory function of the lumbosacral nerve roots should be assessed, although objective neurologic deficits are uncommon.

## Diagnostic Tests

With spondylolisthesis, lateral radiographs demonstrate forward translation of L5 relative to S1 (expressed as percentage of the anterior-posterior width of the vertebral body) (**Figure 3**). If only spondylolysis has occurred, there is no forward translation of L5, but a defect in the pars interarticularis is evident on the oblique views (a "collar" on the Scotty dog) (**Figure 4**).

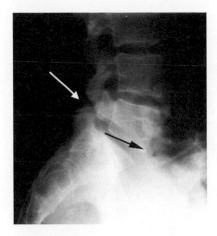

**Figure 3**

Lateral radiograph demonstrating a grade I L5-S1 spondylolisthesis. Black arrow indicates the direction of the slip; white arrow indicates the defect.

# DIFFERENTIAL DIAGNOSIS

Ankylosing spondylitis (HLA antigen, sacroiliac joint changes)

Intervertebral disk injury or herniation (no step-off or slip, and no defect seen on plain radiographs, radiculopathy occasionally present)

Intervertebral diskitis (elevated erythrocyte sedimentation rate and fever, disk space narrowing on radiographs)

Osteoid osteoma (night pain, abnormal bone scan, pain relieved by aspirin)

Spinal cord tumor (sensory findings, upper motor neuron signs)

# ADVERSE OUTCOMES OF THE DISEASE

Progressive or complete slip of the vertebral body, chronic back pain and disability, weakness or paralysis of the lower lumbar nerve roots, or bowel and bladder involvement (cauda equina syndrome) are possible.

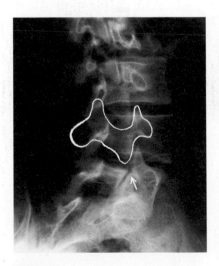

**Figure 4**

Oblique radiograph shows a normal "Scotty dog" appearance (outlined area). In the vertebra below, the Scotty dog has a "collar" (arrow), indicating the pars interarticularis defect of spondylolisthesis.

# TREATMENT

Observation to evaluate the possibility of increasing slippage is indicated until growth is completed. The frequency of evaluation depends on the amount of growth remaining, the degree of slippage, and whether a patient is symptomatic. A weight-bearing spot lateral radiograph is usually adequate for follow-up. In symptomatic patients, activities that aggravate the condition should be discontinued. An exercise problem that targets strengthening of the abdominal and paraspinal muscles, stretching of the hamstring muscles, and postural adaptations may be helpful. A custom-fitted thoracolumbar orthosis may control pain in patients who remain symptomatic despite activity modifications. Spinal fusion is indicated in symptomatic children who have a documented progression and a slip of greater than 50% and significant growth remaining. Patients whose symptoms cannot be relieved through nonsurgical treatment also should be considered for surgery.

## ADVERSE OUTCOMES OF TREATMENT

Despite treatment, the slip may progress. Spinal fusions may be complicated by pseudarthrosis and continued pain.

## REFERRAL DECISIONS/RED FLAGS

Patients with significant pain and/or a confirmed spondylolisthesis need further evaluation.

# TARSAL COALITION

## SYNONYMS
Calcaneal bar
Peroneal spastic flatfoot
Rigid flatfoot
Talocalcaneal bar

ICD-9 Code
**755.67**
Anomalies of the foot, not elsewhere
classified

## DEFINITION
Tarsal coalition is an abnormal connection between any two
tarsal bones. Initially, the coalition may be fibrous or
cartilaginous, but it often ossifies during early adolescence and
restricts hindfoot motion. The two most common locations for a
tarsal coalition are between the calcaneus and navicular
(calcaneonavicular coalition) and between the talus and
calcaneus (talocalcaneal coalition). The condition is bilateral in
approximately 50% of patients and may be found in other
family members who are asymptomatic but have no hindfoot
motion.

## CLINICAL SYMPTOMS
If symptoms develop, they usually occur during adolescence,
when ossification of the bar starts to occur. Calcaneonavicular
coalitions generally become symptomatic in children between
the ages of 9 and 13 years, while symptoms from a
talocalcaneal coalition generally develop later, between the ages
of 13 and 16 years.

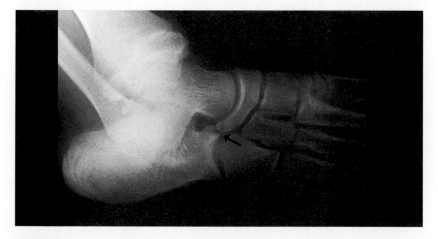

**Figure 1**
Oblique radiograph of a foot with a cartilaginous calcaneonavicular
coalition (arrow).

SECTION 9 ■ PEDIATRIC ORTHOPAEDICS

The onset of pain usually is insidious but can be associated with an injury or change in activity. Parents may observe a limp and the foot turning out. Pain from a talocalcaneal coalition usually is vague and located deep within the hindfoot, while a calcaneonavicular coalition usually causes pain laterally over the area of the coalition.

## TESTS

### Physical Examination

Hindfoot motion (inversion and eversion) is markedly restricted. Spasm of the peroneal muscles is frequent and can be demonstrated by quickly inverting the foot. Peroneal spasm holds the foot in a stiff, everted flatfoot posture; however, regardless of whether peroneal spasm is present, patients with tarsal coalition typically have a rigid flatfoot; the longitudinal arch is absent whether in a weight-bearing position or not.

### Diagnostic Tests

AP, lateral, and oblique radiographs of the foot will delineate a calcaneonavicular coalition (**Figure 1**). Talocalcaneal bars are difficult to see on routine radiographs, even with special views; therefore, CT is necessary to confirm the diagnosis.

## DIFFERENTIAL DIAGNOSIS

Accessory navicular (medial prominence and pain over the navicular)

Congenital vertical talus (rigid flatfoot deformity noted in the neonate)

Flexible flatfoot (no restriction of subtalar motion, usually without pain)

## ADVERSE OUTCOMES OF THE DISEASE

Pain, restricted inversion and eversion of the foot, and limited walking and running are possible consequences.

## TREATMENT

Treatment options include observation, short leg cast immobilization, resection of the coalition, and arthrodesis. Observation or activity modifications are appropriate for children who are asymptomatic or who have minimal symptoms. For more severe symptoms or if milder symptoms persist, a 4- to 6-week trial in a short leg walking cast may be of benefit. For patients with persistent symptoms that do not respond to nonsurgical treatment, resection of the coalition is the preferred treatment. Resection reduces pain in most patients, but this procedure is more reliable for calcaneonavicular coalitions. Hindfoot arthrodesis (joint fusion) is reserved for patients who have not responded to resection procedures or patients who are not candidates for coalition resection (the coalition is too large or arthritic changes are already present).

## Adverse Outcomes of Treatment

Complications include cast sores, postoperative infection, failure of fusion, recurrence of a resected coalition, inadequate pain relief, and arthritic changes.

## Referral Decisions/Red Flags

Significant pain following nonsurgical treatment indicates the need for further evaluation.

Section 9 ■ Pediatric Orthopaedics

# Toe Walking

## DEFINITION

Toe walking can be a normal variation of gait in children as they begin to walk; however, when it persists in children who are older than 18 months and who are otherwise normal and have no underlying neurologic deficit, it is known as idiopathic toe walking. This condition involves both legs and also is referred to as habitual toe walking.

## CLINICAL SYMPTOMS

Children with idiopathic toe walking generally are active, asymptomatic, and have no functional difficulties or other medical problems. Parental concern or a history of a sibling with toe walking usually is the impetus for seeking medical attention.

## TESTS

### Physical Examination

The diagnosis of idiopathic toe walking is one of exclusion; therefore, pathologic causes must be ruled out. Obtaining a thorough history is critical, particularly a detailed birth history. Cerebral palsy is suggested by a history of prematurity, anoxia, hypoxia, or perinatal infection. Muscular dystrophy is suggested by a positive family history and proximal muscle weakness. The time of onset also is important. In children with idiopathic toe walking, the onset of walking is normal, and toe walking begins with the onset of gait. Children with cerebral palsy usually have delayed gross motor milestones. Children with Duchenne muscular dystrophy initially walk with a heel-toe gait but develop toe walking at a later age.

Toe walking varies in severity (**Figure 1**), but children with idiopathic toe walking generally can stand with their feet flat on the floor and can walk heel-toe if reminded. Some will have decreased ankle dorsiflexion, while others do not.

### Diagnostic Tests

Diagnostic tests should be ordered only if the history is unclear or if the examination reveals some abnormality suggestive of another disorder.

## DIFFERENTIAL DIAGNOSIS

Cerebral palsy (delayed developmental milestones, spasticity of gastrocnemius-soleus complex)

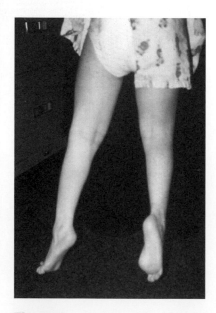

**Figure 1**
Example of a child with idiopathic toe walking.

Intraspinal abnormality (cavus feet, unilateral or asymmetric involvement)

Muscular dystrophy (proximal muscular weakness, positive family history)

Occult hydrocephalus (upper motor neuron signs)

## Adverse Outcomes of the Disease

The prevalence of long-term sequelae has not been documented; however, in some patients, persistent callosities and pain in the forefoot develop during late adolescence.

## Treatment

Treatment depends on the age of the child and the severity of the problem. In the toddler who has just begun to walk, the condition often resolves spontaneously after 3 to 6 months. Observation is appropriate for older toddlers who only occasionally walk on their toes. Stretching exercises may be tried for young children with mild contractures; however, children at this age typically do not tolerate extensive therapy. Serial casting for 6 to 8 weeks is often successful in children 3 to 8 years of age who have persistent toe walking and a persistent equinus. A short leg cast is applied with the ankle in near maximal dorsiflexion, and the casts are changed at 2- to 3-week intervals, with the amount of dorsiflexion increased at each cast change. After casting, many of these children will walk heel-toe, but some will revert to their previous gait pattern. Physical therapy that focuses on heel cord stretching or use of an ankle-foot orthosis may be helpful in preventing recurrence.

Surgical treatment also is an option and typically is indicated for an older child with a fixed heel cord contracture when nonsurgical treatment is ineffective or poorly tolerated. Heel cord lengthening is an outpatient procedure that can be tried after all nonsurgical measures have failed. Postoperatively, approximately 6 weeks of cast immobilization is required.

## Adverse Outcomes of Treatment

Observation and stretching exercises are complicated only by failure or recurrence. Recurrence and skin problems can occur with casting or with heel cord lengthening.

## Referral Decisions/Red Flags

Any child with persistent toe walking despite stretching and physical therapy or with evidence of a neuromuscular impairment requires further evaluation. Unilateral toe walking is

Section 9 ■ Pediatric Orthopaedics

never normal. In these instances, thorough examination is required to identify the underlying pathologic process. The most common causes of unilateral toe walking are limb-length discrepancy, cerebral palsy, and intraspinal abnormality.

# TORTICOLLIS

## SYNONYM
Wry neck

## DEFINITION
Torticollis is a head position characterized by rotation of the chin toward one shoulder combined with tilting of the head to the opposite shoulder. Torticollis is a finding, not a diagnosis. Congenital muscular torticollis and atlanto-axial rotary subluxation are the most common causes.

Congenital muscular torticollis is a unilateral contracture of the sternocleidomastoid (SCM) muscle. Scar tissue in the muscle impedes growth of the SCM muscle. As a result, the involved muscle develops a contracture that causes the head to tilt toward the affected side and rotate toward the unaffected side (**Figure 1**). Facial asymmetry also develops.

Atlanto-axial rotary subluxation (AARS) is a rotational displacement of C1 on C2. Approximately 50% of neck rotation occurs between C1 and C2. Children between 2 and 12 years are most commonly affected. Greater ligamentous laxity in children probably explains its increased incidence in this population. AARS may be associated with minor trauma or develop after an upper respiratory infection (Grisel syndrome).

## CLINICAL SYMPTOMS
Parental concern about the head posture is the usual reason for the visit for both conditions. For congenital muscular torticollis, the parents also may note a lump or swelling in the muscle at 4 to 6 weeks of age. If present, this mass disappears in a few weeks. Children with AARS may report neck pain, but the discomfort typically is minimal.

## TESTS

### Physical Examination
Infants with congenital muscular torticollis hold the head in a "cock robin" position. Contracture of the left SCM muscle directs the chin to the right shoulder and tilts the left ear to the left shoulder and limits neck rotation to the left and lateral tilt to the right. The opposite deformity is seen with contracture of the right SCM muscle. Flattening of the face is noted on the side of the contracted SCM muscle.

SECTION 9 ■ PEDIATRIC ORTHOPAEDICS

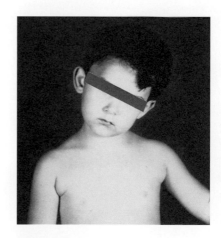

**Figure 1**
Child with congenital muscular torticollis. The chin is rotated to the patient's right and the head inclined to the left.

Patients with AARS hold the head in a similar position. SCM muscle spasm, however, may be noted on the "chin" side. This spasm differs from that of congenital muscular torticollis in which the SCM muscle on the "ear" side is tight.

The examination also should include assessment for ocular or neurologic disorders. Congenital muscular torticollis can be associated with developmental hip dysplasia, and that possibility should be investigated.

### Diagnostic Tests

AP and lateral radiographs of the cervical spine should be obtained in patients with congenital muscular torticollis to rule out underlying congenital bony anomalies. Patients with AARS also should have open mouth views of the odontoid; however, good views are difficult to obtain in this condition. CT with the head maximally rotated to the right and then maximally rotated to the left may be required to document AARS. Before CT, obtain flexion-extension lateral views to rule out upper cervical instability. Despite possible limitation by muscle spasm, these views should be obtained only with active, never passive, motion.

# DIFFERENTIAL DIAGNOSIS

### Congenital muscular torticollis

Benign paroxysmal torticollis (intermittent torticollis)

Congenital anomalies of the base of the skull (rare, evident on radiographs)

Klippel-Feil syndrome (congenital cervical spine anomalies, short neck, low hair line)

Ocular disorders (torticollis may improve when eyes are closed or vision blocked)

### Atlanto-axial rotary subluxation

Fractures of the upper cervical spine (history of trauma, evident on radiographs)

Neoplasms of the cervical spine (indolent onset, pain, evident on radiographs)

Osteomyelitis of the cervical spine (evident on radiographs, laboratory studies)

Posterior fossa or spinal cord tumor (neurologic examination, gentle passive motion may not be as limited, MRI)

# ADVERSE OUTCOMES OF THE DISEASE

Facial asymmetry and persistent limited motion are possible with congenital muscular torticollis. With AARS, persistent limited motion also is possible. Upper cervical instability may be present, which could increase the risk of neurologic injury.

## TREATMENT

Nonsurgical treatment of congenital muscular torticollis consists of frequent stretching exercises that tilt and rotate the head. Supervision by a physical therapist is helpful, but parents must actually do the stretching exercises several times a day. The infant's bed and changing table can be positioned to encourage the infant to look away from the limited side. If the problem persists after 12 to 18 months, surgical release/lengthening of the SCM should be considered.

Initial management of AARS is immobilization in a soft cervical collar and analgesics for pain. Range-of-motion exercises are not helpful. If reduction does not occur in approximately 1 week, cervical traction with a head halter and better pain management should be attempted. Conditions that persist for several months may require upper cervical fusion for relief of symptoms.

## ADVERSE OUTCOMES OF TREATMENT

For patients with congenital muscular torticollis, failure of stretching programs and a persistent deformity are possible. Even with surgical treatment, the contracture may recur with growth.

For patients with AARS, persistent deformity is possible. Recurrence is rare in patients diagnosed and treated promptly. Upper cervical arthrodesis permanently limits neck motion.

## REFERRAL DECISIONS/RED FLAGS

For infants with congenital torticollis, failure to improve following 2 to 3 months of nonsurgical treatment, the presence of anomalies of the skull or cervical spine, or abnormal results of neurologic or eye examination indicate the need for further evaluation.

Children with acquired torticollis who have an abnormal neurologic examination or evidence of instability on lateral radiographs need urgent specialty evaluation. Acquired torticollis that persists for more than 2 or 3 weeks or situations in which initial treatment has failed usually need further evaluation as well.

SECTION 9 ■ PEDIATRIC ORTHOPAEDICS

# TRANSIENT SYNOVITIS OF THE HIP

**ICD-9 Code**

**719.05**
Effusion of joint, pelvic region and thigh

## SYNONYMS

Observation hip
Toxic synovitis

## DEFINITION

Transient synovitis of the hip is a sterile effusion of the joint that resolves without therapy or sequelae. Children 2 to 5 years of age are most commonly affected, and boys are affected two to three times more often than girls. The etiology is unknown, but mild trauma at an age when the socket or acetabulum is not fully developed seems to be the best explanation. This theory fits the demographics. Another theory proposes an infectious etiology, but numerous studies have not demonstrated a bacterial or viral agent. Therefore, the term "toxic synovitis" should not be used to describe this disorder.

## CLINICAL SYMPTOMS

Typically, the child awakens with a limp or refuses to walk. Children who can communicate, typically localize their pain to the groin or proximal thigh. After "loosening up," the limp may improve but will worsen toward the end of the day.

## TESTS

### Physical Examination
Examination reveals a limp and mild restriction of hip motion, particularly abduction. Most children are afebrile.

### Diagnostic Tests
Because transient synovitis is a diagnosis of exclusion, the extent of the evaluation process depends on the degree and duration of symptoms. If a child is seen 1 to 3 days after onset, is afebrile, does not appear ill, has only mildly restricted abduction (movement of at least 25° to 30°), and does not guard when the hip is moved in other directions, then radiographs and laboratory studies are not necessary. However, if the symptoms have been present for several days but the child is afebrile and has only mildly restricted motion, then AP and frog-lateral radiographs of the pelvis are appropriate to rule out a latent osteomyelitis or other chronic process. Diagnostic studies, such as a CBC, erythrocyte sedimentation rate, C-reactive protein, blood cultures, and radiographs, are

indicated if the patient has very limited motion or a temperature that is higher than 99.5°F (37.5°C).

Radiographs usually are normal; however, they may show widening of the joint space. Ultrasound and bone scan often demonstrate changes but are rarely necessary. A joint effusion will be seen on ultrasound, and a bone scan can demonstrate mild uptake.

Aspirate the joint if there are findings compatible with septic arthritis.

## DIFFERENTIAL DIAGNOSIS

Juvenile rheumatoid arthritis (multiple joints, persistent symptoms, systemic symptoms)

Legg-Calvé-Perthes disease (limp worse at the end of the day, present after 2 to 6 weeks of symptoms, abnormal radiographs)

Rheumatic fever (arthralgias progress in a migratory fashion to other joints, systemic symptoms)

Septic arthritis of the hip (primary disorder to exclude: temperature above 99.5°F [37.5°C], erythrocyte sedimentation rate > 20 mm/hr, C-reactive protein > 1.0)

## ADVERSE OUTCOMES OF THE DISEASE

The symptoms and associated limp typically resolve within 3 to 14 days. Recurrence is possible but uncommon. No sequelae have been associated with transient synovitis. Legg-Calvé-Perthes disease subsequently develops in 1% to 3% of patients, but whether the disorders have any association is unclear. A delay in diagnosing septic arthritis also is possible.

## TREATMENT

Most children can be treated by bed rest at home, with the parents periodically checking the temperature. When the diagnosis is equivocal or if the patient is uncomfortable, hospitalization for observation and traction are indicated.

## ADVERSE OUTCOMES OF TREATMENT

None

## REFERRAL DECISIONS/RED FLAGS

A temperature higher than 99.5°F (37.5°C) or an erythrocyte sedimentation rate greater than 20 mm/hr suggests septic arthritis, in which case patients need further evaluation. Also, patients need additional evaluation if radiographs suggest Legg-Calvé-Perthes disease.

# APPENDIX A
## MUSCULOSKELETAL CONDITIONING—HELPING PATIENTS PREVENT INJURY AND STAY FIT

Over the past 50 to 75 years, the United States has experienced a shift in lifestyle. Once a society in which most individuals worked in physically stressful jobs (eg, farming, steelmaking, road and railroad building); walked to work, to visit friends, and to shop; and climbed stairs rather than riding elevators, ours is now a society in which most individuals sit in offices during most of their workday and drive to their activities. The mental stresses may be great, but the physical stresses of most jobs are small. Yard and household chores have also become physically less demanding, thanks to technologic advances: lawnmowers are motorized, and sweepers, floor waxers, dishwashers, and clothes washers have replaced manual activities for these tasks.

Unfortunately, as physical inactivity has become more common, health issues associated with this inactivity have become all too prominent. Obesity and associated diseases such as heart disease, diabetes mellitus, and hypertension have been reported to be "epidemic" in the United States.

One responsibility of a physician is to educate patients on the importance of physical activity as a part of a healthy lifestyle. Such an exercise prescription typically includes not only instruction in a general aerobic exercise program for cardiovascular fitness (such as swimming, cycling, or walking) but also exercise to strengthen areas weakened by injury or inactivity or areas that would be particularly challenged by a new activity. For example, a 50-year-old man who wishes to play tennis or a 45-year-old woman who recently secured a job as a painter would benefit from both cardiovascular exercise to increase endurance and specific exercises for conditioning the shoulders and trunk. A body made fit by musculoskeletal stretching, strengthening, and proprioceptive exercises is less likely to sustain injury during sport, work-related activities, or daily activities such as gardening or housekeeping. This appendix provides examples of these exercises.

A conditioning program for either the body as a whole or a specific targeted anatomic area of the body consists of three basic phases: stretching exercises to restore range of motion, strengthening exercises to improve muscle power, and proprioceptive exercises to enhance balance and agility.

Stretching and strengthening exercises are generally begun first, followed by proprioceptive exercises. Patient handouts are provided here for the stretching and strengthening exercises. Additionally, proprioceptive exercises for beginners are described in the text. Plyometric exercises may also be added for power development after basic strength and flexibility have been achieved. Advanced proprioceptive exercises and plyometric exercises should be done under the supervision of a physical therapist or certified athletic trainer.

The goal of a conditioning program is to enable people to live a fit and healthier lifestyle by being more active. A well-structured conditioning program will also prepare the individual for participation in sports and recreational activities. The greater the intensity of the activity in which the individual wishes to engage, the greater the intensity of the conditioning that will be required. If the individual attends physical therapy for instruction in a conditioning routine rather than using only an exercise handout such as provided here, the focus should be on developing and committing to a home exercise fitness program.

Conditioning exercises follow, arranged by anatomic area. Musculoskeletal conditioning of the shoulder is discussed first, followed by the hip, knee, foot and ankle, and lumbar spine. Each section describes a home exercise program and includes patient exercise handouts that may be printed from the DVD that accompanies this book.

# SHOULDER CONDITIONING

The shoulder is a complex structure that allows movement in many different planes. The muscles of the shoulder most important in overhead sports activities such as tennis, baseball, and swimming are the glenohumeral and scapular rotators. Strengthening the scapular stabilizers, as well as the rotator cuff and deltoid muscles, is important because strong, coordinated function of all shoulder muscle groups helps stabilize the glenohumeral joint and helps prevent injury when the individual engages in activities such as gardening or housekeeping or work- or sport-related activities that involve repetitive upper extremity motion. Also, increased strength in these muscles translates into a higher velocity tennis serve or baseball pitch.

Proprioceptive or balance exercises help train the joints of the upper extremity to perceive joint positions and hence enhance the individual's perception of the position of the body in space. Examples of proprioceptive exercises are scapular retraction done while lying on an exercise ball or push-ups performed on an air mattress or with each hand on a small ball instead of the floor. These exercises should be done only after adequate flexibility and strength have been achieved. Also, instruction and supervision in such exercises is required to ensure that they are performed safely.

For individuals beginning a new sport activity, once the prescribed goals of stretching, strengthening, and proprioceptive conditioning have been met, a period of sport-specific training should begin. During this period, the patient would perform the actions normally required by the sport with gradually increasing intensity and duration.

Forcing stretching or strengthening to the point of pain is always deleterious and should be avoided. Progress is achieved by performing these exercises frequently (2 to 4 times a day, 7 days a week) and making small gains. The patient should be instructed to call the physician if the exercises cause pain.

## Stretching Exercises

The capsule and muscles of the posterior shoulder may be tight, especially in the individual who participates in repetitive overhead activities, including overhead throwing sports. Cross-over arm stretches are helpful to relax these muscles.

## Strengthening Exercises

Exercises to strengthen the deltoid and rotator cuff muscles can be done most easily using commercially available elastic therapy bands. These are available in different thicknesses, which provide different amounts of resistance. The same exercises can also be performed with pulleys or free weights. It usually takes 2 to 3 weeks to progress from one band or weight to the next. For strength training, the patient should perform 2 sets of 8 repetitions, progressing to 3 sets of 12 repetitions. Once 12 repetitions are reached, the resistance should be increased and the repetitions started over at 8. However, the patient should be advised not to progress to the next level of resistance if he or she still has difficulty at the current level or if pain develops when trying the new one. The patient should also be instructed to continue stretching exercises during this stage so that the hard-won gains in range of motion are not lost.

## Proprioceptive Exercises

Proprioceptive exercises for the shoulder involve weight bearing through the arms. For example, push-ups performed with the hands on an exercise ball are an excellent advanced exercise for improving dynamic scapular stabilization. For the novice, standing push-ups done against a wall provide good proprioceptive training. To perform this exercise, the individual should stand several feet away from a wall with a 5″ or 7″ exercise ball in each hand. Leaning toward the wall, place the balls on the wall and move them up and down with the eyes closed to increase position sense. Then do push-ups against the wall with the hands on the balls, bending and extending at the elbow.

# HOME EXERCISE PROGRAM
# FOR SHOULDER CONDITIONING

For the exercises that use a stick, you may use a yardstick or stick of similar size. The exercises should never be performed at a level that causes pain. If the exercises cause pain, call your doctor.

## Stretching and Strengthening Exercises for the Shoulder

| Exercise | Muscle Group | Number of Repetitions/Sets | Number of Days per Week | Number of Weeks |
|---|---|---|---|---|
| **Stretching** | | | | |
| Pendulum | General | 10 repetitions/2 sets, progressing to 15 repetitions/3 sets | 5 to 6 | 2 to 3 |
| Passive internal rotation | Subscapularis Pectoralis major and minor | 4 sets | 5 to 6 | 6 to 8 |
| Passive external rotation | Infraspinatus Teres minor | 4 sets | 5 to 6 | 6 to 8 |
| Cross-over arm stretch | Posterior deltoid | 4 sets | 5 to 6 | 6 to 8 |
| **Strengthening** | | | | |
| External rotation | Infraspinatus Teres minor | 8 repetitions/3 sets, progressing to 12 repetitions/3 sets | 3 | 8 |
| Standing row | Middle trapezius Rhomboid | 8 repetitions/3 sets, progressing to 12 repetitions/3 sets | 3 | 8 |
| Internal rotation | Pectoralis major and minor Subscapularis | 8 repetitions/3 sets, progressing to 12 repetitions/3 sets | 3 | 8 |
| Bent-over horizontal abduction | Middle and lower trapezius | 8 repetitions/3 sets, progressing to 12 repetitions/3 sets | 3 | 8 |
| Elbow flexion | Biceps | 8 repetitions/3 sets, progressing to 12 repetitions/3 sets | 3 | 8 |
| Elbow extension | Triceps | 8 repetitions/3 sets, progressing to 12 repetitions/3 sets | 3 | 8 |

APPENDIX A ■ MUSCULOSKELETAL CONDITIONING

# Stretching Exercises

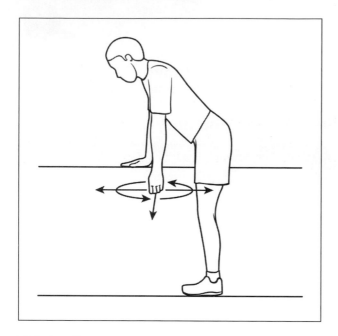

### Pendulum
Lean forward, supporting the body with one arm and relaxing the muscles of the other arm so that it hangs freely. Gently move the arm in forward-and-back, side-to-side, and circular motions. Repeat on the other side.

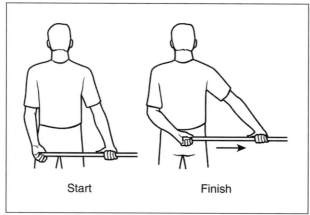

Start    Finish

### Passive Internal Rotation
Behind your back, grasp the stick with one hand and lightly grasp the other end of the stick with the other hand. Pull the stick horizontally as shown so that the arm is passively stretched to the point of feeling a pull without pain. Hold for 30 seconds and then relax for 30 seconds. Repeat on the other side.

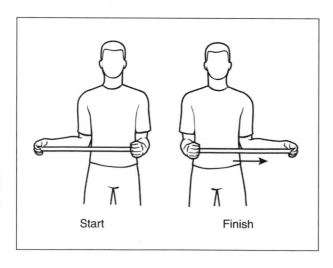

Start    Finish

### Passive External Rotation
Grasp the stick with one hand and cup the other end of the stick with the other hand. Push the stick horizontally as shown, keeping the elbow against the side of the body so that the arm is passively stretched to the point of feeling a pull without pain. Hold for 30 seconds and then relax for 30 seconds. Repeat on the other side.

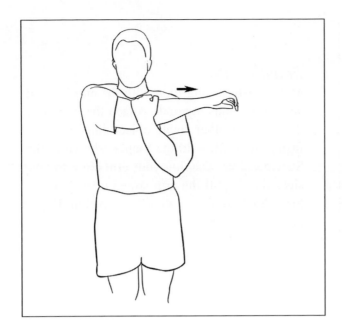

### Cross-Over Arm Stretch

Gently pull the elbow of one arm across the chest as far as possible without feeling pain. Hold the stretch for 30 seconds and then relax for 30 seconds. Repeat on the other side.

## Strengthening Exercises

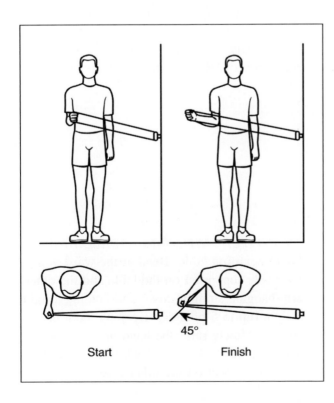

45°

Start     Finish

### External Rotation

Make a 3-foot-long loop with the elastic band and tie the ends together. Attach the loop to a doorknob or other stable object. Standing with your side to the wall, hold the loop as shown in the Start position. Keeping your elbow close to your side, rotate the arm outward slowly and then slowly return to the Start position. Repeat on the other side.

APPENDIX A ■ MUSCULOSKELETAL CONDITIONING

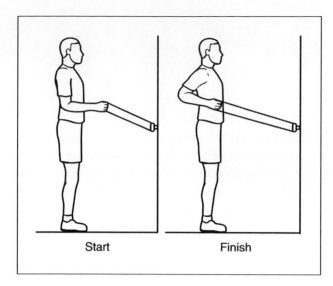

### Standing Row

Make a 3-foot-long loop with the elastic band and tie the ends together. Attach the loop to a doorknob or other stable object. Standing facing the wall, hold the loop as shown in the Start position. Keeping your arm close to your side, slowly pull the arm straight back and then slowly return to the Start position. Repeat on the other side.

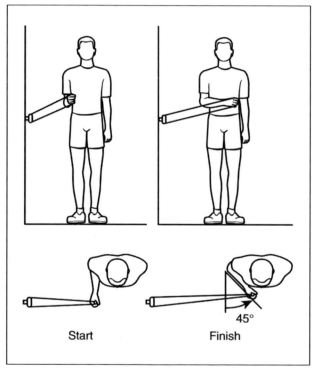

### Internal Rotation

Make a 3-foot-long loop with the elastic band and tie the ends together. Attach the loop to a doorknob or other stable object. Standing with your side to the wall, hold the loop as shown in the Start position. Keeping your elbow close to your side, rotate the arm across your body slowly and then slowly return to the Start position. Repeat on the other side.

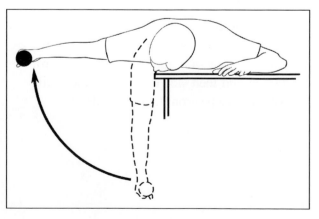

### Bent-Over Horizontal Abduction

Stand next to a table. Bend at the waist with your side supported on the table and the other arm hanging straight down and holding a light weight (up to 5 pounds). Keeping the arm straight, slowly raise the hand up to eye level and then slowly lower it back to the starting position. Repeat on the other side.

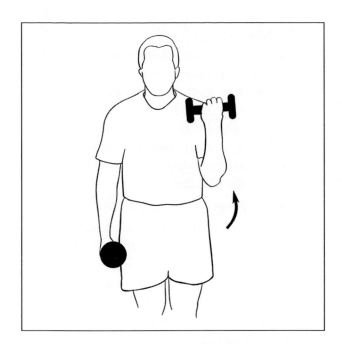

### Elbow Flexion

Stand with your weight evenly distributed over both feet. Holding a light weight (up to 5 pounds) and keeping the arm close to the side, slowly bend the elbow up toward the shoulder as shown; hold for 5 seconds, slowly return to the starting position, and then relax. Repeat on the other side.

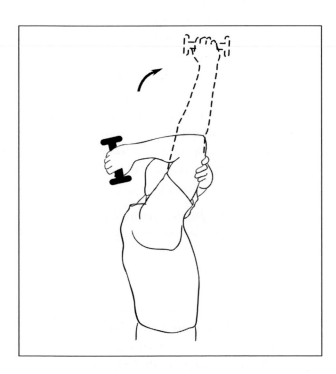

### Elbow Extension

Stand with your weight evenly distributed over both feet. Holding a light weight (up to 5 pounds), raise your arm with the elbow bent and with your opposite hand supporting your elbow. Slowly straighten the elbow overhead, hold for 5 seconds, and then slowly lower the arm to the starting position. Repeat on the other side.

APPENDIX A ■ MUSCULOSKELETAL CONDITIONING

# HIP CONDITIONING

The 35 muscles of the hip and pelvis are important in walking and running activities. Both the shoulder and hip are ball-and-socket joints, but because of its particular anatomy, the hip is more stable than the shoulder.

Conditioning of the hip should consist of stretching, strengthening, and power (plyometric) phases. Proprioceptive conditioning is also important for balance and control of the lower kinetic chain movement patterns.

## Warm-Up and Stretching Exercises

The hip muscle groups are large and require an adequate warm-up, such as riding on a stationary bicycle or jogging for 10 minutes to raise the core body temperature. In addition to or instead of these activities, the patient may perform the stretching exercises described below. The patient should stretch the muscle to the end of the available range of painless motion of the muscle and joint, holding the position of maximum stretch for 30 seconds.

## Strengthening Exercises

Exercises that isolate muscle contraction and do not stimulate co-contractions are important for strengthening the hip muscles. In general, weight-bearing activities produce co-contractions and non–weight-bearing exercises do not. Strengthening of the large hip muscle groups requires heavier weights and fewer (6 to 12) repetitions. After beginning with a weight that allows the patient to perform 6 to 8 repetitions initially, working up to 12 repetitions should be the goal of the strengthening phase. The exercises described below isolate the gluteus medius (posterior fibers), gluteus maximus, and the internal and external rotators, which often are weak and therefore contribute to hip pathology.

## Plyometrics and Proprioceptive Conditioning

In addition to strengthening, the athlete requires power and balance. Neuromuscular training, which improves the communication between the muscles and the proprioceptors, includes plyometrics (for power) as well as balance and perturbation exercises. Jumping exercises, such as jumping forward and backward over a barrier, are a basic form of plyometrics. These should be attempted only by individuals with full range of motion and adequate strength in the hip, pelvic and abdominal, and back muscles. Balance involves three systems: the visual, vestibular, and proprioceptive systems. With balance training, the athlete consciously attempts to hold a posture for 30 to 60 seconds. With perturbation training, the athlete stands on an unstable surface such as a balance board while it is being perturbed by an outside force. These types of plyometric and proprioceptive exercises should be supervised by a physical therapist or certified athletic trainer.

# HOME EXERCISE PROGRAM FOR HIP CONDITIONING

The stretching exercises below may be done in addition to or in place of riding a stationary bicycle or jogging for 10 minutes. When performing the exercises, you should stretch slowly to the limit of motion, taking care to avoid pain. If you experience pain with the exercises, call your doctor.

## Stretching and Strengthening Exercises for the Hip

| Exercise | Muscle Group | Number of Repetitions/Sets | Number of Days per Week |
|---|---|---|---|
| **Stretching** | | | |
| Seat side straddle | Adductor muscles Medial hamstrings Semitendinosus Semimembranosus | 4 repetitions/2 to 3 sets | Daily |
| Modified seat side straddle | Hamstrings Adductor muscles | 4 repetitions/2 to 3 sets | Daily |
| Leg stretch | Hamstrings | 4 repetitions/2 to 3 sets | Daily |
| Sitting rotation stretch | Piriformis External rotators Internal rotators | 4 repetitions/2 to 3 sets | Daily |
| Knee to chest | Posterior hip muscles | 4 repetitions/2 to 3 sets | Daily |
| Leg cross-over | Hamstrings | 4 repetitions/2 to 3 sets | Daily |
| Cross-over stand | Hamstrings | 4 repetitions/2 to 3 sets | Daily |
| Iliotibial band stretch | Tensor fascia | 4 repetitions/2 to 3 sets | Daily |
| Prone quadriceps stretch | Quadriceps | 4 repetitions/2 to 3 sets | Daily |
| **Strengthening** | | | |
| Prone hip extension | Gluteus maximus | 6 to 8 repetitions, progressing to 12 repetitions | 2 to 3 |
| Side-lying hip abduction | Gluteus medius | 6 to 8 repetitions, progressing to 12 repetitions | 2 to 3 |
| Internal hip rotation | Medial hamstrings | 6 to 8 repetitions, progressing to 12 repetitions | 2 to 3 |
| External hip rotation | Piriformis | 6 to 8 repetitions, progressing to 12 repetitions | 2 to 3 |

APPENDIX A ■ MUSCULOSKELETAL CONDITIONING

# Stretching Exercises

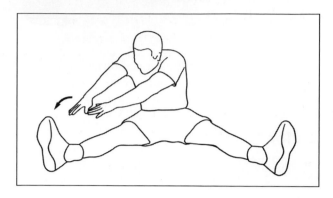

### Seat Side Straddle
Sit on the floor with your legs spread apart. Place both hands on the same ankle and bring your chin as close to your knee as possible. Hold the maximum stretch for 30 seconds and then relax for 30 seconds. Repeat on the other side. Repeat the sequence 4 times.

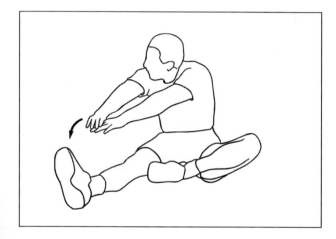

### Modified Seat Side Straddle
Sit on the floor with one leg extended to the side and the other leg bent as shown. Place both hands on the ankle of the extended leg and bring your chin as close to your knee as possible. Hold the maximum stretch for 30 seconds and then relax for 30 seconds. Reverse leg positions and repeat on the other side. Repeat the sequence 4 times.

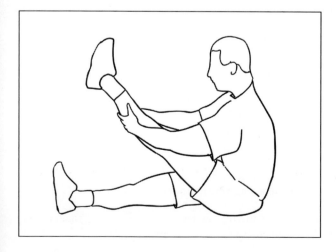

### Leg Stretch
Sit on the floor with your legs straight and your hands grasping the calf of one leg. Slowly lift and pull the leg toward your ear, keeping your back straight and the other leg flat on the floor or bent slightly if necessary for comfort. Hold the maximum stretch for 30 seconds and then relax for 30 seconds. Repeat with the other leg. Repeat the sequence 4 times.

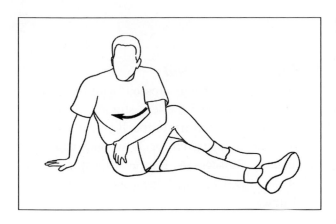

## Sitting Rotation Stretch

Sit on the floor with both legs straight out in front of you. Cross one leg over the other, place the elbow of the opposite arm on the outside of the thigh, and support yourself with your other arm behind you. Rotate your head and body in the direction of the supporting arm. Hold the maximum stretch for 30 seconds and then relax for 30 seconds. Reverse positions and repeat the stretch on the other side. Repeat the sequence 4 times.

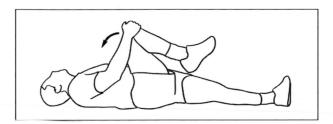

## Knee to Chest

Lie on your back on the floor with your knees bent and your heels flat on the floor. Grasp one knee and slowly bring it toward your chest as far as it will go. Hold the maximum stretch for 30 seconds and then relax for 30 seconds. Repeat with the other leg, then do both legs together. Repeat the sequence 4 times, working up to 3 sets of 10.

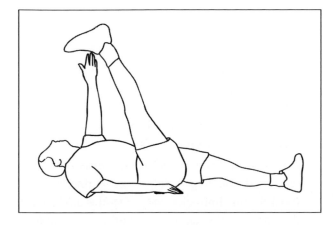

## Leg Cross-Over

Lie on the floor with your legs spread and your arms at your sides. Keeping the leg straight, bring your right toe to your left hand. Try to keep the other leg flat on the floor, but you may bend it slightly if needed for comfort. Hold the maximum stretch for 30 seconds and then relax for 30 seconds. Repeat with the left leg and the right hand. Repeat the sequence 4 times.

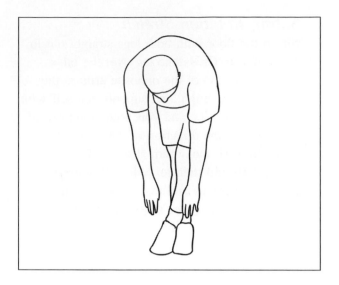

### Cross-Over Stand

Stand with your legs crossed, with the feet close together and the legs straight. Slowly bend forward and try to touch your toes. Hold the maximum stretch for 30 seconds and then relax for 30 seconds. Repeat with the position of the legs reversed. Repeat the sequence 4 times.

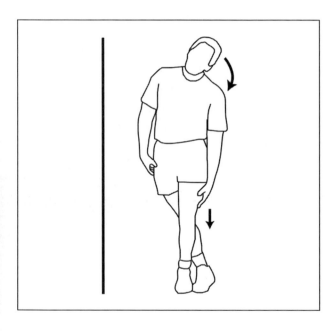

### Iliotibial Band Stretch

Stand next to a wall for support. Begin with your weight distributed evenly over both feet, and then cross one leg behind the other. Lean the hip of the crossed-over leg toward the wall until you feel a stretch on the outside of the leg. Hold the maximum stretch for 30 seconds and then relax for 30 seconds. Repeat the sequence 4 times.

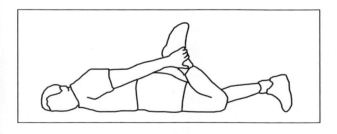

### Prone Quadriceps Stretch

Lie on your stomach with your arms at your sides and your legs straight. Bend one knee up toward your buttocks and grasp the ankle with the hand on the same side. Pull on the ankle and hold at the point of maximum stretch for 30 seconds, then relax for 30 seconds. Repeat on the opposite side. Repeat the sequence 4 times.

# Strengthening Exercises

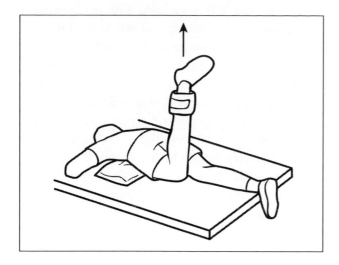

### Prone Hip Extension

Lie face down with a pillow under your hips and the knee on the affected side bent 90°. Elevate the leg off the floor, lifting the leg straight up with the knee bent. Lower the leg to the floor slowly, to a count of 5. Ankle weights should be used, starting with light enough weight to allow 6 to 8 repetitions, working up to 12 repetitions. Then add as much weight as can be lifted only 8 times. Work up to 12 repetitions again. Continue this cycle of adding weight and increasing repetitions.

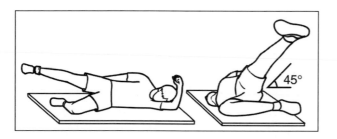

### Side-Lying Hip Abduction

Lie on your side with the affected hip on top, cradling your head in your arm, and the bottom leg bent to provide support. Slowly move the top leg up and back to 45°, keeping the knee straight. Lower the leg slowly, to a count of 5, and relax it for 2 seconds. Ankle weights should be used, starting with light enough weight to allow 6 to 8 repetitions, progressing to 12 repetitions. Then add as much weight as can be lifted only 8 times. Work up to 12 repetitions again. Continue this cycle of adding weight and increasing repetitions.

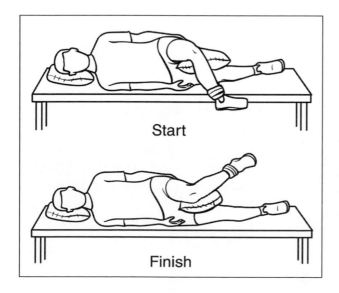

Start

Finish

### Internal Hip Rotation

Lie on your side on a table with a pillow between your thighs. Bend the top leg 90° at the hip and 90° at the knee. Start with the foot of the top leg below the level of the top of the table; lift to the Finish position, which is rotated as high as possible. Lower the leg slowly, to a count of 5. Begin with an ankle weight that allows 6 to 8 repetitions, progressing to 12 repetitions. Then add as much weight as can be lifted only 8 times. Work up to 12 repetitions again. Continue this cycle of adding weight and increasing repetitions.

APPENDIX A ■ MUSCULOSKELETAL CONDITIONING

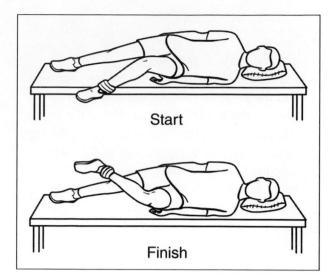

Start

Finish

## External Hip Rotation

Lie on your side on a table with the bottom leg bent 90° at the hip and 90° at the knee. Start with the foot below the level of the top of the table; lift to the Finish position, which is rotated as high as possible. Lower the leg slowly, to a count of 5. Begin with an ankle weight that allows 6 to 8 repetitions, progressing to 12 repetitions. Then add as much weight as can be lifted only 8 times. Work up to 12 repetitions again. Continue this cycle of adding weight and increasing repetitions.

# KNEE CONDITIONING

The knee, like the shoulder, is an unstable joint. Muscles provide stability to the knee joint and the patellofemoral articulation. Strengthening the quadriceps and hamstrings muscle groups provides dynamic stability to the knee. In addition, the hip muscles, such as the gluteus maximus, the gluteus medius, and the internal and external rotators, help to control the movements of the femur and the posture of the patellofemoral articulation. Conditioning of the knee should focus on three phases: stretching, strengthening, and neuromuscular (proprioceptive) training. Plyometrics (power training) would be added for the competitive athlete after basic strength and flexibility have been achieved. Advanced proprioceptive exercises and plyometric exercises should be done under the supervision of a physical therapist or certified athletic trainer.

## Stretching Exercises

The effectiveness of strengthening exercises for the quadriceps muscle group may be compromised if the range of motion of the knee is limited. Stretching the soft tissues to gain range of motion, especially after trauma or periods of immobilization, can be very effective in gaining range of motion. Hamstring stretching exercises such as leg stretches, leg cross-overs, and cross-over standing increase the range of motion at the knee and hip during functional activities such as walking and running.

Once the patient has achieved normal range of motion and strength, sport- or work-specific training should begin. The knee musculature needs to be strong and powerful, and protective reflexes need to be optimized to reduce the risk of injury during sporting maneuvers such as sudden changes in direction while running.

## Strengthening Exercises

Exercises to strengthen the quadriceps and hamstrings can be performed conveniently with progressively heavier ankle weights. The resistance training must be progressive so that the muscle is constantly stimulated to grow. Hamstring curls, supine straight-leg raises (for the quadriceps), prone straight-leg raises (for the hamstrings), wall slides, and forward lunges are good strengthening exercises. The patient should begin with a weight that allows 2 sets of 8 to10 repetitions and should work up to 3 sets of 12 to15 repetitions. After reaching 3 sets of 15 repetitions with a given weight, the patient should add weight and drop back to 2 sets of 8 repetitions. Strengthening of the gluteus medius and gluteus maximus using hip abduction

APPENDIX A ■ MUSCULOSKELETAL CONDITIONING

and extension exercises should also be part of the knee strengthening program.

## Proprioceptive Training

Proprioceptive training is important for balance. Balance, or postural control, is the result of the integration of visual, vestibular, and proprioceptive afferent inputs. The goal of proprioceptive training is to enhance the activity of the proprioceptors, thereby improving their ability to protect ligaments of the knee. Several commercial devices, such as tiltboards and proprioceptive disks, are available for proprioceptive training. Advanced balance training should be performed under the supervision of a physical therapist or certified athletic trainer.

## Plyometric Exercises

Explosive power of the lower leg is necessary for a high level of athletic performance. Plyometrics and explosive weight training facilitate the development of power in the quadriceps and hamstrings muscles. Examples of plyometric exercises are jumping rope and jumping from side to side over a 6-inch-high barrier. More advanced exercises should be performed under the supervision of a physical therapist or certified athletic trainer.

# HOME EXERCISE PROGRAM FOR KNEE CONDITIONING

## Stretching and Strengthening Exercises for the Knee

| Exercise | Muscle Group | Number of Repetitions/Sets | Number of Days per Week | Number of Weeks |
|---|---|---|---|---|
| **Stretching** | | | | |
| Leg stretch | Hamstrings | 3 to 6 repetitions/3 sets | Daily | 6 to 8 |
| Leg cross-over | Hamstrings | 3 to 6 repetitions/3 sets | Daily | 6 to 8 |
| Cross-over stand | Hamstrings | 3 to 6 repetitions/3 sets | Daily | 6 to 8 |
| Straight-leg raise | Quadriceps | Work up to 3 sets of 10 repetitions | Daily | 6 to 8 |
| Straight-leg raise (prone) | Gluteus maximus | Work up to 3 sets of 10 repetitions | Daily | 6 to 8 |
| Wall slide | Quadriceps Hamstrings | Work up to 3 sets of 10 repetitions | Daily | 6 to 8 |
| **Strengthening** | | | | |
| Forward lunge | Quadriceps | Work up to 3 sets of 10 repetitions | 3 | 6 to 8 |
| Hamstring curl | Hamstrings | 10 repetitions/5 sets/3 times a day | 3 | 6 to 8 |
| Side-lying hip abduction | Gluteus medius | 6 to 8 repetitions, progressing to 12 repetitions | 3 | 6 to 8 |
| Hip extension | Gluteus maximus | 6 to 8 repetitions, progressing to 12 repetitions | 3 | 6 to 8 |

APPENDIX A ■ MUSCULOSKELETAL CONDITIONING

# Stretching Exercises

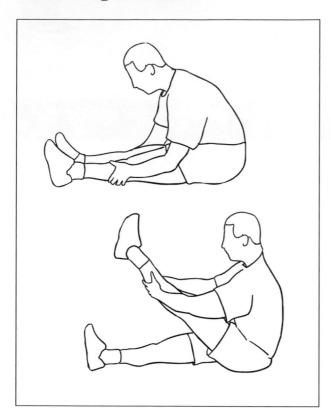

## *Leg Stretch*

Sit on the floor with your legs straight in front of you and place your hands on the backs of your calves. Slowly lift and pull one leg toward your ear, keeping your back straight. Hold the stretch for 5 seconds. Alternate from side to side. Repeat each leg 3 to 6 times. For comfort, you may slightly bend the leg not being stretched.

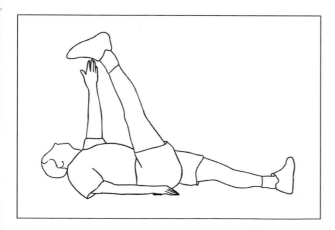

## *Leg Cross-Over*

Lie on the floor with your legs spread and your arms out to the sides. Bring your right toe to your left hand, keeping the leg straight. Hold the stretch for 5 seconds. Alternate from side to side. Repeat each leg 3 to 6 times. For comfort, you may slightly bend the leg not being stretched.

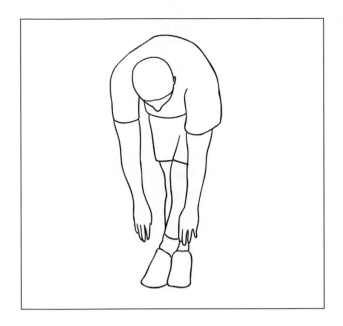

### Cross-Over Stand
Stand with your legs crossed. Keeping your feet close together and your legs straight, slowly bend forward toward your toes. Hold the stretch for 5 seconds. Repeat with the opposite leg crossed in front.

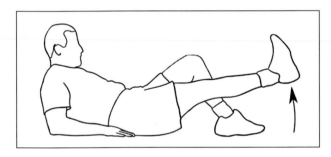

### Straight-Leg Raise
Lie on the floor with one leg straight and the other leg bent. Tighten the thigh muscle of the straight leg and slowly raise it 6 to 10 inches off the floor. Hold this position for 5 seconds. Repeat with the opposite leg. Work up to 3 sets of 10.

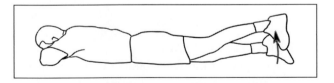

### Straight-Leg Raise (Prone)
Lie on the floor on your stomach with your legs straight. Keeping the leg straight, tighten the hamstrings of one leg and raise the leg as high as you can. Hold this position for 5 seconds. Repeat with the opposite leg. Work up to 3 sets of 10.

APPENDIX A ■ MUSCULOSKELETAL CONDITIONING

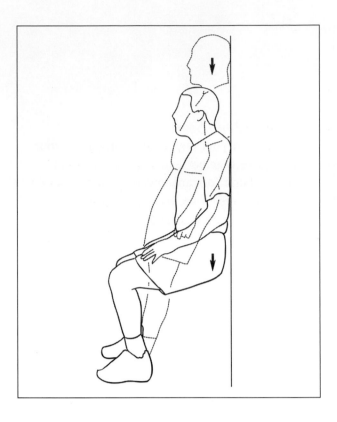

### Wall Slides
Stand with your back against a wall and your feet about 1 foot from the wall. Tuck your pelvis under so that your lower back is flat against the wall. Stop when your knees are bent 90°. Hold for 5 seconds and then relax. Work up to 3 sets of 10.

## Strengthening Exercises

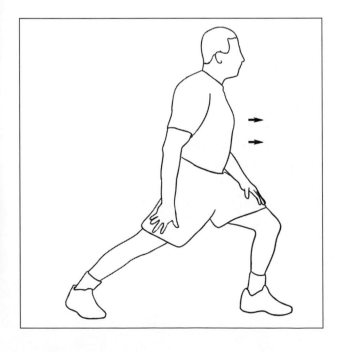

### Forward Lunges
Stand up with the feet about 3 to 4 feet apart and with the forward foot pointing forward and the back foot angled to provide support. Lunge forward, bending the forward knee and keeping the back and the back leg straight. You should feel a slight stretch in the left groin area. Hold the stretch for 5 seconds. Repeat with the opposite leg.

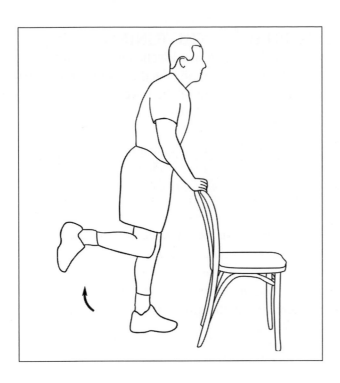

## Hamstring Curls

Stand on a flat surface with your weight evenly distributed over both feet. Hold onto the back of a chair or the wall for balance. Raise the heel of one leg toward the ceiling. Hold this position for 5 seconds and then relax. Perform 5 sets of 10, 3 times a day.

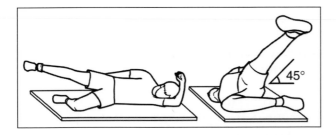

## Side-Lying Hip Abduction

Lie on your side with the affected hip on top, cradling your head in your arm, and the bottom leg bent to provide support. Slowly move the top leg up and back to 45°, keeping the knee straight. Hold this position for 5 seconds. Slowly lower the leg and relax it for 2 seconds. Ankle weights should be used, starting with light enough weight to allow 6 to 8 repetitions, progressing to 12 repetitions. Then return to 6 to 8 repetitions and add weight.

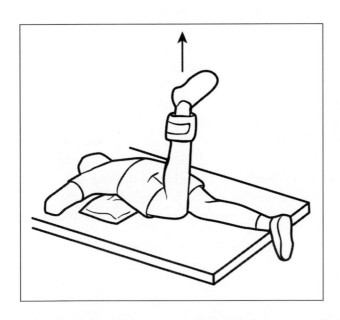

## Hip Extension

Lie face down with a pillow under your hips and the knee on the affected side bent 90°. Elevate the leg off the floor to a count of 5, lifting the leg straight up with the knee bent. Ankle weights should be used, starting with light enough weight to allow 6 to 8 repetitions, working up to 12 repetitions. Then return to 6 to 8 repetitions and add weight.

APPENDIX A ■ MUSCULOSKELETAL CONDITIONING

# FOOT AND ANKLE CONDITIONING

The foot is the first part of the lower kinetic chain to hit the ground during weight-bearing activities and is therefore the first input to the neuromuscular system of the lower kinetic chain. Dynamic joint stability is critical for injury prevention and improved performance during sports activities. Whether an individual experiences a single-episode lateral ankle sprain or develops chronic ankle instability most likely depends on rehabilitation of the individual's proprioception.

## Stretching Exercises

Performing stretching exercises to warm up the muscles prior to athletic activities is important for optimal neuromuscular control and for maintaining normal range of motion. Heel cord stretches performed with the knee both straight and bent are good stretching exercises for the gastrocnemius-soleus muscle complex.

## Strengthening Exercises

Strengthening exercises for the foot and ankle include calf raises, ankle curls, and ankle inversion/eversion exercises.

## Toe Strengthening Exercises

The toe strengthening program is helpful for patients with the particular conditions listed, including bunions, hammer toes, plantar fasciitis, and toe cramps.

## Proprioceptive Exercises

Optimizing the proprioceptive system is important in preventing injuries such as ankle sprains and anterior cruciate ligament tears in both athletes and nonathletes. Balance, or postural control, is the result of the integration of visual, vestibular, and proprioceptive afferent inputs. The goal of proprioceptive training is to enhance the activity of the proprioceptors, thereby improving their ability to protect ligaments of the foot and ankle. Several commercial devices, such as tiltboards and proprioceptive disks, are available for proprioceptive training. Perturbation training is another way to optimize the proprioceptive system, especially in athletes. Perturbation exercises are performed on an unstable surface with perturbing forces applied in all directions. Perturbation training and advanced balance training should be performed under the supervision of a physical therapist or certified athletic trainer.

## Plyometrics

Explosive power is necessary for a high level of athletic performance. Plyometrics facilitate the development of power. Examples of plyometric exercises are jumping rope and jumping from side to side over a 6-inch-high barrier. More advanced exercises should be performed under the supervision of a physical therapist or certified athletic trainer.

APPENDIX A ■ MUSCULOSKELETAL CONDITIONING

# HOME EXERCISE PROGRAM FOR FOOT AND ANKLE CONDITIONING

## Stretching and Strengthening Exercises for the Foot and Ankle

| Exercise | Muscle Group | Number of Repetitions/Sets | Number of Days per Week | Number of Weeks |
|---|---|---|---|---|
| **Stretching** | | | | |
| Heel cord stretch | *Knee straight:* Gastrocnemius *Knee bent:* Soleus | 4 to 5 repetitions/2 to 3 sets | Daily | 6 to 8 |
| **Strengthening** | | | | |
| Calf raises | Gastrocnemius-soleus complex | 10 repetitions/3 sets | 3 | 6 to 8 |
| Ankle curls | Anterior tibialis | 10 repetitions/3 sets | 3 | 6 to 8 |
| Ankle eversion/inversion | Posterior tibialis Peroneus longus Peroneus brevis | 10 repetitions/3 sets | 3 | 6 to 8 |

## Toe Strengthening Program

| Exercise | Recommended for | Repetitions or Duration |
|---|---|---|
| Toe squeeze | Hammer toes, toe cramps | 10 |
| Big toe pulls | Bunions, toe cramps | 10 |
| Toe pulls | Bunions, hammer toes, toe cramps | 10 |
| Golf ball roll | Plantar fasciitis, arch strain, foot cramps | 2 minutes |
| Marble pick-up | Pain in ball of foot, hammer toes, toe cramps | Until all marbles have been picked up |
| Towel curls | Hammer toes, toe cramps, pain in ball of foot | 5 |

# Stretching Exercise

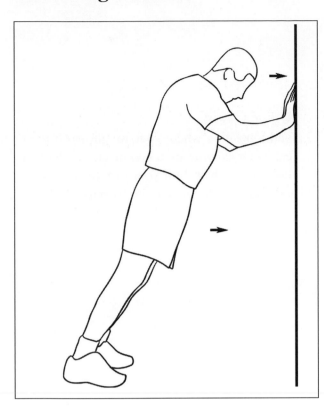

### Heel Cord Stretch

Support yourself against a wall with your feet pointed straight ahead. *Stretch with knee straight:* Keeping the heel in contact with the ground and the knee straight, place the foot as far back as possible until a stretch is felt in the calf. *Stretch with knee extended:* Same position but bend the knee of the leg being stretched. Hold the stretch for 30 seconds, then relax for 30 seconds. Repeat on the other side. Perform 2 to 3 sets of 4 to 5 repetitions of each exercise.

# Strengthening Exercises

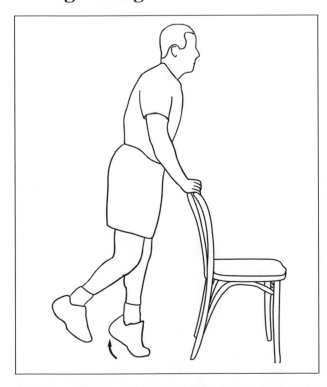

### Calf Raises

Stand with your weight evenly distributed over both feet. Hold onto the back of a chair or the wall for balance. Lift one foot so that all your weight is on the other foot. Then lift the heel off the floor as high as you can. Repeat on the other side. Work up to 3 sets of 10 repetitions.

APPENDIX A ■ MUSCULOSKELETAL CONDITIONING

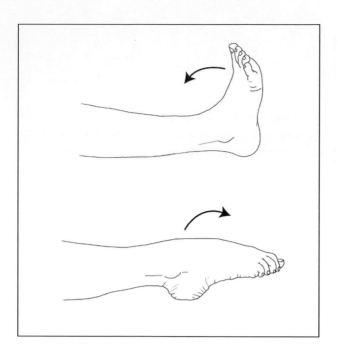

## Ankle Curls

Find a position where your weight is off your feet, such as lying on a bed or on the floor or seated on a chair. Pull your toes toward you and then extend them as far as possible. Perform 2 to 3 sets of 10 repetitions.

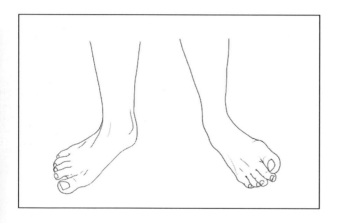

## Ankle Eversion/Inversion

Find a position where your weight is off your feet, such as lying on a bed or on the floor or seated on a chair. Slowly move your foot from side to side, keeping the lower leg motionless and moving only at the ankle. Perform 2 to 3 sets of 10 repetitions.

# Toe Strengthening Exercises

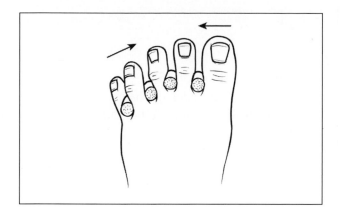

## *Toe Squeeze*
Place small sponges or corks between the toes and hold a squeeze for 5 seconds. Repeat 10 times.

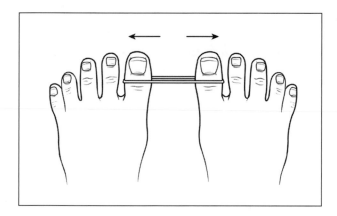

## *Big Toe Pulls*
Place a thick rubber band around both big toes and pull the big toes away from each other and toward the small toes. Hold for 5 seconds. Repeat 10 times.

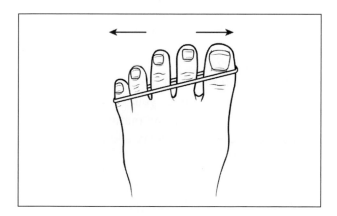

## *Toe Pulls*
Put a thick rubber band around all your toes and spread them. Hold this position for 5 seconds. Repeat 10 times.

Figures adapted from Brochure: *Bunion Surgery.* Rosemont, IL, American Academy of Orthopaedic Surgeons, 1995.

APPENDIX A ■ MUSCULOSKELETAL CONDITIONING

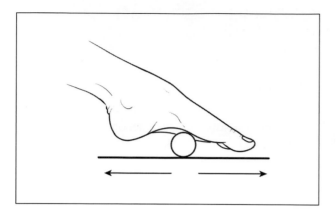

## Golf Ball Roll

Roll a golf ball under the ball of your foot for 2 minutes to massage the bottom of the foot.

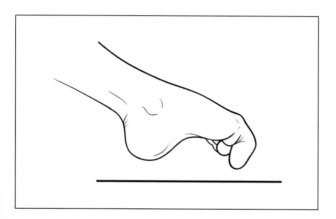

## Marble Pick-up

Place 20 marbles on the floor. Pick up one marble at a time and put it in a small bowl. Repeat until you have picked up all 20 marbles.

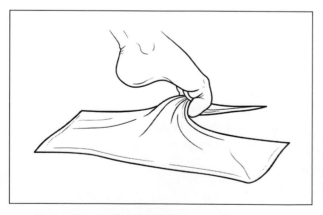

## Towel Curls

Place a small towel on the floor and curl it toward you, using only your toes. You can increase the resistance by putting weight on the end of the towel. Relax and repeat 5 times.

Figures adapted from Brochure: *Bunion Surgery.* Rosemont, IL, American Academy of Orthopaedic Surgeons, 1995.

APPENDIX A ■ MUSCULOSKELETAL CONDITIONING

# LUMBAR SPINE CONDITIONING

The lumbar spine muscles attach to the thoracic spine, the ribs, and the pelvis. Conditioning to prevent low back pain should involve stretching exercises, to improve range of motion, and endurance exercises. The focus of conditioning should be on having the patient understand and commit to a daily home exercise program. Because little or no muscle damage occurs with isometric exercises (unlike the concentric and eccentric exercises involved with strength training), recovery from isometric-endurance training occurs within several hours, and so isometric-endurance exercises may and should be done every day.

## Stretching Exercises

General stretching exercises for the lumbothoracic spine are helpful for improving range of motion. The cat back stretch and the cobra stretch are excellent stretching exercises for the spine in general. Flexibility of the hamstring muscles is also important for improving the mobility of the lumbar spine and reducing stress on the lumbar spine. The seat side straddle, modified seat side straddle, sitting rotation stretch, and leg cross-over are all excellent stretching exercises for the lumbothoracic spine.

## Endurance Exercises

The four muscle groups that protect the spine from daily overuse and trauma include the abdominals; the quadratus lumborum (two groups, one on each side of the spine); and the back extensors. The back extensors are the most important because poor endurance of these muscle groups has been found in patients with low back pain. Isometric-endurance exercises for these muscle groups, such as the bird dog exercise, have an important stabilizing effect on the spine.

The quadratus lumborum is an important lateral stabilizer of the trunk. A good endurance exercise for this muscle is the side bridge, which should be repeated on both sides for maximum and symmetric lateral stability.

The abdominals are important to stabilization of the lumbar and thoracic spine. The four major muscle groups that make up the abdominals are the transverse abdominus, internal and external obliques, and the rectus abdominus. The transverse abdominus muscle is a strong stabilizer of the lumbar spine through its attachment to the thoracolumbar fascia. Traditional sit-ups have been found to greatly increase the load on the lumbar disks and therefore should be avoided by low back pain patients. A safe exercise is abdominal bracing, which activates all the abdominal muscles, including the transverse abdominus, and does not stress the lumbar spine. This exercise does not activate the transverse abdominus if a pelvic tilt is performed.

# HOME EXERCISE PROGRAM FOR LUMBAR SPINE CONDITIONING

Perform the exercises in the order listed. If any of the exercises causes pain, call your doctor.

## Stretching and Endurance Exercises for the Lumbar Spine

| Exercise Type | Muscle Group/ Area Targeted | Number of Repetitions/Sets | Number of Days per Week | Number of Weeks |
|---|---|---|---|---|
| **Stretching** | | | | |
| Cat back stretch | Middle and low back | 10 repetitions | Daily | 3 to 4 |
| Cobra stretch | Low back | 10 repetitions | Daily | 3 to 4 |
| Seat side straddle | Adductor muscles Medial hamstrings Semitendinosus Semimembranosus | 10 repetitions | Daily | 3 to 4 |
| Modified seat side straddle | Adductor muscles Hamstrings | 10 repetitions | Daily | 3 to 4 |
| Sitting rotation stretch | Piriformis External rotators Internal rotators | 10 repetitions | Daily | 3 to 4 |
| Leg cross-over | Hamstrings | 10 repetitions | Daily | 3 to 4 |
| **Endurance** | | | | |
| Bird dog | Back extensors | 5 repetitions | Daily | 3 to 4 |
| Side bridges | Quadratus lumborum | 5 repetitions | Daily | 3 to 4 |
| Abdominal bracing | Abdominals | 5 repetitions | Daily | 3 to 4 |

## Stretching Exercises

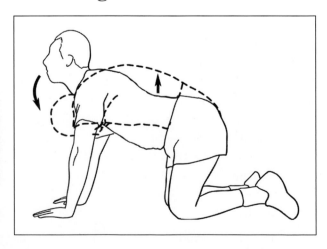

### Cat Back Stretch
Kneel on your hands and knees in a relaxed position. Raise your back up like a cat and hold for 30 seconds. Relax for 30 seconds. Repeat 10 times.

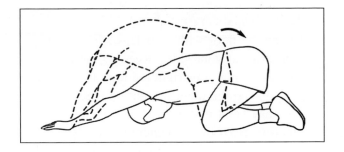

## Cobra Stretch

Crouch on your hands and knees. First rock forward onto your extended arms, allowing your back to sag. Hold for 5 seconds. Then rock back and sit on your bent knees with your arms extended and your head tucked in. Hold for 5 seconds. Repeat 10 times.

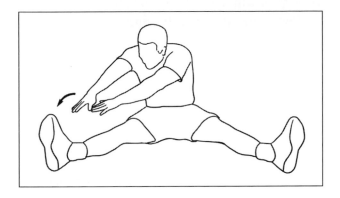

## Seat Side Straddle

Sit on the floor with your legs spread apart. Place both hands on the same ankle and bring your chin as close to your knee as possible. Hold the maximum stretch for 30 seconds and then relax for 30 seconds. Repeat on the other side. Repeat the sequence 10 times.

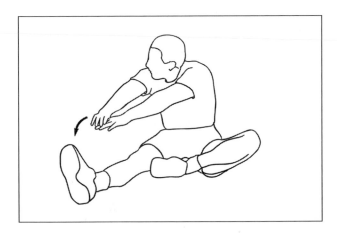

## Modified Seat Side Straddle

Sit on the floor with one leg extended to the side and the other leg bent as shown. Place both hands on the ankle of the extended leg and bring your chin as close to your knee as possible. Hold the maximum stretch for 30 seconds and then relax for 30 seconds. Reverse leg positions and repeat on the other side. Repeat the sequence 10 times.

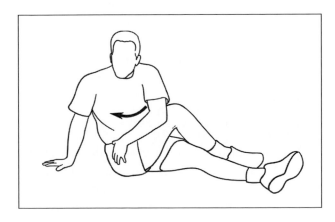

## Sitting Rotation Stretch

Sit on the floor with both legs straight out in front of you. Cross one leg over the other, place the elbow of the opposite arm on the outside of the thigh, and support yourself with your other arm behind you. Rotate your head and body in the direction of the supporting arm. Hold the maximum stretch for 30 seconds and then relax for 30 seconds. Reverse positions and repeat the stretch on the other side. Repeat the sequence 10 times.

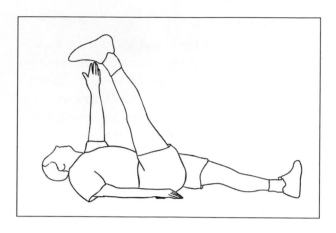

## Leg Cross-Over

Lie on the floor with your legs spread and your arms at your sides. Keeping the leg straight, bring your right toe to your left hand. Try to keep the other leg flat on the floor, but you may bend it slightly if needed for comfort. Hold the maximum stretch for 30 seconds and then relax for 30 seconds. Repeat with the left leg and the right hand. Repeat the sequence 10 times.

# Endurance Exercises

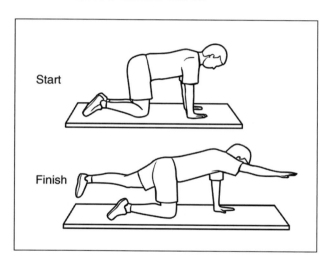

Start

Finish

## Bird Dog

Kneel on the floor on your hands and knees. Lift your right arm straight out from the shoulder, level with your body, at the same time you lift your left leg straight out from the hip. Start by holding the position for 15 seconds. Repeat with the opposite arm and leg. Perform 5 repetitions daily. The goal is to hold this position for 150 seconds (30 years of age or older) or 170 seconds (younger than 30 years).

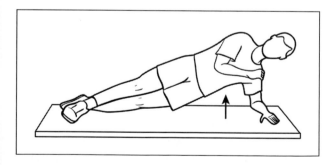

## Side Bridges

Lie on your side on the floor. With your elbow bent at 90°, lift your body off the floor as shown, keeping your body straight. Hold the position for 15 seconds and then repeat on the other side. Perform 5 repetitions daily. The goal is to hold the position for 150 seconds on each side. Note: For beginners, the knees may be bent 90°.

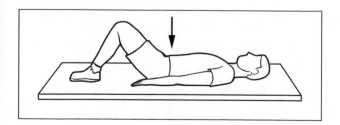

## Abdominal Bracing

Lie on your back on the floor with your arms at your sides, your knees bent, and your feet flat on the floor. Contract your abdominal muscles so that your stomach is pulled away from your waistband. Hold this position for 15 seconds. Perform 5 repetitions daily.

# MEASURING JOINT MOTION—UPPER EXTREMITY

## Shoulder

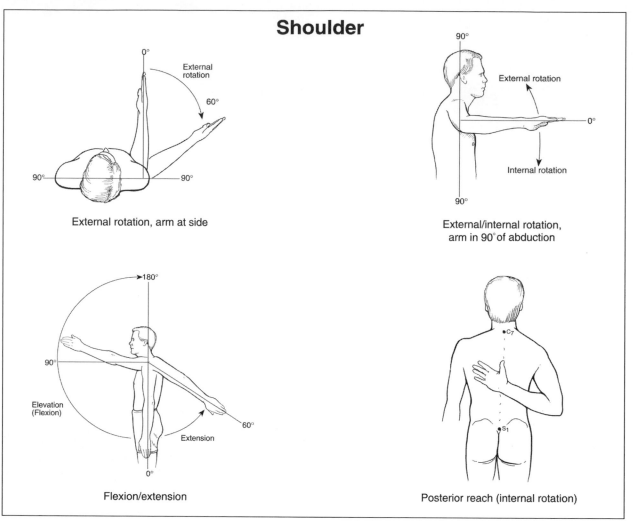

External rotation, arm at side

External/internal rotation, arm in 90° of abduction

Flexion/extension

Posterior reach (internal rotation)

## Wrist and Forearm

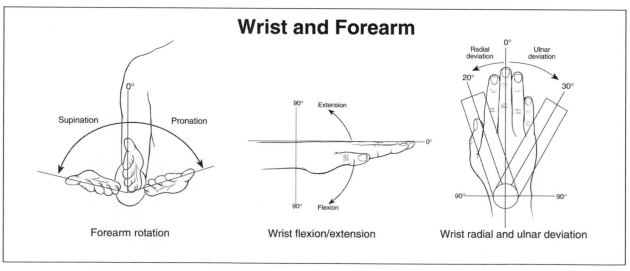

Forearm rotation

Wrist flexion/extension

Wrist radial and ulnar deviation

APPENDIX B ■ MEASURING JOINT MOTION

# MEASURING JOINT MOTION—LOWER EXTREMITY

## Hip

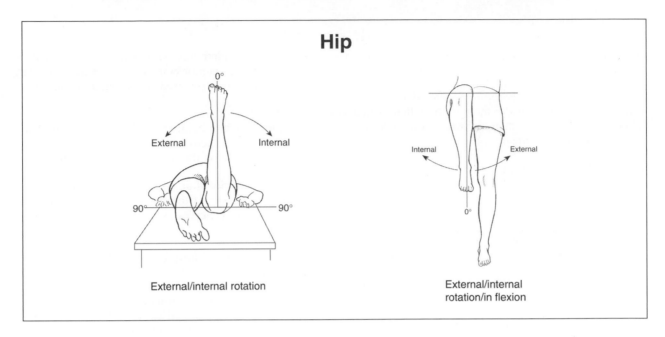

External/internal rotation

External/internal
rotation/in flexion

## Knee

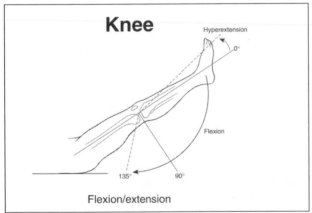

Flexion/extension

## Ankle

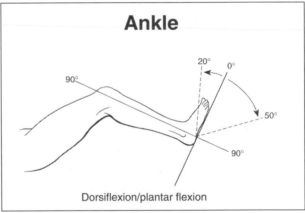

Dorsiflexion/plantar flexion

## Foot

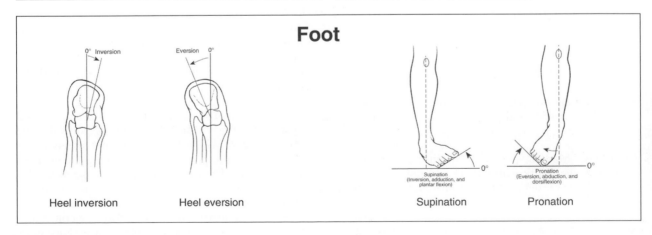

Heel inversion          Heel eversion

Supination          Pronation

# GLOSSARY

**Abduction**   The movement of a body part away from the midline

**Acupuncture**   The insertion of needles into precisely defined points on the body; thought to realign imbalances of yin-yang and qi and thereby bring harmony to the "climate" of an individual

**Adduction**   The movement of a body part toward the midline

**Adhesive capsulitis**   Self-limiting condition resulting from any inflammatory process about the shoulder in which capsular scar tissue is produced, resulting in pain and limited range of motion; also called frozen shoulder

**Aerobic exercise**   Exercise that uses oxidative metabolic pathways to provide energy

**Allograft**   Biologic tissue from a cadaver that is used to surgically replace damaged tissue

**Alternative medicine**   A wide spectrum of treatments—many finding support from collective anecdotal evidence—that is not considered standard therapy because of the lack of a scientific rationale, clinical evidence, or a favorable historic tradition

**Anabolic steroid**   Testosterone, or a steroid hormone resembling testosterone, that stimulates anabolism in the body

**Anaerobic exercise**   Exercise of short duration, not requiring the body's utilization of oxygen to make fuel available

**Anaerobic metabolism**   Oxygen debt; when the cardiovascular system is unable to meet the needs of the working muscles, the anaerobic metabolism is activated

**Analgesia**   The relief of pain

**Ankylosing spondylitis**   An inflammatory disorder that affects the low back and pelvis and produces stiffness and pain

**Ankylosis**   Marked stiffness of a joint typically observed with end-stage arthritis, following a complex intra-articular fracture, delayed treatment of septic arthritis, or severe rheumatoid arthritis

**Anorexia nervosa**   A condition, common in young females, in which the patient takes in less food and may become seriously emaciated and malnourished; a manifestation of a severe underlying psychological disorder

**Anterior compartment syndrome**   Increased soft-tissue pressure in the anterior compartment of the lower leg, resulting in pain, decreased sensation, and muscle paralysis

**Anterior cruciate ligament (ACL)**   Ligament that passes from the lateral intercondylar notch of the femur to attach anteriorly on the articular surface of the tibia

**Anterior superior iliac spine**   Blunt bony projection on the anterior border of the ilium, forming the anterior end of the iliac crest. Serves as the origin of the sartorius muscle.

**Anterior surface**   Surface at the front of the body, facing the examiner

**Anterior talofibular ligament**   One of three lateral ligaments of the ankle; arises from the anterior border of the lateral malleolus to attach to the neck of the talus

**Anterior tibial tendon**   Structure that arises in the anterior compartment of the leg and passes downward and medially to insert on the first cuneiform and the base of the first metatarsal

**Anterior tibiofibular ligament**   Part of tibiofibular syndesmosis; it arises from the anterior calculi on the lateral side of the tibia and blends into the interosseous membrane above the ankle joint

**Anterolateral rotatory instability**   Anterior internal rotational subluxation of the lateral tibial condyle on the femur, reflecting damage to the anterior cruciate ligament and lateral structures

**Anteromedial rotatory instability**   When the medial plateau of the tibia rotates anteriorly and medial joint opening occurs, indicating disruption of the superficial tibia collateral ligament, medial and posteromedial capsular structures, and anterior cruciate ligament

**Anteroposterior drawer test**   Test for anterior and posterior laxity in which the examiner holds the knee in 90° of flexion, stabilizes the thigh, and slowly draws the tibia forward on the fixed femur, noting the degree of displacement. The examiner then attempts to displace the tibia posteriorly on the femur. The test is positive if changes in anteroposterior displacement of the tibia are noted. The injured side should always be compared with the noninjured side. The Lachman test is done similarly but with the knee in 30° of flexion.

**Anulus fibrosus**   The outer ring of fibrous material surrounding the nucleus of the intervertebral disks

**Apophysis**   A cartilaginous structure at the insertion of major muscle groups into bone that may be susceptible to overuse syndromes and acute fractures in pediatric athletes

**Apophysitis**   Inflammation of an apophysis; injury from repetitive traction to the cartilaginous growth plate near the origin or insertion of muscle

**Arcuate ligament**   Posterior third of the lateral capsule, which, together with the popliteus attachments, provides considerable stability to the posterolateral corner of the knee

**Arthrocentesis**   Aspiration of a joint

**Arthrodesis**   The surgical fusion of a joint. The procedure removes any remaining articular cartilage and positions the adjacent bones to promote bone growth across a joint. A successful fusion eliminates the joint and stops motion. The usual purpose is pain relief or stabilization of an undependable joint.

**Arthroplasty**   A procedure to replace or mobilize a joint, typically performed by removing the arthritic surfaces and replacing them with an implant. Total joint arthroplasty is replacement of both sides of the joint. Hemiarthroplasty replaces only one side of a joint.

**Arthroscopy**   A form of minimally invasive surgery in which a fiberoptic camera, the arthroscope, is introduced into an area of the body through a small incision

**Aspiration**   Removal of fluids from a body cavity; often done to obtain specimens for analysis

**Autograft**   Biologic tissue from the patient's own body that is used to surgically replace damaged tissue

**Avascular necrosis**   A condition in which cells die as a result of inadequate blood supply; *See also* osteonecrosis

**Avulsion fracture**   A fracture that occurs when a ligament or tendon pulls off a sliver of the bone

**Axis**   The second cervical vertebra (C2)

**Bankart fracture**   A small chip fracture off the anterior and inferior rims of the glenoid that is seen after an anterior dislocation of the shoulder

**Biceps brachii**   Muscle in the anterior arm, originating from two heads (hence biceps) from the anterior glenoid and the coracoid process of the scapula and inserting into the biceps tuberosity of the radius. It is a powerful flexor of the elbow and supinator of the forearm.

**Biceps muscle**   Large muscle that covers the front of the humerus; functions include forearm flexion and hand supination

**Biceps tendinitis**   Inflammation of the biceps tendon in its subacromial location

**Bisphosphonates**   Potent inhibitors of osteoclasts and bone resorption. May be used to treat osteoporosis and Paget disease.

**Bone infarction**   Bone death that occurs as the result of ischemia

**Bone remodeling**   A process that couples bone resorption by osteoclasts with deposition of osteoblasts (new bone cells)

**Bone scan**   A study used to identify lesions in bone such as fracture, infections, or tumor. A radioisotope is injected into a vein and allowed to circulate through the body. The distribution of radioactivity in the skeleton is measured by a special camera that can detect the emission of gamma rays. Lesions in bone with increased metabolic activity (eg, fracture, tumor, or infection) will show increased uptake of the radioisotope and appear as a dark area in the bone. Also called bone scintigraphy.

**Brachial muscle**   Originates on the humerus, extends anteriorly across the elbow joint, and attaches into the ulna; functions in forearm flexion

**Brachial plexus**   Network of nerves that pass from the lower part of the cervical spine and upper part of the thoracic spine down the arm

**Bucket-handle tear**   Complete longitudinal tear of the central segment of the meniscus with the torn fragment "flipped" into the joint like the handle of a bucket

**Bunion**   Prominence of the first metatarsal head often associated with lateral shift of the great toe (hallux valgus deformity)

**Bursa**   A sac formed by two layers of synovial tissue that is located where there is friction between tendon and bone or skin and bone

**Bursitis**   Inflammation of a bursa

Burst fracture A compression-type fracture of a vertebra that involves posterior displacement of the fragments, often into the spinal canal

**Calcaneofibular ligament**   The longest of the three lateral ligaments of the ankle; inserts on the lateral surface of the calcaneus

**Calcaneus**   Heel bone

**Capsule**   A collagenous structure that surrounds a joint like a sleeve. The capsule allows motion of joints and protects the articular cartilage. The capsule, along with ligaments, tendons, and bony structure, provides stability of the joint.

**Carpal bones**   Bones of the wrist

**Cartilage**   A cellular tissue that, in the adult, is specific to joints, but in children forms a template for bone formation and growth. Hyaline cartilage is a low-friction cellular tissue that coats joint surfaces. Fibrocartilage is tough with high collagen content, such as found in the meniscus of the knee, or the anulus fibrosus portion of the intervertebral disk.

**Cauda equina** The terminal nerve roots of the spinal cord located within the vertebral canal; so named because they resemble the tail of a horse

**Cavus** Excessive height of the longitudinal arch of the foot

**Cellulitis** Inflammation of subcutaneous tissue. Can be caused by trauma or infection.

**Cerebellum** The brain area located posteriorly and attached to the brain stem; functions with the cerebral cortex and brain stem to regulate movement and posture

**Cerebrum** A mass of nerve tissue that makes up the largest part of the brain

**Cervical spine** The upper seven vertebrae, which extend from the base of the occiput to the first thoracic vertebra

**Chondroblasts** The cells that form cartilage

**Chondroitin sulfate** An important class of glucosaminoglycans in articular proteoglycans; the oral form is thought to prevent degradation of joint cartilage and relieve symptoms

**Chondromalacia** Softening of the articular surface that results from exposure of normal cartilage to excessive pressure or shear

**Chondrosarcoma** A primary sarcoma formed from cartilage cells or their precursors but without direct osteoid formation

**Chronic rotator cuff tear** Tear of the rotator cuff of the shoulder resulting from degeneration within the rotator cuff tendon

**Clavicle** The collarbone

**Clavicular epiphyseal fracture** Fracture of the growth plate of the clavicle; may appear clinically as a dislocation, especially if some displacement is present

**Claw toe** Deformity involving hyperextension of the MTP joint and a hyperflexion of the interphalangeal joint

**Closed fracture** A fracture that does not disrupt the integrity of the surrounding skin

**Closed reduction** A procedure to restore normal alignment of a fractured bone or dislocated joint in which the fractured bones are simply manipulated and no incision is needed

**Clubfoot** A complex foot disorder that includes three separate deformities: metatarsus adductus, ankle equinus, and heel varus

**Coccyx** The three to five fused vertebrae distal to the sacrum

**Collagen** A triple helix protein that is the major structural macromolecule of the extracellular matrix of articular cartilage; found also in bone, tendon, and ligament

**Colles fracture** Fracture of the distal radius, with dorsal displacement of the fragments; often caused by a fall on an outstretched arm with the hand extended

**Comminuted fracture** A fracture with more than two fragments

**Common peroneal nerve** Nerve lying below the head of the fibula that controls movement at the ankle and supplies sensation to the top of the foot

**Compartment syndrome** Ischemia of the nerves and muscles within a fascial compartment caused by elevated pressure within the compartment; frequently seen in association with tibial fractures

**Compound fracture** Any fracture in which the overlying skin has been penetrated

**Computed tomography (CT, CAT scan)** A radiographic modality that allows cross-sectional imaging from a series of x-ray beams. The x-ray tube is rotated 360° around the patient, and the computer converts these images into a two-dimensional axial image. CT is capable of imaging bone in three planes: coronal, sagittal, and oblique. This modality is particularly useful in evaluating fractures and bone tumors.

**Concentric contraction** The shortening of a muscle during activation

**Concentric exercises** Exercises in which the muscle shortens while contracting against resistance

**Condyle** A rounded process at the end of a long bone

**Connective tissue** Tissue that connects and supports the structures of the body

**Contusion** Bruise; injury to soft tissue without a break in the skin

**Copper therapy** An as-yet unproved therapy in which any of a number of copper devices are applied to the body to reduce pain and inflammation associated with joint and connective tissue problems

**Coracoacromial ligament** Ligament lying anteromedially and superior to the glenohumeral joint; defines the subacromial space

**Coracoclavicular ligaments** Strong stabilizers of the acromioclavicular joint, consisting of the conoid and trapezial ligaments

**Coronal plane** A coronal plane is any plane of section in the anatomical position that passes vertically through the body and is perpendicular to the median plane. It divides the body into anterior and posterior sections.

**Cortical bone** Dense bone that is responsible for skeletal homeostasis

**Corticosteroids** Cortisone-like medicines that are used to provide relief for inflamed areas of the body. They lessen swelling, redness, itching, and allergic reactions. Often used for a number of other diseases such as asthma or other auto immune diseases.

**Costal arch**   Fused costal cartilages of the sixth to tenth ribs forming the upper border of the abdomen

**Costovertebral angle**   Angle that is formed by the spine and the tenth rib; the kidneys lie beneath the back muscles in the costovertebral angle

**COX-1**   Cyclooxygenase-1 enzyme; an enzyme that is present in most bodily tissues (including platelets and gastrointestinal mucosal tissues) and serves as a "housekeeping" enzyme to form prostaglandins

**COX-2**   Cyclooxygenase-2 enzyme; an enzyme that is thought to be present in the body only when induced in response to injury and is responsible for the formation of prostaglandins that mediate pain and inflammation

**Coxa valgus**   A valgus or abduction deformity of the hip. The neck/shaft angle in increased.

**Coxa magna**   A deformity of the hip in which the ball of the hip joint is enlarged. May be secondary to Legg-Perthes disease or arthritis.

**Crepitus**   A grating or grinding sound

**Cross-table lateral view**   Lateral view of the hip obtained by flexing the opposite hip and directing the x-ray beam "across" the table to image a true lateral of the hip. Used in imaging hip fractures, when a frog lateral view (taken with the hip abducted and rotated) would cause patient discomfort.

**Crush injury**   An injury produced as a result of continuous pressure applied to a part of the body, usually an extremity

**Cryotherapy**   The therapeutic use of cold

**Cubital tunnel syndrome**   Compression of the ulnar nerve at the elbow

**Cubitus (Elbow)**   Cubitus varus is a bowing (or adduction) deformity of the elbow. Cubitus valgus is an elbow aligned in the opposite direction.

**Curettage**   The removal of growths from within cavity walls; in the treatment of musculoskeletal tumors, the scraping of tumor out of bone

**Deep venous thrombosis (DVT)**   Venous clot formation caused by immobilization, hypercoagulation, obstructed venous flow, or endothelial injury, among others

**Degenerative joint disease (DJD)**   Deterioration of the articular cartilage that lines a joint, which results in narrowing of the joint space and pain; osteoarthritis

**Delayed union**   A delay in normal fracture healing; not necessarily a pathologic process

**Deltoid**   The muscle that arises from the inferior surface of the lateral third of the clavicle, the acromion, and the spine of the scapula and inserts into the deltoid tuberosity of the humerus. The anterior fibers assist in flexing and medially rotating the arm, whereas the posterior fibers extend and laterally rotate the arm. Acting as a unit, the deltoid acts to abduct the arm at the glenohumeral joint.

**Deltoid ligament**   One of the major support ligaments of the ankle; originates on the medial malleolus and spreads to attach to the medial border of the talus

**Dermatome**   A localized area of skin that is has its sensation via a single nerve from a single nerve root of the spinal cord

**Diaphysis**   The shaft of a long bone

**Direct bone healing**   Method of healing of a fracture in which the approximated bone ends attach themselves to one another by laying down woven bone

**Discoid meniscus**   A congenital deformity in which the meniscus is discoid in shape rather than semilunar

**Diskectomy**   A surgical decompression procedure in which an intervertebral disk is removed

**Dislocation**   Complete disruption in the normal relationship of two bones forming a joint (ie, no contact of the articular surfaces). The direction of the dislocation is described by the position of the distal bone (eg, with an anterior dislocation of the shoulder, the humerus is displaced anterior to the scapula).

**Displaced fracture**   A fracture that produces deformity of the limb

**Distal**   Location in an extremity nearer the free end; location on the trunk farther from the midline or from the point of reference

**Dorsal**   Toward the posterior surface of the body

**Dorsalis pedis artery**   The continuation of the anterior tibial artery on the anterior surface of the foot

**Dual-energy x-ray absorptiometry (DEXA or DXA)**   A diagnostic imaging technology that uses two different x-ray voltages to assess bone density

**Dynamic strength**   The magnitude of isotonic or isokinetic contraction

**Dysplasia**   A broad term that describes a condition affecting growth or development in which the primary defect is intrinsic to bone or cartilage

**Dystrophy**   A condition resulting from defective or faulty nutrition, broadly construed to include nourishment of tissue by all essential substances, including those normally manufactured by the body itself

**Eccentric contraction**   The lengthening of a muscle during activation

**Eccentric exercises**   Exercises in which the muscle lengthens despite resisting a force, as in slowly lowering a weight

**Ecchymosis**   Bruising or discoloration associated with bleeding within or under the skin

**Edema**   Condition in which fluid escapes into the tissues from vascular or lymphatic spaces and causes local or generalized swelling

**Effusion**   The presence of fluid within a joint

**Electrical muscle stimulation (EMS)**   Treatment in which the biphasic current delivers stimulation to muscles in a variety of ways, including pulse, surged, or tetanizing contractions

**Electromyography (EMG)**   A test that measures the electrical response of muscle contraction

**Enchondral bone healing**   Process in which capillaries grow among mesenchymal cells, forming a fibrovascular tissue known as callus that bridges the gap between bone ends

**Endochondral ossification**   The formation of bone within a cartilage model

**Enthesopathy**   A disease process occurring at the insertion of muscle, tendon, or ligament into bone or joint capsule

**Epiphysis**   A part of a long bone developed from a center of ossification distinct from that of the shaft and separated at first from the latter by a layer of cartilage

**Epiphyseal line**   The part of a long bone that produces growth

**Equinus**   Plantar flexed position of the ankle

**Ewing sarcoma**   A primary sarcoma of the bone that usually arises in the diaphyses of long bones, ribs, and flat bones of children and adolescents

**Exercise-induced compartment syndrome**   A condition in which exertion leads to relative muscle swelling within a restricted fascial compartment, resulting in compression of neurovascular structures, reduced circulation, muscle ischemia, bone death, and the painful buildup of lactic acid

**Extensor**   A muscle, the contraction of which causes movement at a joint with the consequence that the limb or body assumes a more straight line, or so that the distance between the parts proximal and distal to the joint is increased or extended; the antagonist of a flexor

**Extensor digitorum brevis**   Short toe extensor on the dorsum of the foot

**Extensor digitorum longus**   Muscle in the anterior compartment of the muscles of the leg; divides and inserts on the dorsum of the small toes

**Extensor hallucis longus**   Muscle in the anterior compartment of the leg that inserts on the dorsum of the great toe

**Extensor mechanism**   Complex interaction of muscles, ligaments, and tendons that stabilizes the patellofemoral joint and acts to extend the knee

**Extensor supinator muscle group**   Muscle group originating on the lateral epicondyle of the humerus and extending down the forearm dorsally into the wrist and hand that includes the extensor carpi radialis longus, the extensor carpi radialis brevis, and the supinator

**External fixation**   Stabilization of a fracture or unstable joint by inserting pins into bone proximal and distal to the injury that are then attached to an external frame

**Fabella**   Sesamoid bone that is sometimes found in the lateral gastrocnemius muscle tendon

**Fascia**   Sheet or band of tough fibrous connective tissue; lies deep under the skin and forms an outer layer for the muscles

**Fascia lata**   Originates from the lateral crest region and continues over the lateral aspect of the knee, enveloping the lateral aspect of the thigh; iliotibial tract

**Fasciculation**   Involuntary contractions, or twitchings, of groups (fasciculi) of muscle fibers, a coarser form of muscular contraction than fibrillation

**Fast twitch muscle fibers**   Type II muscle fibers

**Fat embolism syndrome**   Respiratory distress and cerebral dysfunction caused by droplets of marrow fat released at a fracture site and deposited in the lungs or brain

**Fatigue fracture**   Microfracture that occurs when the bone is subjected to frequent, repeated stresses, such as in running or marching long distances, and the rate of bone breakdown exceeds the rate of bone repair

**Fat pad**   Specialized soft-tissue structure for weight bearing and absorbing impact

**Fat pad sign**   A sign on a lateral view of the elbow with the elbow flexed 90° that indicates swelling within the joint, often from a fracture with hemorrhage

**Felon**   Infection of the pulp of the distal phalanx of the finger

**Female athlete triad**   The constellation of abnormal or absent menses, eating disorders, and osteoporosis/stress fractures seen in female athletes

**Femoral condyles**   Two surfaces at the distal end of the femur that articulate with the superior surfaces of the tibia

**Femoral head**   Proximal end of the femur, articulating with the acetabulum

**Femoral neck**   The bone connecting the head and the shaft of the femur; fractures frequently occur in this area

**Femur**   The thigh bone; extends from the pelvis to the knee and is the longest and largest bone in the body

**Fibrochondrocytes**   Cells that are able to synthesize fibrous extracellular proteins and have the rounded appearance of chondrocytes

**Fibula**   Outer and smaller of the two bones of the leg, extending from just below the knee to form the lateral portion of the ankle joint

**Fibular collateral ligament**   Ligament that inserts from the femoral condyle to the fibular head

**Flexibility**   The capacity of a muscle to lengthen or stretch

**Flexor**   A muscle the action of which is to flex or bend a joint

**Flexor digitorum longus muscle**   One of the medial stabilizers of the ankle, located in the posterior compartment of the muscles of the leg, that flexes the lateral four toes

**Flexor hallucis longus muscle**   One of the three muscles of the deep portion of the posterior compartment that flexes the great toe

**Flexor pronator muscle group**   A muscle group with a primary role associated with the wrist and hand and a secondary role as elbow flexors

**Floating ribs**   The eleventh and twelfth ribs, which do not connect to the sternum

**Fluoroscopy**   A special type of radiograph that shows continuous motion of the structure, such as wrist motion

**Fracture**   A disruption in the integrity of a bone

**Fracture callus**   Bone developed after a fracture; initially formed from a hematoma at the bleeding edges of bone, it eventually forms a cartilage mass that is remodeled into mature bone

**Fracture-dislocation**   A fracture of bone associated with a dislocation of its adjacent joint.

**Fracture reduction**   The realignment of fracture fragments to restore normal anatomy of the bone

**Freiberg disease**   An osteochondrosis or osteonecrosis of the metatarsal head

**Frequency**   In strength training, the number of workouts completed per unit of time; also refers to number of workouts during 1 week

**Frozen shoulder**   A condition characterized by restricted shoulder movement resulting from acute trauma or a periarticular biceps or rotator cuff tendon injury

**Fusion (arthrodesis)**   The joining of two bones into a single unit, thereby obliterating motion between the two. May be congenital, traumatic, or surgical.

**Galeazzi fracture**   Dislocated ulna with a fractured radius

**Gamekeeper's thumb**   Rupture of the ligament on the ulnar side of the thumb metacarpophalangeal joint that helps to stabilize the joint when pinching

**Ganglion**   A mass of nerve cell bodies usually found lying outside the central nervous system

**Genu (knee)**   Genu valgum is knock-knee deformity; genu varum is bowleg deformity

**Glenohumeral dislocation**   Injury in which the humeral head may displace from the joint; most of these dislocations are anterior and inferior to the glenoid rim

**Glenohumeral joint**   True shoulder joint

**Glenoid labrum**   A soft fibrous rim surrounding the glenoid fossa that deepens the socket and provides stability for the humeral head

**Glenoid labrum tear**   Tear of the glenoid labrum; can result from acute trauma or overuse

**Glucosamine sulfate**   A fundamental component in the synthesis of both hyaluronic acid and chondroitin that is thought to promote cartilage repair and synthesis; the oral form is taken as a dietary supplement to treat arthritis

**Glycosaminoglycans**   Polysaccharides consisting of long-chain, unbranched, repeating disaccharide units, such as keratin and chondroitin sulfate

**Gout**   An inflammatory arthritis associated with deposition of urate in the joint

**Gracilis muscle**   One of the three hamstring muscles of the knee that make up the pes anserine and help protect the knee against rotatory and valgus stress (the other ones are the sartorius and semitendinosus)

**Greater trochanter**   Broad, flat process at the upper end of the lateral surface of the femur to which several muscles are attached

**Greenstick fracture**   A fracture that disrupts only one side of the bone. This fracture pattern is seen in children because of the greater plasticity of their bones.

**Growth factors**   The molecules that stimulate cell growth or activation

**Guarding**   Refusal to use an injured part because motion causes pain; involuntary abdominal muscular contraction reflecting inflammation and pain within the peritoneal cavity

**Hallux**   The great toe

**Hammer toe**   Flexion deformity of the distal interphalangeal joint of the foot

**Hamstring**   One of the large muscle groups at the back of the thigh that flex the knee

**Hangman's fracture**   Fracture of the pedicles of C2

**Head**   The upper or proximal portion of a structure; the head of a bone is the rounded end that allows joint rotation

**Hemarthrosis**   The presence of blood in the joint

**Hematoma**   A collection of blood resulting from injury

**Herniated disk**   Rupture of the nucleus pulposus or anulus fibrosus of the intervertebral disk

**Heterotopic ossification**   The formation of bone in any nonosseous tissue; often occurs following trauma

**Hill-Sachs lesion**   A wedge-shaped impaction fracture of the posterolateral portion of the humeral head seen following anterior dislocations of the shoulder

**Hip pointer**   Painful injury caused by irritation or avulsion of the attachments of the abdominal and thigh muscles at the iliac crest

**Homeopathy**   A system of therapy developed by Samuel Hahnemann based on the "law of similia," from the aphorism, *similia similibus curantur* (likes are cured by likes), which holds that a medicinal substance that can evoke certain symptoms in healthy individuals may be effective in the treatment of illnesses having similar symptoms, if given in very small doses

**ICES**   Ice, compression, elevation, and splinting

**Iliofemoral ligament**   One of three extremely strong ligaments surrounding the hip joint anteriorly and posteriorly, which reinforce the capsule; the other two are the ischiofemoral and the pubofemoral ligaments

**Iliopsoas bursa**   One of the two most important bursae (the other being the trochanteric bursa) about the hip joint; located between the capsule and the iliopsoas muscle anteriorly

**Iliotibial band (ITB)**   Thickening of the iliotibial tract that inserts directly into the lateral tubercle of the tibia

**Ilium**   One of the three bones (ilium, ischium, and pubis) that fuse to form the pelvic bones

**Impacted fracture**   A fracture pattern in which the fragments are pushed together, thus imparting some stability.

**Impingement syndrome**   Shoulder pain caused by tendinosis of the rotator cuff tendon or irritation of the subacromial bursa. *See also* Rotator cuff impingement, external, and Rotator cuff impingement, internal

**Infarct**   An area of tissue that is cut off from its blood supply, becomes ischemic, and dies

**Inflammation**   Heat, redness, swelling, and pain that accompany musculoskeletal injuries; occurs when tissue is crushed, stretched, or torn

**Infraspinatus**   Muscle of the rotator cuff that arises from the dorsal surface of the scapula and inserts on the greater tuberosity

**Instability**   Looseness; unsteadiness

**Intercondylar eminence**   Proximal tibial process; anterior and posterior to the intercondylar eminence are attachment sites for the cruciate ligaments' menisci

**Intercondylar notch**   Bony notch that separates posteriorly the condyles of the femur

**Intercondylar tubercles**   A lateral spur projecting upward from the intercondylar eminence

**Internal fixation**   Surgical insertion of a device that stops motion across a fracture or joint to encourage bony healing or fusion

**Internal impingement**   A condition in the shoulder of throwing athletes that results in tears of the underside of the rotator cuff and the posterior labrum

**Interval throwing program**   A program for shoulder rehabilitation that allows the athlete to get a light workout several times a day at a submaximal level without fatiguing the arm

**Intervertebral disk**   The structure located between two moving vertebrae that stabilizes the spine, helps maintain its alignment, allows motion between vertebral levels, absorbs energy, and distributes load applied to the spine

**Intramedullary nailing or rodding**   A procedure for the fixation of fractures in which a nail or rod is inserted into the intramedullary canal of the bone from one of its two ends

**Intramembranous ossification**   Bone formation characterized by the aggregation of undifferentiated mesenchymal cells, which differentiate into osteoblasts

**Inversion injury**   Ankle injury resulting from landing on the lateral aspect of the foot

**Involucrum**   In osteomyelitis, a sheath of live bone that forms around a piece of dead bone, the sequestrum

**Iontophoresis**   therapeutic modality that uses galvanic electrical current to drive ionized medications through the skin to injured tissues

**Ischemic**   Lacking oxygen, usually as the result of partial or complete blockage of blood flow

**Ischial tuberosity**   The bony prominence felt at the base of each buttock, near the crotch; the major attachment site for the hamstrings and the major weight-bearing structure for sitting

**Ischiofemoral ligament**   One of three extremely strong ligaments surrounding the hip joint anteriorly and posteriorly, which reinforce the capsule; the other two are the iliofemoral and the pubofemoral ligaments

**Ischium**   One of the three bones (ilium, ischium, and pubis) that fuse to form the bony pelvis

**Isokinetic**   Literally, same "speed"; when applied to muscle action, it implies constant velocity of shortening

**Isokinetic exercise**   In isokinetic contractions, the muscle contracts and shortens at constant speed.

**Isometric**   Literally, "same length"; when applied to muscle action, it implies that the muscle length is held constant even with varying loads. Accomplished by contracting the flexors and extensors of a joint at equal loads so that the joint does not move.

**Isotonic**   When applied to muscle action, the condition when a muscle shortens against a constant load, as in lifting a weight

**Isotonic exercise**   Contraction of muscles concentrically or eccentrically against resistance with movement of the part so that the load remains constant

**Jersey finger**   Traumatic rupture of the deep flexor tendon of the ring finger; so named because it often occurs as a result of grabbing an opponent's jersey

**Joint**   Articulation, place of union, or junction between two or more bones of the skeleton

**Joint mobilization**   A manually administered treatment modality in which joints are manipulated to improve flexibility and decrease pain

**Jones fracture**   Stress fracture of the proximal shaft of the fifth metatarsal; a fracture that frequently heals with difficulty

**Jumper's knee**   Chronic tendinosis of the patellar tendon; frequently limited to the distal pole of the patella rather than being diffused throughout the tendon

**Juvenile rheumatoid arthritis**   A chronic inflammatory disease in children that is characterized by pain, swelling, and tenderness in one or more joints and may result in impaired growth and development

**Kohler disease**   Osteochondrosis of the tarsal navicular

**Kyphosis**   Curvature of the spine that is convex posteriorly

**Lamellar bone**   Mature, well-organized form of cortical bone

**Laminectomy**   A surgical decompression procedure in which part of the posterior arch of a vertebra is removed; allows access to the disk

**Lateral**   Lying away from the midline

**Lateral collateral ligament**   Ligament on the lateral side (outside) of three joints—the knee, the elbow, and the ankle

**Lateral condyle**   Forms the lateral border of the upper surface of a joint

**Lateral epicondylitis**   An irritation or partial tear of the extensor tendons of the wrist near their origin at the elbow; also called tennis elbow

**Lateral ligament structure**   The three pairs of the lateral collateral ligament of the ankle: the posterior talofibular ligament, the calcaneofibular ligament, and the anterior talofibular ligament

**Lateral malleolus**   Bony prominence at the end of the fibula that is part of the ankle joint

**Lateral meniscus**   The lateral C-shaped fibrocartilaginous structure of the knee

**Lateral view**   A view that passes from side to side at 90° to an AP or PA view

**Latissimus dorsi**   A muscle of the trunk that originates on the spinous processes and supraspinous ligaments of all lower thoracic, lumbar and sacral vertebrae, lumbar fascia, posterior third iliac crest, last four ribs (interdigitating with external oblique abdominis) and inferior angle of scapula, inserting on the floor of bicipital groove of humerus after spiraling around teres major. Extends, adducts and medially rotates arm. Costal attachment helps with deep inspiration and forced expiration.

**Lavage**   The irrigation or thorough washing of an infected joint with high-volume saline solution

**Lesser trochanter**   Large medial prominence distal to the neck of the femur; the site of the insertion of the iliopsoas tendon

**Ligament**   A collagenous tissue that connects two bones to stabilize a joint

**Limb salvage**   Surgical removal of a tumor without amputation of the affected extremity

**Lisfranc fracture**   A fracture-dislocation of the tarsometatarsal joint

**Longitudinal arch**   Arch along the long axis of the foot formed by the bones of the foot starting at the weight-bearing surface of the calcaneus and ending at the metatarsal heads

**Lordosis**   Curvature of the spine that is convex anteriorly

**Low-molecular-weight heparins (LMWHs)**   Anticoagulants that work by binding to antithrombin-III and catalyze its inactivation of factor Xa

**Magnetic resonance imaging (MRI)**   An imaging modality that depends on the movement of protons in water molecules. When subjected to a magnetic field, protons that are normally randomly aligned become aligned. Radio waves directed at the tissue to be studied are used to change the alignment of these photons. When the radio waves are turned off, the protons emit a signal that is detected and processed by a computer into an image. In the musculoskeletal system, MRI is useful in diagnosing soft-tissue injuries, tumors, stress fractures, and infection.

**Mallet finger**   An injury often caused by direct contact with a ball in which the finger is forced into flexion against resistance and the extensor tendons attaching to the distal phalanx may rupture

**Malunion**   Healing of a fracture in an unacceptable position

**Maximal oxygen consumption ($Vo_{2max}$)**   Reflects the body's ability to maximally extract and use oxygen for aerobic metabolism; measures the lung's ability to extract oxygen

**Mechanism of injury**   A representation of the patterns of energy that cause traumatic injuries

**Medial**   Lying toward the midline

**Medial capsular ligament**   Midthird of the true capsule of the knee joint; ligament extending from the femur to the midportion of the meniscus and then to the tibia

**Medial collateral ligament**   Ligament on the medial aspect of the knee consisting of anterior, posterior, and oblique components and extending from the femur to the tibia

**Medial condyle**   Forms the medial border of the upper surface of a joint

**Medial malleolus**   The bony prominence at the end of the tibia that, together with the lateral malleolus, forms the sides of the ankle joint

**Medial meniscus**   The medial C-shaped fibrocartilaginous structure of the knee

**Medial patellar retinacula**   Extension of the vastus medialis that helps extend the knee joint

**Medial retinaculum**   Structure composed of the aponeurosis of the vastus medial muscle itself; attaching along the medial border of the patella, its primary function is to hold the patella medially

**Median nerve**   Nerve that controls sensation of the central palm, the thumb, and the first three fingers, as well as the ability to oppose the thumb to the little finger

**Medullary canal**   The relatively hollow central core of a long bone that houses blood-forming cells

**Meniscofemoral ligament**   With the meniscotibial ligament, it attaches the midportion of the medial meniscus peripherally to the tibia and the femur

**Meniscotibial (coronary) ligament**   With the meniscofemoral ligament, it attaches the midportion of the medial meniscus peripherally to the tibia and femur

**Meniscus**   A fibrocartilage structure interposed between articular cartilage. In the knee, the medial and lateral meniscus are semicircular structures on the periphery of the joint that act as protective buffers during walking and running activities

**Merchant view**   An axial view of the patella in which the patient lies supine on the x-ray table with the knee flexed 45°. The cassette is held perpendicular to the tibia about halfway between the knee and ankle. The x-ray beam is directed caudally through the patella at an angle of 60° from vertical. This view is useful to evaluate subluxation of the patella and patellofemoral arthritis

**Metacarpal bones**   The five bones of the hand that extend from the wrist to the fingers

**Metaphysis**   The broad portion of a long bone adjacent to a joint. In children, the broad portion of a long bone includes the epiphysis, the physis, and the metaphysis.

**Metastasis**   The transfer of disease from one part of the body to another; tumor metastasis usually occurs via the bloodstream or the lymphatic system

**Metatarsus valgus**   Congenital deformity of the forefoot in which the forefoot is rotated laterally in relation to the hindfoot; also called metatarsus abductus

**Metatarsus varus**   Congenital deformity of the forefoot in which the forefoot is rotated medially in relation to the hindfoot; also called metatarsus adductus

**Microtrauma**   Destruction of a small number of cells caused by additive effects of repetitive forces

**Midline**   Imaginary straight vertical line drawn from midforehead through the nose and the umbilicus to the floor

**Modalities**   Physical agents that can create an optimum environment for injury healing, while reducing pain and discomfort

**Monoarticular**   Affecting a single joint

**Monteggia fracture**   Dislocation of the radial head in association with an ulnar fracture

**Mortise view**   A view of the ankle in which the ankle is rotated internally so that the medial and lateral malleoli are parallel with the plane of the film. This view is used to assess reduction of the ankle joint as well as joint space narrowing

**Morton foot**   Congenital abnormality characterized by a short first metatarsal, which throws weight-bearing stresses to the second metatarsal head, often resulting in pain

**Myelogram**   X-ray study of the spine carried out after injection of a contrast material into the spinal cord sheath; helpful in diagnosing ruptured or bulging disks

**Myelopathy**   An abnormal condition of the spinal cord, whether through disease or compression. The usual consequences are spasticity, impairment of sensation, and impairment of bowel and bladder function.

**Myoblasts**   The embryonic cells that develop into skeletal muscle cells

**Myofascial pain syndrome**   A painful musculoskeletal response that can follow muscle trauma

**Myofibers**   The fibers that constitute a muscle

**Myofibrils**   A slender thread within a muscle fiber that functions in muscle contraction

**Myopathies**   A wide and varied group of primary muscle disorders characterized by weakness

**Myositis ossificans**   Abnormal production of bone within muscle

**Navicular bone**   Bone with which the head of the talus articulates on the medial side of the foot; also a bone in the wrist that articulates with the trapezium, trapezoid, and other carpal bones

**Neck**   The constricted portion of a structure (eg, femoral neck)

**Nerve conduction studies**  Studies that test the speed by which motor, sensory, or mixed (combined motor and sensory) nerves transmit impulses

**Neuralgia**  Pain along the course of a nerve

**Neurapraxia**  A temporary loss of neural function

**Neuritis**  Inflammation or irritation of a nerve

**Neuroma**  A tumor composed of nerve cells

**Neuropathic arthritis**  The chronic, progressive destruction of a joint that is caused by the loss of sensation from an underlying neurologic dysfunction; also known as Charcot arthropathy

**Neuropathy**  An abnormal condition involving a peripheral nerve

**Nocioceptive**  Pain-sensing

**Nondisplaced fracture**  Fracture in which there is no deformity of the limb

**Nonlamellar (woven) bone**  Immature bone

**Nonossifying fibromas**  Osteolytic and sometimes painful proliferative lesions composed of spindle (fibrous) cells

**Nonsteroidal anti-inflammatory drugs (NSAIDs)**  Inhibitors of cyclooxygenase and therefore prostaglandin synthesis

**Nonunion**  Failure of healing of a fracture or osteotomy. With continued motion through a nonunion, a pseudarthrosis will form.

**Nucleus pulposus**  The central core of gelatinous material within intervertebral disks

**Oblique fracture**  A fracture in which the fracture line crosses the bone diagonally

**Oblique view**  A view in which the x-ray beam passes at an angle somewhere between an AP or PA view and a lateral view

**Odontoid view**  An open mouth AP view of the C2 vertebra used to identify fractures of the odontoid (dens) process of C2

**Olecranon bursa**  Bursa in the elbow that separates the skin from the underlying ulna; allows the soft tissue to glide smoothly over the olecranon process

**Olecranon process**  Bony process of the proximal ulna that prevents hyperextension of the elbow

**Open fracture**  A fracture in which the skin is broken, exposing the fracture site to the environment

**Open reduction**  An open surgical procedure in which normal or near-normal relationships are restored to a fractured bone or dislocated joint

**Open reduction and internal fixation (ORIF)**  A procedure that involves incising the skin and soft tissue to repair a fracture under direct visualization

**Origin**  The more fixed end or attachment of a muscle

**Osteitis pubis**  An inflammatory condition of the pubic bones caused by repetitive stress on the symphysis pubis

**Osteoblasts**  The cells that synthesize the organic component of bone; also thought of as the bone-forming cells

**Osteochondral fractures**  Injuries that disrupt articular cartilage and the underlying subchondral bone

**Osteochondritis dissecans (OCD)**  A localized abnormality of a focal portion of the subchondral bone, which can result in loss of support for the overlying articular cartilage

**Osteoclasts**  Large cells that resorb bone matrix when activated

**Osteocytes**  The cells of established bone

**Osteogenesis imperfecta**  A hereditary disorder of connective tissue caused by mutations in the gene for type I collagen

**Osteoid osteoma**  A small, benign, but painful tumor usually found in the long bones or the posterior elements of the spine

**Osteolysis**  Dissolution of bone, particularly as resulting from excessive resorption

**Osteomyelitis**  Infection of bone, either bacterial or mycotic

**Osteonecrosis**  The death of bone, often as a result of obstruction of its blood supply

**Osteophytes**  Overgrowth of bone, common in osteoarthritis and spinal stenosis

**Osteosarcoma**  A primary sarcoma of the bone that is characterized by the direct formation of bone or osteoid tissue by the tumor cells

**Osteosynthesis**  The process of bony union, as in fracture healing. It is a biologic welding process that is sometimes facilitated with grafts of bone from the iliac crest and insertion of fixation devices

**Osteotomy**  Literally, cutting a bone. Used to describe surgical procedures in which bone is cut and realigned.

**Os trigonum**  A bony ossicle posterior to the talus

**Overload principle**  States that strength, power, endurance, and hypertrophy of muscle can only increase when a muscle performs workloads greater than those previously encountered

**Paget disease**  A condition of abnormally increased and disorganized bone remodeling

**Palmar**  The anterior surface of the forearm, wrist, and hand

**Panner disease**  Osteonecrosis of the capitellum seen in teenagers

**Pannus**   A proliferation of synovium beginning at the periphery of the joint surface as seen in rheumatoid arthritis

**Parasympathetic (craniosacral) nervous system**   A part of the autonomic nervous system that causes blood vessels to dilate, slows the heart rate, and relaxes muscle sphincters

**Parathyroid hormone**   The major regulator of calcium homeostasis; promotes increased levels of serum calcium

**Paresthesias**   Abnormal sensations such as tingling, burning, or prickling

**Pars interarticularis**   Part of the vertebra posteriorly between the spinal arch and the pedicle

**Patella**   Kneecap

**Patellar ligament**   *See* patellar tendon

**Patellar plicae**   A synovial fold that may persist into adult life and cause medial knee pain in the absence of trauma

**Patellar tendon**   The extension of the quadriceps mechanism from the patella to the tibia; also called patellar ligament

**Patellectomy**   Surgical excision of the patella

**Patellofemoral groove**   Groove that runs anteriorly between the condyles of the femur; the patella lies in the trochlear groove

**Pathologic fracture**   A fracture caused by a normal load on abnormal bone, which is often weakened by tumor, infection, or metabolic bone disease

**Patient-controlled analgesia (PCA)**   The intravenous or epidural delivery of narcotics via a pump that is controlled by the patient

**Pectoralis major**   A muscle of the upper chest, originating from the anterior surface of the medial half of the clavicle and the anterior surface of the sternum, the superior six costal cartilages, and the aponeurosis of the external oblique muscle and inserting on the lateral lip of the intertubercular groove of the humerus, which adducts and medially rotates the humerus; draws the scapula anteriorly and inferiorly. Acting alone, the clavicular head flexes the humerus and the sternocostal head extends it.

**Pelvic cavity**   Space between the pelvis walls

**Pelvis**   A bony ring, consisting of the sacrum, coccyx, and innominate bones, that connects the trunk to the lower extremities, supports the abdominal contents, and allows passage of the excretory canals

**Percutaneous pinning**   Insertion of pins into bone through small puncture wounds in the skin for stabilization of a fracture or a dislocated joint that was realigned by closed reduction

**Periosteum**   A sleeve of connective tissue that surrounds the shaft of the bone and contributes to fracture healing

**Peritendinitis**   Inflammation of the tendon sheath, marked by pain, swelling, and, occasionally, local crepitus

**Permeative margin**   An indistinct margin visible on radiographic images that signifies the hazy transition between growing tumors and normal bone

**Peroneus brevis muscle**   Muscle in the lateral compartment of the leg that functions to evert the ankle; it passes distal and inferior to the lateral malleolus and inserts on the base of the fifth metatarsal; acts to plantar flex and abduct the foot

**Peroneus longus muscle**   Muscle in the lateral compartment of the leg that functions to evert the ankle; it passes under the cuboid bone and inserts on the inferior surface of the medial cuneiform and base of the first metatarsal; it acts to plantar flex, abduct, and evert the foot

**Phagocytosis**   The process by which white blood cells ingest debris or microorganisms

**Phalanges**   Bones making up the skeleton of the fingers or toes

**Phonophoresis**   The transdermal introduction of a topically applied medication (usually either an anti-inflammatory or analgesic) into soft tissue using ultrasound

**Physis**   The growth plate. Specialized cartilaginous tissue interposed between the metaphysis and epiphysis in long bones in children. Provides growth in length of the bone.

**Pigmented villonodular synovitis**   A proliferative process of the synovial membrane of unknown etiology

**Placebo effect**   The placebo effect is the measurable, observable, or felt improvement in health not attributable to treatment. This effect is believed by many people to be due to the placebo itself in some mysterious way. A placebo (Latin for "I shall please") is a medication or treatment believed by the administrator of the treatment to be inert or innocuous.

**Plantar**   The sole, or flexor surface, of the foot

**Plantar calcaneonavicular ligament**   Sling ligament supporting the longitudinal arch

**Plantar fascia**   Fibrous tissue band that runs from the calcaneal tuberosity to the phalanges and supports the talus

**Plantar fasciitis**   Irritation of the plantar fascia, usually from overuse; the pain is most severe at the calcaneal tuberosity

**Planus**   Flattening of the arch of the foot

**Plyometric exercises**   Exercises that use explosive movements to increase athletic power

**Polyarticular**   Affecting multiple joints

**Polyneuropathies** Neuropathies of several peripheral nerves simultaneously

**Popliteal artery** Continuation of the superficial femoral artery in the popliteal space (posterior surface of the knee); supplies the knee and the calf

**Popliteal fossa** The hollow area on the posterior surface of the knee; popliteal space

**Popliteus muscle** Muscle deep to the popliteal artery with three proximal insertions on the tibia; its primary function is internal rotation of the tibia on the femur

**Portable transcutaneous electrical nerve stimulation (TENS) unit** A portable therapeutic modality that uses electrical stimulation to attempt to modulate pain, strengthen muscles, and enhance soft-tissue healing

**Posterior cruciate ligament (PCL)** Ligament extending from the tibia to the medial surface of the intercondylar notch of the femur that functions with the anterior cruciate ligament in anteroposterior and rotatory stability of the knee

**Posterior glenohumeral dislocation** Disruption of the glenohumeral joint in a posterior direction

**Posterior interosseous nerve** The major terminal branch of the radial nerve that winds around the radius to the dorsal side of the forearm to provide motor and sensory function to the dorsal forearm and wrist

**Posterior process** That part of each vertebra that can be palpated, as it lies just under the skin in the midline of the back

**Posterior sternoclavicular dislocation** Disruption of the sternoclavicular joint posteriorly

**Posterior talofibular ligament** one of the three lateral ligaments of the ankle; the strongest of the three, it helps to resist forward dislocation of the leg on the foot

**Posterior tibial artery** Artery that is just posterior to the medial malleolus; supplies blood to the foot

**Posterior tibial syndrome** Pain along the posterior medial border of the tibia; thought to be secondary to a tight posterior tibial muscle "pulling" on the periosteum in this area; associated with running

**Posterior tibial tendon** One of the structures that creates a dynamic sling supporting the longitudinal arch; attaches directly on the tuberosity of the navicular bone and indirectly on the plantar surface of the navicular and middle cuneiform bones

**Posterior tibiofibular ligament** Part of the talofibular syndesmosis, arises from the posterior calculi on the lateral side of the tibia; helps to hold the fibula snug in its tibial groove

**Posterolateral rotatory instability** The lateral tibial plateau rotates posteriorly in relationship to the femur

**Posteromedial rotatory instability** The medial tibial plateau rotates posteriorly on the femur, with associated medial opening

**Postmenopausal osteoporosis** The most prevalent form of primary osteoporosis

**Postmenopausal osteoporosis** The most prevalent form of primary osteoporosis

**Posttraumatic arthritis** A form of secondary osteoarthritis caused by a loss of joint congruence and normal joint biomechanics

**Preload** Reflection of cardiac muscle quality; an elastic distensible ventricle propels more blood more rapidly than a stiffer, less distensible ventricle

**Primary bone healing** The end-to-end repair process that occurs when the bone ends are anatomically opposed and held together rigidly; no callus forms

**Primary osteoarthritis** Osteoarthritis without an identified cause; characterized by progressive loss of articular cartilage and reactive changes in the bone, leading to the destruction and painful malfunction of the joint

**Proprioception** A sense or perception, usually at a subconscious level, of the movements and position of the body and especially its limbs, independent of vision; this sense is gained primarily from input from sensory nerve terminals in muscles and tendons (muscle spindles) and the fibrous capsule of joints combined with input from the vestibular apparatus

**Proteoglycans** Complex macromolecules that consist of a protein core with covalently bound polysaccharide (glycosaminoglycan) chains

**Proximal** describing structures that are closer to the trunk

**Proximal patellar realignment** Proximal soft-tissue reconstruction designed to align the muscle pull on the patella to enhance the action of the vastus medialis obliquus and to tighten the medial capsule

**Pseudarthrosis** A false joint produced when a fracture or arthrodesis fails to heal

**Pseudofractures** Lines of radiolucency that represent stress fractures with unmineralized osteoid

**Pubic symphysis** Firm fibrocartilaginous joint anteriorly between the two innominate bones

**Pubis** One of the three bones (ilium, ischium, and pubis) that fuse to form the pelvis

**Pulmonary embolism** Migration of a thrombus from a large vein (often in the leg) to the lung, causing obstruction of blood flow, respiratory distress, or even death

**Quadriceps angle (Q angle)**   An angle formed by the intersection of two lines: one line is drawn from the anterosuperior iliac spine to the midpatella; the second is drawn from the midpatella to the anterior tibial tuberosity. These lines parallel the quadriceps and patellar tendons.

**Quadriceps femoris**   Tendon located at the superior border of the patella, or kneecap

**Quadriceps muscle**   Extensor muscle situated at the front of the thigh; composed of four components: the vastus medialis, vastus lateralis, vastus intermedius, and rectus femoris

**Quadriceps tendon**   Convergence of the four muscles of the quadriceps—the rectus femoris, vastus intermedius, vastus medialis, and vastus lateralis; inserts in the superior pole of the patella

**Radial artery**   One of the major arteries of the arm; it can be palpated at the base of the thumb

**Radial nerve**   Nerve carrying sensation to the greater portion of the back of the hand and controlling extension of the hand at the wrist

**Radial styloid**   Bony prominence felt on the lateral (thumb) side of the wrist

**Radiculopathies**   A group of nerve root disorders often caused by nerve root compression or central or neuroforaminal stenosis

**Radius**   Bone on the thumb side of the forearm

**Range of motion (ROM)**   The amount of movement available at a joint

**Reflex**   Fairly fixed pattern of response or behavior similar for any given stimulus; does not involve a conscious action

**Rehabilitation**   Restoration, following disease, illness, or injury, of the ability to function in a normal or near-normal manner

**Resection arthroplasty**   A procedure in which the surfaces of diseased bone are excised, allowing fibrocartilage to grow in its place

**Revascularization**   A procedure to provide an additional blood supply to fractured bone

**Rheumatoid arthritis**   A chronic inflammatory disease that is probably triggered by an antigen-mediated inflammatory reaction against the synovium in the joint

**Rhomboid**   Muscle of the trunk that helps to stabilize and maneuver the shoulder girdle

**RICE method**   A method of treatment of acute injury that is used to counteract the body's initial response to injury; RICE is an acronym for rest, ice, compression, and elevation

**Rickets**   The childhood form of osteomalacia

**Rigid splint**   Splint made from firm material and applied to sides, front, and/or back of an injured extremity to prevent motion at the injury site

**Romberg test**   Used to test for deficits in the sensory systems that provide stability to the trunk. Standing with the feet together, the patient closes his or her eyes. Signs of swaying are a positive sign.

**Rotator cuff**   The rotator cuff is made up of four muscles and their tendons. These combine to form a "cuff" over the head of the humerus. The four muscles—the supraspinatus, infraspinatus, subscapularis, and teres minor—originate from the scapula and together form a single tendon unit that inserts on the greater tuberosity of the humerus. The rotator cuff helps to lift and rotate the arm and to stabilize the ball of the shoulder within the joint.

**Rotator cuff impingement, external**   Impingement of the rotator cuff on the acromion and the coracoacromial ligament; causes microtrauma to the cuff, resulting in local inflammation, edema, cuff softening, pain, and poor function of the cuff

**Rotator cuff impingement, internal**   A condition in the shoulder of throwing athletes that results in tears of the underside of the rotator cuff and the posterior labrum

**Sacroiliac joint**   The joint formed by the articulation of the sacrum and ilium

**Sacrum**   One of the three bones (sacrum and two pelvic bones) that make up the pelvic ring

**Saddle anesthesia**   Decreased sensation around the perineum

**Saddle embolus**   A condition in which one or both of the major pulmonary arteries are totally occluded

**Sarcolemma**   Muscle-cell membrane and its associated basement membrane

**Sarcomeres**   The fundamental components of the contracting unit of the myofibril

**Sarcopenia**   The loss of muscle mass and strength as a result of aging

**Sarcoplasmic reticulum**   A continuous branching network of membrane, which is a specialized form of endoplasmic reticulum unique to muscle

**Sartorius muscle**   One of the medial hamstring muscles that form the pes anserinus and help protect the knee against rotatory and valgus stress (the other pes anserinus muscles are the gracilis and semitendinosus)

**Scapula**   The shoulder blade

**Scapular Y view**   A lateral view of the shoulder taken so that the blade of the scapula, the coracoid process, and the spine of the scapula form a "Y." Used to evaluate anterior and posterior glenohumeral shoulder dislocations. Also called a transscapular view.

**Scapulothoracic joint**   Articulation in which the scapula is suspended from the posterior thoracic wall through muscular attachments to the ribs and spine

**Scheuermann disease**   Osteochondrosis of the vertebral epiphysis resulting in increased thoracic kyphosis in the preteen and early adolescent years

**Schwann cell**   A specialized support cell that encases nerve fibers

**Sclerotic border**   A sharp, geographic margin visible on radiographic images that signifies the transition between inactive or slow-growing tumors and normal bone

**Scoliosis**   Lateral curvature of the spine

**Secondary bone healing**   The repair process that is characterized by the formation of fracture callus, which then remodels to form new bone

**Secondary osteoarthritis**   Osteoarthritis resulting from known precipitants such as bone ischemia, trauma, and neuropathy

**Secondary osteoporosis**   Osteoporosis characterized by conditions in which bone is lost because of the presence of another disease, such as hormonal imbalances, malignancies, or gastrointestinal disorders, or because of corticosteroid use

**Second-degree burns**   Partial-thickness burns that extend down to the dermis; characterized by painful blistering of the skin

**Selective estrogen receptor modulator (SERM)**   A class of drugs that is thought to provide the beneficial effects of hormone replacement therapy without some of its adverse effects

**Semimembranosus muscle**   Muscle extending from the ischial tuberosity to the tibia that acts to flex the leg and extend the thigh; important stabilizing structure to the posterior aspect of the knee

**Semitendinosus muscle**   One of the hamstring muscles that comprise the pes anserinus and help protect the knee against rotatory and valgus stress (the other pes anserinus muscles are the gracilis and sartorius)

**Senile osteoporosis**   Osteoporosis in which an age-related decline in renal production of active vitamin D is the probable cause of bone loss

**Sensory nerve action potential (SNAP)**   The latency, amplitude, and conduction velocity recorded in sensory nerve conduction studies

**Sensory nerves**   Nerves that carry sensations of touch, taste, heat, cold, pain, or other modalities to the spinal cord or brain

**Septic arthritis**   Infection of a joint, either bacterial or mycotic

**Sequestrum**   In osteomyelitis, the dead portion of bone inside and walled off by the involucrum. *See also* involucrum.

**Serratus anterior**   Muscle of the trunk that helps to stabilize and maneuver the shoulder girdle

**Sesamoid bones**   Two small bones located beneath the first metatarsal head that function as extra weight-bearing structures and leverage points for the mechanics of the great toe

**Sesamoiditis**   Inflammation of the sesamoid bones of the great toe

**Sever disease**   Osteochondrosis of the calcaneal apophysis seen in children aged 6 to 10 years

**Shaft**   The long, straight, cylindrical midportion of a bone

**Sharpey's fibers**   The small collagen fibers that attach tendon to bone; in the spine they connect the outer edges of intervertebral disks to the vertebral bodies

**Shin-splints**   Anterior or posterior tibial tendinitis

**Short collateral ligament**   Ligament running parallel to the fibular collateral ligament and attaching to the fibular head posterior to the biceps tendon; also called fabellofibular ligament when it is attached to the fabella; reinforces the posterior capsule and contributes to the lateral stability of the knee

**Shoulder dislocation**   *See* glenohumeral dislocation

**Skeletal homeostasis**   The function of bone that supplies structural support and movement for the body

**Skeletal survey**   Screening radiographs of the entire skeleton

**Skeletal (voluntary) muscle**   Striated muscles that are attached to bones and usually cross at least one joint

**Skeleton**   The skeletal system; the supporting framework of the human body, composed of 206 bones

**Slocum anterolateral rotatory instability test**   Modification of the lateral pivot shift test in which the patient lies on his or her side with the uninvolved leg flexed at the hip and the examiner applies an internal rotation force to the proximal tibia and a valgus stress to the joint; at 20° of flexion the knee visibly, palpably, and audibly reduces

**Slocum external rotation test**   One of the tests for anteromedial-rotatory instability conducted with the hip flexed to approximately 45° and the knee to approximately 80°; a forward motion is applied to the thigh and the degree of anterior drawer is assessed

**Slow twitch muscle fibers**   Type I muscle fibers

**Smooth muscle**   Nonstriated, involuntary muscle that constitutes the bulk of the gastrointestinal tract and is present in nearly every organ to regulate automatic activity

**Soleus muscle**   Muscle, extending from the proximal fibula to the calcaneus, that acts to extend and rotate the foot

**Spinal column**   Central supporting bony structure of the body; vertebral column

**Spinal cord**   Extension of the brain, composed of virtually all the nerves carrying messages between the brain and the rest of the body. It lies inside of and is protected by the vertebrae and the spinal column

**Spinal stenosis**   Narrowing of the canal housing the spinal cord; commonly caused by encroachment of bone

**Spine**   Column of 33 vertebrae extending from the base of the skull to the tip of the coccyx

**Spinous processes**   Palpable prominences in the vertebrae

**Spiral fracture**   A fracture caused by a twisting force that results in a helical fracture line

**Splint**   Device used to immobilize part of the body

**Sprain**   Partial or complete tear of a ligament

**Static stretching**   The passive stretching of a given antagonist muscle by placing it in a position of maximal stretch and holding it there for an extended period

**Stem cells**   Cells with the unlimited ability of self-renewal and regeneration; serve to regenerate tissue

**Stenosis**   A stricture of any canal or orifice. In the spine, a narrowing of the spinal canal secondary to a combination of disk narrowing, thickening of the ligamentum flavum, and osteophytes from arthritis of the facet joints.

**Sternoclavicular dislocation**   Disruption of the articulation that lies between the clavicle and the sternum

**Sternoclavicular joint**   Articulation between the sternum and the clavicle

**Sternocleidomastoid**   Cervical muscle that produces rotation of the head

**Sternum**   Breastbone

**Straight lateral laxity**   Abnormal motion with lateral opening of the joint, or varus laxity; demonstrating injury to the fibular collateral ligament and lateral capsular structures

**Straight medial laxity**   Abnormal motion with medial opening of the joint, or valgus laxity; reflecting damage to the tibial collateral ligament

**Strain**   Partial tear of a muscle

**Stress fracture**   An overuse injury in which the body cannot repair microscopic damage to the bone as quickly as it is induced, leading to painful, weakened bone

**Stryker notch view**   A special view of the shoulder used to demonstrate a Hill-Sachs lesion (a compression fracture of the humeral head on the posterolateral aspect of the articular surface) seen after recurrent anterior dislocations of the shoulder. This view is taken with the patient supine, the hand of the affected shoulder on the top of the head, and the x-ray beam directed 10° cephalad.

**Subacromial bursa**   Bursa that lies in the subacromial space and acts as the protective tissue between the cuff and the bony acromion

**Subacute stage**   Time period between acute and chronic injury

**Subluxation**   An incomplete disruption in the relationship of two bones forming a joint, ie, a partial dislocation. The joint surfaces retain partial contact.

**Supraspinatus**   The most superior muscle that arises from the dorsal surface of the scapula and inserts on the greater tuberosity; part of the rotator cuff

**Sympathetic (thoracolumbar) nervous system**   Part of the autonomic nervous system that causes blood vessels to constrict, stimulates sweating, increases the heart rate, causes the sphincter muscles to constrict, and prepares the body to respond to stress

**Symptom**   Evidence of change in body functions apparent to the patient and expressed to the examiner on questioning

**Synapse**   A specialized site at which an electrical signal is transmitted chemically across a junction to produce a similar electrical impulse on the opposite side

**Syndesmosis**   A form of fibrous joint in which opposing surfaces that are relatively far apart are united by ligaments; eg, the fibrous union between the radius and ulna (radioulnar syndesmosis)

**Synovial fluid**   The straw-colored fluid in the joint that is formed by filtration of capillary plasma

**Synovial joints**   A joint formed by the articulation of two bones, the ends of which are lined with hyaline cartilage and is surrounded by a capsule which is lined with synovium.

**Synoviocytes**   Cells that form the synovial membrane, remove debris, and secrete hyaluronic acid

**Synovitis**   A condition characterized by inflammation of the synovial lining

**Synovium**   The thin membrane that lines a joint capsule. There are two types of synovial cells. Type A act as macrophages and type B produce synovial fluid for joint lubrication. Marked hypertrophy of the synovium occurs with an inflammatory arthritis.

**Tai chi**   A low-impact exercise program that is derived from the martial arts in China and was founded in accordance with the belief that chi (also called qi) is a vital life force flowing through the body

**Talus**   One of the bones forming the ankle joint. It lies below and articulates with the distal tibia.

**Tarsal bones**   Seven bones that make up the rear portion of the foot

**Tarsal coalition**   Fusion of two or more of the major tarsal bones (talus, navicular, calcaneus, and cuboid)

**Tarsal tunnel syndrome**   A neuritis of the posterior tibial nerve resulting in pain and/or numbness along the course of the nerve

**Tendinitis**   Injury to the tendon or musculotendinous unit caused by the application of mechanical loads of high intensity or high frequency

**Tendinosis lesion**   Asymptomatic tendon degeneration caused either by aging or by cumulative microtrauma without inflammation

**Tendon**   A specialized type of collagenous tissue that attaches muscle to bone. Tendons transmit forces of muscular contraction to cause motion across a joint.

**Tennis elbow**   Inflammation of muscle origins at the lateral epicondyle; *also called* lateral epicondylitis

**Tenocytes**   The cells in tendons

**Tenosynovitis**   Inflammation of the thin inner lining of a tendon sheath

**Tenosynovium**   The sheath surrounding a tendon that enhances movement or gliding of the tendon as it transmits muscle forces across joints

**Teres minor**   The most inferior muscle that arises from the dorsal surface of the scapula and inserts on the greater tuberosity; part of the rotator cuff

**Therapeutic ultrasound**   The use of high-energy sound waves for healing purposes. Frequently used by physical therapists to reduce inflammation but increasingly used to heal enthesopathies, such as plantar fasciitis, lateral epicondylitis (tennis elbow), and impingement syndrome of the shoulder, as well as nonunions of fractures.

**Thoracic outlet syndrome**   A constellation of symptoms arising from compression of the vascular or neural components of the brachial plexus in the thoracic outlet

**Thrombus**   A blood clot within a vessel

**Tibia**   Shinbone; the larger of the two leg bones

**Tibial collateral ligament**   One of the major ligamentous support structures of the knee; extends from the medial condyle of the femur to the medial condyle of the tibia and just slightly beyond

**Tibialis anterior muscle**   Muscle located in the anterior compartment of the lower leg; inserts on the medial cuneiform and acts to flex and elevate the foot.

**Tibialis posterior muscle**   One of the three muscles of the deep portion of the posterior compartment of the muscles of the leg; one of the medial stabilizers of the ankle, it acts to invert the foot and extend the ankle.

**Tibial nerve**   Provides motor and sensory function to the lower leg; courses deep to the gastrocnemius muscle

**Tibial plateaus**   The expanded upper ends of the tibia that articulate with the femoral condyles to form the knee joints

**Tibial tubercle**   The bony prominence of the proximal tibia

**Tibiofemoral joint**   Polycentric hinge joint that bears the body's weight during locomotion; joint between each tibial and femoral condyle

**Tibiofibular syndesmosis**   One of the three groups of ankle ligaments; arrangement of dense fibrous tissues between the osseous structures just above the ankle joint that maintains the relationship of the distal tibia and fibula

**Tidemark**   A wavy bluish line visible on histologic staining with hematoxylin and eosin that signifies the border between the deep zone and the zone of calcified cartilage

**Tinel sign**   Percussion of the median nerve at the wrist to demonstrate the degree of nerve irritability by reproducing symptoms of carpal tunnel syndrome

**Tomography**   A radiographic modality that allows visualization of lesions or tissues that are obscured by overlying structures. Structures in front of and behind the level of tissue to be studied are blurred, which allows the object to be studied to be brought into sharp focus. Tomography has been used to evaluate the degree of fracture healing and to evaluate tumors such as osteoid osteoma. Increasingly, CT has replaced tomography as the imaging modality of choice in these circumstances.

**Tonic-clonic**   A generalized seizure involving rigid (tonic) muscular contractions and repetitive (clonic) muscular spasms

**Tophi**   Chalky deposits of urate surrounded by inflammatory cells

**Torus (buckle) fracture**   A fracture that only buckles one side of the cortex. Typically seen in children because of the greater plasticity of their bones.

**Traction**   Action of drawing or pullng on an object

**Traction splint**   Splint that holds a lower extremity fracture or dislocaton immobile; allows steady longitudinal pull on the extremity

**Transcutaneous electrical nerve stimulation (TENS)**   Therapeutic modality in which electrical stimulation is applied to the body with an intact peripheral nervous system; can elicit either sensory or muscular responses by stimulating nerves when electrical current passes across the skin.

**Transverse fracture**   A fracture in which the fracture line is perpendicular to the shaft of the bone

**Transverse plane**   Horizontal section of the body

**Transverse processes**   Together with the posterior processes, the transverse processes allow the attachment of strong intervertebral ligaments that support the spine and also provide anchors for muscles attached to the spinal column

**Trapezius**   Large diamond-shaped muscle lying just beneath the skin of the shoulder girdle lying posteriorly

**Traumatic spondylolysis**   The condition in which one vertebra slips anterior to the one below it secondary to a trauma-induced defect in the right and left pars interarticularis

**Triceps**   The muscle in the back of the upper arm that acts to extend the arm and forearm.

**Trochanter**   Prominence on a bone where tendons insert; specifically, two protuberances, greater and lesser, on the femur

**Trochanteric bursa**   One of the two most important bursae about the hip joint located just behind the greater trochanter and deep to the gluteus maximus and tensor fascia lata muscle

**Trochlea**   A groove in a bone that articulates with another bone, or serves as a channel for a tendon to track in

**T-score**   A score used to express the results of bone density tests derived from the difference between the bone density of the patient being tested and the peak bone density of a healthy, young adult population; a T-score is equivalent to one standard deviation above or below ideal bone mass.

**Tuberculosis**   A chronic granulomatous infection caused by the bacteria *Mycobacterium tuberculosis*

**Tuberosity**   Prominence on a bone where tendons insert

**Turf toe**   A hyperextension injury of the first metatarsophalangeal joint associated with athletic activity on hard surfaces

**Type I muscle fibers (slow twitch)**   Muscle fibersidentified by a slow contraction time and a high resistance to fatigue; helpful with slow movements such as marathons

**Type II muscle fibers (fast twitch)**   Muscle fibers identified by a fast contraction times and rapid fatigue; helpful in rapid movements such as sprints. Type II fibers are further divided in Type II A and Type II B. Type II B fibers have a moderate resistance to fatigue and represent a transition between the two extremes of the slow twitch and type II A fibers.

**Type B synoviocytes**   A type of synovial cell that secretes hyaluronic acid

**Ulnar artery**   Artery originating from the brachial artery and supplying the forearm, wrist, and hand

**Ulnar nerve**   Nerve originating from the brachial plexus and coursing down the ulnar side of the arm, adjacent to the medial condyle of the elbow and into the ulnar side of the forearm; controls sensation over the fifth and ulnar half of the ring fingers and controls much of the muscular function of the hand

**Ulnar shaft**   The long cylindrical portion of the ulna between the olecranon proximally and the styloid distally

**Ulnar styloid**   Bony prominence of the ulna felt on the medial (little finger) side of the wrist

**Ultrasound (Ultrasonography)**   An imaging modality in which images are created from high-frequency sound waves (7.5 to 10 MHz [1 MHz = one million cycles per second]) that reflect off of different tissues. The reflected sound waves are recorded and processed by a computer and then converted into an image. Ultrasound is used to evaluate infant hip disorders and tears of the rotator cuff.

**Valgus**   Angulation of a distal bone away from the midline in relation to its proximal partner. Genu valgum is a knock-knee deformity, with abduction of the tibia in relation to the femur. Can also be used to describe angulation of fractures or bony deformities.

**Varus**   Angulation of a distal bone toward the midline in relation to its proximal partner. Genu varum is a bowleg deformity, with adduction of the tibia in relation to the femur. Can also be used to describe angulation of fractures or bony deformities.

**Vastus intermedius**   A component of the quadriceps muscle that lies in the midline of the thigh and anterior to the femur

**Vastus lateralis**   A component of the quadriceps muscle that lies lateral to the midline of the thigh and anterior and lateral to the femur

**Vastus medialis**   A component of the quadriceps muscle that lies medial to the midline of the thigh and anterior to the femur

**Vastus medialis obliquus (VMO)**   A smaller component of the vastus medialis muscle

**Vertebral arch**   Part of the vertebra composed of the right and left pedicles and the right and left laminae; also called neural arch

**Vertebral body compression**   Compression fracture of the vertebral body without damage to the ligamentous structures; the most common thoracic fracture; also called wedge fracture

**Vertebral column**   Segmented spinal column composed of 24 movable vertebrae, 5 fixed sacral vertebrae, and 4 fixed coccygeal vertebrae

**Vertebrochondral ribs**   Ribs that articulate directly with the sternum via their costal cartilages

**Vertebrosternal ribs**   Ribs that connect the first 10 thoracic vertebrae to the sternum

**Viscoelastic** Having mechanical properties that depend on the loading rate of an applied force

**Viscosupplements** Intra-articular hyaluronic acid preparations commonly used to treat osteoarthritis; thought to increase joint lubrication

**Volar** Toward the anterior surface of the body.

**Volkmann contracture** Volkmann contracture is a deformity of the hand, fingers, and wrist caused by injury to the muscles of the forearm. It is most commonly secondary to compartment syndrome after fracture or other trauma to the forearm. Also sometimes caused by inadvertent injection of caustic material (drugs) into the arterial system of the forearm.

**Voluntary (skeletal) muscle** Muscle, under direct voluntary control of the brain, which can be contracted or relaxed at will

**Warfarin** An anticoagulant drug that reduces the synthesis of vitamin K–dependent clotting factors II, VII, IX, and X in the liver

**West Point axillary view** An axillary view of the shoulder in which the patient is prone on the x-ray table with a pillow placed under the affected shoulder, the arm abducted 90°, and the forearm hanging off the edge of the table. The cassette is placed against the top of the shoulder, and the x-ray beam is then directed at the axilla, angled 25° toward the table surface and 25° toward the patient's midline. Useful to visualize potential damage to the anterior glenoid rim and Hill-Sachs lesions after an anterior dislocation.

**Wolff's law** A law that states that the growth and remodeling of bone is influenced and modulated by mechanical stresses

**Woven bone** Primitive, less-organized form of cortical bone

**X-rays** Radiant energy produced by exposing tungsten to a beam of electrons; useful in imaging many body parts

**Y scapular view** A view taken tangential to the scapula. Normally, the humeral head sits in the convergence of the "Y," which comprises the scapula, acromion, and coracoid. Useful view to identify anterior and posterior dislocations of the glenohumeral joint.

**Yoga** A variety of disciplines designed to bring practitioners into union with mankind and a higher God or life force

**Z-score** Compares the patient's bone mineral density (BMD) with what is expected in someone of the same age and body size. Among older adults, however, low BMD is common, so comparison with age-matched norms can be misleading and therefore the T-score is more important.

# INDEX

# EARN CME CREDIT

## AS YOU BUILD YOUR MUSCULOSKELETAL KNOWLEDGE!

## Essentials of Musculoskeletal Care
## Self-Assessment Examinations

### *Now Available Online at*
### www.aaos.org/essentials_exam

**Earn valuable CME credit as you build your clinical decision-making skills!**
Based on the *Essentials of Musculoskeletal Care, 3rd Edition,* and *Essentials of Musculoskeletal Imaging,* each **Essentials of Musculoskeletal Care Self-Assessment Examination** offers:

- **Twenty-five multiple-choice questions**
- **The opportunity to earn 3** *AMA PRA Category 1 CME Credits*™
- **Convenient online format**
- **Immediate feedback**

Select the topics most relevant to your practice … or challenge yourself with the entire series!

- **Musculoskeletal Problems in Sports Medicine**
- **Musculoskeletal Physical Examination**
- **Common Degenerative Problems of the Musculoskeletal System**
- **Diagnostic Testing and Image Review of the Musculoskeletal System**
- **Common Fractures and Dislocations**
- **General Musculoskeletal Problems in Children**

Take each exam at your convenience – stop and resume as needed.

### *Go online now to* www.aaos.org/essentials_exam

## PLEASE NOTE

If you are a new customer to the American Academy of Orthopaedic Surgeons, you will be asked to create a new account. Once completed, you will receive a "user ID."
**Please make a note of your "user ID" and use it to log in quickly and conveniently in the future.**

If you have any questions about the purchasing process or the examination programs, please contact our AAOS Customer Service Representatives at **800-626-6726** or **custserv@aaos.org.**

**ACCME Accreditation** The American Academy of Orthopaedic Surgeons is accredited by the Accreditation Council for Continuing Medical Education to provide continuing medical education for physicians. The AAOS designates each *Essentials of Musculoskeletal Care Self-Assessment Examination* for a maximum of 3 *AMA PRA Category 1 CME Credits.*™ Physicians should only claim credit commensurate with the extent of their participation in this activity.